AF520915

Handbook of Biotechnology

The Editors

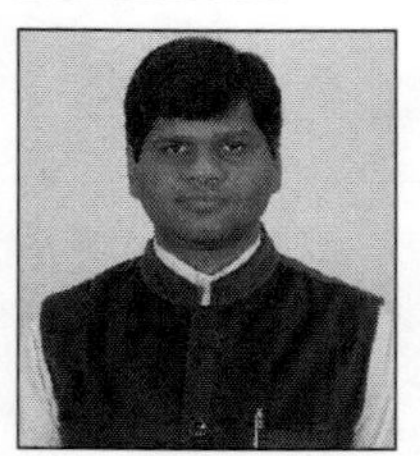

Dr. Saif Hameed is currently Associate Professor at Amity Institute of Biotechnology, Amity University Haryana (AUH). Dr. Hameed did his Bachelors from University of Delhi and Masters from Jamia Hamdard with distinction in 2003 and 2005 respectively. He did his doctoral studies in Life Sciences from Jawaharlal Nehru University in 2010 where he also received CSIR Research Associateship for the one-year postdoctoral work. He has worked as Visiting Scholar in Institut für Mikrobiologie, Heinrich-Heine-Universität, Düsseldorf, Germany in 2008. He has more than 10 years of teaching experience in Biotechnology at both UG and PG levels. Dr. Hameed has received Young Scientist award under Fast Track Scheme from Science and Engineering Research Board, Department of Science and Technology, New Delhi in the year 2012. He is life member of International Society of Infectious Diseases (ISID), Association for Microbiologist (AMI), India and Society of Biological Chemists (SBC), India. Dr. Hameed is actively engaged in research in the field of infectious diseases particularly multidrug resistance (MDR) in pathogenic fungi. He has around 60 peer-reviewed papers to his credit in international journals of repute and five books including three from Springer-Nature. He has successfully convened 5 national conferences as Organizing Secretary. He has supervised 4 Ph.D. students and guided 25 UG & PG level students for their research projects.

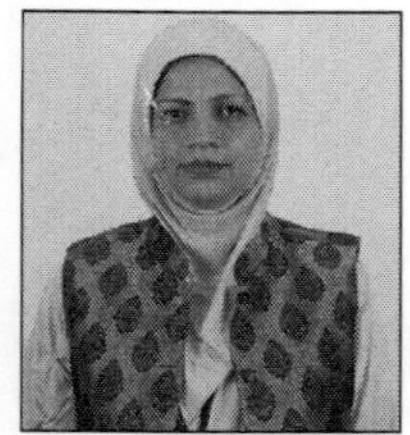

Dr. Zeeshan Fatima is currently Associate Professor at Amity Institute of Biotechnology, Amity University Haryana (AUH). Dr. Fatima did her Bachelors and Masters from Banaras Hindu University in 2000 and 2002 respectively. She earned her doctoral degree in Biochemistry from Aligarh Muslim University in 2008. She has more than 13 years of experience in teaching Biochemistry at UG and PG levels. She has held research positions under nationally and internationally funded research projects which also include her postdoctoral work from University of Cincinnati, Ohio, USA in 2010. Dr. Fatima has received two Young Scientist awards under Fast Track and Women Scientist Schemes respectively from Science and Engineering Research Board, Department of Science and Technology, New Delhi in the year 2012. Additionally, she has bagged extramural projects for funding from Board of Research in Nuclear Sciences (BRNS), Mumbai, Ministry of AYUSH and DBT, New Delhi. She is actively engaged in research in the field of infectious diseases particularly on *Mycobacterium tuberculosis*. She has around 55 peer-reviewed papers to her credit in international journals of repute and five books which includes the ones from Springer-Nature and Elsevier. She has successfully convened four national conferences as Organizing Secretary. She has supervised four Ph.D. students and guided 25 UG & PG level students for their research projects. She is life member of International Society of Infectious Diseases (ISID), Association for Microbiologist (AMI), India and Society of Biological Chemists (SBC), India.

Handbook of Biotechnology

– Editors –

Saif Hameed
Zeeshan Fatima
Associate Professor
Amity Institute of Biotechnology,
Amity University Haryana,
Gurugram (Manesar) – 122 413, Haryana

2022

Daya Publishing House®
A Division of
Astral International Pvt. Ltd.
New Delhi – 110 002

ISBN 978-93-5461-364-7 (HB)

Published by : **Daya Publishing House®**
A Division of
Astral International Pvt. Ltd.
– ISO 9001:2015 Certified Company –
4736/23, Ansari Road, Darya Ganj
New Delhi-110 002
Ph. 011-43549197, 23278134
e-mail: info@astralint.com
Website: www.astralint.com

Printed at : **Replika Press Pvt Ltd**

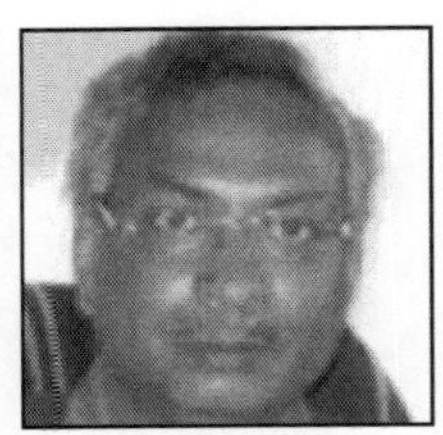

Dr. M. Z. Abdin

Professor of Biotechnology,

Head, Center for Transgenics Plant Development,

School of Chemical and Life Sciences,

Jamia Hamdard, Hamdard Nagar

New Delhi-110062

Foreword

I am happy to endorse the textbook entitled *"Handbook of Biotechnology"* which is being published from student point of view taking into consideration their interest and examination requirements.

The current ongoing pandemic has made us realized that biotechnology is indispensable for studies and research. I am also happy to see that this book is carrying the broad range of topics in the field of biotechnology that are usually covered in two years course of Biotechnology across various Universities in India. This handbook is a valuable resource for the post graduate biotech students particularly from examination point of view.

The book has been compiled from contributors who are teaching diverse topics of biotechnology for many years and aware of the need of students despite numerous biotechnology books available. I congratulate for the efforts taken up by my younger colleagues from Amity University Haryana, Drs. Saif Hameed and Zeeshan Fatima, in compiling this textbook.

I hope the book will have success in the field.

M. Z. Abdin

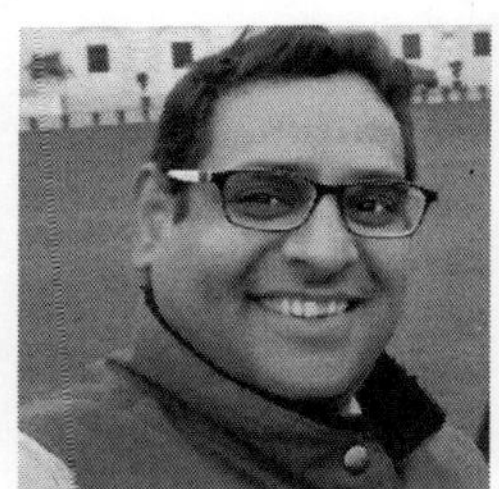

Prof. Pratyoosh Shukla, Ph.D., D.Sc., FNAAS, FAMSc, FBRS
Professor
School of Biotechnology, Institute of Science
Banaras Hindu University, Varanasi-221005, India

Former ASM Indo-US Visiting Research Professor,
University of Cincinnati, College of Medicine, Cincinnati Ohio, USA
Guest Professor, South China University of Technology, Guangzhou, China
Former General Secretary, The Association of Microbiologists of India (AMI) (2014-2020)

Foreword

It gives me immense pleasure to note that the textbook *"Handbook of Biotechnology"* is being published to widely disseminate the current topics and areas in the era of biotechnology being pursued at global level.

Despite numerous biotechnology books available, this handbook is primarily meant for the biotech students of PG levels to attract their interests. The handbook has been written concisely yet in accordance with the recent syllabus of biotechnology courses offered by reputed universities across India. I am sure this book will be useful in creating an interdisciplinary mind set among students and young faculty for biotechnology research and innovations as they will get acquaintance of diverse biotechnology field at single platform. This will also provide an opportunity to the students, faculty and research scholars to enhance their basic knowledge and concepts which will be helpful to plan their prospective research.

I appreciate the efforts taken up by Editors of the book Dr. Saif Hameed and Dr. Zeeshan Fatima, experienced faculty members of Amity University, Haryana in bringing this textbook. Editors have successfully managed to assemble chapters from contributors having considerable command over their respective topics working in diverse areas of biotechnology and touching upon most of the perceivable title points that provide completeness of the offering they made.

I wish the book a great success in the field.

Pratyoosh Shukla

Preface

The book '**Handbook of Biotechnology**' dwells broadly on various topics pertaining to the biotechnology syllabus for PG level. This book intends to cover all the topics of the MSc./M.Tech Biotechnology course syllabus across various Universities in India. It is a compilation of major topics of biotechnology at a single platform and summarizes the matter in the form of capsule notes from examination point of view so that the student need not have to divert to different sources for each individual topic and get the course material in one single book. Faculty and researchers currently engaged in teaching respective subjects of biotechnology with their cumulative efforts have contributed each chapter in nutshell to help compile this biotechnology book targeting PG students.

This unique textbook covers most of the papers of biotechnology syllabus and divided in twenty chapters which are taught throughout the four semesters *viz.* biochemistry, cell biology, microbiology, environmental biotechnology, plant biotechnology, animal biotechnology, recombinant DNA technology, bioinformatics and biostatistics to name few. Moreover, it also covers application-based topics which are present in syllabus as elective subjects *viz.* nanobiotechnogy, pharmaceutical biotechnology, stem cells, IPR *etc.*

The book is comprehensive in scope and concise in approach to ensure vital information pertaining to the topics. The chapters are presented in an impeccable manner to provide fundamental knowledge to the students and research scholars. It is a textbook beneficial mainly for postgraduate students pursuing their degrees in biotechnology but UG students may also be benefitted. Furthermore, students from allied sciences courses (biochemistry, bioengineering, biomedical) can also refer this text- book. Additionally, researchers of the biotechnology doctoral courses may also consult the same to brush up their basics to be applied for research. It provides a forum to foster academic exchange among students across different fields of biotechnology. It will also provide aspirants or job seekers of various examinations and interviews a quick brush-up/revision of biotechnology in nutshell. Considering the promotion of online education, material available on various educational websites and reluctancy for book purchase, it is the demand to make available one book with maximum syllabus coverage. Overall, in view of academic curriculum existing in various universities and institutions for biotechnology courses, the present compilation is appropriate and timely book to meet the requirements and interests of undergraduate and postgraduate students of biotechnology.

We are grateful for the blessings and constant motivation from Dr. Ashok K. Chauhan, President RBEF and Dr. Aseem K. Chauhan, Additional President RBEF and Chancellor, Amity University Haryana (AUH) and Amity University Rajasthan (AUR). Sincere thanks to Dr. P.B. Sharma, VC, AUH, Maj. Gen. B.S. Suhag, DVC, AUH, Dr. Padmakali Banerjee, PVC, AUH and Dr. Rajendra Prasad, Director AIB, AUH for their overall support to enhance our academic rigor. We are grateful to our esteemed contributors for their worthy and timely contributions during the tough times of global pandemic without which this compilation would not become a ready reference for the students in biotechnology field. We take pride to thank Dr. M. Z. Abdin, Professor and Head, Department of Biotechnology, Jamia Hamdard, New Delhi and Dr. Pratyoosh Shukla, Professor, Department of Biotechnology, BHU, Varanasi for endorsing this book by giving their valuable forewords. Patience and support during the manuscript preparation from Astral International Pvt. Ltd is deeply acknowledged.

Saif Hameed

Zeeshan Fatima

Contents

List of Contributors

Akanksha Sharma

Department of Botany, Central University of Jammu, Jammu and Kashmir-181143, India

Amresh Prakash

Amity Institute of Integrative Sciences and Health, Amity University Haryana, Gurugram (Manesar)-122413, India

Anand Singh

Interdisciplinary School of Life Sciences, Banaras Hindu University, Varanasi-221005, India

Anil Kumar

Department of Engineering and Sciences, GD Goenka University, Gurugram-122103, India

Anjali Priyadarshini

Department of Biomedical Engineering, SRM University, Sonepat-131029, India

Aradhana Khare

Amity School of Applied Sciences, Amity University Mumbai, Mumbai- 410206, India

Archana Gupta

Department of Biomedical Engineering, SRM University, Sonepat-131029, India

Babita Khosla

Department of Environmental Sciences, Maharshi Dayanand University, Rohtak-124001, India

Bhuvnesh Yadav

Amity School of Applied Sciences, Amity University Haryana, Gurugram (Manesar)-122413, India

Deepak Kumar

Department of Botany, Institute of Sciences, Banaras Hindu University, Varanasi-221005, India

Ghousepeer

Department of Biomedical Engineering, SRM University, Sonepat-131029, India

Jinny Tomar

Amity Institute of Biotechnology, Amity University Haryana, Gurugram (Manesar)-122413, India

Jyotsna Balaji

Department of Biomedical Engineering, SRM University, Sonepat-131029, India

Kumar Gaurav

Amity Institute of Biotechnology, Amity University Haryana, Gurugram (Manesar)-122413, India

Kusuma Kumari Panda

Amity Institute of Biotechnology, Amity University Uttar Pradesh, Noida-201313, India

Machiavelli Singh

Amity Institute of Biotechnology, Amity University Haryana, Gurugram (Manesar)-122413, India

Manish Shandilya

Amity School of Applied Sciences, Amity University Haryana, Gurugram (Manesar)-122413, India

Ramendra Pati Pandey

Center for Drug, Design, Discovery and Development, SRM University, Sonepat-131029, India.

Ravneet Chug

Amity Institute of Biotechnology, Amity University Rajasthan, Jaipur-302015, India

Ritu Pasrija

Department of Biochemistry, Maharshi Dayanand University, Rohtak-124001, India.

Riya Mukherjee

Center for Drug, Design, Discovery and Development, SRM University, Sonepat-131029, India

Rizwanul Haque

Department of Biotechnology, Central University of South Bihar, Gaya-824236, India

Ruby Dhiman

Department of Microbiology, SRM University, Sonepat-131029, India

Saif Hameed

Amity Institute of Biotechnology, Amity University Haryana, Gurugram (Manesar)-122413, India

Sanchi Gupta

Department of Botany, Institute of Sciences, Banaras Hindu University, Varanasi-221005, India

Sangeeta Kumari

Amity Institute of Biotechnology, Amity University Haryana, Gurugram (Manesar)-122413, India

Sarika Chaturvedi

Amity Institute of Biotechnology, Amity University Haryana, Gurugram (Manesar)-122413, India

Shweta Singh

Amity Institute of Biotechnology, Amity University Haryana, Gurugram (Manesar)-122413, India

Sneh Shalini

Molecular Oncology Laboratory, National Institute of Cancer Prevention and Research, Noida- 201301, India.

Sonika Charak

National Brain Research Center, Gurugram (Manesar)-122052, India

Sunil Kumar

Department of Biological Sciences, Science Research Center (SRC) for Immune Research on Non-lymphoid Organ (CIRNO), Sungkyunkwan University, Jangan-gu, Suwon, Gyeonggi-do 16419, South Korea

Suvarna Chatterjee

Department of Biotechnology, Era Medical College, Era University, Lucknow-226003, India

Syed Shadab Raza

Department of Stem Cell Biology and Regenerative Medicine, Era University, Lucknow-226003,

Zeeshan Fatima

Amity Institute of Biotechnology, Amity University Haryana, Gurgaon (Manesar)-122413, India

Chapter 1

Cell Biology

Ruby Dhiman[1], Jyotsna Balaji[2], Archana Gupta[1,2] and Anjali Priyadarshini*[1,2]

[1]Department of Microbiology; [2]Department of Biomedical Engineering; SRM University, Delhi-NCR, Sonepat, Haryana, India
*e-mail: anjalipriyadarshini1@gmail.com

ABSTRACT

Cell biology is a very vast area dealing with the cell organelles, cell division, cellular trafficking and metabolism. In this chapter we have tried to deal with various aspects of cell biology and the latest research done in this field. It would be preposterous to say that this chapter includes all the domain of cell biology, but we have tried our best to give a comprehensive information about the relevant topics.

Keywords: *Cell cycle, G-protein, Endoplasmic reticulum, Cell trafficking, Cell division, Cyclin, Golgi apparatus, Protein folding.*

1. Introduction

The plasma membrane is the interface between the cytosol and the external environment. The proteins that reside and function on the plasma membrane regulate the cellular entrance and exit of bioactive molecules, actuate signaling cascades in response to external stimuli, and potentiate interactions between cells. The presence and abundance of proteins on the plasma membrane is regulated by anterograde and retrograde intracellular vesicular trafficking, exocytosis, and endocytosis. Cell division requires a dramatic reshaping of the plasma membrane: First, cells retract their processes to round up before division. Second, ingression of the cytokinetic furrow occurs at the cellular equator. Finally, membrane abscission at the level of the cytokinetic midbody separates the two sister cells. All three events depend on a tightly regulated use of the endocytic machinery. The cytoskeleton is an integral component of cellular trafficking mechanisms, as the vesicles and endosomes move on actin filaments or microtubules. Selection and movement of the protein cargo to be trafficked to and from the plasma membrane depends to a great extent on signature organellar targeting motifs within the proteins themselves as well as interactions with various adaptor proteins. Endocytosis is essential not only to the recycling/turnover of plasma membrane proteins, but it also functions in dynamic processes that recycle proteins back to the plasma membrane. Some evidence suggests that transcytosis trafficking mechanisms function in plants.

2. Membrane Structure

Cells allow certain substances to enter and prevent the entry of others, meaning the cell membrane must be very flexible the way red and white blood cells are as they change their shape while passing through the narrow capillaries. The cell membrane is a physical and chemical barrier that separates the inside components of the cell from the external environment.

The fluid mosaic model was first proposed by using S.J. Singer and Garth L. Nicolson in 1972 to explain the structure of the plasma membrane. The fluid mosaic model describes the structure of the plasma membrane as a mosaic of components –including phospholipids, ldl cholesterol, proteins, and carbohydrates–that gives the membrane a fluid character. Plasma membranes range from five to ten nm in thickness. The proportions of proteins, lipids, and carbohydrates in the plasma membrane range with each cell type. For example, myelin contains 18 per cent protein and 76 per cent lipid. The mitochondrial internal membrane includes 76 per cent protein and 24 per cent lipid.

The cell membrane consists of a lipid bi-layer containing integral and peripheral proteins. The lipids that are present in the membrane are in the form of phospholipids with hydrophobic core (tail) and polar head group on both sides; head group faces the aqueous environment, the tail in the interior of the bi-layer.

2.1 Properties of Cell Membrane

2.1.1 Physical Properties of Membrane

- ☆ The plasma membranes allow only certain molecules, such as ions and small organic molecules, into and out of the cell. The ability to allow only certain molecules in or out of the cell is referred to as *selective permeability* or *semi-permeability*. This characteristic helps the cell to regulate its interactions between the internal machinery and the external surroundings, helping to maintain homeostasis.
- ☆ It also acts as the attachment point for both the intracellular cytoskeleton and, if present, the cell wall.
- ☆ It is held together by non-covalent interactions.

2.1.2 Chemical Composition and Properties of Membrane

The cell membrane is composed of three main types of components:

- Lipids (50 per cent)
- Proteins (50 per cent)
- Carbohydrate portions of glycolipids and glycoproteins (10 per cent)

In addition to it:

- Water is present in the membrane
- Ions are associated with it

Lipid Component of the Cell Membrane

The lipid bilayer consists of:

- Outer half of the bilayer:
  - Phosphatidylcholine (most numerous: **60 per cent by weight**)
  - Sphingomyelin
- Inner half of the bilayer:
  - Phosphatidylethanolamine
  - Phosphatidylserine
  - Phosphatidylinositol

Cholesterol is present in eukaryotic membranes in a fairly variable amount and maintains membrane fluidity at a variety of temperatures.

Protein Component of the Cell Membrane

The cell membrane has 50 per cent of proteins by mass. They can be classified as:

- Integral proteins
  - Transmembrane proteins which span over both sides of the membrane
  - Lipid-anchored proteins which are confined to only one side of the membrane
- Peripheral proteins (surface) which do not interact with the hydrophobic core of the membrane
- The third type of membrane protein is the glycophosphatidylinositol (GPI) glycan-anchored proteins. For example, prion protein in the neural membrane.

Polysaccharide Component of the Cell Membrane

Carbohydrate components in the cell membrane are generally embedded into the lipid or protein components of the membrane, *i.e.* as glycolipids or glycoproteins. The glycosylated bits of proteins and lipids protrude the extracellular surface of the membrane, forming a carbohydrate layer on the outer surface of the cell. This is known as cellular glycocalyx.

Generally, if the cell is surrounded by some layer of mucous, there is a high possibility that it has a thick layer of glycocalyx around it. For example, vascular endothelial cell

Water in the Cell Membrane

The water in the cell membrane is present in two main forms:

- "Organized" water, *i.e.* complexed with the hydrophilic heads of the phospholipid molecules.
- Bulk water, *i.e.* chemically normal water flowing through protein channels and pores.

Ions Associated with the Cell Membrane

The cell membrane has dissolved ions helping in the interaction between the membrane and ionic constituents of extracellular and intracellular fluid. Much of these interactions are due to the intrinsic surface charge of the membrane components:

2.2 Integral and Peripheral Membrane Proteins

Membrane proteins can be classified into two broad categories–integral (intrinsic) and peripheral (extrinsic)–based on the nature of the membrane-protein interactions Most cell membranes contain both types of membrane proteins.

Integral membrane proteins, also called intrinsic proteins, have one or more segments that are embedded in the phospholipid bilayer. Most integral proteins contain residues with hydrophobic side chains that interact with fatty acyl groups of the membrane phospholipids, thus anchoring the protein to the membrane. Most integral proteins span the entire phospholipid bilayer. These transmembrane proteins contain one or more membrane-spanning domains as well as domains, from four to several hundred residues long, extending into the aqueous medium on each side of the bilayer. They span the enter lipid bi-layer, typically in α-helix formation.

Peripheral membrane proteins, or extrinsic proteins, do not interact with the hydrophobic core of the phospholipid bilayer. Instead, they are usually bound to the membrane indirectly by interactions with integral membrane proteins or directly by interactions with lipid polar head groups.

2.3 Membrane Lipid

2.3.1 Biosynthesis of Membrane (Lipid Bilayer Biosynthesis)

Phospholipids are a class of lipids that consist of two fatty acyl molecules esterified at the sn-1 and sn-2 positions of glycerol, and contain a head group linked by a phosphate residue at the sn-3 position.

The head group forms a hydrophilic region and determines the type of phospholipid. The fatty acyl side chains are hydrophobic. **Phospholipids** are the main constituent of biological membranes. Phospholipids are involved in stabilizing proteins within the membrane, facilitating the active conformational structure of proteins, and as cofactors in enzymatic reactions. Phospholipids are essential for the absorption, transport and storage of lipids. Phospholipids are secreted into the bile to aid in the digestion and absorption of dietary fat. They form the monolayer on the surface of lipoproteins which function to transport neutral lipids throughout the body. Finally, phospholipids serve as a reservoir for signaling molecules, such as arachidonic acid, phosphatidate, diacylglycerol and inositol trisphosphate. The most abundant phospholipids found in mammalian cells are namely; phosphatidylcholine, phosphatidylethanolamine and phosphatidylserine (Figure 1.1).

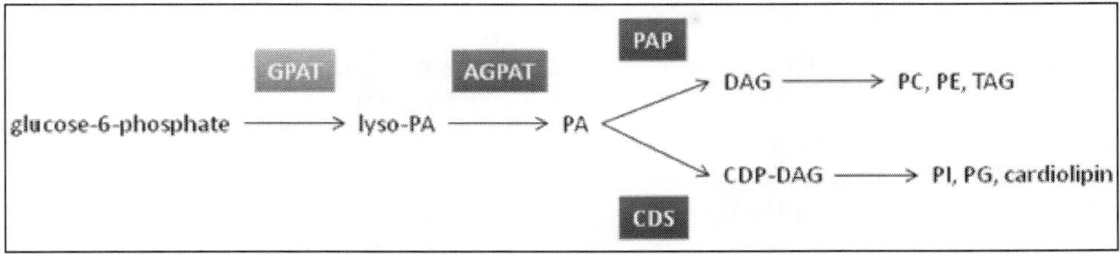

Figure 1.1: Phospholipid Biosynthesis.

2.3.2 Phosphatidic Acid Biosynthesis

Phosphatidic acid forms the backbone on which the synthesis of other phospholipid species and triacylglycerol is based. Phosphatidic acid synthesis begins with the addition of a fatty acyl-CoA, usually saturated, to glycerol 3-phosphate at the sn-1 position to produce lysophosphatidic acid. This reaction is catalyzed by glycerol 3-phosphate acyltransferase and is rate limiting for phosphatidic acid synthesis. There are two forms of this enzyme; one is found in the outer mitochondrial membrane, while the other is found in the endoplasmic reticulum. A second fatty acyl-CoA, often unsaturated, is added to lysophosphatidic acid at the sn-2 position by acylglycerol-3-acyltransferase to form phosphatidic acid. This occurs primarily in the endoplasmic reticulum.

2.3.3 Phosphatidylcholine (PC) Biosynthesis

All nucleated mammalian cells synthesize PC via the CDP-choline pathway. Choline entering the cell is rapidly phosphorylated by choline kinase, converting choline to phosphocholine. Two genes encode the proteins, choline kinase α and β, that are responsible for this phosphorylation. These cytosolic proteins interact to form homo- or heterodimers with increasing levels of activity in the order of: β/β, α/β, α/α.

The second enzyme in this pathway, CTP:phosphocholine cytidylyltransferase (CT), facilitates the conversion of phosphocholine to CDP-choline. There are two isoforms of CTP:phosphocholine cytidylyltransferase, CTα and CTβ, which are encoded by two different genes.

2.3.4 Phosphatidylethanolamine (PE) Biosynthesis

PE is synthesized in the cell through the phosphatidylserine decarboxylation pathway and the CDP-ethanolamine pathway. Phosphatidylserine decarboxylase (PSD) is produced as a 42 kDa protein that undergoes proteolytic cleavage to yield the active enzyme. A mitochondrial targeting sequence is located at the amino terminus of the full-length peptide. The adjacent functional domain is an inner mitochondrial membrane signal. Each of these regions is cleaved, leaving the two functional subunits, a small α-subunit and a larger β-subunit, within the inner mitochondrial membrane. The decarboxylation of phosphatidylserine is the main route for the production of PE found in mitochondrial membranes. PE produced in the mitochondria is also efficiently transported to other membranes within the cell.

2.4 Nuclear Envelope

The nuclear envelope, also known as the nuclear membrane is a structure made up of lipids containing the hereditary material of the eukaryotic cells. It is a permeable structure that encompasses the nucleus. It is found in both animal and plant cells. A cell is involved in many different functions, such as building proteins, converting molecules into energy, and removing waste products. The nuclear envelope protects the cell's genetic material from the chemical reactions that take place outside the nucleus. It also contains many proteins that are used in organizing DNA and regulating genes.

2.4.1 Structure of Nuclear Envelope

The nuclear envelope, made up of two layers encloses the contents of the nucleus during most of the cell's life cycle. The outer membrane of the nucleus is continuous with the membrane of the rough endoplasmic reticulum (RER), and has large number of ribosomes attached to its surface 9Fo. The inner nuclear membrane is compositionally distinct from the outer nuclear membrane and in many cells is lined with a fibrous nuclear lamina on its nucleoplasmic face. The nuclear lamina is a lattice-like sheet of variable width, consisting mainly of polymers of filamentous lamin protein, and is thought to contribute to the structural integrity of the envelope. The outer membrane is also continuous with the inner nuclear membrane since the two layers are fused together at numerous tiny holes called nuclear pores that penetrate the nuclear envelope. These pores regulate the movement of molecules between the nucleus and cytoplasm, allowing some molecules to pass through the membrane, but not others. The space between the outer and inner membranes is known as the perinuclear space and is connected with the lumen of the RER. The nuclear lamina is also thought play to play a role in directing materials inside the nucleus toward the nuclear pores for export and in the disintegration of the nuclear envelope during cell division and its subsequent reformation at the end of the process.

2.4.2 Nuclear Pore Complex (NPC)

The nuclear envelope is perforated with tiny holes known as nuclear pores, which were first discovered in the mid-twentieth century. These pores regulate the passage of molecules between the nucleus and cytoplasm, permitting some to pass through the membrane but not others. DNA and RNA is formed within nucleus and ribosomal sub units in the nucleosomes must leave the nucleus. Nuclear pores are fully permeable to small molecules up to the size of the smallest proteins but form a barrier keeping most large molecules out of the nucleus. The nuclear pore complex is comprised of several subunits Surrounding the inside of the pore is a non-membranous material organized into an annulus that extends spoke-like structures toward the center of the small channel.

3. Cell Trafficking

For a cell to survive, it requires a continuous flow of nutrients. It takes place through the cell membrane, where proteins are trafficked inside the cell to their desired locations, and unwanted and already utilized waste is removed from time to time. So, this is termed as endocytosis and exocytosis. These cellular trafficking pathways are necessary and very crucial for survival and growth. Also, to maintain cellular functions and regulate the chemical and physical environment in the cell.

3.1 Targeting Protein to the Endoplasmic Reticulum

The endoplasmic reticulum is a membrane-bound organelle that is the continuation of the outer nuclear membrane. It is a protein-synthesizing and regulating factory providing proper protein folding and modification. Proteins after manufacturing in cytosol has to be transported to their respective targets for functioning. The endoplasmic reticulum is the significant route for entry of proteins into the secretory endomembrane system-like Golgi apparatus, Lysosomes, and peroxisomes, and inner nuclear membrane. Therefore, more than 30 per cent of the gene coding for proteins is translocated to the endoplasmic reticulum. These secretory proteins have specific characteristic features to them. They carry amino acid sequences at the N-terminal called signal sequence or signal peptide (Figure 1.2).

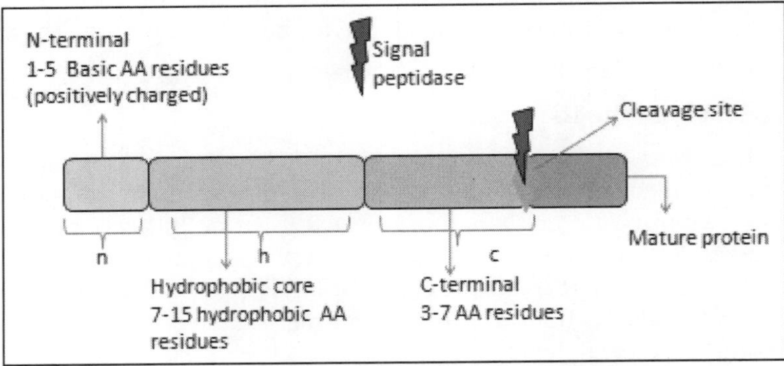

Figure 1.2: Mature Secretory Protein with Signal Peptide.

3.2 Protein Export from the Endoplasmic Reticulum

When proteins are synthesized, folded, assembled, and glycosylated need to be transported from the ER to the Golgi apparatus. This transportation occurs through a Coated transport vesicle called COP 2, a Cup-shaped region in the endoplasmic reticulum that forms a budlike structure called ERES (ER exit sites). They are later transported to the golgi complex for further modifications and sorting. If COP 2 protein undergoes any mutation, COP 2 related diseases are caused, which suggests ER related export defects. Latest studies have revealed that COP 2 mutations can be corrected with the help of genome editing tools.

3.3 Protein Sorting in Golgi Operators and Export from Golgi Apparatus

Golgi apparatus is responsible for protein sorting and post-translational modification, but it also plays a crucial role in maintaining cellular homeostasis. Various enzymes are found in golgi apparatus like kinases, glycosyltransferases, glycosidases, responsible for post-translational modifications of proteins. Golgi also helps in lipid metabolism. A typical Golgi has two faces: the cis face that lies towards the endoplasmic reticulum; proteins destined for secretory pathway enter via Cis Golgi later to medial then to trans Golgi cisternae. These are various functional regions of Golgi.

Proteins, after translation and folding, attain their subsequent structure and function translation. However, once the translation is over, the sequence of amino acids in the protein cannot be revised. After post-translational modification proteins become more efficient in responding to a specific stimulus. Different types of modifications are there; addition of phosphate, phosphorylation, the addition of methyl; methylation, the addition of acetyl group; acetylation in the Golgi. Finally, the protein reaches the Trans Golgi network (TGN) after post-translational modifications.

Endosomes are another membrane-bound organelle, originated from trans-Golgi-network, keeps receiving the membrane proteins and hydrolytic enzymes via secretory vesicles from trans- Golgi-networks. It is essential for the endosomal maturation into late endosome then to lysosome; which is the degradation compartment of cell. while some endosomes do the recycling of the cargo protein back to the plasma membrane.

3.4 SNARE Hypothesis

SNARE derives the Fusion of two membranes mainly meant for the Fusion of neurotransmitters containing vesicles with the plasma membrane for synaptic transmission. Here two complementary SNARES come into the picture, *i.e.*, T-SNARE, and V- SNARE. Fusion of T-SNARE with associated or complementary V-SNARE forms a SNARE complex.[32]V-SNARE protein is confined to the vesicle, and T-SNARE is bound to the target membrane. Thus, transmitting the neurotransmitter carrying inside.

3.5 Protein Import from Mitochondria

Mitochondria contribute to ATP synthesis with the help of the tricarboxylic acid cycle and oxidative phosphorylation. Mitochondria do not just produce energy for cells but also maintains the calcium ion homeostasis response and activation of the ER stress response. More than 1500 mitochondrial proteins were encoded by nuclear DNA, which are synthesized in the cytosol and imported post-translationally in the mitochondrial matrix. Proteins imported into the mitochondrial matrix consist of a targeting sequence of 20-30 amino acids at the N-terminal. These are positively charged amphipathic, alpha helix called pre-sequences. TOM complex plays an important role in recognizing these proteins. Proteins enter inside the intermembrane space via Tom 40 complex present on the outer membrane of mitochondria. Then protein is taken from intermembrane space to matrix via Tim 23 complex, present on the inner mitochondrial membrane. Here MPP (mitochondrial processing peptidase) releases the pre-sequence.

3.6 Import and Sorting of Chloroplast Protein

Chloroplast is a cell organelle in plants. Plants need chloroplast for their photosynthesis. Proteins to be translocated into chloroplasts are called pre-proteins. These pre-proteins to be translocated to chloroplasts are marked with **chloroplast transit peptides (CTP)**, chloroplasts targeting amino acid sequence. Chaperones present in cytosol help navigate these pre-proteins and maintain their unfolded state for easy import. Pre-proteins translocation into the chloroplast occurs through the translocons present on the outer envelope membrane of the chloroplast called the TOC complex. The translocon present on the inner envelope membrane is called the TIC complex. The chaperones generating driving force for protein import into chloroplast are HSP 93, HSP 70, HS P90, and YC f2/FtSHi. In this way, all these proteins help import the proteins into chloroplasts via TIC, TOC, and chaperones.

3.7 Mechanism of Transport of Small Molecules Across the Membrane

There are two processes for the transportation of molecules across any biological membrane (Figure 1.3)

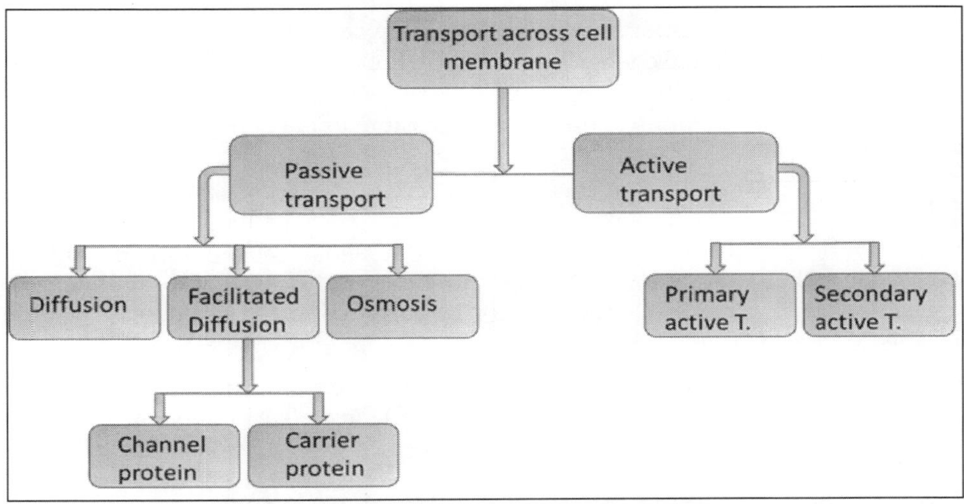

Figure 1.3: Flow Chart Showing Transport of Molecules across Membrane.

1. Diffusion

The molecules move across the membrane from a region of higher concentration to a region of low concentration due to the concentration gradient. It includes the movement of water, gases and lipid-soluble molecules *etc.*

2. Facilitated Diffusion

Molecules move across the membrane due to concentration gradient with the help of other proteins called carrier proteins and channel proteins. **Carrier proteins** undergo a conformational change to transport the molecules. Non- covalent interactions are seen between the transporter and the molecule. Example; GLUT, glucose-mediated transporter. In contrast, **channel protein**-mediated transport is specifically for inorganic ion transport. These are called ion channels, which forms pores through the membrane. They are voltage-gated and ligand-gated channels. Very specific for the transportation of ions. They are used in the transportation of water called aquaporins.

3. Osmosis

Osmosis is the diffusion of water through a selectively permeable membrane water moves from a high concentration to an area of low concentration through the semipermeable membrane.

4. Active Transport

Active transport is the movement of molecules from low to high concentration. This process requires energy to pump the molecules against the concentration gradient. For example, the movement of carbon dioxide from blood vessels.

Primary Active Transport

Primary active transport involves using energy at the membrane protein itself to cause a conformational change that results in the transport of molecules through the proteins embedded in membranes: Eg, Na+-K+ pump. ATP hydrolysis occurs for the movement of sodium ions out and Potassium ions against the concentration gradient.

Secondary Active Transport

Secondary active transport involves using energy to establish a gradient across the cell membrane and utilizing it to transport the desired molecule up its concentration gradient. *e.g.*, transportation of lactose coupled protons at the lactose permease transmembrane protein.

There are other active transport mechanisms called Uniport for transportation of one ion in one particular direction. Symport, all ions move in the same direction, and in Antiport, molecules move in opposite directions.

3.8 NPC and Transport Across the Nuclear Envelope

The cytoplasm and nuclear material are separated by the nuclear envelope consisting of two membranes, the outer membrane and the inner membrane; these membranes fuse, forming a nuclear pore. These are pores made by assembling more than 500 proteins; multiple copies of 30 different proteins make these nucleoporins (Figure 1.4).

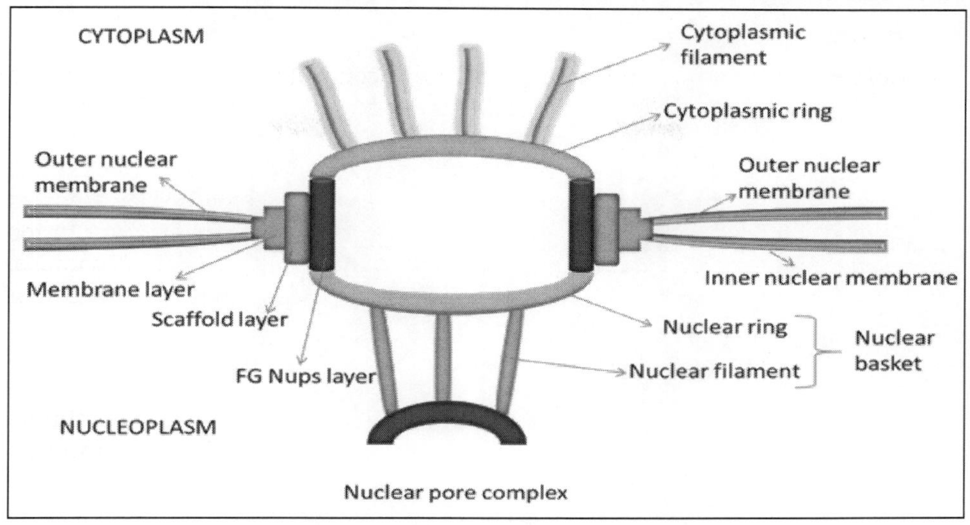

Figure 1.4: Nuclear Pore Complex.

The nuclear pore complex acts as a barrier that selectively let some molecules pass and non-permeable for unwanted molecules. Cargoes up to 40 KDa, and some larger molecules can pass through NPC by passive diffusion while even larger molecules cross via active transport with the help of nuclear transport receptors. These receptors recognize the atomic localization signals. Any signal lacking NLS is denied entry or exit from the nucleus. There are two types of NTR, exportins for bringing the cargo from inner nuclear space to outer nuclear space. These are exportin for bringing cargo from inner nuclear space to outer nuclear space and importin, required for the entry of protein molecules into the nucleus; example α,β and Ran are important and significant Importin examples. Exp-1 is most common exportin.

Nuclear power is made up of nucleoproteins. The nuclear power complex consists of four major components, the core scaffold assembled from the outer ring complex and the inner ring complex. The nuclear basket in the membrane ring contains transmembrane nucleoporins, and the barrier made up of Phenylanaline – glycine (FG). Nucleoporins are attached to the core scaffold with the help of linker nucleoporins (Figure 1.5).

Regulation of Nuclear Import

Nuclear gene expression can be controlled with the help of transcription factors. NF- Kappa B, a transcription factor, is in an inactive form when the I- kappa B is attached. With an appropriate extracellular signal, phosphorylation of I- kappa B takes place, which leads to its proteolytic degradation. Thus, the active NF- Kappa B can be transported to the nucleus now. So, masking of transcription factor while in cytoplasm helps in regulation of nuclear protein import.

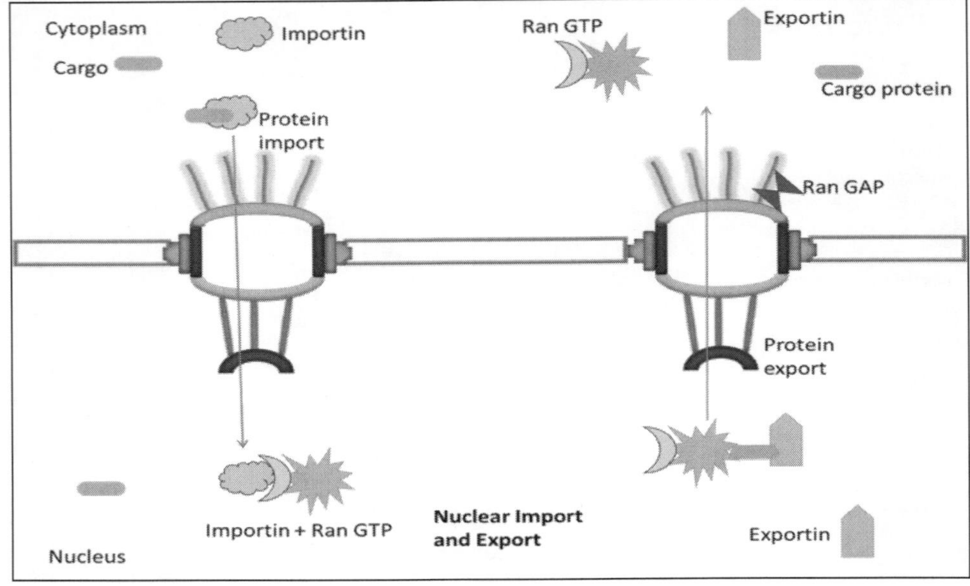

Figure 1.5: Transport Across Nuclear Pore Complex.

4. Intracellular Signaling

Cell signaling is a biological mechanism that occurs in cells which gives cells an ability to receive or generate the signals in response to their surrounding environment. Cell to cell communication between cells is mediated by extracellular signaling molecules. Some of these may operate over long distances.

Receptors play a key role in cell signaling. Receptors help in recognizing the signal molecule (ligand). Receptor molecules are generally proteins. Receptors may be located at cell surface, or interior of the cell such as cytosol, the organelles and nucleus (especially the transcription factors). Usually the cell surface receptors bind membrane-impermeable signal molecules, but sometimes they also interact with membrane permeable signal molecules. A key step in signaling is removal and degradation of the signal molecule. Sometimes the receptor is also degraded. Neurotransmitter re uptake is a mechanism of signaling molecule removal that is commonly seen in nervous system, and is a target of some class of prescription psychiatric medications.

4.1 Importance of Communication between Cells

1. Control of cell division and death
2. Maintenance of homeostasis
3. Adaption to environmental conditions
4. Control of growth and development
5. Regulation of metabolism

At the highest level there are two kinds of communication in the world of living cells. Communication between cells is called **intercellular signaling**, and communication within a cell is called **intracellular signaling**. Often the intracellular communication processes initially are triggered by extracellular signals. Intracellular signaling is the transmission of molecular signals from a cell's exterior to its interior. In intracellular signaling the signals are transmitted across the membrane of cells. These signals act as messengers, hormones, proteins and other biological molecules which are identified by the receptors present on the cell surface which arbitrate their reaction to peptides and proteins like transcription factors which act as intracellular signaling molecules.

External signals such as hormones, sensory signals or electrical signals are specifically recognized by receptors that transduce the external signal into an intracellular signaling chain. The intracellular signaling paths control all functions of the cell such as intermediary metabolism, cell division activity, morphology, and the transcription program.

4.2 Modes of Cell Signaling

There are four categories of cell signaling found in multicellular organisms namely paracrine signaling, endocrine signaling, autocrine signaling, and direct signaling across gap junctions. Each mode of signaling varies from the other because of the distance that the signal travels through the organism to reach the target cell and moreover, not all cells are affected by the same signals.

4.2.1 Paracrine Signaling

When cells are near one another, they often communicate though the release of chemical messenger (ligands that can diffuse through the space between the cells). This type of signaling in which cells communicate over relatively short distances, is known as paracrine signaling. One unique example of paracrine signaling is synaptic signaling, in which nerve cells transmits signals. This process is named for the synapse, the junction between two nerve cells where signal transmission occurs. The neurotransmitters that are released into the chemical synapse are quickly degraded or are taken back up by the sending cell. This "resets" the system so they synapse is prepared to respond quickly to the next signal.

4.2.2 Autocrine Signaling

In autocrine signaling, a cell signals to itself, releasing a ligand that binds to receptors on its own surface (or, depending on the type of signal, to receptors inside of the cell). Autocrine signaling plays an important role in many processes. For example, autocrine signaling is important during development, helping cells take on and reinforce their correct identities. In medicine, autocrine signaling is important in cancer and is thought to play a key role in metastasis (the spread of cancer from its original site to other parts of the body. In many cases, a signal may have both autocrine and paracrine effects, binding to the sending cell as well as other similar cells in the area.

4.2.3 Endocrine Signaling

When cells need to transmit signals over long distances, they often use the circulatory system is used for signal transduction. In endocrine signaling, signals are produced by specialized cells and released into the bloodstream, which carries them to target cells in distant parts of the body. Signals that are produced in one part of the body and travel through the circulation to reach far-away targets are known as hormones. In humans, endocrine glands that release hormones include thyroid, pituitary, pancreas *etc.* Every endocrine gland release one or more types of hormones, many of which regulate the growth and development.

4.3 Direct Signaling through Gap Junctions (Juxtacrine Signaling)

Juxtracrine signaling involves communication between cells that are in direct contact with each other. This communication is often mediated by gap junctions in animal cells and plasmodesmata in plant cells. These tiny channels directly connect neighboring cells. These water-filled channels allow small signaling molecules, called intracellular mediators, to diffuse between the two cells. Small molecules, such as calcium (Ca^{2+}), are able to move between cells, but large molecules like proteins and DNA cannot fit through the channels without special assistance. The transfer of signaling molecules transmits the current state of one cell to its neighbor. This allows a group of cells to coordinate their response to a signal that only one of them may have received. In plants, there are plasmodesmata between almost all cells, making the entire plant into one huge network.

4.4 Steroid Hormone Receptors

Steroid hormone receptors are proteins that have a binding site for a particular steroid molecule. They are found in cytosol and also in the nucleus of target cells. They belong to the Nuclear Receptor family. They are ligand- activated proteins that regulate transcription of certain genes. Their response elements are DNA sequences that are bound by the Hormone-Receptor complex (Figure 1.6).

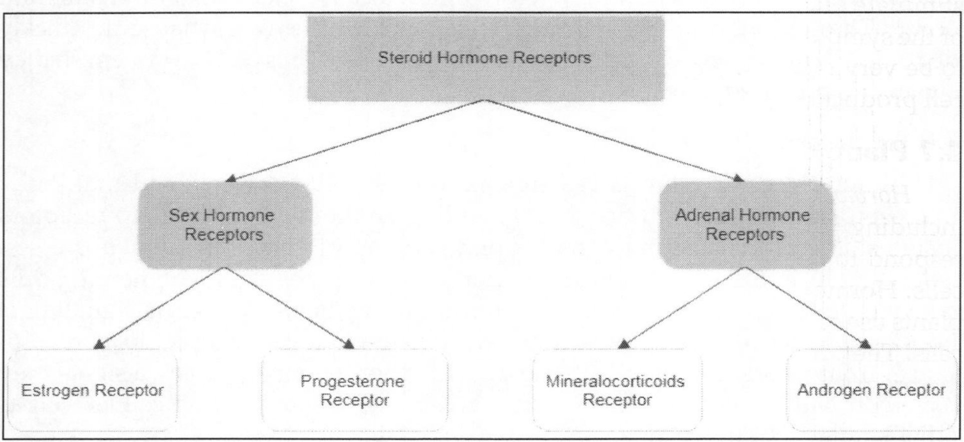

Figure 1.6: Types of Steroid Hormone Receptors

4.5 Peptide Hormones and Growth Factors

Peptide hormones, also known as protein hormones have molecules made up of peptides or proteins, respectively. These hormones have an effect on the endocrine system of animals, including humans. Most hormones can be classified as either amino acid–based hormones (amine, peptide, or protein) or steroid hormones. The former are water-soluble and act on the surface of target cells via second messengers; the latter, being lipid-soluble, move through the plasma membranes of target cells (both cytoplasmic and nuclear) to act within their nuclei.

Insulin is one of the most commonly known peptide hormones. Insulin is one of many peptide hormones found in animals which helps regulate the amount of glucose within cells and the blood. Insulin acts on all cells of the body, binding to receptor proteins on the surface of cells and enabling the uptake of glucose. Most importantly, in healthy individuals, insulin is self-regulating because its release is cause by a high level of glucose in the blood. The other examples include prolactin, a hormone responsible for acting on the mammary glands, and growth hormone, which is responsible for growth and development of the human body.

4.6 Growth Factors

A growth factor is a naturally occurring substance capable of stimulating cell proliferation, wound healing, and occasionally cellular differentiation. Usually it is a secreted protein or a steroid hormone. Growth factors are important for regulating a variety of cellular processes. It typically acts as signaling molecules between cells. Examples are cytokines and hormones that bind to specific receptors on the surface of their target cells.

Growth factors bind to receptors on the cell surface, with the result of activating cellular proliferation and/or differentiation. They are very versatile, stimulating cellular division in numerous different cell types; while others are specific to a particular cell-type. Examples for Growth Factors are EGF, FGF, NGF, PDGF, VEGF, HGF *etc.* Hematopoietic growth factors are hormone-like substances that stimulate bone marrow to produce blood cells. Shortage of blood cells cause most of the symptoms in people with MDS and the the use of growth factors has proven to be very effective. Erythropoietin is a growth factor which promotes red blood cell production.

4.7 Plant Hormones

Hormones are special chemical messengers molecules that help organisms, including plants, respond to stimuli in their environment. In order for plants to respond to the environment, their cells must be able to communicate with other cells. Hormones send messages between the cells. Plant hormones are chemicals plants use for communication, coordination, and development between their many cells. They control everything from the length between nodes on the branches to the programmed death, or senescence seen in many annual plants.

4.8 G-protein Coupled Receptor (GPRC)

GPCR comprises a large protein family of transmembrane receptors that sense molecules outside the cell and activate inside signal transduction pathways and ultimately, cellular responses. G protein-coupled receptors are restricted to eukaryotes, including yeast, choanoflagellates and animals. The ligands that bind and activate these receptors include light-sensitive compounds, odors, pheromones, hormones, and neurotransmitters, and vary in size from small molecules to peptides to large proteins. The actual size of GPRC remains unknown, though nearly 800 different human genes (or ≈ 4 per cent of the entire protein-coding genome) have been predicted from genome sequence analysis. In general, GPCRs can be classified into 5 classes based on sequence homology and functional similarity (Figure 1.7).

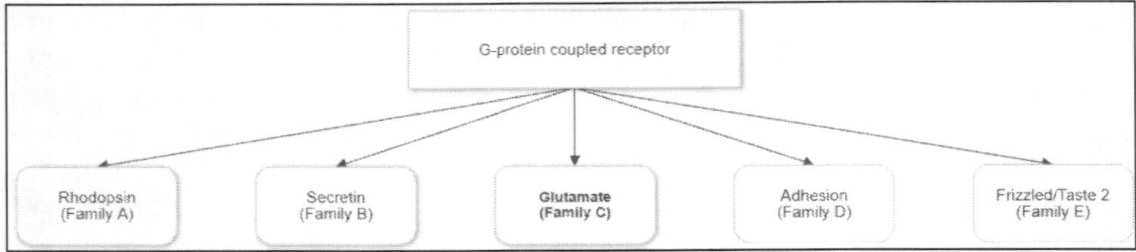

Figure 1.7: Classification of G-protein.

Role of G-protein Coupled Receptor

GPCRs are involved in a wide variety of physiological processes. Some of which are as follows:

1. The visual sense: Rhodopsine which is complex of opsins and chromophore 11- cis retinal, use a photoisomerization reaction to translate electromagnetic radiation into cellular signals due to the conversion of 11-cis-retinal to all-trans-retinal.
2. The sense of smell: receptors of the olfactory epithelium bind odorants (olfactory receptors) and pheromones (vomeronasal receptors)
3. Behavioral and mood regulation: receptors in the mammalian brain bind several different neurotransmitters, including serotonin, dopamine, GABA, and glutamate
4. Regulation of immune system activity and inflammation: Chemokine receptors bind ligands that mediate intercellular communication between cells of the immune system; receptors such as histamine receptors bind inflammatory mediators and engage target cell types in the inflammatory response
5. Autonomic nervous system transmission: Both the sympathetic and parasympathetic nervous systems are regulated by GPCR pathways, responsible for control of many automatic functions of the body such as blood pressure, heart rate, and digestive processes
6. Homeostasis modulation (water balance).

4.9 Receptor-protein Tyrosine Kinase

Tyrosine kinase is an enzyme that can transfer a phosphate group from the ATP to a tyrosine residue in a protein. Receptor tyrosine kinases mediate responses to a large number of signals, including peptide hormones like insulin and growth factors like epidermal growth factor. Like the GPCRs, receptor tyrosine kinases bind a signal, then pass the message on through a series of intracellular molecules, the last of which acts on target proteins to change the state of the cell. RTK is a cell surface receptor that also has a tyrosine kinase activity. The signal binding domain of the receptor tyrosine kinase is on the cell surface, while the tyrosine kinase enzymatic activity resides in the cytoplasmic part of the protein. A transmembrane alpha helix connects these two regions of the receptor.

3.10 c-AMP Pathway of Signal Transduction

Second messengers are molecules that relay signals received at receptors on the cell surface such as hormones, growth factors, *etc.* to appropriate target molecules in the cytosol and/or nucleus. They also serve to amplify the strength of the signal. Binding of a ligand to a single receptor at the cell surface may end up causing massive changes in the biochemical activities within the cell.

There are 3 major classes of second messengers:

1. Cyclic nucleotides (cAMP and cGMP)
2. Inositol trisphosphate (IP3) and diacylglycerol (DAG)
3. Calcium ions (Ca2+)

In this section, we are going to talk about cyclic nucleotides.

cAMP Signal Tranduction Pathway

cAMP stands for cyclic adenosine monophosphate. It is an important second messenger involved in large amounts of cellular effects and biological roles by regulating various metabolic process and mediating the effects of many hormones that binds to a specific receptor on the cell membrane of target cells including catecholamines, ACTH, and vasopressin. It also plays an imperative role in the transcription of some genes.

[Compositions of cAMP - Adenine base + Ribose sugar + 3′, 5′-cyclic phosphate]

Adenosine in cAMP is a nucleoside composed of the pentose sugar D-ribose and adenine, a base. Cyclic AMP contains an ester linkage between the phosphate and ribose units. Some of the hormones that achieve their effects through cAMP as a second messenger (Figure 1.8):

- ☆ Adrenaline
- ☆ Glucagon
- ☆ Luteinizing hormone (LH)

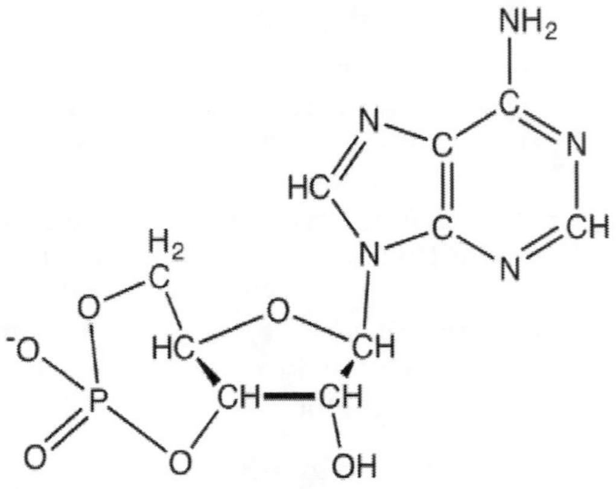

Figure 1.8: Structure of Cyclic Adenosine Monophosphate or 3'-5'-cyclic Adenosine Monophosphate.

Binding of the hormone to its receptor activates a G protein which, in turn, activates adenylyl cyclase. The resulting rise in cAMP turns on the appropriate response in the cell by either (or both): changing the molecular activities in the cytosol, often using Protein Kinase A (PKA) – a cAMP-dependent protein kinase that phosphorylates target proteins; turning on a new pattern of gene transcription.

Functions of cAMP

1. **cAMP as a second messenger**: cAMP is a second messenger, used for intracellular signal transduction. It is involved in transmitting signal from outside the cell to the interior via the process of binding of hormones like glucagon and epinephrine or other signal molecules to cell membrane receptor. It is involved in the activation of protein kinases and regulates the effects of adrenaline and glucagon. cAMP also binds to and regulates the function of ion channels such as the HCN channels and a few other cyclic nucleotide-binding proteins such as Epac1.
2. **In eukaryotic cells:** cAMP and its associated kinases play key role in numerous biochemical processes, including the regulation of glycogen, sugar, and lipid metabolism. There are several minor PKA-independent functions of cAMP like activation of calcium channels, providing a minor pathway by which growth hormone-releasing hormone causes a release of growth hormone. The GEF (guanine nucleotide exchange factor) domain is usually covered by the N-terminal region containing the cAMP binding domain. When cAMP binds, the domain dissociates and exposes the active GEF domain, allowing Epac to activate small Ras-like GTPase proteins, such as Rap1.
3. **In bacteria:** In bacteria, cAMP plays a crucial role and its level varies depending on the medium used for growth. In *E. coli,* cAMP involves in the positive regulation of the lac-operon. cAMP is synthesized from ATP by adenylyl cyclase, as a result increase in the level of cAMP causes

decrease in glucose concentration which is the carbon source. cAMP then binds to the transcriptional regulatory protein, cAMP receptor protein (CRP) also called catabolic activator protein (CAP). After binding of cAMP to CAP enhance the binding capacity of CAP to its binding site (CAP binding site) on target DNA sequence which in lac operon located 60 nucleotides upstream of transcription start site, making it easier for RNA polymerase to bind to the adjacent promoter to start transcription of the lac-operon, increasing the rate of lac-operon transcription. With a high glucose concentration, the cAMP concentration decreases, and the CRP disengages from the lac-operon.

Mechanism of Regulation of cAMP

When stimulatory hormone binds to G-protein coupled receptor, some conformational changes occur in the receptor by which its unexposed catalytic part gets exposed due to which it can interact and activate G-protein with exchange of GDP by GTP at Gα subunit. Now Gα subunit goes and activates membrane bound adenylyl cyclase that facilitates the conversion of ATP to cAMP. This cAMP is now ready to activate protein kinase A which is involved in phosphorylation of several proteins that takes part in the further cellular responses. At the same time of cAMP production by adenylyl cyclase, the cAMP level is controlled by other enzyme that is called cAMP phosphodiesterase which converts cAMP into 5′-AMP. In this process, the adenylyl cyclase is inhibited because GPCR activates the G protein that contains inhibitory alpha subunit which binds to enzyme and inhibits cAMP production.

Synthesis and Degradation of cAMP

cAMP is a cyclic nucleotide which serves as an intracellular and in some cases extracellular secondary messenger. It is derived from adenosine triphosphate (ATP) by adenylyl cyclase located on inner side of plasma membrane and used for intracellular signal transduction in many different organisms, conveying the cAMP-dependent pathway. The elevated cAMP level is regulated by degradation pathway which takes place by cAMP phosphodiesterase enzyme.

4.11 cGMP Signaling Transduction Pathway

Cyclic Guanosine monophosphate or cGMP, is a cyclic nucleotide derived from guanosine triphosphate (GTP). cGMP is a multi-functional second messenger molecule, similar in action to cAMP but generally producing opposite effects on cell function. It has molecular formula of $C_{10}H_{12}N_5O_7P$ and has molecular weight of 345.2 g/mol. It has composition of Guanine nucleotide base, ribose sugar and cyclic phosphate between 3′ and 5′ positions of ribose sugar (Figure 1.9). Cyclic GMP is synthesized from the nucleotide GTP using the enzyme guanylyl cyclase.

Functions of cGMP

1. cGMP is an important molecule of the cell that takes part in various activities in cellular system. When guanylyl cyclase stimulation leads to elevated levels of cGMP, it then mediates biological responses, such as blood vessel dilation which increases blood flow.

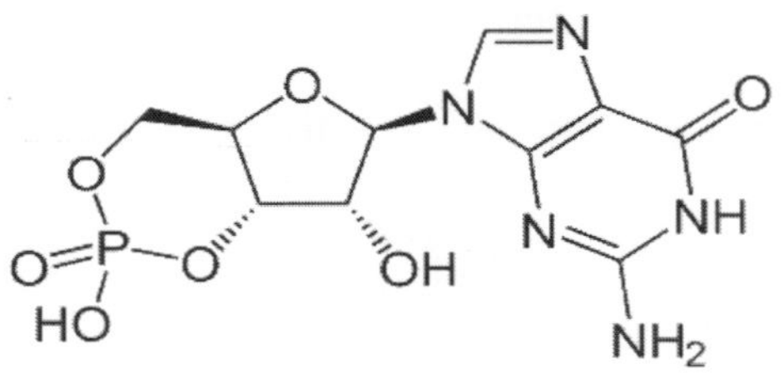

Figure 1.9: Guanosine 3',5'-cyclic Phosphate.

2. The action of cGMP is regularly facilitated by stimulation of cGMP dependent protein kinases, although cGMP is a common regulator of ion channel conductance, glycogenolysis, cellular apoptosis and phosphodiesterases.
3. Another well-known role of cGMP is in the vertebrate eye, where it serves as the second messenger responsible for converting the visual signals received as light to nerve impulses. The photoreceptor in rod cells of the retina is a G protein-coupled receptor called rhodopsin. When light falls on the extracellular side of rhodopsin, then some conformational changes occurs in it by which its bounded chromophore 11-cis retinal is converted to all-trans retinal form, ultimately rhodopsine's unexposed catalytic cytoplasmic side gets exposed which interacts with the G protein transducin and activates them by replacement of GDP by GTP on its α- subunit. The activated Gα then activates cGMP phosphodiesterase 6 which converts all cGMP into 5′ GMP. Due to this cGMP level gradually decreases, the cGMP dependent sodium ion-channel becomes closed. channel is also entry site of calcium ions so Ca^{++} level also decrease. This critical situation created in the cell is called hyperpolarization. But after decreasing Ca^{++} level, guanylyl cyclase is activated and again cGMP synthesis starts. Thus, we can summarize the whole phenomenon as change in cGMP level in retinal rod cells is translated to a nerve impulse by a direct effect of cGMP on ion channels in the plasma membrane.

Regulation Pathway of cGMP

In animals, most of the actions of cGMP are to be mediated by cGMP-dependent protein kinase, which is also called protein kinase G, abbreviated as PKG. After activation of PKG by cGMP, phosphorylates Ser and Thr residues in target proteins. PKG has catalytic and regulatory domains on a single polypeptide chain (Mr, 80,000). A part of regulatory domains fit comfortably in substrate-binding site. After binding of cGMP forces this part of regulatory domain out of the binding site, activating the catalytic domain.

4.12 Phospholipids and Calcium Ions

Calcium ions are very important intracellular messengers. They are probably the most widely used intracellular messengers. Calcium (Ca^{2+}) plays an essential role in the physiology and biochemistry of organisms and the cell. It plays role in common signaling mechanism because once it enters the cytoplasm it exerts allosteric regulatory effects on many enzymes and proteins. Calcium is a second messenger produced by indirect signal transduction pathways such as G-protein coupled receptors. Calcium ions (Ca2+) impact nearly every aspect of cellular life. The principles of Ca^{2+} signaling, from changes in protein conformations driven by Ca^{2+} to the mechanisms that control Ca^{2+} levels in the cytoplasm and organelles. The highly localized nature of Ca^{2+}-mediated signal transduction and its specific roles in excitability, exocytosis, motility, apoptosis, and transcription. Normally, cytosolic calcium (Ca^{2+}) ions is kept very low (10-7 M) by the action of Ca^{2+} pumps in the ER, mitochondria and plasma membrane. Hormonal, neural, or other stimuli cause either an influx of Ca2+ into the cell through specific Ca^{2+} channels in the plasma membrane or the release of sequestered Ca^{2+} from the ER or mitochondria, in either case raising the cytosolic [Ca^{2+}] and triggering a cellular response. This phenomenon is called Calcium ion flux.

Role of Calcium in Cell Signaling

In response to many different signals, a rise in the concentration of Ca^{2+} in the cytosol triggers many types of events such as:

- Muscle contraction
- Exocytosis
    a) Release of neurotransmitters at synapses (and essential for the long-term synaptic changes that produce Long-Term Potentiation (LTP) and Long-Term Depression (LTD)
    b) Secretion of hormones like insulin
- Activation of T cells and B cells when they bind antigen with their antigen receptors (TCRs and BCRs respectively)
- Adhesion of cells to the extracellular matrix (ECM)
- Apoptosis
- A variety of biochemical changes mediated by Protein Kinase C (PKC)

Function of Ca^{2+} in Cell

- Protein function is governed by shape and charge. Ca^{2+} binding triggers changes in protein shape and charge. Similarly, phosphorylation imparts a negative charge, altering protein conformations and their interactions. Protein kinases, comprising ~2 per cent of eukaryotic genomes, remove phosphate from ATP and covalently attach it to the free hydroxyl groups of serine, threonine, or tyrosine residues. The abilities of Ca^{2+} and phosphate ions to alter local electrostatic fields and protein conformations are the two universal tools of signal transduction.
- It carries the information necessary for the contraction of heart.
- Changes in intracellular [Ca^{2+}] are detected by Ca^{2+} -binding proteins that regulate a variety of Ca^{2+} -dependent enzymes exapmle Calmodulin.

4.13 Ras,Raf, MAP Kinase Pathway

Ras/Raf/MAPK pathway the best characterized signal transduction pathway in cell biology. The function of this pathway is to transduce signals from the extracellular environment to the cell nucleus where specific genes are activated for cell growth, division and differentiation. The Ras/Raf/MAPK pathway is also involved in cell cycle regulation, wound healing and tissue repair, integrin signaling and cell migration. It is also able to stimulate angiogenesis through changes in expression of genes directly involved in the formation of new blood vessels.

Thus, signaling through the Ras/Raf/MAPK regulates a variety of cellular functions that are important for tumorigenesis. Dysregulation of this pathway is a common event in cancer as Ras is the most frequently mutated oncogene in human cancer. The ras superfamily of genes encodes small GTP-binding proteins that are responsible for regulation of many cellular processes, including differentiation, cytoskeletal organization, and protein trafficking. Oncogenic ras genes in human cells include H-ras, N-ras and K-ras.

4.14 JAK-STAT Pathway

The JAK-STAT (Janus Kinase-signal transducer and activator of transcription) signaling pathway transmites information from chemical signals outside the cell, which causes DNA transcription and activity in the cell. The JAK-STAT system is a major signaling alternative to the second messenger system.

It consists of three components, namely:

1. A receptor
2. Janus Kinase (JAK)
3. Signal Transducer and Activator of Transcription (STAT)

The JAK-STAT signaling mediates the transfer of message or signal from the cell exterior to the nucleus through a large number of cytokines, hormones and growth factors causing alteration in the transcription of specific genes. The pathway consists of cytokine receptors, a subtype of enzyme linked receptors that depends on cytoplasmic kinases to transfer signals into the cell. Intracellular activation and multimerization of the receptors occur when ligand such as interferon, interleukins bind with the receptor. As a result, Jaks (a cytoplasmic tyrosine kinase) associated with the receptor gets activated.

STATs (Signal Transducer and Activator of Transcription) are latent transcription factor that are confined to the cytoplasm when inactive. There are many types of STATs each with a SH2 domain that plays a crucial role in signal transduction. The SH2 domain of the STAT binds with the phosphotyrosine residue of the activated cytokine receptor. Further, the Jak phosphorylate the STAT on tyrosine residue at the C-terminus, leading to its release from the receptor. The SH2 domain of the dissociated STAT facilitates its binding with a phosphotyrosine residue of the second STAT protein resulting in the formation of either a homodimer or a heterodimer. The STAT dimer translocate into the nucleus, where in it binds to the specific regulatory sequences and stimulates their transcription for the survival, proliferation and differentiation of cell.

4.15 Apoptosis-Role of Caspases

Apoptosis is a biological mechanism which is one type of programmed cell death. Apoptosis is used by multicellular organisms to remove cells that are not needed by the body. Apoptosis has distinctive morphological characteristics such as plasma membrane blebbing, cell shrinkage, chromatin condensation and DNA fragmentation, and begins with the enzymes of the caspase proteases and form a complex group of Cysteine protease activation of multi sub-unit called **apoptosome.**

Caspases

The machinery responsible for apoptosis depends on the family of proteases that have a cysteine at their active site and cleave their target proteins at specific aspartic acids. The activation of a group of enzymes belonging to the cysteine protease family named caspases. The "c" of "caspase" refers to a **cysteine protease** family, while the "Caspase" refers to the enzyme's unique property to cleave after aspartic acid residues.

- ✰ Caspases, or cysteine-aspartic proteases or cysteine-dependent aspartate-directed proteases are a family of cysteine proteases that play essential roles in apoptosis (programmed cell death), necrosis, and inflammation.
- ✰ Caspases are essential in cells for apoptosis, or programmed cell death, in development and most other stages of adult life, and have been termed "executioner" proteins for their roles in the cell. Some caspases are also required in the immune system for the maturation of lymphocytes. Failure of apoptosis is one of the main contributions to tumor development and autoimmune diseases.

5. Cell Division and Regulation of Cell Cycle

The cell cycle is a systematic series of events necessary for cell growth, and cell division result in two new daughter cells. Cell Division is exclusively intended to Duplicate the existing cell to perform cell growth, development, reproduction, and tissue renewal. In prokaryotes, a cell divides by binary fission. Whereas, in eukaryotes, cell division takes place in two ways; Meiosis and Mitosis. Sex cells like ova and sperms; gamete cells divide by meiosis for reproduction purposes to reduce the no. of chromosomes. The somatic cells (all cells other than gamete cells) divide by mitosis for growth, development, maintenance, and recovery purpose.

5.1 Control of Cell Cycle and the Proteins Involved

Cells undergoing cell division passes through accurately timed and discretely regulated growth stages, DNA replication, and division that generates two identical daughter cells. In multicellular organisms, cell division can be broadly divided into two phases; Interphase and the mitotic phase. Interphase has three further subphases called G1, S, and G2 phases (Figure 1.10).

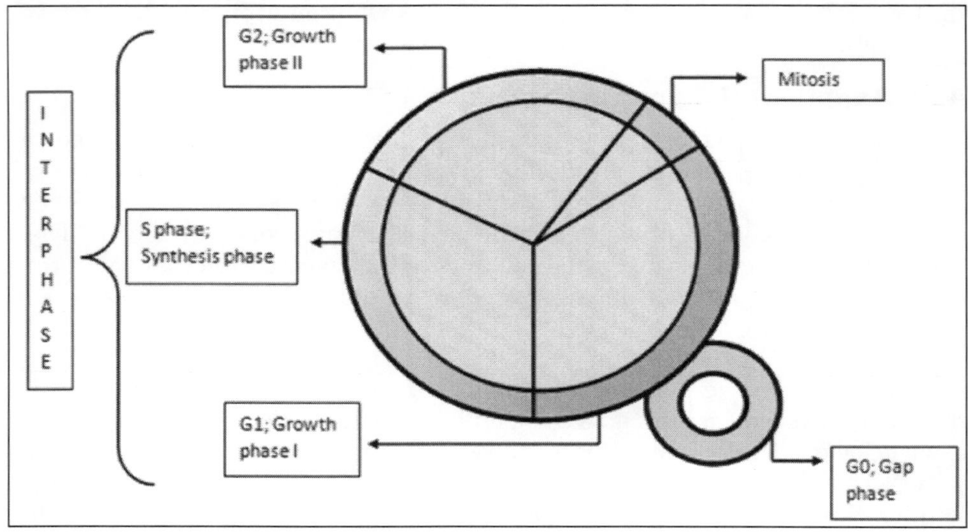

Figure 1.10: Cell Cycle and its Phases.

Interphase: During this phase, the cell undergoes usual processes and prepares itself for cell division. It happens in three different stages of the Interphase.

G1 Phase is the First Gap. In this stage, the cell's biochemical activity is high, but more significant changes are not detectable. The cell has to prepare itself with raw materials like Building blocks of DNA, proteins required for replication, and sufficient energy resources necessary to synthesize DNA. **S phase** is known for the synthesis of DNA. The duplication of chromosomes takes place. So, the synthesis of DNA completes by the activation of Cyclin-Dependent Kinase. **G2 Phase** follows the s phase. Cell, after replication of DNA, restores its energy reserves. Duplication of cell organelles starts as the cell prepares itself for the mitotic phase. Cell growth can be observed during the G2 phase.

G0 phase, cells not dividing actively enters this phase. Any unfavorable environmental conditions like nutrient deficiency, heat shock will temporarily make the cell enter the G0 resting phase until the situation becomes favorable for division. Cells like Nerve cells, Cardiac muscle cells remain in the resting phase permanently.

The cell now enters **Mitosis** phase, here the division of the nucleus takes place called Karyokinesis and cytokinesis occurs. Different stages of Karyokinesis are below;

Karyokinesis

1. Prophase

- ☆ Chromosomes condense
- ☆ Visible spindle fibers emerge from centromere
- ☆ Nuclear membrane dissolves
- ☆ Nucleolus disappears

2. *Prometaphase*

- ✰ Chromosomes condense even more
- ✰ Kinetochore visible at the centromere
- ✰ Spindle microtubules attach to the kinetochore
- ✰ Centrosomes move on respective equatorial positions

3. *Metaphase*

- ✰ Chromosomes align themselves at the metaphase plate
- ✰ It can be easily visualized under the microscope
- ✰ Each sister chromatid is attached to a spindle fiber emerging from equatorial positions

4. *Anaphase*

- ✰ Cohesion proteins binding the sister chromatids together break down
- ✰ Sister chromatids (now chromosomes) are pulled toward the opposite pole (Figure 11)

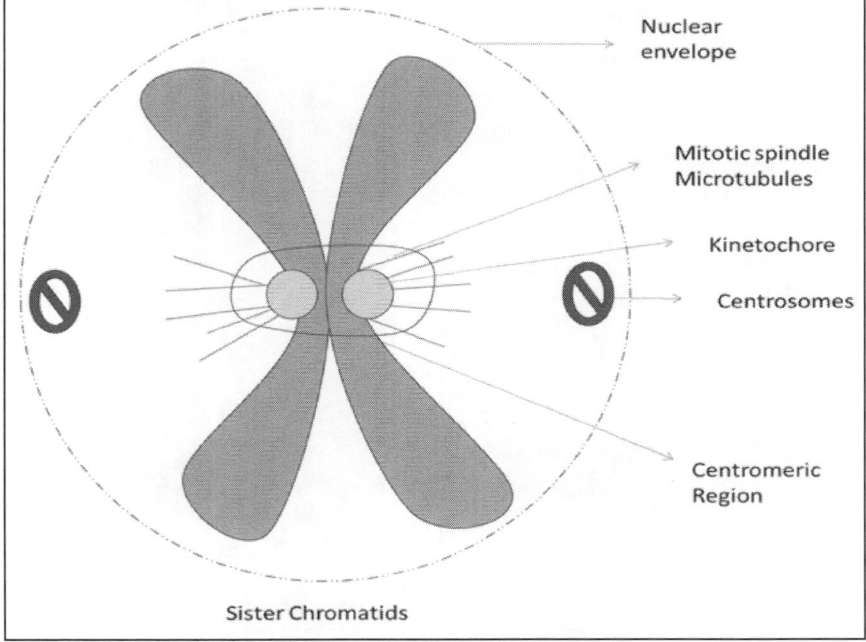

Figure 1.11: Sister Chromatids.

5. *Telophase*

- ✰ Chromosomes arrive at the opposite poles and decondensed
- ✰ Nuclear envelope appears
- ✰ Mitotic spindles break down

Cytokinesis

- ☆ A cleavage furrow separates the two daughter cells (in the animal cell)
- ☆ Cell plate separates the two-cells (in plant cells).

The cell cycle is an irreversible process, and crucial proteins help regulate the cell cycle like Cyclin-Dependent Kinases (CDKs);. So far, More than 20 CDKs have been identified in yeast and eukaryotic cells.

Two proteins play an essential role in cell cycle regulation.

- ☆ **Cyclin proteins**
- ☆ **Cyclin-dependent kinases**

CDKs are the protein enzymes capable of activating and deactivating other proteins by Dephosphorylation. These proteins combine with cyclins to become active. CDKs are expressed throughout the cycle. However, cyclins are manufactured and degraded according to the respective cell cycle phase requirements. The traditional model suggests that cyclin D forms a complex with CDK 4/6. Here cyclins D is a regulatory protein complex for entry into the G1 phase. This complex further phosphorylates retinoblastoma protein (Rb) and liberates the E2F transcription factor. E2 factor successively activates cyclin A and E (Figure 1.12).

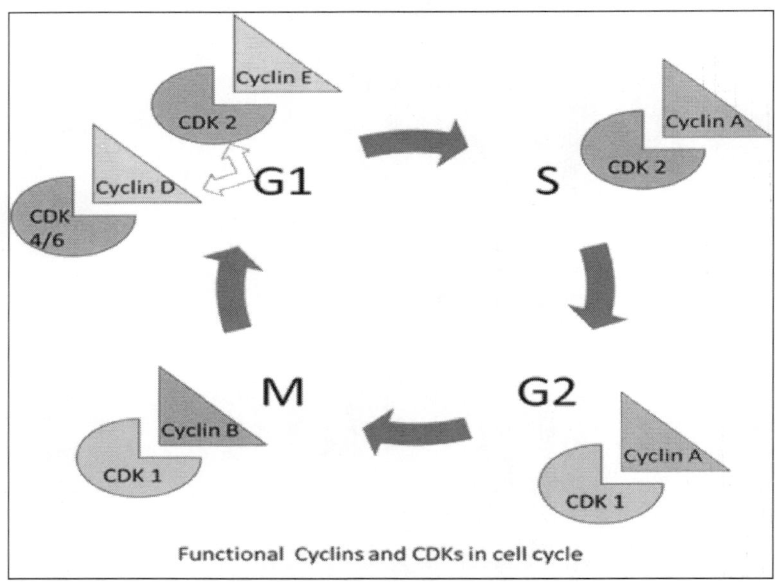

Figure 1.12: Cell Cycle Regulatory Proteins.

5.2 Cell Cycle Check Points

Cell division is a highly regulated Process; any deregulation may lead to cancer-like disease. Certain checkpoints play an essential role in eliminating any deregulation during the cell division (Figure 1.13). Activation of checkpoints suggest any error in the previous cell cycle phase;

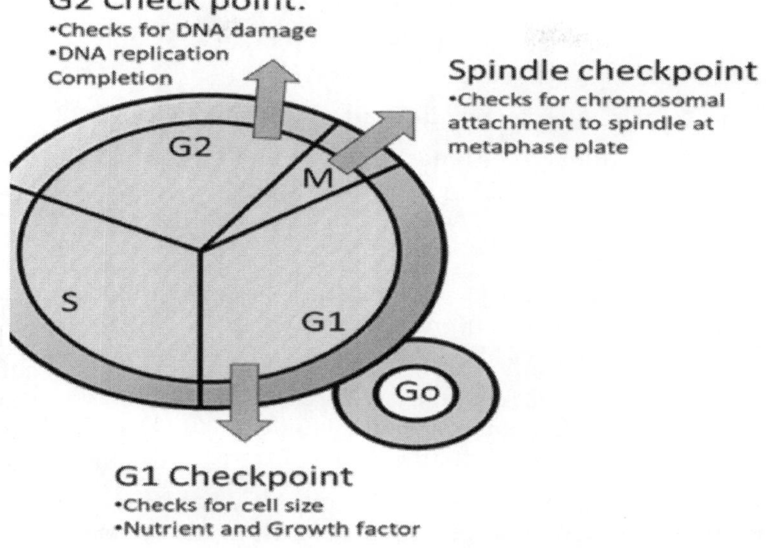

Figure 1.13: Cell Cycle Check Points.

The **G1/S checkpoint**: It is also known as the restriction point. It is a point in the G1 at which removing the growth factors cannot go backsliding to the G0 state. This marks the confirmation of the beginning of cell division. Proteins like Rb/E2F Troll this restriction checkpoint. Thus, this promotes DNA replication as E2F protein will activate all replication promoting genes. The G1/S checkpoint is chiefly induced by the size of the cell, growth factors, nutrition, and DNA damage. The cell size should be large enough to divide, and it should have enough growth factors and energy resources for division. **G2 checkpoint or G2 M checkpoint**; it is also known as DNA replication checkpoint. This checkpoint is instigated by any DNA replication error and DNA damage or destruction. As soon as the DNA damage signal is detected, CDKS is inhibited, leading to cell cycle arrest **Metaphase/ Anaphase Checkpoint**; this Checkpoint is also known as the spindle apparatus checkpoint. The wrong attachment microtubules activate this checkpoint So, The cell temporarily arrests in the metaphase. Some important checkpoint proteins are Mad 1, Mad2, BUB1,BUBRB, BUB3, MPS1.

REFERENCES

1. Garth L. Nicolson: The Fluid–Mosaic Model of Membrane Structure: Still relevant to understanding the structure, function and dynamics of biological membranes after more than 40 years (2013)
2. Tomas Blom et al: Synthesis and Biosynthetic Trafficking of Membrane Lipids(2011)

3. Rosemrie Ungricht *et al*: Mechanisms and functions of nuclear envelope remodeling(2017)

4. Daniel H. Lin: The Structure of the Nuclear Pore Complex (An Update)(2019)

5. Daniel M. Rosenbaum, Soren G. F. Rasmussen,Brian K. Kobilka: The structure and function of G-protein-coupled receptors(2014)

6. Shigekazu Nagata: Apoptosis and Clearance of Apoptotic Cells(2018)

7. Kumar A 2020 Kumar A, Ahmad A, Vyawahare A, Khan R. Membrane Trafficking and Subcellular Drug Targeting Pathways. Front Pharmacol. 2020 May 27;11: 629. doi: 10.3389/fphar.2020.00629. PMID: 32536862; PMCID: PMC7267071.

8. Koch B 2019 Koch B, Yu HG. Regulation of inner nuclear membrane associated protein degradation. Nucleus. 2019 Dec;10(1): 169-180. doi: 10.1080/19491034.2019.1644593. PMID: 31313624; PMCID: PMC6682350.

9. Aviram N 2017 Aviram N, Schuldiner M. Targeting and translocation of proteins to the endoplasmic reticulum at a glance. J Cell Sci. 2017 Dec 15;130(24): 4079-4085. doi: 10.1242/jcs.204396. PMID: 29246967.

10. Wang Y 2019 Wang Y, Mousley CJ, Lete MG, Bankaitis VA. An equal opportunity collaboration between lipid metabolism and proteins in the control of membrane trafficking in the trans-Golgi and endosomal systems. Curr Opin Cell Biol. 2019 Aug;59: 58-72. doi: 10.1016/j.ceb.2019.03.012. Epub 2019 Apr 28. PMID: 31039522; PMCID: PMC7198063.

11. Yoon TY 2018 Yoon TY, Munson M. SNARE complex assembly and disassembly. Curr Biol. 2018 Apr 23;28(8): R397-R401. doi: 10.1016/j.cub.2018.01.005. PMID: 29689222.

12. Priesnitz C 2018 Priesnitz C, Becker T. Pathways to balance mitochondrial translation and protein import. Genes Dev. 2018 Oct 1;32(19-20): 1285-1296. doi: 10.1101/gad.316547.118. PMID: 30275044; PMCID: PMC6169841.

13. Sjuts I 2017 Sjuts I, Soll J, Bölter B. Import of Soluble Proteins into Chloroplasts and Potential Regulatory Mechanisms. Front Plant Sci. 2017 Feb 8;8: 168. doi: 10.3389/fpls.2017.00168. PMID: 28228773; PMCID: PMC5296341.

14. Chen I, 2020 Chen I, Lui F. Physiology, Active Transport. 2020 Sep 13. In: StatPearls [Internet]. Treasure Island (FL): StatPearls Publishing; 2021 Jan–. PMID: 31613498.

15. Glosse P 2018 Glosse P, Föller M. AMP-Activated Protein Kinase (AMPK)-Dependent Regulation of Renal Transport. Int J Mol Sci. 2018 Nov 6;19(11): 3481. doi: 10.3390/ijms19113481. PMID: 30404151; PMCID: PMC6274953.

16. Kim YH 2017 Kim YH, Han ME, Oh SO. The molecular mechanism for nuclear transport and its application. Anat Cell Biol. 2017 Jun;50(2): 77-85. doi: 10.5115/acb.2017.50.2.77. Epub 2017 Jun 27. PMID: 28713609; PMCID: PMC5509903.

17. Jimi E, Fei H, Nakatomi C. NF-κB Signaling Regulates Physiological and Pathological Chondrogenesis. Int J Mol Sci. 2019 Dec 12;20(24): 6275. doi: 10.3390/ijms20246275. PMID: 31842396; PMCID: PMC6941088.

18. L Bartee.2017. Principles of biology. Subtitle Biology 211, 212 and 213, Authors; Lisa Bartee, Walter shriner, and Catherine Creech. L Bartee, W Shriner, C Creech - Principles of Biology, 2017 - openoregon.pressbooks.pub

19. Blackford, A. N., and Stucki, M. (2020). *How Cells Respond to DNA Breaks in Mitosis. Trends in Biochemical Sciences.* doi: 10.1016/j.tibs.2019.12.010 Mitosis labster virtual lab experiment. Trends in Biochemical Sciences, Month 2020

20. Anand, S K., Sharma, A., Singh, N., and Kakkar, P. (2019). *Entrenching role of cell cycle checkpoints and autophagy for maintenance of genomic integrity. DNA Repair, 102748.* doi: 10.1016/j.dnarep.2019.102748

Chapter 2

Biochemistry

*Saif Hameed, Shweta Singh and Zeeshan Fatima**

Amity Institute of Biotechnology, Amity University Haryana,
Gurugram (Manesar) – 122 413, Haryana, India
e-mail: drzeeshanfatima@gmail.com

ABSTRACT

The biochemistry course is aimed to impart an in-depth understanding into the dynamic processes with which various biomolecules undergo in a living system. The major focus of this course is metabolic regulation of carbohydrates, lipids and nitrogenous compounds. The understanding of above has its ramifications in medicine, nutrition, agriculture, fermentation and natural products chemistry.

Keywords: *Water, Biomolecules, Carbohydrates, Proteins, Lipids, Nucleotides.*

Water

Water is generally known as universal solvent because of its ability to dissolve many, but not all, molecules. It can dissolve the molecules that are ionic or polar, but non-polar substances dissolve poorly in water. Oil, for example is non-polar and gets separated from water when mixed with it. On the other hand the electrolytes for example sodium chloride, are able to dissolve quickly in water.

A buffer solution contains a mixture of a weak acid and its conjugate base (or a weak base and its conjugate acid). The equilibrium between the weak acid and its conjugate base allows the solution to resist changes to pH when small amounts of strong acid or base are added.

Henderson-Hasselbalch equation "pH = pKa + log [Base]/[Acid]"

This equation determines the status of acid base balance of the body and preparation of buffers. The pH of human blood or plasma is maintained by bicarbonate buffer (HCO_3/CO_2) *i.e.* carbonic acid (H_2CO_3), bicarbonate ion (HCO_3^-), and carbon dioxide (CO_2). Bicarbonate ions combine with free hydrogen ions and become carbonic acid; hydrogen ions are removed, moderating pH changes. Similarly, excess carbonic acid can be converted into carbon dioxide gas and exhaled through the lungs; this prevents too many free hydrogen ions from building up in the blood and dangerously reducing its pH; likewise, if too much OH^- is introduced into the system, carbonic acid will combine with it to create bicarbonate, lowering the pH.

$$H_2O+CO_2 \leftrightharpoons H_2CO_3 \leftrightharpoons H^++CO^{-3}$$

Isoelectric pH is the pH at which molecule is neutral or do NOT carry any charge. It directly affects the solubility. Neutral molecules are not soluble in water.

Acid-base balance is regulation of body fluids pH which is important for normal physiology of body and cellular metabolism. Acid is a compound which gives H^+ ions in solution (proton donor) whereas Base is a compound which accepts H^+ ions (proton acceptor). The normal pH of blood or plasma is ~7.4 and tightly regulated in the range of 7.36-7.44.

Acidosis is a process causing increased acidity of blood or low blood pH (increased H^+ concentration) or plasma or other body tissues. There are two types of acidosis; respiratory acidosis and metabolic acidosis. It occurs due to retention of CO_2, production of non-volatile acids or organic molecules, loss of bicarbonate ions in urine or feces, intake of acid or acid precursors. ***Acidosis*** $\leq$ ***pH 7.35***

Alkalosis is a process causing increased basicity of blood or high blood pH (reduced H^+ concentration) or plasma or other body tissues. There are two types of alkalosis; respiratory alkalosis and Metabolic alkalosis. It occurs due to loss of acid in vomitus or urine, severe diarrhea, CO_2 loss, gastric aspiration in hospitals. ***Alkalosis*** $\geq$ ***pH 7.45***

Carbohydrates and Metabolism

Definition

Out of the four biomolecules of life, carbohydrates represent one of the most abundant and major class of biomolecules. Biochemically, carbohydrates are polyhydroxy aldehydes or ketones, or substances that yield such compounds upon hydrolysis. They have empirical formula (CH_2O)n composed of carbon (*carbo-*), and hydrogen and oxygen (*-hydrate*); although few carbohydrates also contain nitrogen, phosphorus or sulfur.

Types

Based on the number of monomeric units carbohydrates can be classified into following categories:

1. Monosaccharides

They are the simplest carbohydrates or simple sugars (*saccharide*), which consist of a single polyhydroxy aldehyde or ketone unit. They can be further classified into two types based on the functional group present or number of carbon atoms present. A sugar that bears an aldehyde group is called an **aldose** whereas a sugar with a ketone group is a **ketose**. Similarly the carbohydrates for which n=3, are called **trioses**, **tetroses** (n=4 *e.g.* erythrose, erythrulose), **pentoses** (n=5 *e.g.* ribose, ribulose, xylulose), **hexoses** (n=6 *e.g.* glucose, fructose, galactose, mannose), **heptoses** (n=7 *e.g.* aldoheptose, sedoheptulose). The terms can be combined as well. Thus, glyceraldehyde is a triose that has an aldehyde group and so is an aldose. Hence it can also be referred as an **aldotriose**. Similarly, dihydroxyacetone is a **ketotriose**.

2. Disaccharides

They consist of two monosaccharides joined together by a characteristic **glycosidic bond.** For example, sucrose (glucose and fructose), maltose (glucose and glucose), lactose (glucose and galactose) and trehalose (glucose and glucose).

3. Oligosaccharides

They consist of short chains (3 to 10) of monsaccharides joined by glycosidic bond. For example, maltotriose and raffinose (trisaccharide), stachyose (tetrasaccharide), verbascose (pentasaccharide).

4. Polysaccharides

They consist of more than ten units of monsaccharides joined by glycosidic bond. Depending upon type of monsaccharide units attached, they can be further classified into two categories.

a. Homopolysaccharides

Only one type of monosaccharide units. For example, starch (glucose), cellulose (glucose), glycogen (glucose) and inulin (fructose), chitin (N-acetyl glucosamine), dextran (glucose)

- ☆ **Starch:** In most plants excess glucose is stored as large branched polysaccharide called starch made up of glucose. Further, can be structurally two kind: **Amylose** (13-20 per cent) having glucose units linked by α (1-4) glycosidic bond and **amylopectin** (80-87 per cent) having glucose units linked by α (1-4) glycosidic bond but branched after 24-30 residues with α (1-6) glycosidic bond.
- ☆ **Cellulose:** Structural polysaccharide use to make plant cell walls having glucose units linked by β (1-4) glycosidic bond with no branches. *Not digested by humans due to absence of cellulose.*
- ☆ **Glycogen:** In animals, excess glucose is stored as large branched polysaccharide called glycogen. It consists of glucose units linked by α (1-4) glycosidic bond with branching at every 10 units by the formation of α (1-6) glycosidic bond. *Similar to amylopectin but have more branches.*
- ☆ **Inulin:** Made up of fructose units linked by β (2-1) bonds. *Used in kidney function test to assess glomerular filtration rate.*
- ☆ **Chitin:** made up of N-acetyl glucosamine linked by β (1-4) glycosidic bond.

- ☆ **Dextran:** made up of highly branched monomeric units of glucose having α (1-6), α (1-4), α (1-3) linear and α (1-3), α (1-2) branched glycosidic bonds in bacteria or yeasts.

b. *Heteropolysaccharides*

More than one type of monosaccharides. For example, agar, mucopolysaccharides (hylauronic acid, heparin).

Agar: Made up of agarose (disaccharide made up of D-galactose and 3,6-anhydro-L-galactopyranose) and agaropectin (alternating units of sulfated galactose and glucose molecules).

Mucoploysaccharide: Also referred as glycosaminoglycans (GAG) are composed of repeating disaccharide units of amino sugars and uronic acids.

- ☆ Large numbers of anionic groups (carboxyl and sulfate) confer high holding capacity of cations and water to increase viscosity.
- ☆ They provide elasticity to the connective tissue.
- ☆ Mostly they are structural components of connective tissue, so they act as lubricants and are good shock absorber against mechanical shock.
- ☆ Hyaluronic acid (*only non-sulfated GAG*) in synovial fluids of joints and vitreous humor of eye prevents bacterial attack.
- ☆ Heparin acts as natural anticoagulant.

Functions of Carbohydrates

1. **Energy source:** Carbohydrates represent one of the major and instant sources of energy. For instance, glucose is required for rapidly metabolizing cells such as neuron and RBCs.
2. **Energy storage:** Carbohydrates represent important storage molecules for energy. For example, starch in plants and glycogen in animals.
3. **Structural components:** Carbohydrates serves as structural components of the cell. For example, cellulose in plants, glycolipids in cell membranes.
4. **General roles:** Carbohydrates also serves some general functions as follows:
   - **a.** Ribose sugars serves as components of nucleic acids.
   - **b.** Heparin serves as anticoagulant.
   - **c.** Glucose serves as precursors for synthesis of fats and amino acids.
   - **d.** Glucuronic acid is involved in detoxification process.

Structural Features of Carbohydrates

Stereoisomerism

Stereoisomerism refers to the spatial differences (arrangement of atoms in space) between the isomers having same structural and molecular formula. All monosaccharides except dihydroxyacetone have one or more asymmetric (chiral) carbon atom (having four different attached functional groups) and thus exist as optically active isoforms. The simplest monosaccharide glyceraldehydes contains one chiral center thus its two isoforms are mirror images and referred as D (dextro) and L (levo) depending upon the ability of the molecule to rotate the plane polarized light to either right or left respectively. In other words, when the hydroxyl group on the reference (asymmetric) carbon is on the right in the projection formula, the sugar is the D isomer; when on the left, it is the L isomer. *The convention of numbering and naming carbon atoms follows two rules. Firstly, the carbon atoms are numbered from the end of the carbon chain starting with the aldehyde or ketone group, which is carbon 1 (C-1) and secondly the symbols D and L refer to the configuration of the asymmetric carbon atom farthest from the aldehyde or ketone group*. For example, in glucose, the farthest asymmetric carbon from the aldehyde group is C-5. D-Glucose is called D because the configuration of the atoms bonded to C-5 is the same as for D-glyceraldehyde. Similarly, D-fructose is designated D because the configuration at C-5 matches that for D-glyceraldehyde.

Enantiomers

D and L stereoisomers are referred as enantiomers. For example, D-glucose and L-glucose are enantiomers. These are mirror images of each other.

Epimers

D sugars that differ in configuration at only a single asymmetric carbon atom other than farthest asymmetric carbon atom are called epimers. D-glucose and D-galactose are epimers because they differ in their configuration at C-4 only. Similarly, D-glucose and D-mannose are epimers because they differ in their configuration at C-2 only. These are not mirror images of each other.

Diastereoisomers

D sugars that differ in configuration at one or more asymmetric carbon atoms other than farthest asymmetric carbon atom are called diastereoisomers. D-galactose and D-mannose are diastereoisomers because they differ in their configuration at C-2 and C-4 both. These are not mirror images of each other. All epimers are diastereomers but all diastereomers are not epimers.

Anomers

The aldehyde or ketone group can react with a hydroxyl group to form a covalent bond leading to the formation of a new asymmetric center during cyclization, at C-1 for aldoses (hemiacetalization) and C-2 for ketoses (hemiketalization). This carbon is called hemiacetal or hemiketal carbon and generally referred as anomeric carbon atom. The orientation of OH and H around anomeric carbon results in two isomers called as anomers. If OH group at anomeric carbon lies below the plane of the ring, then it is referred as α **form** and if OH group at anomeric carbon lies above the plane of the ring, then referred as β **form**. All anomers are epimers but all epimers are not anomers.

Mutarotation

The interconversion of both α and β forms in aqueous solutions to give an equilibrium mixture is called as mutarotation. For example, equilibrium mixture of glucose has 36 per cent α form and 63 per cent β form and less than 1 per cent in open chain configuration.

Reducing Sugars

Sugars that have free aldehyde or ketone group at the end are called as reducing sugars hence can reduce either cupric or ferric ions which forms the basis of Fehling's and Benedict's tests. Only reducing sugars (*e.g.* glucose and fructose) exhibit mutarotation since the sugar must have free anomeric carbon atom to exhibit mutarotation. Non-reducing sugars (*e.g.* sucrose and trehalose) does not have any free anomeric carbon hence does not exhibit mutarotation.

Glycosidic Bond

The covalent bond formed when OH group of one sugar reacts with anomeric carbon of other sugar. For instance, lactose is a disaccharide formed between anomeric (C-1) carbon in β confirmation of D-galactose and C-4 of D-glucose, hence referred as β(1-4) D-lactose. Similarly, maltose is a disaccharide formed between the α form of C-1 and C-4 positions of two glucose units, hence referred as α (1-4) D-maltose. For lactose and maltose, one of the anomeric carbons has been used to form the glycosidic bond, leaving the second anomeric carbon free. Thus, both lactose and maltose have a reducing end and therefore are reducing sugars. In contrast, sucrose is a disaccharide formed by bond formation between the anomeric C-1 of glucose and the anomeric C-2 of fructose such that a free reducing group is lacking making sucrose as non-reducing sugar.

Carbohydrate Metabolism

Glycolysis

Overview

Among the four biomolecules of life, carbohydrates occupy the pivotal position in energy metabolism. All the carbohydrates metabolism pathways are linked with glucose. For instance, dietary starch and lactose from milk catabolizes to glucose in the body. Glycolysis is the process of breakdown of glucose to yield energy.

Synonyms

It is also known as Embden-Meyerhoff pathway or EMP after the name of the discoverer.

Definition

The series of reactions involving breakdown of one molecule of glucose into two molecules of pyruvate (in aerobic conditions) and two molecules of lactate (in anaerobic conditions) along with production of two molecules of ATP (Figure 2.1).

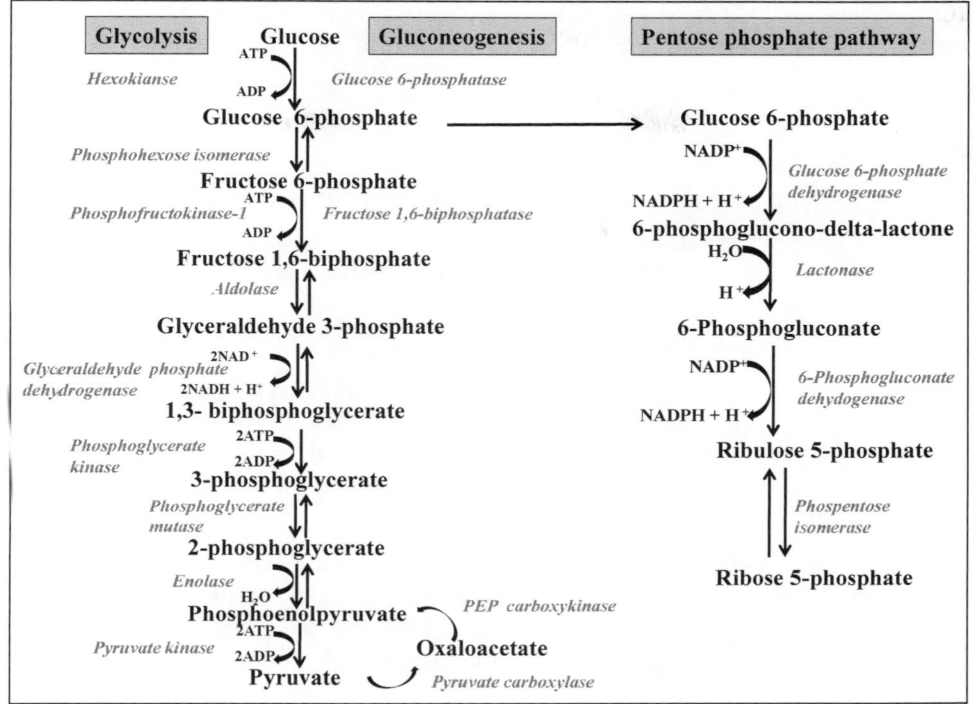

Figure 2.1: Overview of Carbohydrate Metabolism.

Occurrence

This universal cycle occurs in cytosol of all the cells inside the body.

Function

Glycolysis serves two important purposes.

- ☆ Energy production in the form of ATP
- ☆ Intermediate metabolite precursor required for other biosynthetic pathways. *e.g.* Acetyl Co A needed for fatty acid biosynthesis.

Pathway

The breakdown of the six-carbon glucose into two molecules of the three-carbon pyruvate occurs in ten steps in two phases. The first is preparatory phase where the energy of ATP is invested and the carbon chains of all the metabolized hexoses are converted into a common product, glyceraldehyde 3-phosphate. The other is the payoff phase where the energy gain takes place.

Phosphorylation

It is the process of synthesis of ATP. In **oxidative phosphorylation**, involving the electron transport chain, ATP synthesis is linked to the oxidation of NADH and $FADH_2$ to NAD^+ and FAD respectively and occurs via the generation of a proton gradient across the inner mitochondrial membrane. In **substrate-level phosphorylation**, the direct transfer of a phosphate from a sugar–phosphate intermediate to ADP occurs.

Fates of Pyruvate

There are four fates of pyruvate depending upon the body needs:

Entry into the citric acid cycle: Under aerobic conditions, pyruvate is oxidized into acetyl CoA with the help of enzyme pyruvate dehydrogenase which enter citric acid cycle to yield carbon dioxide and water.

$$\text{Pyruvate} + NAD^+ + \text{CoA} \rightarrow \text{acetyl CoA} + CO_2 + \text{NADH}$$

Conversion to lactate: Under anaerobic conditions, pyruvate is reduced to lactate by lactate dehydrogenase to replenish the supply of NAD^+ for continuation of glycolysis which gets depleted due to lack of oxidative phosphorylation. For example, in vigorously contracting skeletal muscles during exercise.

$$\text{Pyruvate} + \text{NADH} + H^+ \rightarrow \text{lactate} + NAD^+$$

Conversion to ethanol: Under anaerobic conditions in yeast and some other microorganisms, the NAD^+ required for the continuation of glycolysis is regenerated by a process called alcoholic fermentation. The pyruvate is converted to acetaldehyde (by pyruvate decarboxylase) and then to ethanol (by alcohol dehydrogenase), NADH is converted to NAD^+:

$$\text{Pyruvate} + H^+ \rightarrow \text{acetaldehyde} + CO_2$$

$$\text{Acetaldehyde} + \text{NADH} + H^+ \rightarrow \text{ethanol} + NAD^+$$

Conversion to fatty acid: Under high energy level when ATP is in excess, the anabolic reaction overtakes the catabolic reactions and acetyl CoA begins to accumulate. Under these conditions, acetyl CoA can be used for fatty acid synthesis or the synthesis of ketone bodies.

Energetics

The energetics of glycolysis can be calculated under two conditions:

- *Anaerobic*: Two ATPs are consumed in the preparatory phase of glycolysis. Four ATPs are generated in the payoff phase in giving rise to pyruvate giving a net yield of two ATPs per glucose molecule.
- *Aerobic*: Apart from above gain in two ATPs, the two NADH molecules that are synthesized are reoxidized via the electron transport chain generating six more ATPs during oxidative phosphorylation. Thus, the net gain of ATP per glucose molecule becomes eights ATPs.

The overall reaction is:

$$\text{Glucose} + 2\text{Pi} + 2\text{ADP} + 2NAD^+ \rightarrow 2\text{pyruvate} + 2\text{ATP} + 2\text{NADH} + 2H^+ + 2H_2O$$

Regulation

Glycolysis is regulated at three irreversible steps of the pathway catalyzed by hexokinase, phosphofructokinase and pyruvate kinase enzymes by feedback inhibition. Under the fed state when energy levels are optimal and there is no requirement of ATP synthesis then glycolysis is inhibited by fructose 2, 6 bisphosphate, citrate, ATP and H^+ ions (acidity). All these factors signal that there is energy replete conditions and no further breakdown of glucose is needed hence glucose is utilized for anabolic reactions. Under the starvation conditions, anabolic reactions involving glucose is halted and glucose breakdown via glycolysis is initiated.

Gluconeogenesis

Definition

The synthesis of glucose from non-carbohydrate precursors such as lactate, pyruvate, alanine, glycerol.

Occurrence

Gluconeogenesis occurs in liver.

Significance

The glucose reserves in our body are sufficient for only half a day during fasting conditions. Hence sites such as brain, erythrocytes and skeletal muscles which requires constant source of energy in the form of glucose relies on this pathway. In addition, gluconeogenesis also serves as a detoxification pathway to clear the byproducts of metabolism. For instance, lactate produced in muscle and erythrocytes, alanine in muscles, glycerol produced in adipose tissue or propionyl CoA produced from fatty acid oxidation.

Reactions

Glycolysis is the conversion of glucose into pyruvate while gluconeogenesis involves conversion of pyruvate into glucose. In principle, gluconeogenesis is the reverse of glycolysis however, the irreversible steps of glycolysis are catalyzed by different enzymes in gluconeogenesis namely pyruvate carboxylase, phosphoenol pyruvate carboxykinase, fructose 1,6 bisphosphatase and glucose 6 phosphatase (Figure 2.1).

Energetics

Two molecules of pyruvate are required to produce one molecule of glucose. Hence the number of ATPs invested are as follows:

Pyruvate carboxylase 1ATP x 2 = 2 ATP

PEP carboxykinase 1GTP x 2 = 2 GTP

Phophoglycerate kinase 1 ATP x 2 = 2 ATP

Total 6 ATP

This contrasts with only 2 ATP gain for glycolysis, hence an extra 4ATPs are required to reverse the glycolysis by gluconeogenesis.

Regulation

Since both glycolysis and gluconeogenesis are reversible in nature in majority of steps where ATPs are either generated or utilized hence if both cycles are operating simultaneously then it would lead to a 'futile cycle'. Hence any condition that requires energy production and glucose breakdown such as insulin, AMP will lead to enhance glycolysis. Alternatively, under conditions of fed state H^+, citrate, acetyl CoA, fructose 2,6 bisphosphate, glucagon and cortisol where energy requirement is minimal then gluconeogenesis is induced.

Cori Cycle (Lactic Acid Cycle)

Gluconeogenesis from lactate is called as Cori's cycle after name of the discoverer. In vigorous contracting muscles lactate is produced from glycolysis which is a metabolic dead-end product. Hence lactate diffuses out of the muscle cells and carried to liver via blood where it is converted back to pyruvate by lactate dehydrogenase which is subsequently converted to glucose via gluconeogenesis steps. This glucose is released back to muscle via blood and these cyclic events are known as Cori cycle.

Pentose Phosphate Pathway (PPP)

Synonyms

Hexose monophosphate shunt, phosphogluconate pathway

Overview

Reducing power of the cell is available in the form of NADH and NADPH. Although similar in structure both are metabolically non-interchangeable hence these need to be synthesized independently. The set of reactions that synthesizes NADPH are known as PPP (Figure 2.1). The cycle begins with glycolytic intermediate glucose 6 phosphate and ends with other sets of glycolytic intermediates namely fructose 6 phosphate and glyceraldehyde 3 phosphate, hence is known as 'shunt'.

Occurrence

PPP occurs in cytosol of all living tissue such as liver, adrenal cortex, RBC, adipose tissue and mammary glands that actively synthesizes fatty acids and sterols which require NADPH.

Reactions

The pathway involves two phases namely oxidative and non-oxidative.

Oxidative phase involves conversion of glucose 6 phosphate into ribulose 5 phosphate via oxidative decarboxylation reaction with an intermediate formation of phosphogluconate and formation of two molecules of NADPH.

Non-oxidative phase involves series of rearrangement reactions of three molecules of ribulose 5 phosphate into two molecules of fructose 6 phosphate and one molecule of glyceraldehyde 3 phosphate (which enters glycolysis) with the help of enzymes transaldolase and transketolase.

Significance

PPP mainly serves two purpose:

1. Generation of NADPH which is required for synthesis of fatty acids, steroids, phagocytosis and RBC membrane integrity. *G6PD deficiency leads to increased hemolysis as NADPH is required for maintaining RBC membrane integrity.*
2. Generation of ribose sugars which is required for nucleotide synthesis.

Regulation

The oxidative phase reaction is irreversible hence the rate limiting step governed by the NADPH levels. The reactions for the non-oxidative phase are reversible in nature hence can me directed according to the need of the cells as follows:

1. In rapidly dividing cells requiring more ribose than NADPH, the flux is directed from fructose 6 phosphate and glyceraldehyde 3 phosphate in synthesis of ribose sugars.
2. When need for NADPH and ribose are balanced then the cycle takes place for the generation of both NADPH and ribose.
3. When adipose tissue synthesizing fatty acids require more NADPH than ribose then oxidative phase reaction is enhanced while non-oxidative phase reactions enters the glycolysis to produce more glucose 6 phosphate.
4. When cells require both NADPH and ATP then oxidative phase reaction is enhanced while non-oxidative phase reactions enter the glycolysis to produce pyruvate.

Glycogenolysis

Overview

Glycogen breakdown to produce glucose is known as glycogenolysis. Liver and skeletal muscles are the major storage sites for glycogen to serve two contrasting roles. Glycogen stored in liver is used to maintain blood glucose levels for tissues such as brain while in skeletal muscles it serves as source of energy for muscle contraction.

Glycogen Breakdown

It involves two enzymes glycogen phosphorylase and glycogen debranching enzyme. Glycogen phosphorylase removes one glucose unit by breaking α1–4 glycosidic bonds from non-reducing end (free 4′ OH) in the form of glucose 1 phosphate. The reaction also involves Pi since it requires a covalent bond formation with phosphate group. Glucose 1phosphate formed gets converted by phosphoglucomutase to glucose 6 phosphate.

Glycogen (n residues) + Pi ⟶ Glycogen (n-1) + glucose 1 phosphate

Glucose 1 phosphate ⟶ glucose 6 phosphate

The fate of glucose 6 phosphate depends upon the tissue. For instance, in liver tissues, glucose 6 phosphatase converts it to glucose for maintenance of blood glucose levels for other tissues.

Glucose 6 phosphate + H_2O ⟶ Glucose + Pi

Contrary, in muscle tissue due to absence of glucose 6 phosphatase and different role, glucose 6 phosphate is immediately metabolized via glycolysis to yield instant energy.

Glycogen phosphorylase can break single glucose residues from non-reducing ends upto four residues away from a branch point involving α 1–6 glycosidic bonds due to steric hindrance. Glycogen debranching enzyme removes the branches thereby allowing glycogen phosphorylase to continue the glycogen degradation. Glycogen debranching enzyme have both transferase and α1–6 glucosidase activity which transfer the branched residues (three) to the original linear chain and cleaves the branch point. Thus, with the help of these enzymes, complete breakdown of glycogen molecule yields glucose 1 phosphate (90 per cent) and glucose (10 per cent).

Regulation

Glycogen phosphorylase is the regulatory enzyme for glycogenolysis which is regulated by covalent modification where phosphorylated form is the active form and dephosphorylated form is the inactive form. The enzyme activity is inhibited by insulin and activated by glucagon and adrenalin.

Glycogenesis

Overview

Glycogenesis is the formation of glycogen from glucose but requires separate set of reactions by utilizing UDP-glucose which is the activated form of glucose (acetyl CoA and AA-tRNA are activated form of acetate and amino acids).

Occurrence

It occurs in cytosol of liver and muscle tissues.

Reaction

It takes place in two steps:

1. Activation of glucose to form UDP-glucose by UDP-glucose pyrophosphorylase which is the donor of glucose in glycogen synthesis.
   UTP + Glucose 1 phosphate ⟶ UDP-Glucose + PPi
2. Chain extension and formation of glycogen with the help of glycogen synthase and branching enzyme. Glycogen synthase transfer the glucose units to non-reducing ends of the existing chain (primer) known as glycogenin made of eight residues. After enough residues are attached, the branching enzyme (amylo 1-4 to 106 transglycosylase) transfers about seven residues by breaking the α 1–4 glycosidic bonds and re attaching at more interior site with α 1–6 glycosidic bond to produce branches.

Significance of Branching

Since the glycogen degrading and synthesizing enzymes work only at the ends hence existence of many termini allows enhanced rate of synthesis and degradation than would have been possible with non-branched molecule. Additionally, branches increase the solubility of the glycogen molecule.

Regulation

Glycogen synthase is the regulatory enzyme which is also regulated by covalent modification. The phosphorylated form is inactive while the dephosphorylated form is active. The enzyme activity is decreased by adrenaline and enhanced by insulin.

TCA Cycle

Overview

Tricarboxylic acid (TCA) cycle or citric acid cycle or Kreb cycle after the name of the discoverer in 1937 occurs in mitochondria of eukaryote (except RBC and lens) and cytosol of prokaryotes. The function of TCA cycle is to oxidize the pyruvate formed during glycolysis into CO_2 and H_20 and generate energy in the form of ATP. Additionally, it also helps in oxidation of acetyl CoA generated during fatty acid oxidation.

Reactions

The overall reaction occurs in three phases.

1. Oxidation of pyruvate to acetyl CoA: Pyruvate formed during glycolytic breakdown is oxidized to acetyl CoA with a multi enzyme complex pyruvate dehydrogenase. Since this reaction also generates CO_2 hence is also known as oxidative decarboxylation.
2. The citric acid cycle: The acetyl group is oxidized by series of eight reactions to generate CO_2 and electrons stored in NADH and $FADH_2$.
3. Oxidation of NADH and $FADH_2$: These are reoxidized and energy released is used for ATP synthesis by oxidative phosphorylation.

Energetics

Each of the NADH and $FADH_2$ formed during TCA cycle generates 3 and 2ATP molecules respectively by oxidative phosphorylation. One GTP formed is equivalent to ATP molecule. Thus, the complete breakdown of one molecule of glucose from TCA cycle generates 30 ATP molecules.

Regulation

Since the major role of TCA cycle is provision of energy hence the cycle is induced when cellular energy levels are low (high ADP concentration, low ATP and NADH) and impeded as ATP (and then $NADH_2$, succinyl CoA and citrate) accumulates.

Functions

TCA cycle serves two significant amphibolic functions:

1. The catabolic nature is primary function that deals with the provision of energy.
2. Anabolic role of TCA cycle involves many intermediates that are used to synthesize other compounds. For instance, Succinyl CoA is used for heme synthesis, oxaloacetate and alpha ketoglutarate is used for production of aminoacids.

Electron Transport Chain and Oxidative Phosphorylation

Overview

The reducing equivalents in the form of NADH and $FADH_2$ produced during glycolysis and TCA cycle needs to be re-oxidized to generate ATP and NAD and FAD for fresh cycles to continue. This involves specialized set of electron carriers located on mitochondrial membrane known as Electron transport chain (ETC) or respiratory chain since oxygen is the terminal electron acceptor converting to water. During these oxidation reactions, the part of the free energy is utilized to produce ATP by ATP synthase thus known as oxidative phosphorylation. Rest of the free energy is used to generate heat required to maintain body temperature.

ETC

This oxidation reaction for NADH and $FADH_2$ occurs via sequence of complex enzymes which accepts electron and transfer to oxygen producing water. This involves four enzyme complexes (NADH dehydrogenase, succinate dehydrogenase, cytochrome bc1 complex and cytochrome oxidase complex) embedded in the inner mitochondrial membrane and two mobile electron carriers (ubiquinone or CoQ and cytochrome c) to link these large enzyme complexes (Figure 2.2).

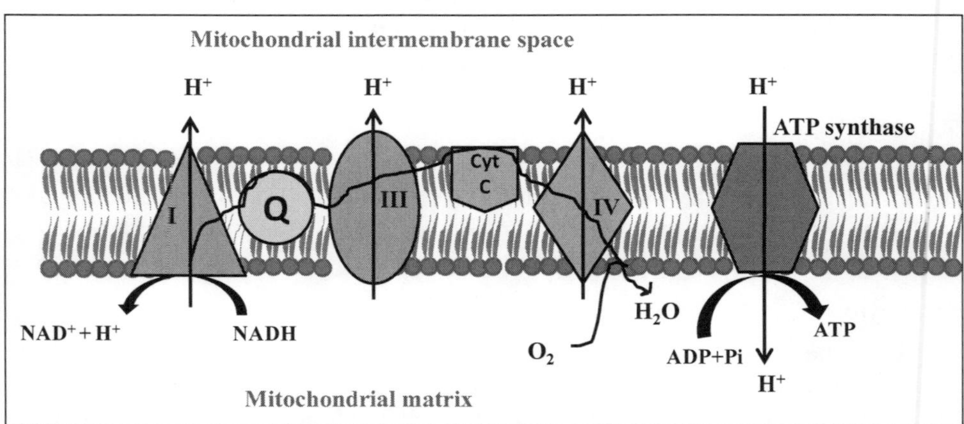

Figure 2.2. Overview of ETC and Oxidative Phosphorylation.

H^+ Gradient

There is a net flow of electrons from NADH (most negative redox potential or least affinity for electron) to oxygen (most positive redox potential or highest affinity for electrons) via all the enzyme complexes and electron carriers. Each NADH donates two electrons however each electron carrier comprising cytochrome, FeS center and copper atom can carry only one electron. Additionally, each molecule of oxygen requires four electrons to get reduce to form one molecule of H_2O. This causes a fall (more positive) in redox potential throughout the *etc.* mainly at the three major complexes (NADH dehydrogenase, cytochrome bc1 and cytochrome oxidase) leading to pump H^+ ions from matrix to intermembranous space thereby creating a H^+ gradient. Similarly, electron transport from $FADH_2$ occurs from succinate dehydrogenase complex leading to H^+ ions to be pumped, however, succinate dehydrogenase itself is not an H^+ pump hence the gradient is only created at two complexes (bc1 and cytochrome oxidase).

Oxidative Phosphorylation

The synthesis of ATP (phosphorylation) that occurs by oxidation of NADH and $FADH_2$ from *etc.* This mechanism for proposed by Peter Mitchell in 1961 (Nobel prize winner) and the hypothesis is known as Chemiosmotic hypothesis. This states that the energy liberated during electron movements create proton gradient that is used to drive ATP synthesis. The pumping out of protons generates a higher concentration of H^+ ions in the intermembranous space with positive electrical potential towards the side facing the intermembrane space thereby creating an electrochemical proton gradient. These protons when flow back into the matrix through enzyme ATP synthase (complex 5) drives the ATP synthesis. Since the pumping of electrons take place only at two positions during $FADH_2$ oxidation contrary to three positions during NADH oxidation, the amount of ATP formation from $FADH_2$ is less (two ATP) than that of NADH (three ATP).

Uncouplers

Few chemicals like 2,4, dinitro phenol, 2,4, dinitro cresol, dicumarol, thyroxine, gramicidin A, valinomycin and nigercin binds to the H^+ ions (proton ionophores) and dissipate the proton gradient leading to inhibition of ATP synthesis with no effect on electron movement and oxygen consumption. This is known as uncoupling action and the agents are known as uncouplers. The production of heat during uncoupling is known as thermogenesis. This phenomenon is important in brown adipose tissues in new borns and hibernating animals which contain uncoupler thermogenin and the heat generated provides protection from cold conditions.

Glyoxylate Cycle

Overview

It is a variation of the tricarboxylic acid cycle and anabolic pathway for the conversion of acetyl-CoA to succinate to synthesize carbohydrates.

Occurrence

It occurs in glyoxysomes of plants, bacteria, protists and fungi.

Significance

In microorganisms, the glyoxylate cycle allows cells to utilize simple carbon compounds as a carbon source when complex sources such as glucose are not available. The cycle is generally assumed to be absent in animals, with the exception of nematodes at the early stages of embryogenesis. Isocitrate lyase and malate synthase are the key enzymes of glyoxylate cycle (Figure 2.3).

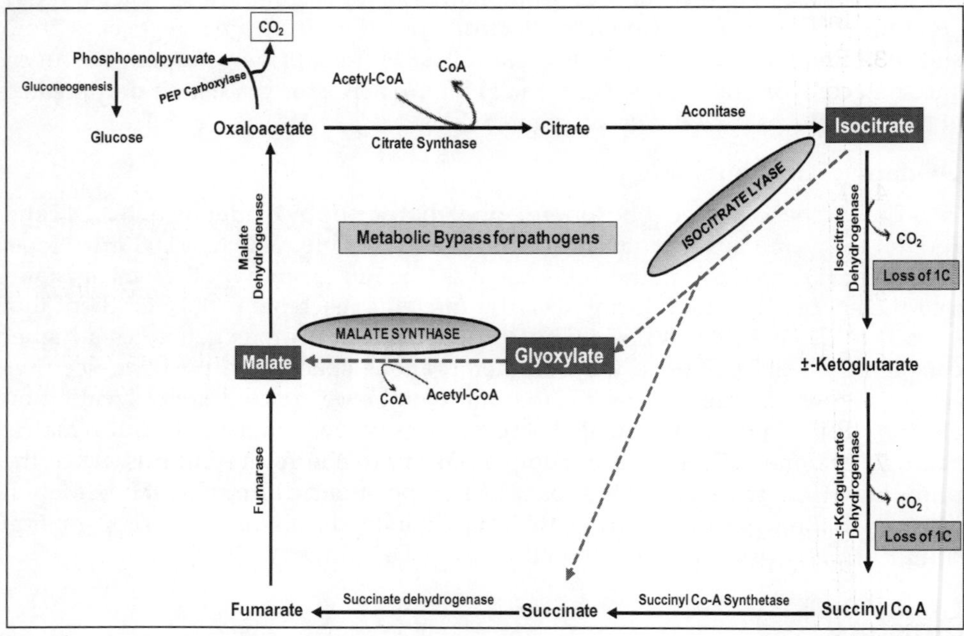

Figure 2.3: Overview of Glyoxylate Cycle.

Reaction

The glyoxylate cycle results in the net conversion of two acetyl-CoA to succinate instead of 4 CO_2 as in citric acid cycle. Succinate is transferred to mitochondrion where it can be converted to OAA (TCA) for gluconeogenesis.

$$2\ \text{acetyl-CoA} + 2\ NAD^+ + FAD \rightarrow OAA + 2\ CoA + 2\ NADH + FADH_2 + 2\ H^+$$

Amino Acids and Proteins

Definition

They are macromolecules or defined as polymers, which are comprised of one or more long chains of amino acid residues. They are one of the most abundant macromolecules playing diverse roles in living systems structurally and functionally.

They have different shapes and molecular weight that is decided by amino acids sequences.

Functions of Proteins

They serve many essential functions, which are as follows:

1. **Structural proteins:** Proteins serve in making structure of the cytoskeleton and other different structures. For *e.g.* actin, tubulin, keratin.
2. **Hormones:** Hormones are chemically signaling molecules which are sometimes composed of small proteins secreted by endocrine gland. They help in coordination of various activities throughout the body. For *e.g.* Insulin, thyroxin, glucagon.
3. **Enzymes:** Enzymes catalyzes the biochemical reaction composed of complex or conjugated proteins. Digestive enzymes such as amylase, pepsin, trypsin helps in digestion of complex molecules into monomer units which can be absorbed by the cells.
4. **Transport:** Proteins also helps in transportation of important molecules across the cell membrane. They also carry important substances in the blood or lymph in the body. For *e.g.* Hemoglobin, albumin.
5. **Contraction:** Proteins also play important role in muscle contraction in human body. For *e.g.* Myosin, Actin.
6. **Storage:** Proteins also gets stored for the nourishment of embryo and seedlings during early development. For *e.g.* Albumin, legume storage proteins.
7. **Defense:** Proteins also plays important role in form of immunoglobins, which protect the body from foreign pathogens. For *e.g.* Antibodies
8. **Synthesis and Repair:** Proteins also helps in synthesis and repair of DNA by transmitting the signals and acting as anchor for their synthesis.

Structure of Proteins

Proteins are classified structurally into four levels:

1. **Primary structure:** It is the simplest and basic level of protein structure. There is a linear sequence of amino acids forming a polypeptide chain. For *e.g.* Insulin hormone has two polypeptide chain of amino acids interconnected. The A and B chains in this structure are called as linear sequence of amino acids and sets an example of primary structure.
2. **Secondary structure:** It is the second level of protein structure, which is formed by the interaction of atoms within the polypeptide chain and results into folded structures. The two types of structures are α-helix and β-pleated sheets. These structures formed by hydrogen bonds, which is formed between carbonyl O of one amino acid and other H atom of other amino acid.
3. **Tertiary structure:** This three-dimensional structure of polypeptide chain represents the tertiary level of structure formed by the interaction between

the R groups of the amino acids that make up the protein structure. There are hydrophobic interactions in which R groups of amino acids having nonpolar groups cluster together on the inside of protein and hydrophilic amino acids goes outside and interact with water molecules. In tertiary structures, there are also disulfide bonds, covalent linkages formed between the sulfur containing side chains of amino acid cysteine, which are said to be stronger bonds than the other types of bonds.

4. **Quaternary structure:** This level of structure is formed when two or more polypeptide chains come together to form a quaternary structure of protein. For *e.g.* Hemoglobin protein, which carries blood in human body, consists of four units, 2 α-units and 2 β sheets.

Amino acids are structural and functional unit of proteins. The proteins formed by the attachment of two amino acids by peptide bond (with release of water molecule) in a linear manner forming a long chain. They are organic molecules composed of basic amino group (-NH_2), an acidic carboxyl group (-COOH), H atom and R group as a side chain. The general structure of amino acid (Figure 2.4) is as follows:

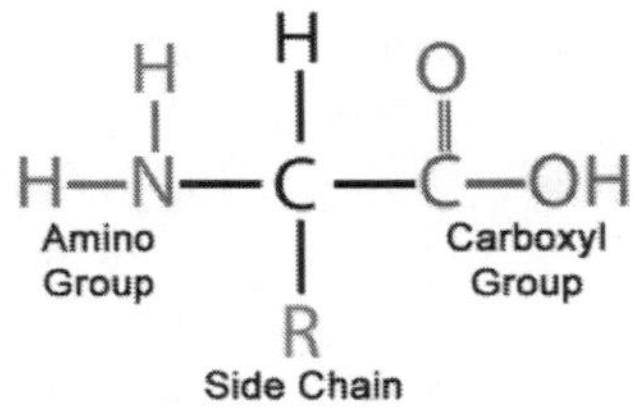

Figure 2.4: General Structure of Amino Acid.

Amino acids are the best-known examples of zwitterions. A zwitterion is a molecule with functional groups in which at least one has a positive and one has a negative electrical charge, resulting in net charge of zero. As amino acids contain amine group (basic) and a carboxylic group (acidic). The -NH_2 group is the stronger base, and so it takes up H+ from the -COOH group to leave a zwitterion. Zwitterion exists in solution at neutral pH.

Exceptions

1. Amino acid glycine, does not have R group and contains α-carbon attached with two hydrogens and is the simplest amino acid.
2. Amino acid proline does not have amino group, instead it has imino group (nitrogen is part of a ring) and forms bends and kinks in protein sequence.
3. Cysteine amino acid contains a thiol (-SH) group which enable to form covalent bonds with other cysteines.
4. All of the 20 amino acids except glycine are of the L-configuration, as glycine does not contain an asymmetric carbon atom, since it is

not optically active. As for all but one amino acid the α-carbon is an asymmetric carbon.

Amino Acids Classification:

There are 20 amino acids (Figure 2.5), which have been categorized into essential and non-essential amino acids. The bifurcation is based on the criteria that the amino acids which our body cannot synthesize and needed through our diet are called as essential amino acids. For *e.g.* Isoleucine, Leucine Methionine, Phenyl alanine, Threonine, Valine, Tryptophan and Histidine. Non-essential amino acids are the amino acids which are synthesized in our body and not required to take through diet. For *e.g.* Aspartate, Alanine, Aspargine, Arginine, Cystine, Glycine, Proline Glutamic acid, Serine and Tyrosine.

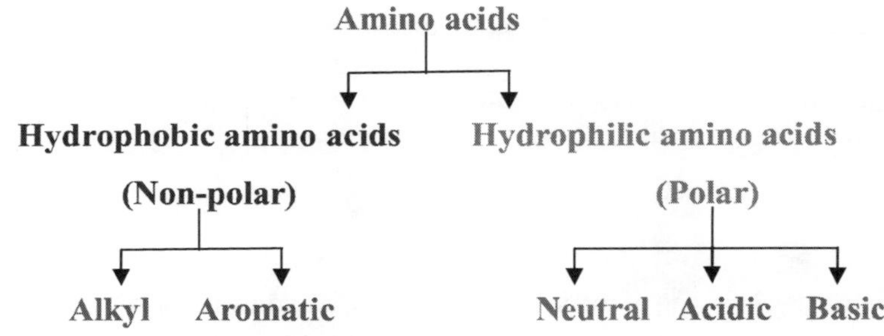

Alkyl R group	Aromatic R group	Neutral R group	Acidic R group	Basic R group
Glycine	Tryptophan	Asparagine	Glutamic acid	Arginine
Valine	Phenyalanine	Cysteine	Aspartic acid	Histidine
Alanine	Tyrosine	Glutamine		Lysine
Proline		Serine		
Leucine		Threonine		
Isoleucine				
Methionine				

Figure 2.5: Classification of Amino Acid Based on Polarity of R Groups.

Amino Acid Biosynthesis

Overview

All amino acids are derivative of intermediates formed in important pathways such as glycolysis, the citric acid cycle, or the pentose phosphate pathway. Nitrogen atom enters in these pathways through glutamate and glutamine. Ten of the amino acids have only one or a few enzymatic steps removed from their precursors. The pathways for others, such as the aromatic amino acids, are more complex.

Biosynthesis of Phenylalanine, Tryptophan and Tyrosine

Phenylalanine hydroxylase converts phenylalanine to tyrosine. Phenylalanine hydroxylase reaction is irreversible, dietary tyrosine cannot replace phenylalanine. Catalysis by this mixed-function oxidase incorporates one atom of O_2 into phenylalanine and reduces other atom to water. Reducing power, provided as tetrahydrobiopterin derives ultimately from NADPH.

Biosynthesis of Valine, Leucine and Isoleucine Amino Acids

While leucine, valine, and isoleucine are all nutritionally essential amino acids, tissue aminotransferases reversibly interconvert all three amino acids and their corresponding α-keto acids. The valine and isoleucine pathways share four enzymes. Pyruvate gives rise to valine and isoleucine in pathways that begin with the condensation of two carbons of pyruvate with another molecule of pyruvate (valine path) or with α-ketobutyrate (isoleucine path). The α-ketobutyrate is derived from threonine in a reaction that requires pyridoxal phosphate. An intermediate in the valine pathway, a-ketoisovalerate, is the starting point for a four-step branch pathway leading to leucine.

Urea Cycle

Overview

The urea cycle is one of the key pathways for the removal of nitrogen in humans. Ammonia is resultant from a variety of precursor protein sources. Approximately, 90 per cent percent of ingested protein is metabolized to urea which is excreted through the urine.

Synonyms

It is also known as Krebs-Henseleit cycle or ornithine cycle.

Definition

Urea cycle is important for converting ammonia (toxic by-product of nitrogen metabolism) into urea as humans and mammals excretes the ammonia in form of urea. Urea enters blood stream, which is filtered by kidneys and excreted in the urine.

Occurrence

It occurs in cytosol and mitochondrial matrix of liver cells.

Pathway

Urea cycle consists of 5 steps involving several key enzymes and involving two organelles (Figure 2.6). The first step occurs in mitochondria where ammonia coverts into carbamoyl phosphate. It is further along with ornithine forms citrulline, which is further released into cytosol to form arginosuccinate with the aspartate. Arginosuccinate is cleaved into fumarate and arginine. In the last step of this cycle, arginine is converted into ornithine with release of Urea and water molecule.

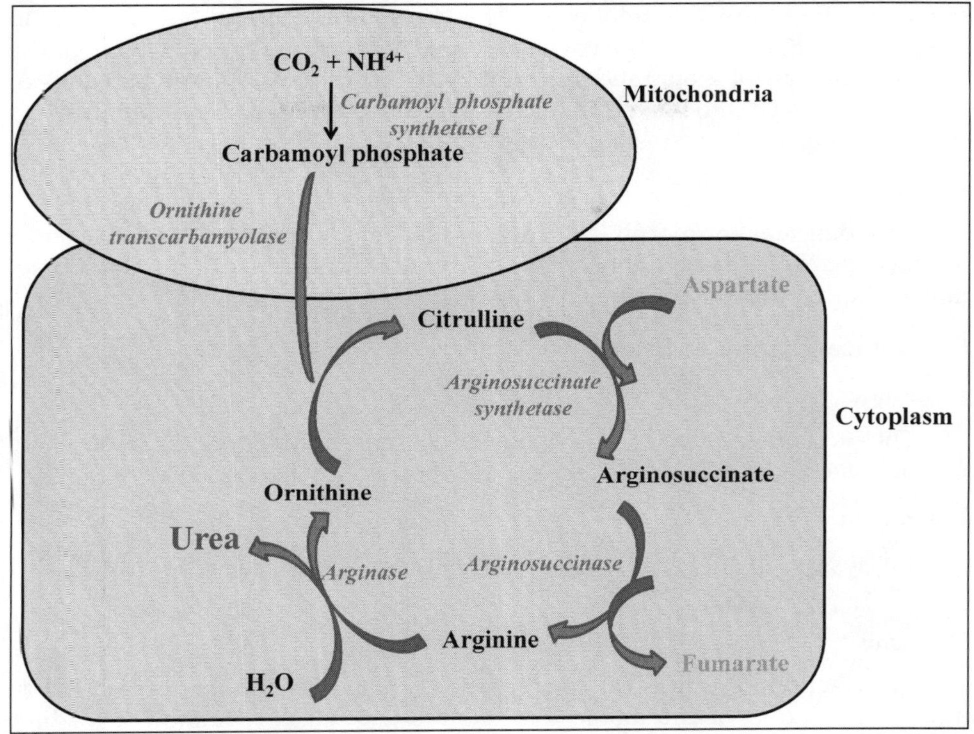

Figure 2.6: Overview of Urea Cycle.

Significance

The main significance of the urea cycle is to remove toxic ammonia from the body. A nonfunctional urea cycle would unable to remove excess amount of ammonia in the body, which can lead to hyperammonemia and other related diseases. Even the deficit of one or more of the key enzymes catalyzing reactions in the urea cycle can cause several disorders related to the cycle.

Porphyrin and Heme Metabolism

Overview

Porphyrins are known as precursors of heme, important component of hemoglobin, myoglobin. Heme consists of porphyrin ring carrying iron as central ion. Its main functions are binding O_2, electron transfer in energy reactions, taking part in oxidative reactions.

Occurrence

Heme synthesis occurs in liver and bone marrow.

Reactions

The initial and final steps of reaction occur in mitochondria and an intermediate step occurs in cytosol. Degradation of heme occurs inside macrophages present in spleen, which removes damaged or old erythrocytes from the blood circulation. The amino acids from the globin and iron are recycled while the porphyrin is degraded. Heme is converted into Biliverdin, which is further converted into Bilirubin and is the end-product of heme metabolism.

Significance

Any deficiency in porphyrin leads to inadequate heme production results in other metabolic complications. The disruption of heme synthesis results into microcytic, hypochromic anemia.

Succinate-glycine Pathway

Overview

The succinate-glycine cycle is analogous to the citric acid cycle, in that they are both involved with the metabolism of a 2-carbon compound.

Definition

It is the group of reactions called succinate-glycine cycle in which the glycine is converted to carbon dioxide.

Pathway

The reaction starts from the condensation of active" succinate on the α-carbon atom of glycine to yield α-amino-β-ketoadipic acid. Then, α-amino-β-ketoadipic acid further on decarboxylation yields δ-aminolevulinic acid. In this cycle, carboxyl group of glycine is converted to carbon dioxide on decarboxylation of α-amino-β-ketoadipic acid, and the α-carbon atom of the glycine is converted to carbon dioxide following the conversion of the

δ-aminolevulinic Acid to α-ketoglutaric Acid

Significance

It is significant for synthesis of porphyrin as it is precursor for heme synthesis.

Major Metabolic Disorders of Amino Acid Metabolism

As we know, amino acids are building blocks of proteins which have diverse functions in our body. Any defect in the gene or protein leads to defects in the functionality of that protein and enzyme which leads to metabolic disorders. Some of metabolic disorders of amino acids metabolism are as follows:

1. **Phenylketonuria:** It is inherited autosomal recessive disorder caused by defects in phenylalanine hydroxylase (PAH) gene, which results in low levels of the enzyme PAH. This leads to decreased metabolism of phenylalanine. This results in intellectual disability, behavioral problems, seizures, and mental disorders.
2. **Hawkinsinuria:** This disorder occurs due to deficiency of the 4-hydroxyphenylpyruvate dioxygenase enzyme, due to defects in the

HPD gene. A compound Hawkinsin (4-dihydroxy-cyclohexyl acetic acid) is formed from tyrosine metabolite precursors. The affected patients experience metabolic acidosis.

3. **Alkaptonuria:** It is a recessive disorder caused by mutations in the HGD gene, which encodes for homogentisate dioxygenase. The disorder leads to homogentisic acid accumulation in patients which results in pigmentation of connective tissue, arthritis of joints and spine, kidney and prostate stones. In children, it can be diagnosed easily as urine turns to dark color when exposed to air.
4. **Tyrosinemia type I:** It is a life-threatening disorder of tyrosine metabolism which is caused by variation in FAH gene, which encodes fumarylacetoacetase involved in tyrosine degradation. The enzyme defect causes the accumulation of precursors maleylacetoacetate and fumarylacetoacetate, and their by-products which are toxic to cells, liver and kidney.
5. **Tyrosinemia type II**: It is also known as Richner-Hanhart syndrome. This disorder is autosomal recessive disorder which is caused by defects of the first step of tyrosine degradation in the enzyme tyrosine aminotransferase. This results into increased levels of tyrosine and its metabolites in blood, Cerebral Fluid and urine. The patients develop skin and neurological problems.
6. **Maple Syrup Urine Disease: It** occurs due to disorder of branched chained amino acid catabolism. It is an autosomal recessive inborn error of metabolism which is caused by mutations in the subunits of the enzyme branched-chain alpha-keto acid dehydrogenase complex (BCKAD), leads to accumulation of the branched-chain amino acids (leucine, isoleucine, and valine. This disorder causes elevated leucine levels which results into cerebral edema and intoxication, irritability, lethargy, cerebral edema, coma and death.
7. **Homocystinuria:** It is an autosomal recessive disorder caused by defects in CBS gene which encodes for cystathionine beta-synthase. It is characterized by developmental delays and intellectual disability, with progressive myopia, defects in skeletal system such as scoliosis, pectus, stiff joints and thromboembolism.

Biological Nitrogen Fixation

Overview

Biological nitrogen fixation is a process in which nitrogen gas (N_2) from the atmosphere is integrated into the tissue of certain plants with the help of soil microorganisms, which are not able to obtain nitrogen directly.

Definition

It was discovered by Beijerinck in 1901 and known to be carried out by a specialized group of prokaryotes. These organisms have the capacity to utilize the nitrogenase which catalyze the conversion of atmospheric nitrogen (N_2) to ammonia (NH_3). Plants can readily assimilate NH_3 to produce nitrogenous biomolecules.

Occurrence

It can occur in non-leguminous as well as leguminous plants in which symbiont bacteria such as *Azotobacter* species resides in root nodules of these plants.

Reactions

It is high activation reaction. It is carried out by protein complex called as nitrogenase complex which consists of dinitrogenase reductase and dinitrogenase. The process is coupled to the hydrolysis of 16 equivalents of ATP, accompanied by the conformation of one equivalent of H_2. The conversion of N_2 into ammonia occurs at a metal cluster. As nitrogenase is degraded by oxygen, hence, it is scavenged by oxygen binding protein called leghaemoglobin.

The overall reaction is:

$$N_2 + 16\ ATP + 8\ H^+ + 8\ e^- \longrightarrow 2\ NH_3 + H_2 + 16\ ADP + 16\ Pi$$

It is following types:

1. **Non-Symbiotic/asymbiotic Biological Nitrogen Fixation**: Biological nitrogen fixation by microorganisms living freely or staying out of plant cell is called non-symbiotic Biological Nitrogen Fixation. *e.g. Chlorobium, Nostoc.*
2. **Associative Biological Nitrogen Fixation:** Some bacteria living in secure contact with the roots of plants, fix nitrogen. This association is a loose mutualism, called associative symbiosis. Fixed nitrogen is absorbed by the roots and the bacteria get nourishment from the carbohydrates released by the roots. *e.g. Azospirillum brasilense* in association with cereal roots
3. **Symbiotic Biological Nitrogen Fixation:** Symbiotic nitrogen fixation is *e.g.* of mutualistic relationship in which plants provide a niche and fixed carbon to bacteria in exchange for fixed nitrogen. *e.g. Bradyrhizobium japonicum* is a slow growing symbiont of Soybeans.

Structure and Functions of Vitamins

Vitamins: These are organic compounds required by the body in small amounts for performing various functions. They cannot be synthesized in our body and obtained through sources like diet, rumen of bacteria and sun. Vitamins are of diverse nature such as alcohols, aldehydes, organic acids, their derivatives and nucleotide derivatives.

Functions of Vitamins

1. They are required for metabolism.
2. They are required for protection.
3. They are essential for maintenance of health and proper growth.

4. They assist in the formation of hormones, blood vessels, chemicals and genetic materials.
5. They act as catalysts by combining with proteins to activate enzymes that are essential for biological reactions.

Classification of Vitamins

They have been classified based on their ability to be absorbed in fat or water.

Fat Soluble Vitamins

They are hydrophobic compounds which are stored in the liver and generally not excreted out of the body. For their absorption, bile salts and fats are required. Common examples are Vitamins A,D,E and K.

1. **Vitamin A:** It is a yellow primary alcohol derived from carotene. Its deficiency causes night blindness.
2. **Vitamin D:** It is important for bones. The two major physiological forms of vitamin D are D2 (ergocalciferol) and D3 (cholecalciferol).
3. **Vitamin E:** It is also called Tocopherol. It exists in the diet as a mixture of eight closely related compounds called tocopherols. Its def
4. **Vitamin K:** It is also called phylloquinone or anti-hemorrhagic vitamin or coagulation vitamin. Vitamin K is a complex unsaturated hydrocarbon which is found in two forms, vitamin K1 (phylloquinone) and vitamin K2 (Menaquinone).

Water Soluble Vitamins

They are water soluble vitamins which are not stored in body. Common example is Vitamin B complex and Vitamin C. They are readily excreted in the urine. Most of vitamins belonging to this class act as coenzymes.

Vitamin B Complex

1. **Vitamin B1:** It is colorless and crystalline substance. The addition of a pyrophosphate (ppi) from ATP converts it to thiamine pyrophosphate (TPP), the coenzyme for all decarboxylation of alpha keto acids.
2. **Vitamin B2:** component of the flavin coenzymes, FAD and FMN. It is composed of an isoalloxazane ring system linked to ribitol. It is mainly used in energy metabolism of sugars and lipids.
3. **Vitamin B3:** Niacin can be synthesized from tryptophan. Niacin contains a substituted pyridine ring and when NAD^+ activated forms NAD^+ and its phosphorylated derivative $NADP^+$, which are coenzymes of many dehydrogenases.
4. **Vitamin B5:** It is also called pantothenic acid that forms an essential part of acyl groups including the acetyl group derived from pyruvate. The coenzyme is derived metabolically from ATP, the vitamin pantothenic acid and β-mercaptoethylamine.

5) **Vitamin B6:** It exists in three forms: Pyridoxine, Pyridoxal and Pyridoxamine and their corresponding phosphates. Pyridoxal phosphate participates in transamination, decarboxylation, racemization reactions and numerous modification of amino acid sequence side chains.
6) **Vitamin B7:** It is also called Biotin which works as a coenzyme commonly associated with enzyme performing carboxylation reactions. Biotin is also known as "anti-egg white injury factor" or as H-factor.
7) **Vitamin B9:** It is also called Folic acid. The active form acid is tetrahydrofolate (THF). Coenzymes derived from the vitamin folic acid participates in the generation and utilization of single – carbon functional groups, methyl, methylene and formyl.
8) **Vitamin B12:** The metal cobalt in vitamin B12 is coordinated with a tetrapyrole ring system, which is like the porphyrin ring of heme compounds. The reactions requiring B12 involves methyl group transfer and adenosyl cobalamin dependent isomerization.

Vitamin C

It is commonly called as ascorbic acid. It is essential for the hydroxylation of proline and lysine in the formation of collagen. Collagen is a fibrous-protein with myriad connective and supportive functions. Its deficiency causes Scurvy.

Vitamin Derivative Co-factors

A cofactor is a non-protein chemical compound or metallic ion that is required for an enzyme's activity as a catalyst. Cofactors can be divided into two types: inorganic ions and complex organic molecules called coenzymes. Coenzymes are mostly derived from vitamins and other organic essential nutrients in small amounts (Table 2.1). The most common vitamin derived cofactors are thiamine (Vit B1), Riboflavin (B2), Niacin, Pantothenic acid (Vit B5), Vitamin B6 (Pyridoxine), Biotin, Vitamin B12 (Cobalamin) and folic acid.

Table 2.1: Vitamins and their Coenzyme Derivatives

Coenzyme	*Related Vitamin*	*Chemical Reaction*
NAD^+, $NADP^+$	Niacin	Oxidation-reduction
FAD	Riboflavin (B_2)	Oxidation-reduction
Thiamine pyrophosphate	Thiamine (B_1)	Transfer of aldehyde group
Coenzyme A	Pantothenate	Transfer of acyl group
Tetrahydrofolate	Folate	Transfer of one carbon group
Biotin	Biotin	Carboxylation
Pyridoxal phosphate	Pyridoxal (B_6)	Transamination

Lipids and Metabolism

Introduction

Lipids are organic compounds which are generally insoluble in water (polar solvents) and soluble in organic solvent (non-polar) such as chloroform, alcohol *etc.* Fats and oils are storage form in most organisms while phospholipids and sterols are structural components of most biological membranes.

Types

Based on their composition lipids can be classified as

1. **Simple lipids**: Esters of fatty acids with alcohol. Fats and oil are esters of fatty acids with glycerol hence acylglycerols. Fats are solid while oil are liquid at room temperatures. Similarly, waxes are fatty acids with higher alcohol such as bees wax, spermaceti wax, lanolin *etc.*
2. **Complex lipids**: Esters of fatty acids with alcohol along with a conjugate group that can be phosphate, carbohydrate and protein.
    a. **Phospholipids**: The conjugate group is phosphate. Based on nature of alcohol can be:
        i. **Glycerophospholipids**: The alcohol is glycerol. *e.g.* Lecithin, plasmalogen.
        ii. **Sphingophospholipids**: The alcohol is sphingosine. *e.g.* Sphingomyelin.
    b. **Glycolipids**: The conjugate group is carbohydrate. Based on types of carbohydrate:
        i. **Cerebrosides**: Carbohydrate residue is glucose or galactose. *e.g.* kerasin, cerebron.
        ii. **Gangliosides**: Carbohydrate residue is oligosaccharide. *e.g.* GM1, GM2.
    c. Other compound lipids:
        i. **Sulpholipids**: The conjugate group is sulphate. *e.g.* Globosides
        ii. **Aminolipids**: The conjugate group is amino acid. *e.g.* Lipoproteins (LDL, HDL).
3. **Derived lipids**: These are precursors of simple lipids. *e.g.* Fatty acids, cholesterol, steroid hormones, ketone bodies *etc.*

Fatty Acids

Overview

Fatty acids (FA) are aliphatic carboxylic acid having general formula R-COOH where R is the hydrocarbon chain and COOH is the carboxyl group.

Types

Based on nature of hydrocarbon chain:

1. **Saturated FA**: They do not contain any double bond. *e.g.* Acetic acid (2C), propionic acid (3C), butyric acid (4C), valeric acid (5C), lauric acid (12C), palmitic acid (16C), arachidic acid (20C). Based on number of carbon atoms can be two types:
   a. **Even chain FA**: Having even number of carbon atoms. *e.g.* Acetic acid (2C), butyric acid (4C), lauric acid (12C), palmitic acid (16C), arachidic acid (20C).
   b. **Odd chain FA**: Having odd number of carbon atoms. *e.g.* propionic acid (3C), valeric acid (5C).
2. **Unsaturated FA**: They contain double bond in the hydrocarbon chain. *e.g.* Based on number of double bonds can be two types:
   a. **Monounsaturated FA (MUFA):** Contain only single double bond. *e.g.* Palmitoleic acid, oleic acid.
   b. **Polyunsaturated FA (PUFA):** Contain more than one double bond. *e.g.* Linoleic acid (2), linolenic acid (3), arachidonic acid (4).

Nomenclature of FA

Numbering: The numbering of carbon atoms starts from COOH group which is C1 while the adjacent carbon is C2 and so on.

Naming: The next carbon (C2) from COOH group is the α carbon, while C3 becomes the β carbon, C4 becomes the ¥ carbon and so on. The farthest methyl carbon is known as þ or n carbon.

Double bond position: It is denoted from COOH group either by delta (most common) or þ carbon end by þ or n. *e.g.* Palmitoleic acid has one double bond which can be as delta 9 or þ 7 means that double bond is present between 9th and 10th carbon from COOH group or 7th and 8th carbon atom counting from þ end.

Shorthand depiction of FA: Being long structures FA are usually represented in shorthand style. *e.g.* Palmitic acid is written as 16:0 which means it has 16 carbon atoms and no double bonds. Similarly, oleic acid is written as 18:1 which means it has 18 carbon atoms and one double bond.

Short chain FA: 2 to 6 carbon atoms.

Medium chain FA: 8 to 14 carbon atoms.

Long chain FA: 16 or more carbon atoms. Most FA belongs to this category.

Cis-trans FA: If the orientation of hydrogen atoms at the double bond are on same side then it is called as 'cis' form while orientation on opposite sides are called as 'trans' form.

Essential FA: Those FA which are not synthesized in our body and need to be supplied with diet. *e.g.* Linoleic acid, arachidonic acid.

Functions of FA

1. FA helps in formation of phospholipids.
2. FA helps in lipid transport.

3. FA helps in hormones synthesis like eicosinaoids.
4. FA helps in cholesterol level regulation.
5. FA helps in reproduction being constituents of gonads.
6. FA helps in epidermal growth.

Triacylglycerol

Overview

Triacylglycerol (TAG) or neutral fat or simply fat are esters of FA with glycerol. Upon the hydrolysis (lipolysis) of TAG one molecule of glycerol and three molecules of FA are released with the help of lipase enzyme. This process is important during the mobilization of fats from adipose tissue or digestion of fats from diets.

Functions

TAG is the major storage form of fats in the adipose tissue which serves several functions:

1. Fats are storage form of energy.
2. Fats are concentrated form of energy in comparison to carbohydrates.
3. Fat acts as heat insulators.
4. Fat acts as shock absorbers.

Rancidity

It refers to the tendency to become stale or appearance of unpleasant odor or taste of fats/oils. This could be due to partial hydrolysis of naturally occurring lipases (hydrolytic rancidity) or oxidation of unsaturated FA (oxidative rancidity) to form peroxides by lipid peroxidation.

Cholesterol

Definition

Cholesterol is an animal sterol which is chemically 3-hydroxy 5,6 cholestene.

Function

It serves various functions:

1. Constituent of cell membrane.
2. Synthesis of bile acid or bile salts.
3. Synthesis of vitamin D3
4. Synthesis of steroid hormones such as cortisol, aldosterone, testosterone.

FA Oxidation

Overview

The breakdown of FA involves oxidation of long chain FA by conversion into their acyl coenzyme (CoA) derivatives followed by successive removal of 2C units in the form of acetyl CoA. This process involves production of NADH and $FADH_2$ that can be further oxidized by *etc.* to yield energy in the form of ATP.

Location

FA oxidation occurs in cytosol of prokaryotes and mitochondria of eukaryotes mainly in adipose tissue and adrenal cortex.

Formation of Acyl CoA

FA is activated by thioester link with CoA by enzymes acyl CoA synthase (FA thiokinase) and consumption of ATP molecule.

$$R\text{-}COO^- + HS\text{-}CoA + ATP \longrightarrow R\text{-}CO\text{-}S\text{-}CoA + AMP + PPi$$

Carnitine Shuttle

Acyl CoA derivatives usually upto 10 C can readily diffuse the mitochondrial membrane by diffusion however for higher carbon derivatives role of a shuttle molecule carnitine comes into play. At the outer face of inner mitochondrial membrane, the enzyme carnitine acyl transferase I removes the CoA group and replace with carnitine molecule. This acylcarnitine is then transported across the inner membrane by acylcarnitine translocase which release the carnitine molecule in the matrix. Carnitine acyl transferase II enzyme located on the matrix side transfer the acyl group into CoA and this cycle continues.

β-oxidation of FA

The combination of four reactions comprises one round of FA breakdown resulting in removal of 2C units in the form of acetyl CoA. Since the cleavage involves β bond of the FA chain hence this oxidation reaction is also known as β-oxidation. The series of reactions involving the breakdown of FA comprises:

1. Oxidation of fatty acyl CoA to form a trans double bond producing enoyl CoA and $FADH_2$ by enzyme acyl CoA dehydrogenase.
2. Hydration of trans enoyl CoA to form 3-ketoacyl CoA by the enzyme enoyl CoA hydratase.
3. Oxidation of 3-hydroxy acyl CoA to 3-ketoacyl CoA by enzyme hydroxy acyl CoA dehydrogenase and formation of NADH.
4. Thiolysis of 3-ketoacyl CoA by the enzyme ketothiolase producing acetyl CoA and acyl CoA shortened by 2C units and start further cycle until the last cycle when acyl CoA with 4C units are cleaved into two molecules of 2C acetyl CoA. For odd chain FA the last 5C is split into 3C propionyl CoA and 2C acetyl CoA.

Energetics

For instance, as β-oxidation of 16C acyl CoA like palmitoyl CoA will give eight molecules of acetyl CoA after seven rounds of cycle:

Palmitoyl CoA + 7 FAD + 7 NAD^+ + 7 CoA + 7 H_2O ⟶ 8 acetyl CoA + 7 $FADH_2$ + 7 NADH + 7 H^+

Five molecules of ATP are produced from one NADH (3) and $FADH_2$ (2) respectively from one round of degradation. Hence the total number of ATPs generated from 7 rounds are as follows:

7 rounds NADH and $FADH_2$ oxidation	5ATP x 7 = 35 ATP
8 Acetyl CoA oxidation	12ATP x 8 = 96 ATP
Palmitate activation	—1 ATP x 2 = 2 ATP
Total	129 ATP

Ketone Bodies

Under normal metabolic condition, acetyl CoA formed during FA breakdown enters the TCA cycle to yield energy. However, under abnormal state when level of acetyl CoA increases more than the rate of consumption in TCA cycle then it is converted to acetoacetate, D-3-hydroxybutyrate and acetone by **ketogenesis** and these products are commonly referred as ketone bodies which are excreted in urine in a condition known as **ketonuria**. Under diabetic conditions, acetoacetate is formed faster than the consumption hence diabetics have high levels of ketone bodies and acetone can be detected even in their breadth.

Fatty Acid Synthesis

Overview

FA synthesis takes place in cytosol by different sets of enzymatic reactions by condensation of 2C units from acetyl CoA.

Transport of Acetyl CoA

Since FA synthesis occurs inside cytosol hence acetyl CoA which is otherwise impermeable to mitochondrial membrane has to be transported from mitochondria to cytosol. This is achieved by condensation of acetyl CoA with OAA by enzyme citrate synthase to citric acid which traverses the membrane. The citric acid is cleaved by citrate lyase to regenerate acetyl CoA and OAA with consumption of energy. OAA is further converted to malate by malate dehydrogenase and then to pyruvate which returns inside mitochondria by a reaction involving NADP linked malate enzyme to produce NADPH which is particle source of NADPH for FA synthesis. The other source is from PPP.

FA Synthesis Reactions

The FA synthesis mainly involves two enzyme systems:

1. Acetyl CoA carboxylase system: Acetyl CoA is carboxylated to form malonyl CoA (for even no FA) or propionyl CoA (for odd no FA) by CO_2 in the form of bicarbonate by enzyme acetyl CoA carboxylase with consumption of one ATP molecule. Then acyl carrier protein (ACP) is added by transacetylase enzymes to form acetyl-ACP and malonyl-ACP.

2. FA synthase complex: The elongation of FA takes place by following reactions:
   a. **Condensation** of acetyl –ACP and malonyl-ACP to form acetoacetyl-ACP by enzyme acyl-malonyl-ACP condensing enzyme.
   b. **Reduction** of acetoacetyl-ACP to form 3-hydroxybutryl-ACP using NADPH and enzyme ketoacyl-ACP reductase.
   c. **Dehydration** of 3-hydroxybutryl-ACP to produce crotonyl-ACP catalysed by 3-hydroxyacyl-ACP dehydratase.
   d. **Reduction** of crotonyl-ACP by second NADPH to give butyryl ACP by enoyl-ACP reductase.

This first round of elongation reactions produces the 4C butyryl-ACP. The cycle now repeats with malonyl-ACP adding 2C units in each cycle to the lengthening acyl-ACP chain. This continues until the 16-carbon **palmitoyl-ACP** is formed. For each of the seven rounds one ATP and two NADPH are used in the reduction reactions.

$$8\text{ acetyl CoA} + 7\text{ ATP} + 14\text{ NADPH} + 6\text{ H}^+ \longrightarrow \text{palmitate} + 14\text{ NADP}^+ + 8\text{ CoA} + 6\text{ H}_2\text{O} + 7\text{ ADP} + 7\text{ Pi}$$

Formation of Double Bonds

In eukaryotes the double bonds are introduced in saturated FA by the enzyme **desaturase** which requires NADH and oxygen. In mammals the double bonds cannot be introduced beyond C9 hence cannot form linoleic and linolenic acids therefore are considered as **essential FA** and must be obtained with diets.

Regulation

The synthesis and breakdown of FA must be coordinated in a manner such that futile cycle is prevented. Hence FA synthesis occurs when carbohydrate and energy are plentiful and while FAs are scarce. The key enzyme in the regulation of FA synthesis is **acetyl CoA carboxylase** which synthesizes malonyl CoA.

Triacylglycerol (TAG)

Overview

Triacylglycerols (also called as triglycerides or simply fat) comprises three FA chains esterified to glycerol backbone. Simple TAGs have identical FA chains, while mixed TAG have two or three different FA chains. TAG are the major dietary lipids and major fuel store in humans that yield around three times more energy than carbohydrate or proteins. TAGs are stored in specialized tissue known as adipose or fat tissue and transported to all parts of body in large lipid protein body known as lipoproteins.

Synthesis

TAGs are synthesized with the help of FA CoA and glycerol 3 phosphate. The latter is derived from glycolytic intermediate DHAP hence TAG synthesis only occurs when glycolysis is activated i.e under fed state. The synthesis occurs via series of reactions involving formation of lysophosphatidic acid and phosphatidic acid leading to TAG synthesis. This pathway does not involve ATP but driven by cleavage of high energy thioester bond between acyl moiety and CoA.

Breakdown

Both the stored or dietary fats are hydrolysed by lipases into respective FA chains from glycerol backbone. FA can be further broken down by β-oxidation to liberate energy while glycerol backbone is converted to DHAP which enters glycolysis. Dietary lipids are hydrolyzed in similar ways by pancreatic lipases to release FA which are taken up by intestinal cells and aided by detergent properties of bile salts.

Regulation

The catabolic hormones glucagon, epinephrine and norepinephrine stimulate hydrolysis of TAGs and thereby oxidation of FA and inhibits FA synthesis. Contrary the anabolic hormone insulin has opposite effect hence stimulating the TAG synthesis and preventing the FA breakdown to avoid any futile cycle.

Cholesterol

Overview

Cholesterol is an important constituent of cell membrane in humans and precursor of steroid hormones (oestrogen, progesterone, testosterone, cortisol) and bile salts.

Synthesis

Cholesterol is mainly synthesized de novo in liver and also obtained rom diet. The 27 carbon atoms of cholesterol are derived from acetyl CoA via series of reaction involving formation of mevalonate by HMG Co A reductase, geranyl pyrophosphate, farnesyl pyrophosphate, lanosterol leading to formation of cholesterol.

Regulation

Cholesterol synthesis is mainly governed by the cellular cholesterol level which is transported round the body in lipoprotein. The enzyme HMG CoA reductase is regulated by feed back inhibition mechanism and regulates the cholesterol synthesis. This enzyme is also competitively inhibited by drugs lovastatin and compactin routinely used to treat hypercholesterolemia (high blood cholesterol).

Module V: Nucleotide Metabolism

Structure and Functions of Nucleic Acids DNA and RNA

Definition

Nucleic acids consist of phosphoric acid, sugars and organic bases. DNA (Deoxyribonucleic acid) and RNA (Ribonucleic acid) are building blocks of life as they carry genetic information. The unique structure of DNA double helix permits the information to be copied and pass on to next generation. DNA and RNA are polymers of monomeric units called nucleotides.

Structure

Nucleic acids are polynucleotides and each nucleotide consists of nitrogen containing aromatic base that is attached to pentose sugar, which in turn is attached to a phosphate group. Each nucleic acid consists of four or five possible nitrogen-containing bases: adenine (A), guanine (G), cytosine (C), thymine (T), and uracil (U). A and G are categorized as purines, and C, T, and U are collectively called pyrimidines. All nucleic acids contain the bases A, C, and G; T is found only in DNA, whereas U is found in RNA. The pentose sugar in DNA (22 -deoxyribose) differs from the sugar in RNA (ribose) by the absence of a hydroxyl group (-OH) on the 22 carbon of the sugar ring (Figure 2.7).

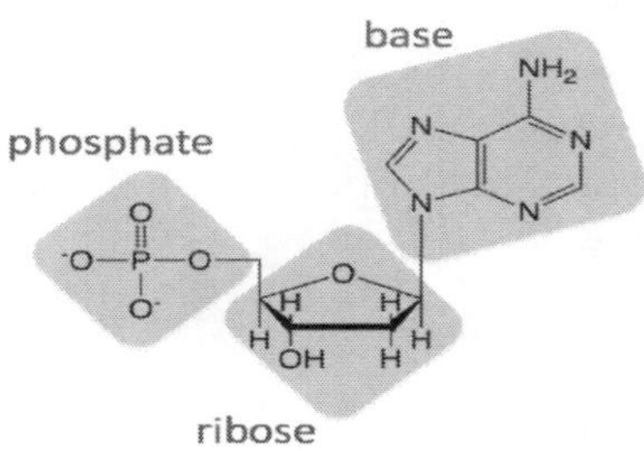

Figure 2.7: Structure of RNA.

DNA is double helical structure whose two strands runs in antiparallel direction held together by hydrogen bonds. The DNA helix has a repeat of 10.5 base pairs per turn, with sugars and phosphate forms the phosphodiester backbone (covalent) of the molecule and the nitrogenous bases oriented in the middle. DNA is formed by dNTPs by the formation of a phosphodiester bond, reaction catalyzed by DNA polymerase enzyme, between the 3′OH of one nucleotide and the 5′ phosphate of the next. The strand has a free 5′ phosphate at one end and the other has a free 3′ hydroxyl group which are designated as the 5′ and 3′ ends of the strand.

RNA is single stranded, which has ribonucleotides joined by the phosphodiester bonds except, it has uracil in place of thymine. RNA is chemically less stable than DNA. It has small molecular mass. RNA is of three types which are as follows:

1. **Messenger RNA (mRNA):** It acts as an intermediate between protein-coding gene and its protein.
2. **Ribosomal RNA (rRNA):** It is a major component of ribosomes and helps mRNA bind in the right part so its sequence information can be coded in a precise manner.
3. **Transfer RNA (tRNA):** It acts as a carrier that transfers the information for protein synthesis by carrying amino acids to ribosome.

Functions

1. They store genetic information that passes from one generation to another.
2. They also serve as energy carrier such as ATP and GTP.

3. They also play role as components of co-enzymes (FAD and NAD).
4. They also took part in cellular signal transduction such as cAMP as secondary messengers.

Nucleotide Biosynthesis

It occurs through two pathways:

1. **De novo pathways:** It represents the nucleotide synthesis from the scratch using simple molecules such as CO_2, amino acids and tetrahydrofolate in which synthesis starts from simple precursor molecules. In this pathway, there is a use of 5-phosphoribosyl-1-pyrophosphate (PRPP) and required a high requirement for energy as compared with the salvage pathway. The synthesis of purine nucleotides AMP and GMP begins with the transfer of an amido group from glutamine to PRPP.
2. **Salvage pathways:** It represents the synthesis from recycling of nucleotides that are available from degradation of DNA and RNA. Primary pathway consists of a single reaction which is catalyzed by enzyme adenosine phosphoribosyl transferase. Free adenine reacts with PRPP to yield the adenine nucleotide:

$$\text{Adenine + PRPP} \longrightarrow \text{AMP + PPi}$$

Then free guanine and hypoxanthine (the deamination product of adenine) are salvaged in the same way by a different enzyme, hypoxanthine-guanine phosphoribosyl transferase.

Purine Degradation, Pyrimidine Breakdown

The purine nucleotides are degraded via a pathway in which the phosphate group is vanished by the action of 5′-nucleotidase. Adenylate yields adenosine, which is deaminated to inosine by adenosine deaminase. Inosine is hydrolyzed to yield its purine base hypoxanthine and D-ribose. Hypoxanthine is oxidized to xanthine and uric acid by flavoenzyme xanthine oxidase. GMP is hydrolyzed to yield the nucleoside guanosine, which is then cleaved to free guanine and Guanine undergoes hydrolytic removal of its amino group to yield xanthine, which is converted into uric acid by xanthine oxidase. GMP catabolism yields uric acid. The end product of purine degradation is uric acid

Pyrimidine degradation leads to formation of urea. For instance, thymine is degraded to methylmalonyl semialdehyde, which is an intermediate in the valine degradation pathway. Further, it is degraded to methylmalonyl-CoA and then to succinyl-CoA.

Reduction of Ribonucleotides to Deoxyribonucleotides

Overview

The reduction of ribonucleotides to deoxyribonucleotides is important for synthesis of DNA by using deoxyribonucleotides. This reaction is catalyzed by ribonucleotide reductase; it removes the 2′-hydroxyl group of the ribose ring of nucleoside diphosphates, which results in reduction, and production of deoxyribonucleotides. The R1 subunit of ribonucleotide reductase contains the active site as well as two allosteric sites. This subunit contains three conserved cysteine residues and a glutamate residue, which participate in the reduction of ribose to deoxyribose. Other R2 subunit has a role in catalysis and generates a free radical in each of its two chains and contains a stable tyrosyl radical.

Reaction

It is series of reactions through radical mechanism:

1. The reaction begins with the transfer of an electron from a cysteine residue on R1 to the tyrosyl radical on R2. Electron loss create a reactive cysteine thiol radical lying in the active site of R1.
2. This radical interacts with a hydrogen atom from C-32 of the ribose unit, generated as radical at carbon atom.
3. This promotes the release of the hydroxide ion on the carbon-2 atom. Second cysteine residue is protonated and hydroxide ion leaves as a water molecule.
4. A hydride ion (a proton on two electrons) transferred from a third cysteine residue to complete the reduction of the C-22 position forms a disulfide bond, and reforms a C-32 radical.
5. This C-32 radical captures the same hydrogen atom originally abstracted by the first cysteine residue that free the deoxyribonucleotide to leave the enzyme.
6. Disulfide bond which is generated in the enzyme's active site is further reduced by disulfide-containing proteins like thioredoxin for regeneration of the active enzyme.

Thymidylate Synthetase – as Target Enzyme for Chemotherapy

During DNA synthesis, thymidylate synthase acts as a key enzyme in the synthesis of essential precursor called as 2′-deoxythymidine-5′-monophosphate. It acts by catalyzing the conversion of deoxyuridine monophosphate (dUMP) to deoxythymidine monophosphate. DNA damage occurs on daily basis through various reasons like environmental factors such as UV radiation, or habits such as smoking. The maintenance of healthy DNA is important for normal body functioning and evasion of the cancerous activity. Hence, thymidylate synthase become vital target for cancer treatment through chemotherapy. It is useful for treatment of breast, colorectal, gastric pancreatic, ovarian cancers. Several drugs are used as thymidylate synthase inhibitors in chemotherapy. The first used inhibitor was 5-fluorouracil (5-FU) used for treatment of the breast colorectal, gastric pancreatic, head and neck and ovarian cancers. 5-FU converts to FdUMP that binds irreversibly to thymidylate synthase in a competitive mode. Methotrexate is also an inhibitor of thymidylate synthase which is structural analogue of tetrahydrofolate.

Major Metabolic Disorders of Nucleotide Metabolism

The major metabolic disorders of nucleotide metabolism involve abnormalities resulting into common diseases such as hyperuricemia to deficiency of enzymes leading to defective purine and pyrimidine metabolism. Some metabolic disorders have been discussed here:

1. **Gout**: It occurs due to increased accumulation of uric acid in blood and tissues, which results in joints swelling, pain, and inflammation which results in abnormal deposition of sodium urate crystals. The genetic deficiency of important enzyme in purine metabolism is one of the causes of Gout. This disease affects the kidneys as excess uric acid deposited in kidney tubules.
2. **Lesch-Nyhan syndrome:** A genetic absence of hypoxanthine-guanine phosphoribosyltransferase activity leads to Lesch-Nyhan syndrome, mostly affects male children. Nucleic acids breakdown leads to hypoxanthine and guanine accumulation and the absence of hypoxanthine-guanine phosphoribosyltransferase enzyme results into rise in PRPP levels. This leads to high levels of uric acid. Patients with Lesch-Nyhan syndrome have mental retardation and poor co-ordination.
3. **Adenosine deaminase (ADA) deficiency:** Genetic mutations causes disturbances in purine metabolism which causes ADA deficiency. This condition leads to severe immunodeficiency diseases in which T lymphocytes and B lymphocytes do not develop properly. Lack of ADA enzyme results in increased cellular dATP, which is an inhibitor of ribonucleotide reductase. High levels of dATPs results in deficiency of dNTPs in T lymphocytes. Thus, patients suffering from ADA do not have effective immune system.

REFERENCES

1. Minchin, S., and Lodge, J. (2019). Understanding biochemistry: structure and function of nucleic acids. Essays in biochemistry, 63(4), 433–456.
2. Jinnah, H.A., Sabina, R.L., Van Den Berghe, G. (2013). Metabolic disorders of purine metabolism affecting the nervous system. Handb Clin Neurol.113: 1827-1836.
3. Rose, M. G., Farrell, M. P., and Schmitz, J. C. (2002). Thymidylate synthase: a critical target for cancer chemotherapy. Clinical colorectal cancer, 1(4), 220–229.
4. Berg JM, Tymoczko JL, Stryer L. (2002). Biochemistry. (5th edition). W H Freeman: New York.
5. Shemin, D., Russell, C. S., and Abramsky, T. (1955). The succinate-glycine cycle. I. The mechanism of pyrrole synthesis. The Journal of biological chemistry, 215(2), 613–626.
6. Cox M, Lehninger AL, Nelson DR (2008). Lehninger principles of biochemistry (5th edition.) Palgrave Macmillan: London.

7. Al Hafid N., Christodoulou J. (2015). Phenylketonuria: a review of current and future treatments". Translational Pediatrics. 4 (4): 304–17.
8. Santi, C., Bogusz, D., and Franche, C. (2013). Biological nitrogen fixation in non-legume plants. Annals of botany, 111(5), 743–767.
9. Rodwell, V. W., Botham, K. M., Kennelly, P. J., Weil, P. A., and Bender, D. A. (2015). Harper's illustrated biochemistry (30th edition.). McGraw-Hill Education LLC: New York.
10. Pelley, J.W. and Goljan, E.F. (2011). Biochemistry. (3rd edition). Philadelphia: USA.
11. Smith, C. M., Marks, A. D., Lieberman, M. A., Marks, D. B., and Marks, D. B. (2005). Marks' basic medical biochemistry: A clinical approach. Lippincott Williams and Wilkins: Philadelphia.
12. Baron, S.J. and Lee, C.I. (2013). Biochemistry and Genetics. (2nd edition). Mc Graw Hill Education LLC: New York.
13. Hames, D. and Hooper, N. (2005). Biochemistry. (3rd edition). Taylor and Francis Group Education LLC: New York.

Chapter 3

Microbiology

Sarika Chaturvedi and Aradhana Khare*

Amity Institute of Biotechnology, Amity University Haryana, Gurugram (Manesar) – 122 413, Haryana, India
**Amity School of Applied Sciences, Amity University, Mumbai, Maharashtra, India*
e-mail: schaturvedi@ggn.amity.edu

ABSTRACT

Microbes are the smallest living organisms, present as oldest form of life on the Earth that affects all the flora and fauna. Microbiology is an ancient biological science in which identification and characterization of microorganisms and their interactions with the surrounding environment are studied. This science brings collectively all microbiological disciplines and from around the world. Microbiology deals with the current global aspirations and challenges, such as maintaining food, water, and energy security for a healthy population on a habitable earth. It develops 'how diverse is life on Earth? and 'does life exist elsewhere in the Universe'? Microbes can be put to work in many ways for current global challenges, such as food safety, making life-saving drugs, health, and environmental sustainability, the manufacture of biofuels, cleaning up pollution, and producing/processing food and drink. This chapter focuses on key concepts of microbiology, aseptic techniques, infectious diseases, biogeochemical cycles, microbiological process for the purification of water, the characteristics of antibiotics with a focus on applications in various fields.

Keywords: *Microbiology, Archaebacteria, Bioremediation, Extremophile, Epidemiology, Opsonin and Psychrophiles*

1. Introduction

Micro-biology is the study of microscopic organisms which are either a single cell (unicellular), a cell cluster (multicellular), or has no cells at all (acellular), algae, and protozoa such as bacteria, fungi, viruses rotifers, planarians.

Based on cells and nucleus there are two types of microorganisms:

A) **Prokaryotic** – These are simple cell structure without nucleus and sub-cellular organelles. eg; Blue green algae

B) **Eukaryotic** – These are complex cell structure with nucleus and specialized membrane-bound organelles such as mitochondria, lysosomes, endoplasmic reticulum and golgi bodies.

Microorganisms present in all parts of the biosphere including liquid water, soil, hot springs, on the ocean floor, high in the atmosphere, deep inside rocks within the Earth's crust and human body.

Microbes have an important in biotechnology, molecular biology, immunology, food technology, beverage industry, genetic engineering, Virology *etc.*

2. Origin of Life

The origin of life is a result of a supernatural event and according to different hypothesis of the origin of life will fall into two categories

A) Abiogenesis

According to this theory LIFE can come from NON-LIVING things or decomposing material *i.e.* SPONTANEOUS GENERATION. This theory supported by Aristotle, John Needham, Lazarro Spallanzani and Felix Pouchet.

Table 3.1: Discovery of Microorganisms and Scientist Involved in Microbiology

Name of the Scientists	*Findings*
Antonie van Leeuwenhoek	Father of Microbiology, Designed first Microscope. First one to observe microorganisms
Louis Pasteur	Disproved the theory of Spontaneous generation, Devised the process of pasteurization, Made vaccines for chicken cholera, anthrax and rabies
Ferdinand Julius Cohn	Classified bacteria as sphericals, short rods, threads, and spirals
Robert Hooke	First used the word cell
Robert Koch	Father of Modern Bacteriology, proved that anthrax is caused by the bacterium *Bacillus anthrasis* Established Koch's Postulates i) The causative (etiological) agent must be present in allaffected organisms but absent in healthy individuals ii) The agent must be capable of being isolated and cultured inpure form iii) When the cultured agent is introduced to a healthy organism,the same disease must occur iv) The same causative agent must be isolated again from theaffected host

B) Biogenesis

This theory says that complex living things come only from other living things, by means of reproduction. This theory is supported by Francesco Redi, Schwann, Friedrich Schroder, Von Dusch and John Tyndall

3. Pure Culture Techniques

Pure culture techniques also known as axenic culture refer to "selectively growing" a specific kind of microorganism in the lab. It is defined as a population of cells or multicellular organisms growing in the absence of other species or types. It may originate from a single cell or single organism, in which case the cells are genetic clones of one another.

Generally, the primary culture obtained from natural source is normally a mixed culture containing microbes of different kinds.

There are Five I's, used to locate, grow, observe, and characterize microorganisms.

i) **Inoculations**: Producing a pure culture
ii) **Isolation**: Colony on media, one kind of microbe, pure culture
iii) **Incubation**: Growing microbes under proper conditions
iv) **Inspection**: Observation of characteristics (data
v) **Identification**: Use of data, correaltion, to ID organism to exact species.

There are techniques employed to obtain pure cultures of microorganisms.

A) Aerobic culture method

i) Streak culture
ii) Lawn culture
iii) Pour plate vs Spread culture method
iv) Serial Dilution method
v) Liquid culture

B) Anaerobic culture method

C) Special Techniques

A) Aerobic Culture Method

i) **Streak culture** pure culture is developed by using platinum wire or nichrome wire.

The inoculum is streaked over the agar surface of a well dried plate and spread over a small area at the periphery.

On incubation, separated colonies are obtained over the last series of streaks.

ii) **Lawn culture/Carpet Culture** It provides a uniform layer of bacterial growth on a solid medium.

It is prepared by flooding the surface of the plate with a liquid suspension of the bacterium and incubating the plate overnight at 37°C.

This is useful for bacteriophage typing and antibiotic sensitivity testing and in the preparation of bacterial antigens and vaccines.

iii) Pour plate or Spread Plate Method (Willey *et al.*, 2007)

Table 3.2: Differences between Pour Plate and Spread Plate Method

Pour Plate Method	*Spread Plate Method*
A plate is prepared by mixing the inoculums with molten agar medium before pouring in the plate.	Inoculum is spread on the solidified agar medium with spreader.
Colony growth is in and on the medium	Colony growth is only on the surface of the plate.
More area to grow	Less area to grow
Count the number of colony forming bacteria in a sample	Isolate specific clonal colony
Allows the identification of microorganisms	Used to isolate specific colonies

iv) Serial dilution method It involves the process of taking a sample and diluting it through a series of standard volumes of distilled water or 0.9 per cent saline. Then, a small measured volume of each dilution is used to make a series of pour or spread plates.

v) Liquid culture Liquid cultures are inoculated by touching with a charged loop or by adding the inoculum with pipettes or syringes.

Uses

Blood culture, Sterility tests, Continuous culture methods

Disadvantage

It does not provide a pure culture from mixed inoculum.

B) Anaerobic Culture Methods

Anaerobic condition can be achieved by

i) **Displacement of O_2** O_2 is replaced with other gases like hydrogen, nitrogen, helium or CO_2 e.g: Candle jar method

ii) **Absorption of O_2** O_2 is absorbed by chemical as Alkaline pyrogallol, *McIntosh – Fildes' anaerobic jar* and Gaspak and biologically by incubation with aerobic bacteria, germinating seeds or chopped vegetables.

iii) **Reduction of $O_2$by** using reducing agents – 1 per cent glucose, 0.1 per cent Thioglycolate

iv) **Production of vacuum** using vacuum desiccator.

C) Special Methods

i) **Capillary pipette method**: In this methods several small drops of a suitably diluted culture medium are put on a sterile glass-coverslip by a sterile pipette drawn to a capillary. After that each drop examine under the microscope until one finds such a drop, which contains only one microorganism. This drop is removed with a sterile capillary pipette to fresh medium. The individual microorganism present in the drop starts multiplying to yield a pure culture.

ii) **Micromanipulator method**: In this instrument is used in conjunction with a microscope to pick a single cell (particularly bacterial cell) from a hanging drop preparation. It is used to pick out a single cell from a mixed culture. The micro-manipulator has micrometer adjustments by means of which its micropipette can be moved right and left, forward, and backward, and up and down. A series of hanging drops of a diluted culture are placed on a special sterile cover-slip by a micropipette.

4. Preservation of Pure Cultures

It's necessary to maintain the continuous growth, viability and purity of the microorganism by keeping the pure cultures free from contamination.

i) **Refrigeration** Pure cultures can be successfully stored at 0-4°C either in refrigerators or in cold-rooms. This method is applied for short duration (2-3 weeks for bacteria and 1-1.5 months for fungi) because the metabolic activities of the microorganisms are greatly **slowed down** but not stopped. Thus their growth continues slowly, nutrients are utilized and waste products released in medium. Therefore after some time death of the microbes occurs.

ii) **Paraffin Method** This is a simple and most economical method using liquid paraffin that is poured over the slant (slope) of culture and stored upright at room temperature. The layer of paraffin ensures anaerobic conditions and prevents dehydration of the medium. This condition helps microorganisms or pure culture to remain in a dormant state and, therefore, the culture is preserved for several years.

iii) **Cryopreservation** This technique used for storage of pure cultures for long times and the microorganisms of culture are rapidly frozen in liquid nitrogen at -196°C in the presence of stabilizing agents such as glycerol and dimethyl sulphoxide that prevent the formation of ice crystals and promote cell survival.

iv) **Lyophilization (Freeze-Drying)** In this culture is rapidly frozen at a very low temperature (-70°C) and then dehydrated by vacuum. Therefore the metabolic activities of microorganisms are stopped and the microbes go into dormant state and retain viability for years and stored in the dark at 4°C in refrigerators. This is the most frequently used technique by culture collection centers.

5. Measurement of Microbial Growth

i) **Petroff-Hausser counting chamber/Haemocytometer** can be useful for organisms that can't be cultured. Special stains (*e.g.* serological stains or stains for viable cells) can be used for specific purposes

ii) **Serial dilution and colony counting** Also known as "viable cell counts" Concentrated samples are diluted by serial dilution

$$\frac{\text{CFU}}{\text{ml}} \text{ in original sample} = \frac{\text{colonies counted}}{(\text{dilution factor})(\text{volume plated, in ml})}$$

iii) **Membrane Filtration** Used for samples with low microbial concentration

A measured volume (usually 1 to 100 ml) of sample is filtered through a membrane filter (typically with a 0.45 µm pore size). The filter is placed on a nutrient agar medium and incubated. Colonies grow on the filter and can be counted.

iv) **Turbidity** Light scattering is measured as optical absorbance in a spectrophotometer. Optical absorbance is directly proportional to the concentration of bacteria in the suspension

$$\text{OD} \propto \text{Conc. of Bacteria}$$

v) **Mass determination** Cells are removed from a broth culture by centrifugation and weighed to determine the "wet mass."The cells can be dried out and weighed to determine the "dry mass."

6 Sterilization

Sterilization is a process of destruction of all forms of living microorganisms from a substance.

The Methods of Sterilization there are two type of sterilization as: Physical and chemical sterilization.

- ☆ **Physical Sterilization Heat** is the most common method of sterilization. The heat used kills the microbes in the substance. The temperature of the heat and duration of heating are the factors that affect the extent of sterilization.
- ☆ **Pasteurization** is the process of heating the milk at a temperature of 6o°C for 30 minute or 72°C for 15 sec.
- ☆ **Autoclave** The process is carried out at a temperature 121°C for 20 min at 15psi pressure.
- ☆ **Flaming** is the process of exposing metallic device like the needle, scalpels, and scissors to flame for few minutes.
- ☆ **Incineration** is used for inoculating loops used in microbe cultures. The metallic end of the loop is heated to red hot on the flame. This exposure kills all the germs.

☆ **Hot air oven** is suitable for het sterilization of dry material like powders, metal devices, glassware, and other such laboratory stocks. Dry heat destroys microorganisms by dehydration and oxidation or even incineration.

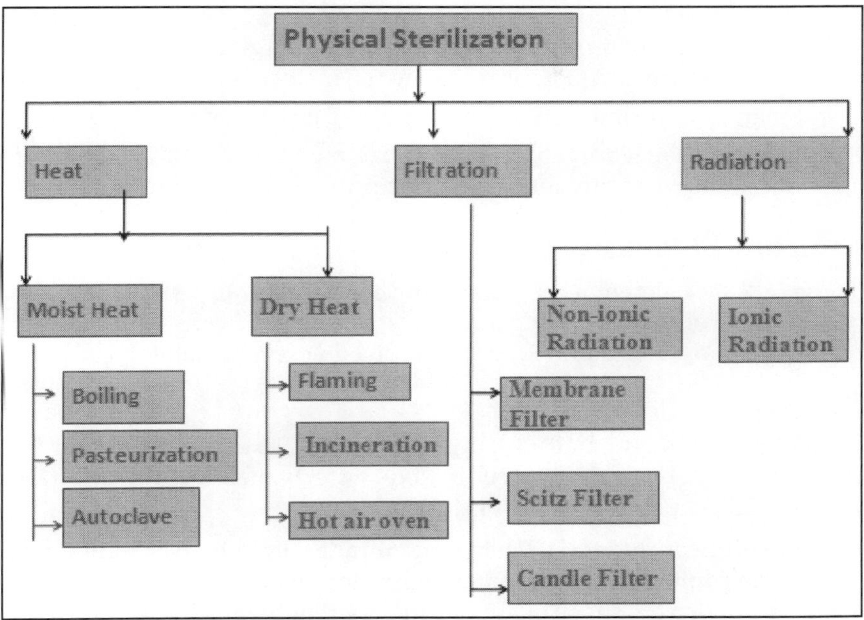

Figure 3.1: Different Types of Physical Sterilization.

☆ **Non-ionic radiations** like Ultra Violet radiations, they can be used even at the door entrances to prevent entry of live microbes through the air.

☆ **Ionizing radiation** X-rays, γ-rays, *etc.*

☆ **Filtration** In this method, liquids are filtered through bacterial filters to remove any microbes present. This method is very effective for sterilization of heat sensitive liquids.

☆ **Chemical Sterilization: Ethylene oxide, gluteraldehyde, formaldehyde, H_2O_2, peracetic acid are chemicals used for sterilization.** These penetrates quickly into the material like steam so, the sterilization is effective.

☆ **Ethylene oxide** is used for sterilization but it is very poisonous. Therefore **Carbon dioxide** is added to minimize the chances of an explosion.

☆ **Hydrogen Peroxide** is a low temperature sterilization process, used to sterilize heat-sensitive devices. A hydrogen peroxide sterilization process involves H_2O_2 vapor filling the sterilizer chamber, contacting and sterilizing exposed device surfaces. Once the sterilization cycle has completed, the vapor is vacuumed from the chamber and converted to water and oxygen.

7. Cell Structure

A cell is the smallest structural and functional unit of all organisms, size ranges from one millimeter to one micrometer. It originates from pre-existing cells.

- Detailed study of cell was done by the biologist Schleiden and Schwan in 1838-39.
- With the growth of the cells, they need a large surface area of plasma membrane to adequately exchange the materials.
- Small **cells** are more efficient at diffusion as they have a HIGH SA:V **ratio**.
- Cells specialized in absorption utilize membrane modifications such as microvilli to greatly increase surface area per unit volume.

A) Structure of Prokaryotic Cells

These cells lack a membrane-bound nucleus, structurally smaller and simpler than eukaryotic cells (which have a nucleus).Prokaryotic cells are placed in two taxonomic domains: 1. Bacteria 2. Archaea (Live in extreme habitats)

i) Bacteria

Bacteria is extremely small - 1–1.5 μm wide and 2–6 μm long. It occur in three basic shapes: a) Spherical called coccus b) Rod-shaped called bacillus c) Spiral called spirillum (if rigid) or spirochete (if flexible).

Cell Envelope includes: **i) Plasma membrane** - lipid bilayer with imbedded and peripheral protein. **ii) Mesosomes-** Form internal pouches (mesosomes) **iii) Cell wall** - maintains the shape of the cell and is strengthened by peptidoglycan **iv) Glycocalyx**- layer of polysaccharides on the outside of the cell wall **v)Capsule**-Well organized and resistant to removal **vi)Cytoplasm-**Semifluid solution, Bounded by plasma membrane, Contains water, inorganic and organic molecules, and enzymes. **vii)Nucleoid-** is a region that contains the single, circular DNA molecule. **viii) Plasmids-** are small accessory (extra-chromosomal) rings of DNA **ix)Appendages** Flagella – Provide motility, Fimbriae – small, bristle-like fibers that sprout from the cell surface, Sex pili – rigid tubular structures used to pass DNA from cell to cell.

ii) Archaea Bacteria

Archaea are prokaryotic cells with no true nucleus (nucleoid in the cytoplasm), able to survive in extreme environments, including very salty, acidic, and very hot surroundings and include both aerobic and anaerobic species. They have unique cell membrane chemistry with cell wall without peptidoglycan and cytoplasmic membrane, ether linked lipids to glycerol, 70S ribosomes and 16S r-RNA, Histones-like proteins associated with the DNA. These are capable of methanogenesis that produces methane. *e.g. Crenarchaeota, Euryarchaeota* Methanogens.

B) Structure of Eukaryotic Cells

These cells contain membrane-bound nucleus that houses DNA, Specialized organelles, Plasma membrane. Some cells (*e.g.*, plant cells) have a **cell wall.** Domain Eukarya includes: Protists, Fungi, Plants and Animals

i) Protists

Protists are the simplest eukaryotic organisms, derived from the Greek word "protistos", meaning "*the very first*".

- ✰ Most protists live in water, damp terrestrial environments or even as parasites.
- ✰ Neither plants nor animals or fungi so they may be autotrophic or heterotrophic in nature.
- ✰ Unicellular in nature but also found as a colony of cells and contains a nucleus which is bound to the organelles. e.g; Protozoans, Dinoflagellates, Euglenoids, Slime molds.

ii) Fungi

The term fungus comes from the Latin word for mushrooms, are heterotrophic and multicellular.

- ✰ Cell walls of fungi are made up of chitin, a complex polysaccharide, a polymer of N-acetylglucosamine.
- ✰ Fungi multiply either asexually, sexually, or both and most of them produce spores.
- ✰ Fungi interact with other organisms by either forming associations beneficial or mutualistic (mycorrhizae, lichens) or by causing serious infections.
- ✰ Commercial applications in food industry as baking, brewing, and cheese and wine making. *e.g. Penicillium notatum, Aspergillus* (Spore-bearing structures)

iii) Plants

Plants belong to kingdom plantae, are multicellular eukaryotic organisms with cell walls made of cellulose.

- ✰ Plant cells have chloroplasts, make food by photosynthesis, have specialized reproductive organs.
- ✰ Plants undergo a life cycle that is called the alternation of generations through both haploid and diploid generations. e.g; Green algae, Mosses, ferns **iv) Animals** Animals are eukaryotic, multi-cellular, heterotrophs with complex tissue structure with differentiated and specialized tissues.
- ✰ Animal cells don't have cell walls; their cells may be embedded in an extracellular matrix.
- ✰ They can be carnivores, herbivores, omnivores, or parasites.

- ✰ Most animals have complex tissue structure with differentiated and specialized tissue.
- ✰ Mostly are motile and reproduce sexually.
- ✰ Animals vary in complexity and are classified based on anatomy, morphology, genetic makeup, and evolutionary history.

7. Taxonomy

Taxonomy is the science of biological classification of living and extinct organisms. A taxon is referred to as a group of organisms classified as a unit. According to Mayr **(1982),** "Taxonomy is the theory and practice of classifying organisms". It is an information system comprising of classification, nomenclature, description, and identification of organisms.

i) Taxonomy Hierarchy

It is the process of arranging various organisms into successive levels of the biological classification either in a decreasing or an increasing order. Each of this level of the hierarchy is called the taxonomic category.

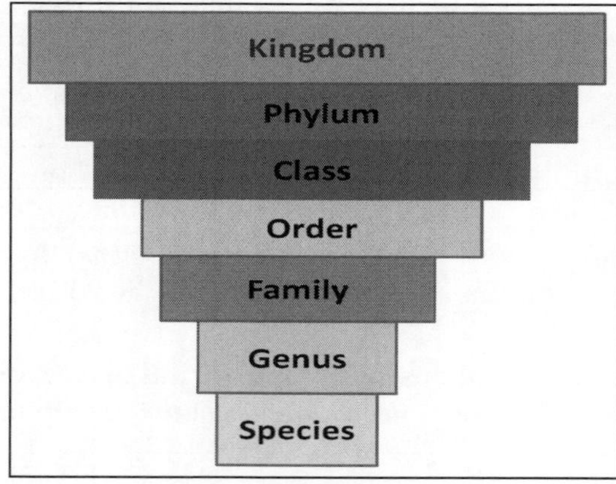

Figure 3.2: Hierachy of Taxonomy.

ii) Objectives of Taxonomy

A) To classify organisms into taxa based on similarities in phenotypic characteristics.

B) To assign each Taxon a name, known as nomenclature. Each scientific name has two parts a genus name and a species name. Both name must be in Latinized form. This is a binomial nomenclature, was introduced by Carl Linneaus (1753) *e.g. Mycobacterium tuberculosis.*

C) Third objective is to serve as an instrument for identification.

iii) Types of Taxonomy

A) Classical Taxonomy

This is based on selected stable characteristics like phenotypic characteristics, morphological features, cultural characteristics, biochemical properties, pathogenicity, antibiotic sensitivity, serological relationship.

B) Molecular Taxonomy

This classification is based on use of proteins and nucleic acid an indicator for evolution because sequences of monomers changes slowly and randomly. Taxonomically important morphological, cultural, and physiological- biochemical characteristics are shown in Table 3.3 respectively.

Table 3.3: Morphological, Cultural Characteristics and Physiological and Biochemical Properties of Microorganisms

Morphological Characteristics of Taxonomic Value	
Characteristics	*Variations*
Cell Morphology: Unicellular	Cocci, Bacilli, Vibrios, Spirilli, Spirochaetes, Stalked, Sheathed
Cell Morphology: Multicellular	Mycelia, Filamentous
Cell Arrangement	Single, Pairs, Chains, Bunches, Packets
Gram staining	Gram Positive, Gram Negative
Flagellation	Monotrichous, Lophotrichous, Amphitrichous, Penitrichous or Nonflagellte
Motility	Non-motile, Flagellar locomotion
Spores	Non-sporing, Endospore, Exospores, Myxospores
Cell inclusion	Poly β-hydroxybutyrate, volutin, polysaccharides, protein crystal
Cultural Characteristics	
Oxygen relationship	Aerobic, micro aerobic, facultative anaerobic, obligatory anaerobic
Temperature relationship	Psychrophilic, Mesophilic, Facultative thermophilic, Obligately thermophilic, Hyperthermophilic
pH Relationship	Acidophilic, Alkalophilic
Colony morphology	Discrete, surface texture, colour, elevation margin, soluble and insoluble pigments, color of pigments
Physiological and biochemical properties	
Nutrition type	Chemo-organotrophic, Chemo-lithotrophic, Phototrophic, Photo-organotrophic
Mode of Energy Metabolism	Respiration, Fermentation, Photosynthesis, Oxidation
Nitrogen Source Utilization	Molecular Nitrogen, Ammonium salts, Nitrate, Organic nitrogenous compounds
Carbon Source Utilization	CO_2, sugars, sugar acids, Sugar alcohols, Organic acid, Polysaccharides

iv) Microbial Evolution and Systematic

Microbial evolution refers to the genetically driven changes that occur in microorganisms and that are retained over time. (Bergey *et al.*, 1994)

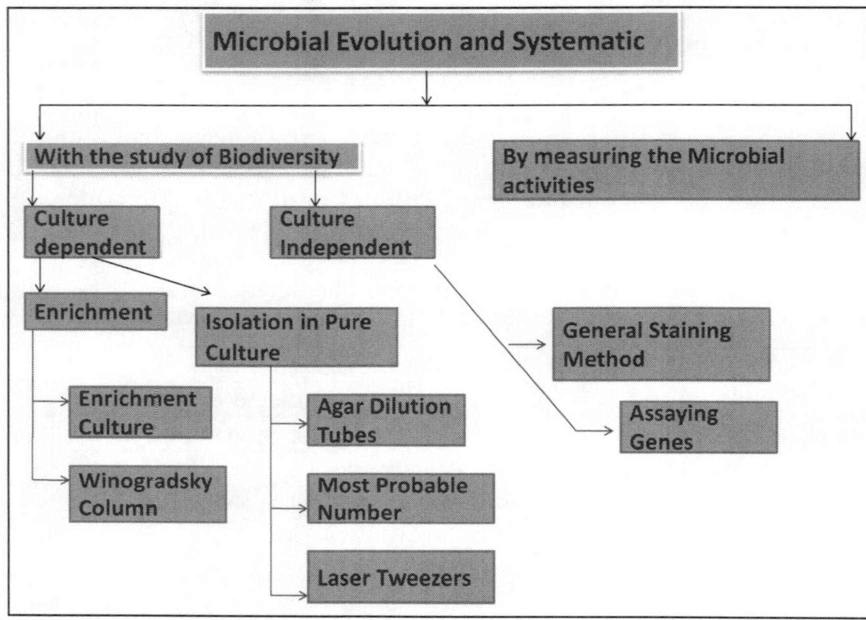

Figure 3.3: Microbial Evolution and Systematic.

9. Microbial Growth

A microbial culture is a method of multiplying microbial organism by letting them reproduce in predetermined culture medium under controlled laboratory conditions and growth refers to production of biomass leading to cell division, or reproduction.

A) Types of Microbial Growth

i) Batch Culture

A "batch culture" is a closed system in broth medium, where no additional nutrient is added after inoculation of the broth. In batch culture, medium was prepared, sterilized, and then inoculate into the bioreactor. It allows the cells to grow and produce the product. Once the product formation reaches maximum harvest the fermentation broth.

The biomass at different time intervals can be measured in four different phases.

i) Lag phase

ii) Log phase (exponential phase)

iii) Stationary phase

iv) Death phase

a) Lag Phase

Initial period of cultivation. The change of cell number is zero or negligible. The cells may grow during this period but not able to divide. During this phase of bacterial growth, synthesis of RNA, enzymes and other molecules take place. This period can last from 1 hour to several days. Cells are not dormant in this phase.

b) Log Phase or Exponential Phase

This period is characterized by cell doubling. The number of new bacteria appearing per unit time is proportional to the present population. If growth is not limited, doubling will continue at a constant rate so both the number of cells and the rate of population increase doubles with each consecutive time period.

For this type of exponential growth, plotting the natural logarithm of cell number against time produces a straight line. The slope of this line is the specific growth rate of the organism, which is a measure of the number of divisions per cell per unit time.

The exponential growth is expressed as

$$dX/dt = \mu X \qquad (1)$$

where μ= Specific growth rate, X = cell dry weight

If μ is constant w.r.t. (which in most cases it is, on rearranging and integrating, equation (1) gives

$$\int_{X_0}^{X} \frac{dX}{X} = \int_{0}^{t} \mu dt$$

$$X = X_0 e^{\mu t}$$

where x_0 is the original biomass concentration, x is the biomass concentration after the time interval, t hours, e is the base of the natural logarithm.

On taking natural logarithms, it becomes:

$$\ln X = \ln X_0 + \mu t \qquad (2)$$

Mean Generation Time

The mean generation time (doubling time) is the **amount of time** required for the concentration of **cells to double** during the log stage. It is expressed in units of **minutes**.

Mean generation time can be determined directly from a semilog plot of **bacterial concentration vs time** after inoculation.

Doubling Time

It is the time required to double the quantity of biomass, that is growing exponentially.

X: $X_0 \rightarrow 2X_0$ (The amount of biomass at the start must double)

t: $0 \rightarrow td$ (Within a finite time, td, or doubling time)

$$td = \frac{\ln 2}{\mu} = \frac{0.693}{\mu}$$

c) *Stationary Phase*

Stationary phase results from a situation in which growth rate becomes equal to death rate and overall no population growth takes place. It results in a horizontal line. It happens because over a period, the available nutrients become depleted and waste products start to accumulate and the cells become less metabolically active. In this phase, spore forming bacteria produce spores and pathogenic bacteria begin to generate substances and causes diseases.

d) *Death Phase/Decline Phase*

In this phase, no. of living cells decreases due to less availability of nutrients, change on environmental temperature above and below the tolerance band of species and other injurious conditions.

ii) Continuous Culture

Continuous culture is an open system in which fresh media is continuously added to the culture at a constant rate, and old broth is removed at the same rate.

This can be done if:

1. Fresh nutrients are constantly supplied.
2. Accumulated cells and waste products are removed at the same time.
3. Conditions such as temperature and pH are kept at their optimum values.

Advantages

1. Growth rate, biomass concentration can be controlled and maintained.
2. Uniformity of operation
3. Process demands are constant
4. Constant product quality.
5. Continuous cycle of sterilisation, fermentation, harvesting, extraction

Disadvantages

1. Susceptibility to contamination
2. Duration of run is longer/increased chance of contamination
3. Strain degeneration arising from large number of generations
4. Contamination with "fitter" competitor *e.g.* lower Ks

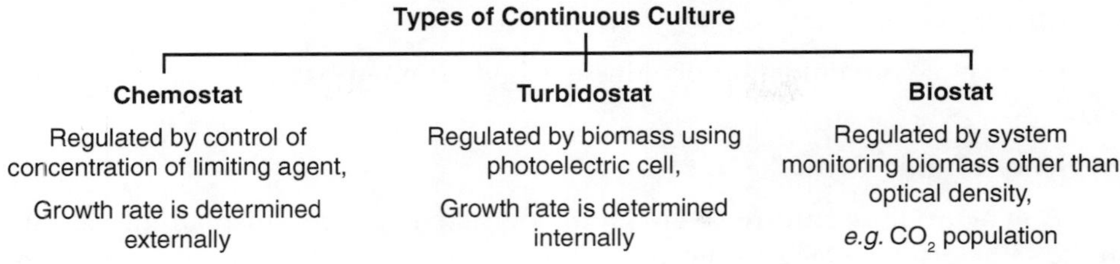

Figure 3.4: Types of Continuous Culture

Kinetics for Continuous Culture

Relationship between growth rate or specific growth rate and medium flow can be described mathematically (Tortora *et al.*, 2016)

The medium flow through the system is represented by the term dilution rate

$$D = F/V$$

where, D = dilution rate (h^{-1}), V = culture volume (l),

F = flow rate ($l\ h^{-1}$)

Mass balance or the rate of change of cells in reactor = RATE of ACCUMULATION minus RATE of LOSS

$$dX/dt = m.X - D.x$$

where, X = Total biomass, x = Biomass concentration

Application of Continuous Culture

In industry, Waste-treatment, Single-cell protein, Continuous beer production, Continuous amino acids, organic acids production, ethanol, baker's yeast

iii) Fed-batch Culture

Fed-batch culture is also called as semi-closed system of cultivation. In this technique, fresh culture media is prepared and it is inoculated with culture organism and then incubated for particulate time. During the course of incubation a particular nutrient is added at intervals without removing the used up media. So the volume of culture increases continuously.

Addition of medium prolongs both the log and stationary phases that increasing biomass and amount of metabolites.

Increases the yield from 25 per cent to more than 1000 per cent compared with batch fermentation.

Fed batch culture technique is applied in many types of fermentation process.

Advantage

Fed batch culture gives greater product yields than batch culture technique.

Disadvantage

Chance of contamination of culture is higher in fed-batch than batch culture technique.

iv) Synchronous Growth Culture

A **synchronous culture** is a microbiological culture in which all the cells are in the same growth stage.Numerous factors influence the cell cycle, some of them stochastic (random), normal, non-synchronous cultures have cells in all stages of the cell cycle.

External conditions can be changed, essential nutrient can also be eleminated, chemical growth inhibitors can be added so as to arrest the growth of all cells in the culture.After growth has completely stopped for all the cells, the inhibitor can be easily removed from the culture and the cells then begin to grow synchronously.

For example, for photosynthetic cells light can be eliminated for several hours and then re-introduced.

Cells in different growth stages have diferent physical properties, thus can be physically separated based on their density or size using centrifugation (for density) or filtration (for size).

v) Diauxic Growth Culture

The meaning of Diauxic growth is double growt, and is caused by the presence of **two sugars** on a culture growth media, one of which is easier for the target bacterium to metabolize.

The preferred sugar is consumed first, which leads to rapid growth, followed by a **lag phase**, where the cellular machinery used to metabolize the second sugar gets activated. After that, the bacterium experiences a slower growth phase, during which the second sugar is metabolized. Generally, glucose is used as a first sugar.

10. Microbial Fermentation

Fermentation refers to the process of chemical transformation of organic substrate using enzymes of microorganisms. It is an extracellular process resembling to anaerobic respiration to some extent.

Industries producing medicine, organic acids (butaric acid, latic acid, oxalic acid *etc.*), organic solvent, amino acids, enzymes are all based on the application of certain microorganisms for fermentation based processes. (Stanbury *et al.*, 2016)

A) Requirement for Fermentation Process

Specific strain of microoganisms or its mutants capable of showing fermentation efficiently at a much faster rate.

Sutiable substrate for the microorganisms which can easily be fermented.

Proper environment for optical rate of fermentation.

B) Type of Fermentaion

i) Solid State Fermentation

In this microbial growth and product formation occur at the surface of solid substrates. *e.g.* mushroom cultivation,mold-ripened cheeses,starter cultures *etc.*

This approch has been used for the production of extracellular enzymes, certain valuable chemical, fungual toxic, and fungal spores.

Traditional substrates used are several agricultural products *e.g.*, rice, maize, soyabean *etc.* which selectively supports mycelial organisms.

ii) Submerged

Liquid Fermentations It is traditionally used to produce microbially derived enzymes and involves submersion of the microorganism in an aqueous solution containing all the nutrients needed for growth.

The fermentation media is based on renewable raw materials like maize, sugars, and soya. For Antibiotics and enzymes (aerobic fermentation) butanol (anaerobic fermentation)

The main advantage of SmF process is that it can be easily scaled up with ease of automation and do not suffer from the heat mass transfer limitations. However, the major drawbacks associated, are the low productivity, high production cost, and complexity of the medium.

Batch-fed and continuous fermentation processes are common for SmF.

For harvesting products different techniques as centrifugation and concentrated by evaporation, membrane filtration or crystallization. If pure product preparations are required, they are usually isolated by gel or ion exchange chromatography.

11. Role of Microbes in Food Industry

Microbes like bacteria, molds and yeast are used in the production of various food products and are also responsible for food spoilage during the processing plant, storage, transport and distribution or before consumption, thereby causing intoxication and diseases. (Naduka Okafor 2007)

- ☆ Different food products provide different conditions for the growth of microorganisms, which is controlled by factors like nutrients, pH, moisture content, temperature, relative humidity, gases (CO_2, O_2).
- ☆ Meat and dairy products are rich in protein and fat than vegetables and fruits hence microbial spoilage resulting in proteolysis and putrefaction of the food products.

Examples of Microbes Used in Food Industry

Strains of Streptococcus, *Lactobacillus Bifidobacterium*, Erwiniaetc. are used in the production of fermented food and dairy products.

- ☆ *Streptococcus thermophilus* and *Lactobacillus bulgaricus* are used to produce yogurt.

- Food spoilage infections and disease causing bacteria are *Acinetobacter, Aeromonas, Escherichia, Proteus, Alcaligenes, Flavobacterium, Pseudomonas, Arcobacter, Salmonella, Lactococcus, Serratia, Campylobacter, Shigella, Citrobacter, Listeria, Staphylococcus, Micrococcus, Corynebacterium, Vibrio Enterobacter, Paenibacillus, Weissella, Enterococcus, Yersinia.*
- The pathogenic or disease causing bacteria are usually gram negative, and Gram-positive *Clostridium botulinum, C.perfringens* and *Bacillus cereus* are known to cause food intoxications.
- *Saccharomyces carlsbergensis* is most commonly used in fermentation of most beers.
- Mushrooms (*Agaricus bisporus*) are one of the most important fungi used as a food source.
- Yeasts as *Brettanomyces, Schizosaccharomyce, Candida, Cryptococcus, Debaryomyces, Zygosaccharomyces, Hanseniaspora, Saccharomyces.* These have the ability to ferment sugars to ethanol and carbon-dioxide and used in industrially production of the baker's yeast.
- Molds are used in ripening of various types of food products as Roquefort, Camembert cheese.
- Molds are employed to produce enzymes like amylase used in making bread or citric acid used in soft drinks.
- Molds are used in ripening of many oriental foods. *Bothrytiscinerea,* is used in rotting of grape for production of wine. Lactic fermentations using molds results in a unique Finnish fermented milk called viili.
- Lactic acid bacteria are used for coagulation of milk that can be processed to yield a wide variety of cheeses, including soft unripened, soft ripened, semisoft, hard, and very hard types.
- *Spirulina,* a *cyanobacterium,* also is a popular food source sold in specialty stores.

i) Wine Production (Enology)

Wine in an alcoholic beverage made from the fermentation of grape juice (*Vitis vinifera*). Industries producing wine called wineries. Wine can be made by using naturally occurring mo'son grapes surface (wild yeast and bacteria) as *Saccharomyces ellipsoideus.*

ii) Single Cell Proteins

Single-cell proteins (SCP) or microbial proteins refer to edible unicellular microorganisms.

The biomass or protein extract from pure or mixed culture of algae, yeasts, fungi or bacteria may be used as an ingredient or a substitute for protein-rich foods and is suitable for human consumption or as animal feeds.SCP develops when microbes ferment waste materials (including wood, straw, cannery, and food-processing wastes, residues, hydrocarbons). They are found in very low concentrations, usually less than 5 per cent.Microorganisms usually have a much higher protein content of 30–70 per cent in the dry mass than vegetables or grains.

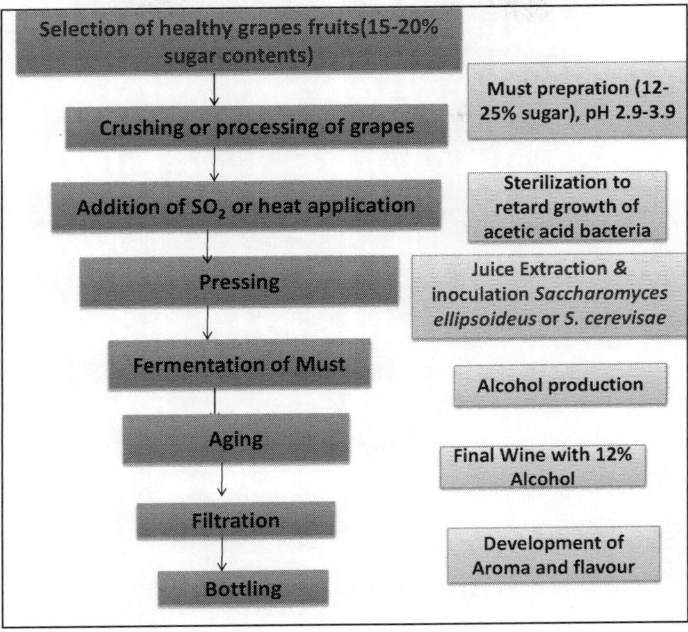

Figure 3.5: Flow Diagram of Wine Production.

Examples

Yeast: *Saccharomyces cerevisiae, Pichia pastoris, Candida utilis, Torulopsis coralline, Geotrichumcandidum*

Fungi (Mycoprotein): *Aspergillus oryzae, Fusarium venenatum, Sclerotium rolfsii, Polyporus, Trichoderma, Scytalidiumacidophilum*

Bacteria: *Rhodobacter capsulatus*

Algae: Spirulina (dietary supplement), *Chlorella*

12. Production of Dairy Products (Fermented Milks and Cheese)

Milk is a whitish liquid containing proteins (2.5 per cent), lactose (5 per cent), fats (3.6 per cent), water (87.5 per cent) and various minerals and vitamins (0.7 per cent) produced by the mammary glands. Milk is extremely perishable and various methods are employed to preserve it, the most prominent being fermentation. Fermentation is a metabolic process in which an organism converts a carbohydrate such as starch and sugar into alcohol and/or acid. Fermented Milk Products Cheese, Yoghurt, Cultured buttermilk, Acidophilus milk Kefir.

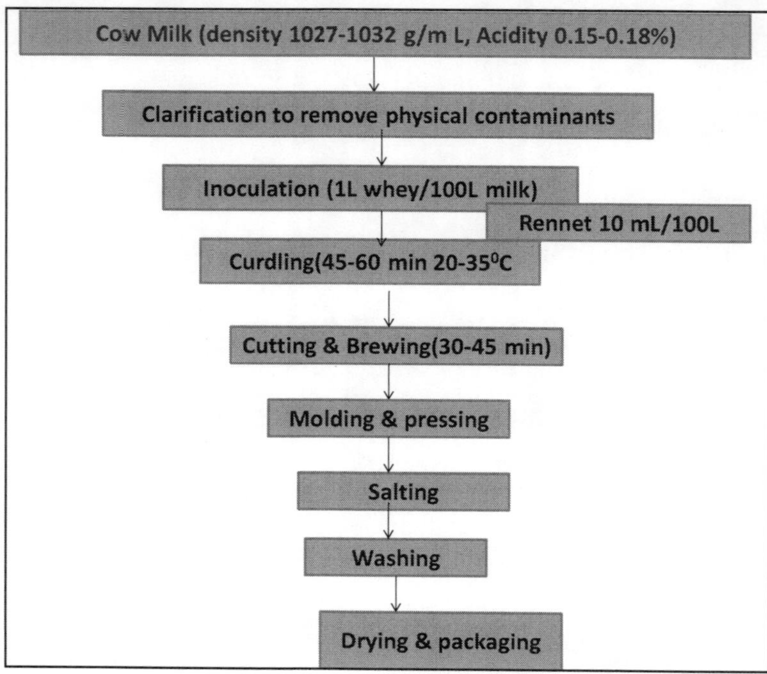

Figure 3.6: Cheese Production.

13. Microbial Stress-Response

A changing environment creates conditions that can be stressful for microorganisms, and they are neither immortal, nor impervious to stress. Ability to sense and respond to potentially lethal changes in the environment is important for survival of microorganisms.The bacterial stress response enables bacteria to survive in adverse and fluctuating conditions in the immediate surroundings. (Stanier *et al.*, 2015)

Microbes must have physiological acclimation mechanisms to survive and remain active in the phase of stress, else they will die. These adaptation startegies can alter the composition of the active microbial community creating shifts in ecosystem-level C, energy, and nutrient flows.Different regulatory networks designed to suvive stress *e.g.* acid stress is the combined biological effect of H^+ions and weak acid concentrations

A) Microbial Stress

Microbes grow at maximum rate with sufficient nutrients and optimal growth temperature, pH, oxygen levels, nutrients and solute concentrations. Changes in these parmeters can affect the maximum growth of microbes is callled environemnt stress.

Maximum Growth rate = Minimum Genration Time

Variations (Deviation) from Optimum Growth Conditions = Envirnmental Stress

Microbial Stress response = Adaptation

B) Types of stress

i) Physicochemical and chemical
ii) Nutritional deprivation
iii) Toxic Compounds
iv) Interaction with other cells

C) Adaptation (Strategies)

Eliminate stressor, Repair damage, Escape

D) Examples of Bacterial Stress Responses

1. Heat and cold Shock
2. Envelope and oxidative stress
3. Oxygen and amino acid scarcity
4. SOS response to DNA damage
5. Mettaloregulation
6. Sporulation
7. DNA uptake

14. Virology

The study of virus known as virology. Virus is a Latin word, which means poisonous fluid or venom.

A) Characteristic Features of Viruses

1. They are sub or ultramicroscopic.
2. They have either DNA or RNA,never both.
3. Apart from DNA few viruses contain protein coat called as envelope.
4. Retain by molecular filter.
5. They depend on post machinery for the synthesis of their body parts.
6. They can be transmitted from one host to another either directly or indirectly.
7. Inside the host cell they do not go any kind of division.
8. They are host specific.
9. They are inert outside their host cell in crystalline form.

Table 3.4: Properties of Virus Showing Difference between Living and Non-living Characteristics

As Living	*As Non Living*
Genetic material and protein	Non cellular
Replicate only inside a host.	Absence of cell organelle.
It is infectious, can cause disease.	It can crystallized and store indefinitely.
It can cause mutation.	They are metabolically inert.
It is susceptible to heat and chemicals *etc.*	They have no energy synthesizing enzyme.
It can bring enzymatic changes(in vitro).	They don't have functional autonomy.

B) Morphology and Structure of Viruses

i) Nucleic Acid

Either DNA or RNA.

The nucleic acid may be single- or double-stranded, circular or linear.

Generally plant viruses,ssRNA is present but in **Couliflower mosaic viruses** ds DNA is present.

ii) Protein Coat

It is known as **capsid** and made up of small subunit known as **capsomeres.**

An additional covering is also present in some viruses around capsid known as **envelope.** Such type of viruse known as **enveloped virus**.

C) Replication of Viruses

Viral replication involves six steps: attachment, penetration, uncoating, replication, assembly, and release.

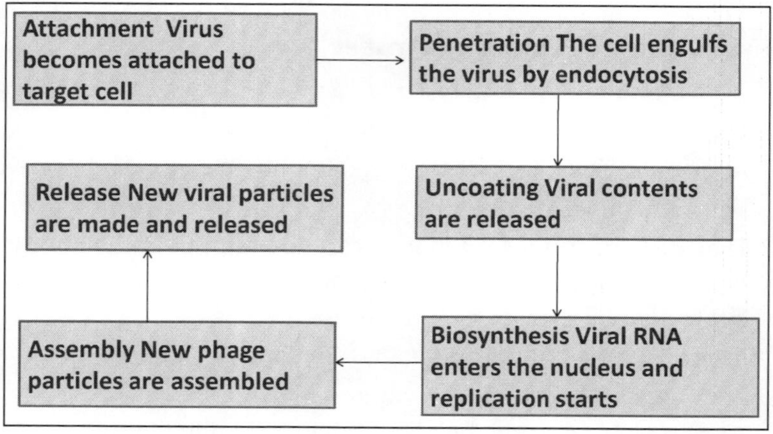

Figure 3.7: Steps for Replication of Virus.

During attachment and penetration, the virus attaches itself to a host cell and injects its genetic material into it.

During uncoating, replication, and assembly, the viral DNA or RNA incorporates itself into the host cell's genetic material and induces it to replicate the viral genome.

During release, the newly-created viruses are released from the host cell, either by causing the cell to break apart, waiting for the cell to die, or by budding off through the cell membrane

15. Virion

The virion shell or capsid protects the interior core that includes the genome and other proteins. After the virion binds to the surface of a specific host cell, its DNA or RNA is injected into the host cell and viral replication occurs, resulting in the spread of the infection to other host cells.

A virion is the infectious particle that is designed for transmitting the nucleic acid genome among hosts or host cells.

Virions are produced in the cytoplasm of complex viral 'factories,' the viruses.

It is a complete, infective form of virus outside a host cell, with a core of RNA and capsid.

16. Viroids

Theodor O. Diener

Potato spindle tuber and at least 15 other crop diseases are caused by viroids, an entity that nobody had ever heard of before 1971, its official date of discovery.

Theodor O. Diener, the Agricultural Research Service plant pathologist who discovered the pathogen, named it the "viroid," because it is "like a virus."

It is smaller than viruses. It contains only low molecular weight RNA (ssRNA) and not protein coat.

Found only in plants.

17. Prions

It was discovered by Stanley D. Prusiner

The term "**prions**" refers to abnormal, pathogenic agents that are transmissible and are able to induce abnormal folding of specific normal cellular proteins called **prion** proteins that are **found** most abundantly in the brain. The functions of these normal **prion** proteins are still not completely understood.

They are misfolded protein.(sc)

They are not self replicating and synthesize.

Some diseases caused by prions are

Kuru disease in human(laughing death disease)

Creutzfeldt jakob disease in human and animals.

Scrapie disease of sheep and goats

Mad cow disease(Bovine spongiform encephalopathy)

18. Plant Microbe Interaction

Plants are non-motile but they constantly require both the biotic and abiotic stress. Plants secrete various organic compounds resulting in a nutritionally enriched environment favorable for microbial growth. As a result, plants are heavily colonized with a diversity of microbes, which are called either epiphytes (colonize plant surface) or endophytes (colonize plants interior) influence plants in direct and indirect ways.

Plants and microbes can have variety of interactions including Ecological, pathogenic, symbiotic and associative.

A) Ecological Relationship

Bacteria, fungi, viruses and oomycetes that colonize the living plant tissues are encased in this narrow region in the initial step of infection. Different region is believed to be an interface which mediates the first crosstalk between host and pathogen. Different types of pathogen based on effects are classified as:

i) **Necrotrophy:** plant cells are killed

ii) **Biotrophy:** plant cells remain alive

iii) **Hemibiotrophy**: plant cells initially alive later killed.

There is a different type of relationship between plant and pathogens

I) Symbiotic Relationships

It is referred as a neutral, antagonistic or synergistic relationship between two dissimilar organisms (SYMBIOTES, SYMBIONTS) living in close association with each other.

It provides at least one of the participating species with a nutritional advantage.

Three types of symbiosis have been recognized depending on the nature of relationship. Mutualism, Commensalism, Ammensalism and Parasitism

i) Mutualism (+/+)

Mutualism is a biological interaction between two species wherein both species benefit from each other. They exchange food or provide shelter or protection, but may still be able to live independent life. *e.g.* Plants and Microbes *e.g.* Rhizobium in root nodules. Protists and Fungi *e.g.* Lichen

ii) Commensalism (+/0)

Commensalism is the relationship between two different species where one species is benefited from the relationship and the other is neither affected positively or negatively. *e.g.* Barnacles adhere to the skin of a whale or shark. The barnacle benefits from the relationship and does not harm or help its host. Barnacle Shark.

iii) Ammensalism

It is the ecological interaction in which an individual species harm another without obtaining benefit. *e.g.* Algal blooms can lead to the death of many species of fish and other animals, however the algae do not benefit from the deaths of these individuals. Black walnut trees secretes a chemical from its roots which prevents the growth of neighboring trees.

Parasitism (+/-)

It is a relationship between two species in which one benefits (**parasite**) from the other (**host**).

19. Animal-Microbes Interactions

The human host is regularly in contact with microorganisms but only a few of these can establish themselves within the host tissue and the host responds to the microorganism by assembling a series of defense mechanisms like resistance and susceptibility. Host resistance to parasite invasion is divided in to

a) **Non specific resistance** and

b) **Specific/acquired resistance**.

There are a group of microorganism associated with human body and form association-ship as

i) Normal Flora

These are microorganisms that are frequently found on/within the body of a healthy person or in the environment and influences the anatomy, physiology, susceptibility to pathogens, and morbidity of the host. Vast majority of normal flora are bacteria, which are found in skin, respiratory tract nose and nasopharynx; mouth and oropharynx, eye(conjunctivae) and outer ear, intestinal tract stomach and small intestine, large intestine, intestinal tract of newborn, Genitourinary tract external genitalia and anterior urethra, vagina, blood and tissues.

ii) Sterile Sites in the Human Body

Colonization of one of these sites generally involves a defect or breach in the natural defenses that creates a portal of entry

Brain; Central nervous system

Blood; Tissues; Organ systems

Sinuses; Inner and Middle Ear

Lower Respiratory Tract: Larynx; Trachea; Bronchioles (bronchi); Lungs; Alveoli

Kidneys; Ureters; Urinary Bladder; Posterior Urethra

Uterus; Endometrium (Inner mucous membrane of uterus); Fallopian Tubes; Cervix and Endocervix

iii) Skin Flora

It refers to the microorganisms preferably residue on the human skin. Most skin microorganisms are found in the most superficial layers of the epidermis and the upper parts of the hair follicles. Fatty acids secreted by the glands of the skin inhibit the microbial growth. Neither profuse sweating nor washing and bathing can eliminate or significantly modify the normal resident flora. (Greenwood *et al.*, 2012)

There are four main groups of bacteria that predominate almost everywhere on the skin:

1. Diphtheroids (*e.g.* corynebacteria like Corynebacterium diphtheria;
2. Propioniobacterium acnes was once classified as a Corynebacterium is considered part of this group),
3. Micrococci (which include the staphylococci such as Staphylococcus epidermidis),
4. Streptococci (either (α) or (γ) hemolytic, and the enterococci.

Besides bacteria the skin also is the home to yeast (like Candida) and fungi.

20. Nutrient Cycling

Nutrient cycles are natural pathways by which movement of essential elements takes place from the abiotic and biotic compartments of the Earth to be recycled and reutilized.

In this process, nutrients get absorbed, transferred, released, and reabsorbed.

Soil microbes play an important role in nutrient recycling. They decompose organic matter to release nutrients, which can be taken up by plant roots.

Nutrient cycling rate depends on various biotic, physical, and chemical factors.

Example are carbon cycle, nitrogen cycle, water cycle, oxygen cycle, which occur in water, air and soil, whereas calcium, phosphorus, potassium, *etc.* are recycled mainly in soil and are available locally.

These cycles also include unidirectional energy flow from one trophic level to another

A) Carbon Cycle

Carbon is the main constituent of all the living cells. All the organic matter and bio-molecules contain carbon.

Carbon is present mainly as carbon dioxide and methane in the atmosphere

There is a continuous exchange of carbon between biotic and abiotic components by the process of photosynthesis and respiration

Atmospheric carbon dioxide is fixed by plants in the process of photosynthesis

All the living organisms release carbon dioxide during respiration

Carbon is released into the atmosphere by burning of fossil fuels and auto emissions

Organic carbon from dead and decaying organisms and waste products is released into the atmosphere after decomposition

B) Nitrogen Cycle

Nitrogen is also an essential component of life. Nitrogen cannot be directly utilised by living organisms and has to be converted to other forms.

By the process of nitrogen fixation, nitrogen-fixing bacteria fix atmospheric nitrogen to ammonia and nitrifying bacteria convert ammonia to nitrate. It is then taken up by plants

Atmospheric nitrogen is converted to nitrates directly by lightning and assimilated by plants

Decomposers break down proteins and amino acids of dead and decaying organic matters and waste product

Denitrifying bacteria convert ammonia and nitrates to nitrogen and nitrous oxide by the process of denitrification. In this way, nitrogen is released back into the atmosphere

Importance of Nutrient Cycling

For the transformation of nutrients from one form to another so that it can be readily utilized by different organisms, *e.g.* plants cannot take atmospheric nitrogen and it must be fixed and converted to ammonium and nitrate for uptake.

Transfer of nutrients from one place to another for utilization, *e.g.* air to soil or water

It keeps the ecosystem in equilibrium and help in storing nutrients for future uptake

Through nutrient cycling, living organisms interact with the abiotic components of their surroundings.

21. Bioremediation

Bioremediation is a viable, environment friendly technology for cleaning-up the contaminated sites, pollutants, and toxins from soil, and water using microorganisms. Two types of microorganisms are used in bioremediation process

(i) **Indigenous microorganisms** these are found already at a given site. Their growth can be stimulated by maintain proper soil temperature and level of oxygen, and other nutrients.

(ii) **Exogenous microorganisms** these are not found at the site to degrade a particular contaminant but are added to the site. The soil conditions at the new site may need to be adjusted to ensure that the exogenous microorganisms will thrive.

Basic Essential Conditions

1. Oxygen at a residual level of 1 ppm. or more

2. Essential inorganic nutrients
3. Microbes and substrate must be in contact
4. Water - either salt or fresh
5. Other conditions such as pH, temperature, salinity, type of contaminant,

Bioremediation Techniques

A) *In situ* Treatment

In situ bioremediation involves treating the contaminated material at the site.

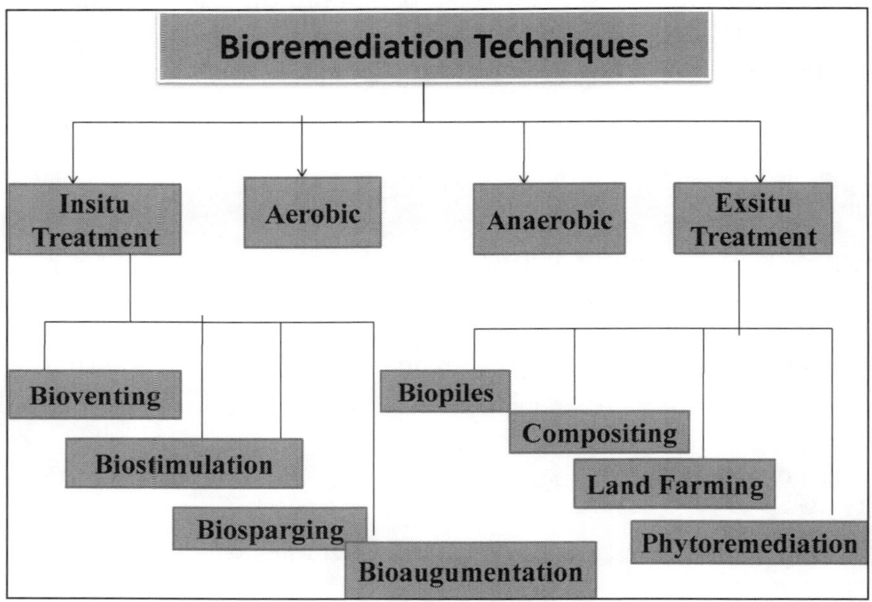

Figure 3.8: Different Types of Bioremediation Techniques.

i) Bioventing

In this process microbial activity is increased by introducing oxygen into the soil using forced air and used to biodegrade organic constituents adsorbed in the groundwater.

Nitrogen and phosphorus as nutrients are also added into soil to increase the growth rate of indigenous microorganisms.

ii) Biostimulation

It involves pumping of Oxygen Releasing Compounds (ORCs)into the soil to encourage microbial activity. It is used in groundwater contamination as ORCs are present in liquid form only.

iii) Biosparging

In this process air is injected into the groundwater to enhance increase the biological activity of the indigenous microorganisms.

iv) Bioaugumentation

It involves the addition of naturally occurring specific microbes to the contaminated sites. It costs less money, time, and disruption.

B) Aerobic Treatment

This process is normally used for groundwater, Oxygen Releasing Compounds ORC and H_2O_2 as amendments are introduced either by injection or water recirculating systems to the site. This process transforms organic contaminants into carbon dioxide and water at a very fast rate.

C) Anaerobic Treatment

Carbon sources such as molasses or Hydrogen Releasing Compounds (HRC) as amendments are introduced by injection or water recirculating systems. In this process contaminants are converted into methane, carbon dioxide and traces of hydrogen.

D) *Ex situ* Treatment

Ex situ involves the removal of the contaminated material to be treated elsewhere.

i) Biopiles

In this process the soil is excavated and mixed with necessary amendments after which the loads are placed in an enclosed building and aerated using blowers and/or pumps.

ii) Compositing

In this method, contaminated soil is excavated and combined with bulking agents and organic amendments such as hay, wood chips, vegetative and manure, at 54 to 65°Cto convert organic contaminants into mild stabilized byproducts. Compost is used as a key ingredient in organic farming. Aerobic bacteria manage the chemical process by converting the inputs into heat, carbon dioxide and ammonium. The ammonium is further converted by bacteria into plant-nourishing nitrites and nitrates through the process of nitrification.

Three types of designs used in his process

1. Aerated static pile composting (compost is formed into piles and aerated with blowers or vacuum pumps),
2. Mechanically agitated in-vessel composting (compost is placed in a reactor vessel where it is mixed and aerated),
3. Windrow composting (compost is placed in long piles known as windrows and periodically mixed with mobile equipment). a) Open windrow system in which the compost stacks in elongated piles and aerated it by tearing

down and rebuilding piles. b)Static windrows systems in this aerate the compost piles by a forced air system.

Among these windrow composting is usually considered to be the most cost-effective composting alternative.

iii) Land Farming

Soil is excavated and spread in lined treatment beds and amendments are not necessarily added but the soil is tilled to aerate to increase the microbial activity. This treatment is enhanced from photo-oxidation by the sun.

iv) Phytoremediation

It consists of mitigating pollutant concentrations in contaminated soils, water, or air, with plants able to contain, degrade, or eliminate metals, pesticides, solvents, explosives, crude oil and its derivatives, and various other contaminants from the media that contain them.

22. Wastewater Treatment

It is the process of removing contaminants from wastewater, both runoff and domestic, also known as sewage treatment. There are 6 steps in the process of Wastewater treatment.

1. **Preliminary treatment** physical treatment and clarification of large particles.
2. **Primary treatment** physical treatment of smaller particles occurs, gravitational force is used and water flow is also reduced.
3. **Secondary treatment** bacteria, fungi, protozoa take up the organic compound.
4. **Tertiary treatment** chemical treatment occurs in this stage with the help of ozone, chlorine and all these chemicals help in removing odour and kill microorganisms used in secondary stage. Reverse osmosis is also done.
5. **Sludge processing** involves biological, chemical and physical treatment. It involves sludge thickening, sludge digestion by heating the sludge and dehydration of sludge to produce solid cakes of sludge. Sludge can be used for increasing the fertility of the land.
6. **Effluent discharge**

1. Preliminary Treatment

i) Screening

Bar screeners are used to protect downstream structures from the arrival of large objects that could cause blockages in connecting pipelines.

ii) Grit Chambers

Also called primary clarifiers, uses long narrow tanks wheresolids such as sand, coffee grounds, and eggshells get settle out of the water under gravity. The settled solid known as raw or primary sludge are moved along the tank bottom by mechanical scrapers. Sludge is collected in a hopper, where it is pumped out for removal.

2. Primary Treatment

Approximately 25 to 50 per cent of the incoming biochemical oxygen demand (BOD), 50 to 70 per cent of the total suspended solid (SS), and 65 per cent of the oil and grease are removed during primary treatment. Typical materials that are removed during primary treatment are fats, oils, grease, gravels rocks, larger settleable solids including human waste and floating materials.

Sedimentation tank is used in the primary process. It has 2 arms of rotor. One is used for separating scum (grease and oil) present on the top or on the surface of water and other arm is used in bottom for sludge separation and later moves to sludge handling facility. Sedimentation tank also includes Settling zone and Sludge zone.

3. Secondary Treatment

In the secondary treatment microorganisms are used for the removal of organic matter. The microorganism uptake the soluble organic carbon and nutrients present in the wastewater and generate new cells which gradually settle down as sludge. Protozoa act as predator and help in controlling bacterial population.

Trickling filter is an aerobic treatment system that utilizes microorganisms to remove organic matter from wastewater. It involves mass transfer, adsorption, variety of biochemical and genetic reactions. There are various enzymes that are secreted to catalyze these processes and then the production of the subsequent biomass or the biogas, rate of that depends on the kind of enzyme kinetics which is being followed.

Autotrophic microorganisms derive the energy for synthesis either from the inorganic substances which is of the form of chemo-autotrophs or from the photosynthesis which are from the photo-autotrophs.If there is no source of organic carbon available, then microorganisms derive this energy through the oxidation of their own protoplasm and that is why this process is known as endogenous respiration.

The biological treatment systems typically have two distinct stages, one is the biological reactor where the different reactions take place including oxidation, formation of the new cellular mass, and formation of the gasses and various end products or byproducts. Another stage is sedimentation where this mass which is produced gets settle down.

4. Tertiary Treatment

Tertiary treatment is the final cleaning process that removes bacteria, viruses, and parasites to improve wastewater quality before it is reused, recycled, or discharged to the environment. It also removes the inorganic compounds, and substances, such as the nitrogen and phosphorus using chemical as alum. Addition of alum, makes tiny particles cluster together in masses called floc. Floc is trapped by the sand, whereas the clear water fed to the chlorine contact tank to disinfect the tertiary treated wastewater using microorganisms *Giardia and Cryptosporidium.* Unused chlorine is removed by adding sodium bi-sulphite just before it is discharged since it can be harmful to water quality and aquatic life when in high concentrations.

5. Sludge Processing

i) Sludge Thickening

In this step, the sewage sludge is thickened in a gravity thickener or dissolved air flotation (air bubbles)to reduce its overall volume, thus enabling the easy handling of the sludge.

ii) Sludge Digestion

This is a biological process in which the organic solids present in the sludge are decomposed into stable substances to reduce the total mass of solids, while destroying any present pathogens to enable easy dewatering.

It is a two-phase process.

i) the dry solid sludge is heated and mixed in a closed tank to enable anaerobic digestion by acid-forming bacteria. These bacteria hydrolyze the large molecules of proteins and lipids present in the sludge and break them down into smaller water-soluble molecules, which they then ferment into various fatty acids.

ii) The sludge is converted by other bacteria to produce a mixture of carbon dioxide (CO_2) and methane, after which the methane is collected and reused to power the digestion tank and generate power.

iii) Dewatering

The sludge is dewatered before final disposal. 70 percent, water is removed by using Sludge-drying beds, solid-liquid separation devices, centrifugation, rotary drum vacuum filter and the belt filter press to carry out this process.

REFERENCES

1. Bergey, David H., John G.H., Noel R. Krieg; Peter H.A. Sneath (1994). Bergey's Manual of Determinative Bacteriology 9th Edition Lippincott Williams and Wilkins. ISBN 0- 683-00603-7.

2. Willey J, Sherwood L. M., Woolverton C. (2007) Prescott's Microbiology 7th Edition McGraw-Hill Science Engineering ISBN-13: 978-0072992915.

3. Tortora G. J., Berdell R. F., Christine L. C. (2016) Microbiology: An Introduction, 12th Edition Cloth ISBN-13: 9780321929150

4. Stanbury P., Whitaker A. S. J. (2016) Hall Principles of Fermentation Technology Butterworth-Heinemann **ISBN-13:** 9780080999531

5. Okafor N (2007) Modern Industrial Microbiology and Biotechnology Science Publisher, Enfield, NH, USA ISBN 978157808434.

6. Greenwood D., Slack, R.B., Peutherer, J.F. (2012) Medical microbiology. 12th Edition. Churchill Livingstone, London ISBN 9780702040092.

7. Stanier R.Y., Ingraham J.L., Wheelis M.L., Painter P.R. (2005). General Microbiology. 5th edition. McMillan. ISBN 10: 0333417682

Chapter 4

Immunology

Riya Mukherjee and Ramendra Pati Pandey*

Centre for Drug Design Discovery and Development (C4D), SRM University, Delhi-NCR, Rajiv Gandhi Education City, Sonepat – 131 029, Haryana, India
****e-mail: ramendra.pandey@gmail.com***

ABSTRACT

Immunology is the branch of science which deals with the immune response to foreign invaders. All the multicellular organisms have evolved their immune system massively to increase protection from pathogens. The inordinate number of variations have been formed by the immune system in terms of different cells and molecules which consist of immense potential in specifically recognizing the foreign substances and also eradicating them from the system. The immune system has an interesting property of self-nonself discrimination and besides, it can able to recognize the altered host cells which can give rise to cancer. The presence of multiple constituents of the system enables to convert, the recognization of foreign invaders into different effector responses that specifically eliminate the pathogens of a particular type. Typically, the immune system generates the memory response in certain pathogen exposures which proves to be an amazing property as it prevents the host from getting attacked for the second time. This amazing property of memory response is the key for the vaccination as this indicates that the immune system is being educated to prepare it for further attacks. Immunity has been divided into two types, innate immunity, and adaptive immunity which together play a major role in protection. Innate immunity, non-specific but the first line of defense prevents many infections in the beginning by eliminating them within few hours of coming in contact with this immune system. On the other hand, adaptive immunity develops a response to infection by recognizing it, then eliminates it, and also remember the foreign invaders. Somehow, if the foreign invaders manage to evade the innate immune system, adaptive immunity catches them and makes an effective attack on the invaders. If any closely related or similar pathogen tends to attack the same host, induced memory cells show effective results in eradicating the pathogens. This chapter highlights the study of immunology in a broader aspect to provide a piece of deep knowledge about highly applied aspects of immunology in terms of immune responses, regulation of immunoglobulin gene expression, major histocompatibility complexes, vaccines along with immunodiagnostic techniques.

Keywords: *Immune system, Innate immunity, Adaptive immunity, Pathogens, Immunoglobulin, Major histocompatibility complexes, Vaccines.*

Components of Mammalian Immune System

The main component of the immune system is the innate immune system and adaptive immune system. In addition, the main goal of the immune system is to protect the host from foreign invaders, and this defensive mechanism in the host gives rise to a wide number of cells, tissues, and organs that help in recognizing the pathogens and neutralize them. The specific, as well as non-specific immunity, is induced by the white blood cells or the leukocytes. The presence of different parts of the immune system has been taken into count for the components of the immune system. The white blood cells, the complement system, the lymphatic system, antibodies, *etc.* are a major part of the immune system. Below, a schematic diagram explains the components of the mammalian immune system.

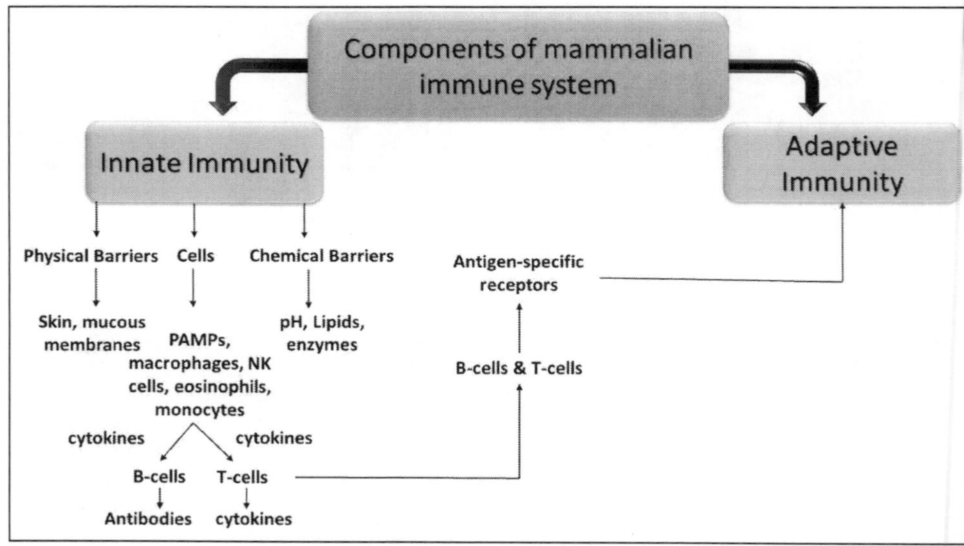

Figure 4.1: Components of the Mammalian Immune System. Modified from Life Sciences (Fundamentals and Practice I) Sixth edition by Pranav Kumar I Usha Mina.

Innate Immunity

Innate immunity is called the first line of defense against any foreign invaders. The presence of innate immunity is from birth, in every individual and is considered to be non-specific in nature. This native immunity is functional against all foreign invaders or pathogens since birth without creating any memory. There are different elements of innate immunity, cellular and molecular elements that help to encounter the pathogens.

Physical Barriers

Most of the foreign invaders try to penetrate through the skin and mucous membrane for attacking the body by damaging the former. These are the physical barriers that are called the first line of defense against any infection. The mucous

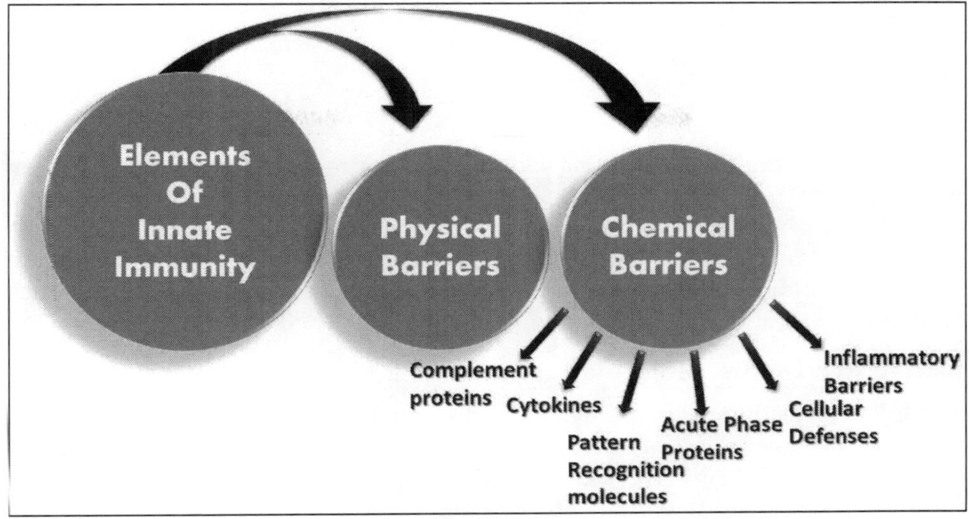

Figure 4.2: Elements of Innate Immunity.

membrane is present in the mucosal epithelia which line the respiratory tract, urogenital tract, and gastrointestinal tract which protects the interior of the body from foreign invaders. Similarly, the skin of our body can be divided into two layers, the epidermis, the outer thin layer, and the dermis, a thicker one. The sweat is acidic in pH, sebaceous secretions, different fatty acids, and hydrolytic enzymes inhibit the growth of many microorganisms. There is the presence of different biochemical defenses which are synthesized with excellent antimicrobial activity. One of them is psoriasin, a small protein synthesized by human skin that shows potent antibacterial activity against the Gram-Negative Bacteria *E.coli.*

The ability of the mucous membrane is to entrap foreign invaders or pathogens. The presence of cilia in the respiratory tract helps to throw the pathogens out of the tract. Likewise, tears consist of lysozyme, lactoferrin, IgA that provides protection to the eyes from pathogens[1-5].

Chemical Barriers

Chemical Barriers consists of complement proteins, cytokines, pattern recognition molecules, acute-phase proteins, cationic peptides, *etc.* These protect against the pathogen just before the adaptive system of the body develops.

Complement Proteins

There are numerous soluble proteins produced by the liver and are circulated further in the blood and extracellular fluid of the body, these proteins are termed complement proteins. The proteins are composed of an innumerable amount of serum proteins and once activated, the main function is to follow the controlled cascade for the destruction of the pathogens. They tend to lyse the outer membrane of the pathogen or make the pathogen captivating for the phagocytic cells. The opsonization of the pathogens arises by the specific molecules that recognize PAMPs (innate) or by the antibodies (adaptive) that go and binds to specific foreign antigens. Due to this activation of the complement system, there can be inflammation at the site of infection.

Cytokines

Cytokines are low molecular weight soluble proteins that are activated for immunoregulation of both adaptive and innate immunity. There are different cytokine-producing cells that upon activation synthesize cytokines such as monokines, lymphokines, interleukins, interferons, tumor necrosis factor-alpha (TNF-α). Cytokines are generally redundant, multifunctional, and pleiotropic. They bind with specific receptors of cytokines for the activity.

Pattern Recognition Molecule

Initial detection of the pathogen is the prime aspect of immunity and there are different molecules that have the ability to acknowledge Pathogen-Associated Molecular Pattern (PAMP). These PAMPs are recognized by the pattern-recognition receptors. There are different pattern recognition receptors(PRRs) such as Nod-like receptors (NLRs), RIG-I-like receptors (RLRs), Toll-like receptors (TLRs), Aim2-like receptors (ALRs), and C-type lectin receptors (CLRs). Toll-Like Receptors (TLRs) function as signaling receptors. TLRs are the type-I integral transmembrane proteins which are composed of intracellular C-terminal region and extracellular N-terminal domain, that constitute around 16-28 leucine-rich repeats(LRRs) and can recognize the PAMPs. Generally, human TLRs are approximately 700-1100 amino acids long. TLRs are broadly expressed in the innate immune cells along with other non-immune cells. TLRs mainly localize to the cell surface or different intracellular parts such as lysosomes, ER, endosomes, *etc.*, and helps in recognizing PAMPs.

There is a distinct general signaling mechanism or pathway followed by the TLR but two separate pathways have been observed. A pathway that guides in the production of ample inflammatory cytokines known as the MyD88-dependent pathway, and a MyD88-independent pathway along with IFN-α stimulation with the maturation of dendritic cells.

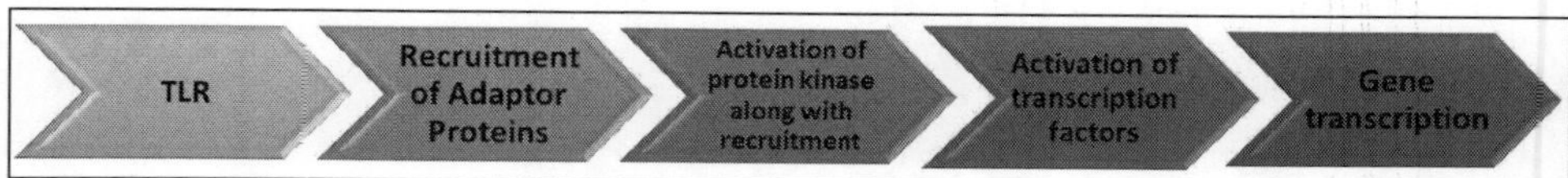

Figure 4.3: TLR Basic Signaling Mechanisms.

Acute-Phase Proteins

Acute-phase proteins are another set of plasma proteins synthesized in the liver upon the attack by the foreign invaders. After the release of the cytokines by macrophages, the liver rapidly starts secreting these acute-phase proteins. These acute-phase proteins include serum amyloid protein A (SAA), mannose-binding protein (MBP), C-reactive protein (CRP). These proteins help to recognize the molecular patterns present on the surface of the microbes for further directing the destruction of the microbes.

Cellular Defenses

Cellular defenses are the special cells that direct the innate host defense mechanisms. The cells like neutrophils, NK cells, monocytes, and macrophages play a major role in protection by destroying the foreign invaders through the process called phagocytosis. This foreign particle remains entrapped in the phagosome after the ingestion through phagocytosis and enters into the lysosomes forming phagolysosomes. These are further destroyed through two distinct mechanisms, such as Oxygen-dependent killing mechanisms and Oxygen-independent killing mechanisms.

During the process of phagocytosis, there is a metabolic process that takes place in the activated phagocytes named respiratory burst which requires high consumption of oxygen by the cells. Therefore, these activated phagocytes secrete toxic substances such as reactive oxygen and reactive nitrogen intermediates that show high antimicrobial activity. Likewise, the oxygen-independent killing mechanism includes activated macrophages that synthesize defensins, lysozyme, and other hydrolytic enzymes that show degradative properties, thereby killing the microbes.

Inflammatory Barriers

Inflammation is a non-specific defense mechanism. The inflammatory response is mediated by a variety of signaling molecules. Two prime mediators of the inflammatory response are histamine that is released by a variety of cells in the response to some tissue injury and kinins that are present in the blood plasma in an inactive form.

Adaptive Immunity

Unlike innate immunity, adaptive immunity is specific in nature and has the capability of recognizing and eliminating selectively all the specific foreign invaders. It has antigenic specificity, also the ability to recall the earlier foreign particle and respond more largely and rapidly. It also possesses the self and non-self recognition ability. Adaptive immunity has been further divided into active and passive immunity. The main goal of the adaptive immune system or acquired immunity is to eliminate the antigen and it is being executed in two ways. Humoral immunity and cell-mediated immunity. The B lymphocytes mature and produce antibodies that circulate in the blood, known as humoral immunity. The other type of immunity is mediated by T-cells, which do not produce antibodies but helps in synthesizing numerous cytokines that eventually help in the destruction of the foreign particle, and is known as cell-mediated immunity. The T-cells show specificity against the foreign invaders via T-cell receptors (TCRs) performing many effector functions when the antigen-presenting cells (APCs) bring the invaders into the lymphoid organs for destruction. Both the adaptive and innate immune system works together cooperatively to fight against the pathogens.

Specific Cell Types of Innate Immunity

Innate immunity is capable of inducing a potent immune response with the help of various cell types. Among them, the most common cell types are neutrophils, macrophages, dendritic cells, natural killer cells.

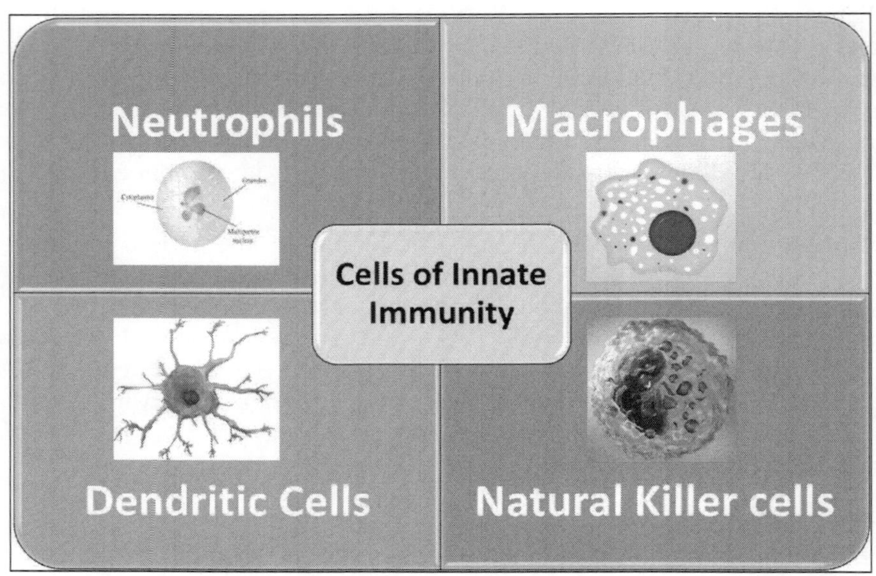

Figure 4.4: Specific Cell Types of Innate Immunity

Neutrophils are those cells that arrive at the site of infection at first from the blood. They consist of many TLRs on their surfaces. Like, TLR2 helps to detect the peptidoglycan of gram-positive bacteria, and TLR4 helps to detect the lipopolysaccharide on the cell wall of gram-negative bacteria. Binding with the foreign invader occurs and the particle is eventually phagocytosed. Other than phagocytosis, neutrophils can oxidatively and non-oxidatively attack the invaders that contribute to a multipronged, coordinated, and effective destruction of the pathogens. This mechanism employs reactive oxygen species (ROS) and reactive nitrogen species (RNS) along with antimicrobial peptides for eliminating the pathogens.

Macrophages, when activated by stimuli exhibit a larger phagocytic activity to kill the pathogens, they secrete different inflammatory mediators. Macrophages also show two antimicrobial devices just like neutrophils that is ROS and RNS. Activated macrophages also produce cytokines and complement proteins for the destruction of the invaders.

Dendritic cells, like macrophages, use all the agents to cause phagocytosis of the pathogens. Dendritic cells can also generate ROS and RNS which secrets antimicrobial peptides for causing the destruction. They are also a potent producer of interferons. Plasmacytoid dendritic cells produce type I interferons which are antiviral cytokines.

Natural Killer cells (NK cells) are the first line of defense against mainly viral infections. It causes the lysis of viral-infected cells. It has been observed that NK cells produce interferon-γ and TNF-α, the most important immunoregulatory cytokines for eliminating pathogens. Nk cells direct the adaptive immune system by mediating the macrophage activation thereby developing the T_H cells.

Cells of the Immune System

The immune system consists of cells, tissues, and organs that help to recognize foreign particles and neutralize or destroy them. Among them, white blood cells or leukocytes are responsible for both specific and non-specific immunity. All these leukocytes arise from a hematopoietic stem cell. When the hematopoietic cell undergoes hematopoiesis, two pathways arise that give rise to a common lymphoid progenitor cell and a common myeloid progenitor cell. The lymphoid progenitor cell gives rise to the B-cells, T-cells, some dendritic cells, and NK cells. The myeloid progenitor cells give rise to red blood cells (erythrocytes), white blood cells (neutrophils, eosinophils, basophils, monocytes, mast cells, dendritic cells), and platelets. Below, **Figure 4.5,** the schematic diagram gives a brief idea about the cells of the immune system [6-10].

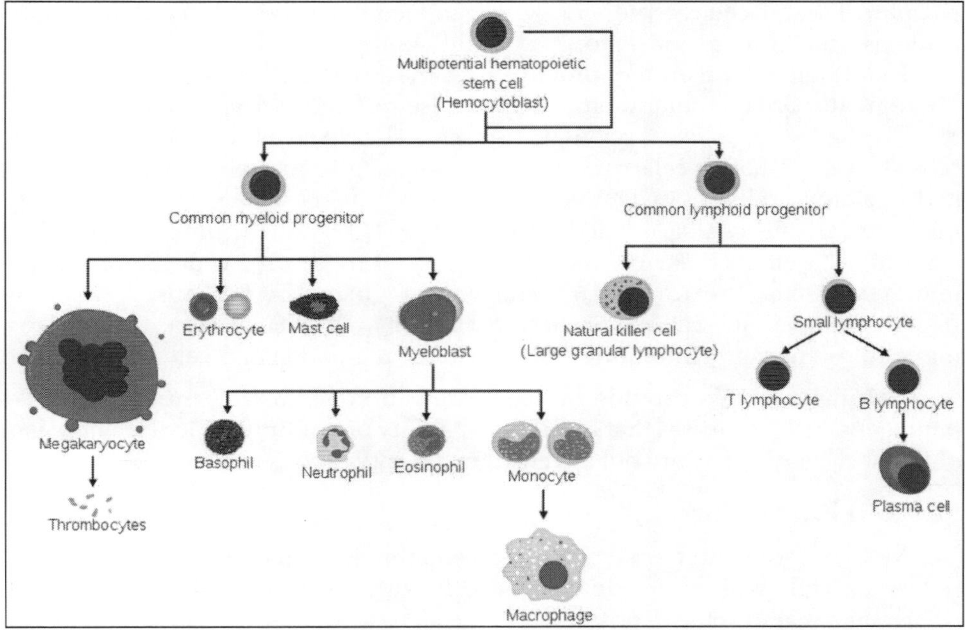

Figure 4.5: Cells of the Immune System.

(Adapted from A. Rad and Mikael Haggstrom, M.D. - Author info - Reusig images Example citation (in caption or footnote): By A. Rad and M. Haggstrom, CC-BY-SA 3.0 license. Image: Hematopoiesis (human) diagram.png by A. Rad.)

Lymphoid Progenitor

Lymphocytes with antigen receptors are the main cells for adaptive immunity and are responsible for multiple features such as specificity, memory, and diversity.

These lymphocytes add up to 20 per cent -40 per cent of the body's white blood cells and 99 per cent of the cells in the lymph. They are mainly found circulating in the blood, lymph and are capable of migrating into the lymphoid organs as well such as the thymus, lymph nodes, spleen, *etc.*

B-lymphocytes

B-lymphocytes get mature in the bone marrow and are responsible for expressing membrane-bound antibodies. The naive B-cells once when interacting with the antigen for the first time, the cells tend to divide further into effector cells also called plasma cells, and into memory cells. Because of the antibodies production capabilities, B-cells are the major part of the humoral immune response. B-cells also act as Antigen Presenting Cells (APCs).

T-lymphocytes

T-lymphocytes generally arise in the bone marrow but the maturation of the T-lymphocytes takes place in the thymus gland. During the process of maturation, T-cell membranes start expressing antigen-binding molecules known as the Tcell receptor. These T-cell receptors recognize antigen that is bound to cell membrane proteins known as major histocompatibility complex molecules (MHC). When the T-cell detects the antigen bound with the MHC molecule, it immediately differentiates after proliferation and gives rise to effector T cells and memory T cells. These T-cells have subpopulations such as T helper cells ($T_{H)}$, and T cytotoxic cells ($T_{C)}$ cells. T helper cells carry $CD4^+$ membrane glycoproteins on their surfaces and T cytotoxic cells carry $CD8^+$ membrane glycoproteins on their surfaces. Further, the T helper cells can be divided into T_H1, T_H2, T_H17, and $T_{FH.}$ Immune response arises due to intracellular pathogens is regulated by the T_H1 cells. Similarly, the immune response to extracellular pathogens is regulated by T_H2 cells. T_H17 secrete IL-17 which mediates cell-mediated immunity. T_{FH} (T follicular helper cells) play a major role in humoral immunity and help in the regulation of B-cell development.

Cytotoxic T-cells provide massive protection against all the intracellular pathogens such as viruses that have the capability of multiplying in the cytoplasm of the host cells as they are not attacked by the antibodies.

Myeloid Progenitor

Myeloid progenitor arises from the hematopoietic stem cells and it includes red blood cells and other white blood cells such as granulocytes, monocytes, macrophages, and some dendritic cells.

Granulocytes

Granulocytes have the cytoplasmic matrix which consists of granules that specifically contain reactive elements that trigger the elimination of the pathogens and enhance inflammation. Granulocytes are known as polymorphonuclear leukocytes (irregular-shaped nuclei with two or more lobes). Granulocytes are further divided into neutrophils, eosinophils, basophils, and mast cells.

Monocytes

Monocytes are mononuclear. They circulate in the bloodstream for 8 hours and get enlarged, then they migrate into the tissues where they differentiate themselves into macrophages or dendritic cells.

Macrophages

During an infection, when blood monocytes migrate into the tissues, they differentiate into specific tissue macrophages. Following are the properties of macrophages.

1. Antigen Presentation
2. Phagocytosis
3. Huge synthesis of cytokines such as TNF-α, IL-12, IL-10, IL-6, fibroblast growth factor
4. Presence of membrane receptors

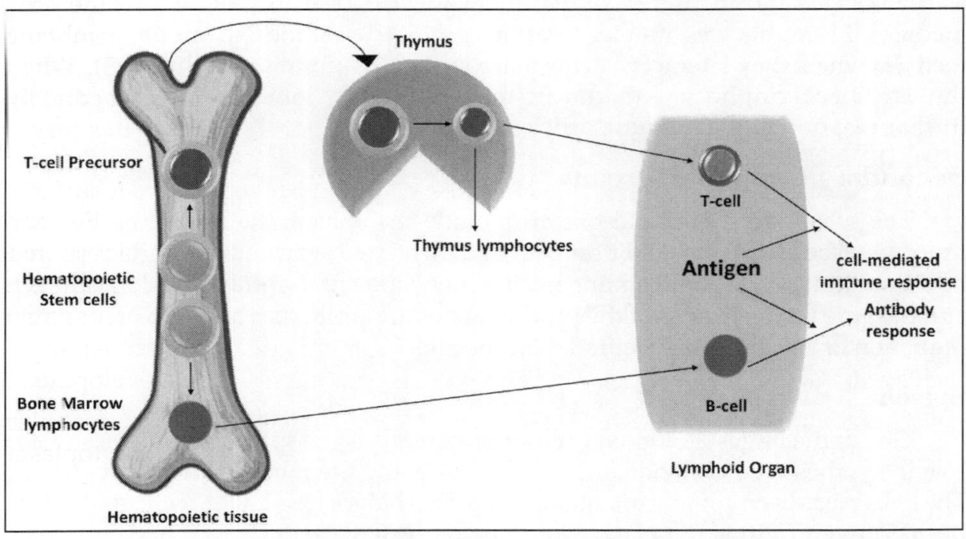

Figure 4.6: Activation and Development of Cells.

Role of Organs in the Adaptive Immune System

The organs of the adaptive immune system have been divided into primary and secondary lymphoid organs. The maturation of lymphocytes takes place in the thymus and bone marrow, which are termed primary lymphoid organs. The differentiation and proliferation of the lymphocytes take place in the secondary lymphoid organs that include lymph nodes, spleen, *etc.*

Primary Lymphoid Organs

Bone Marrow

B-cells are synthesized and get mature in the bone marrow. Following the maturation, B-cells are circulated in the bloodstream and are transported to the secondary lymphoid organs where they eventually interact with the foreign antigens. These B-cells solely exhibit the antibody response in the body. Bone marrow B-cells are the origin of approximately 90 per cent of the immunoglobulins IgG and IgA in plasma.

Thymus

The maturation of the T-cells takes place in the thymus. The thymus is a flat, bilobed organ that is situated just above the heart. Each lobe is encircled by a capsule and is further divided into lobules that are separated by the connective tissue called trabeculae. Each lobule is cleaved into two compartments; the outer compartment termed cortex that is densely packed with immature T-cells known as thymocytes and the inner compartment consists of scanty thymocytes termed medulla. T lymphocytes after maturation in the cortex of the thymus move into the medulla where they interact with the macrophages. Here, after the thymic selection; the functional lymphocytes migrate to the secondary lymphoid organs where they further respond to the foreign particles.

Secondary Lymphoid Organs

The secondary lymphoid organs include the spleen, the lymph nodes, and mucosa-associated lymphoid tissue (MALT). The two very important roles played by the secondary lymphoid organs are, it is highly potent in entrapping the pathogen and they are the main sites of the production of the antibodies and also helps in the induction of the antigen-specific T-lymphocytes.

Spleen

One of the largest secondary lymphoid organs is the spleen and plays a major role in synthesizing antibodies, thereafter releasing them in the blood circulation. The spleen has been compartmentalized into two halves termed Red pulp and White pulp. The red pulp is the place where the old RBCs are destroyed and removed. On the other hand, White pulp is a place that is rich in T-cells. It is been studied that 30-40 per cent of the spleen cells are T-lymphocytes and 50 per cent of spleen cells are B-lymphocytes.

Lymph Nodes

Lymph nodes are the bean-shaped structure which is composed of the medulla and cortex. Lymph nodes are loaded with macrophages, lymphocytes, and dendritic cells. Lymph nodes are efficient in trapping the foreign antigen, then they get interacted with the macrophages, T-cells, and B-cells which together arise an immune response thereby generating the required antibodies and antigen-specific T cells.

Mucosa-Associated Lymphoid Tissue (MALT)

The secondary lymphoid tissues are majorly located in the digestive, respiratory, and gastrointestinal tracts that are together called MALT. The main functional importance of this MALT is the production of a large amount of antibody-producing plasma cells.

Antigens

Antigens are those substances that induce the ability to generate antibody responses. They are the agents who can bind specifically with the T-cell receptors (TCRs) or an antibody molecule. There is a functional variation in two terms antigenicity and immunogenicity. Antigenicity refers to the process in which any agents or compounds can bind with either the TCR or the antibody molecule whereas, in the case of immunogenicity, the agents or the compounds termed immunogen is capable of inducing an immune response in the body. Thus, it is being said that all immunogens are antigens but all antigens are not immunogens.

Haptens

Haptens are low molecular weight substances that are chemically very simple and cannot induce an immune response in their native state. Haptens are the perfect example for all immunogens are antigens but all antigens are not immunogens as haptens are antigenic in nature but are not immunogenic. Despite that, haptens can be transformed immunogenic when they are conjugated to some high molecular weight complex termed carriers.

Immunogen Properties Required for Immunogenicity

Foreignness

The immunogen should be a foreign body for the host. The adaptive immune system can induce the immunogenicity or immune response only when there is a presence of a foreign element inside the body (non-self).

Size

The immunogenicity of an immunogen also depends on the size or molecular weight of the agent. Small compounds having molecular weight <1000 Da are generally not immunogenic, compounds of molecular weight 1000 and 6000 Da may or may not be immunogenic, and the substances having molecular weight >6000 Da are generally immunogenic. Generally, the larger agents or immunogens have increased immunogenicity.

Chemical Complexity

All proteins are immunogenic but the greater is the complexity of the protein, the more will be the immune response to that particular protein. The studies thus have proved that heteropolymers exhibit greater immunogenicity than homopolymers due to the structural complexity.

Dosage and Route of Administration

The quantity of the immunogen also plays a major role in stimulating the immune response. The insufficient dose of the immunogens might not be able to stimulate an immune response so a definite amount of immunogens are required to induce the immunogenicity. Along with that, the route of administration decides the outcome of the immunization. Normally, immunogens are administered through some routes such as intravenous, intradermal, intramuscular, subcutaneous. The antigens which are administered subcutaneously are found to be the strongest immunogens as they show a greater immune response.

Epitopes

Immune cells of the body do not detect the whole antigen or immunogen instead, the lymphocytes detect specific sites on the immunogen termed epitopes, also known as antigenic determinants. The research has presented that on the same antigenic molecule, different epitopes are identified or detected by B and T cells.

Epitope Properties of B-cells

- Generally, the B-cells epitopes found on the protein molecule are composed of hydrophilic amino acids and are able to bind with antibodies.
- B-cell epitopes have mobile peptides that contain sequential and non-sequential amino acids.
- Also, B-cell epitopes often get located in the flexible region of an immunogen and exhibit site mobility.
- Complex proteins consist of multiple overlapping B-cell epitopes, among which some are immunodominant.

Immunoglobulins: Structure and Properties

As studied above, B-cells massively indulge in synthesizing immunoglobulins (Ig), which are also called antibodies. Antibodies are glycoproteins which are consisting of different amino acid sequences and also have different antigen-binding sites. They are exclusively present on the membrane of the B-cells and are secreted by the plasma cells.

Structure of the Antibody Molecule

- The antibody structure is made up of 4 polypeptide chains.
- The antibody is referred to as heterodimer.
- The structure of the antibody molecule consists of two identical heavy (H) chains (containing 440 amino acid residues each having 50000 MW) and two identical light (L) chains (containing 220 amino acid residues each having 25000 MW).
- These light chains and heavy chains are bound to each other by the disulfide linkage and other non-covalent linkages.
- Generally, there are two major classes of light chains further named kappa (κ) and lambda (γ) and five different types of heavy chains μ, γ, α, δ, ε.

- These different types of heavy chains decide the class of the antibody. Thus, the immunoglobulins have been further classified into IgM (μ), IgG (γ), IgA (α), IgD (δ), and IgE (ε).
- Both the light and heavy chains have two definite sequences, the variable sequence at their N-terminal ends and a constant sequence at their C-terminal ends.
- The light chain having the constant region ($C_{L)}$ contains 110 amino acids and the variable region ($V_{L)}$ contains the same number of amino acids.
- Similarly, the heavy region having the variable region contains the same number of amino acids just like the variable region of the light chain and the constant region of the heavy chain contains 330-440 amino acids.
- The variable region of both the light and heavy chains have a diversified region of about approximately 10 amino acid residue that is termed hypervariable regions and each chain having that region is called complementarity determining regions (CDR).

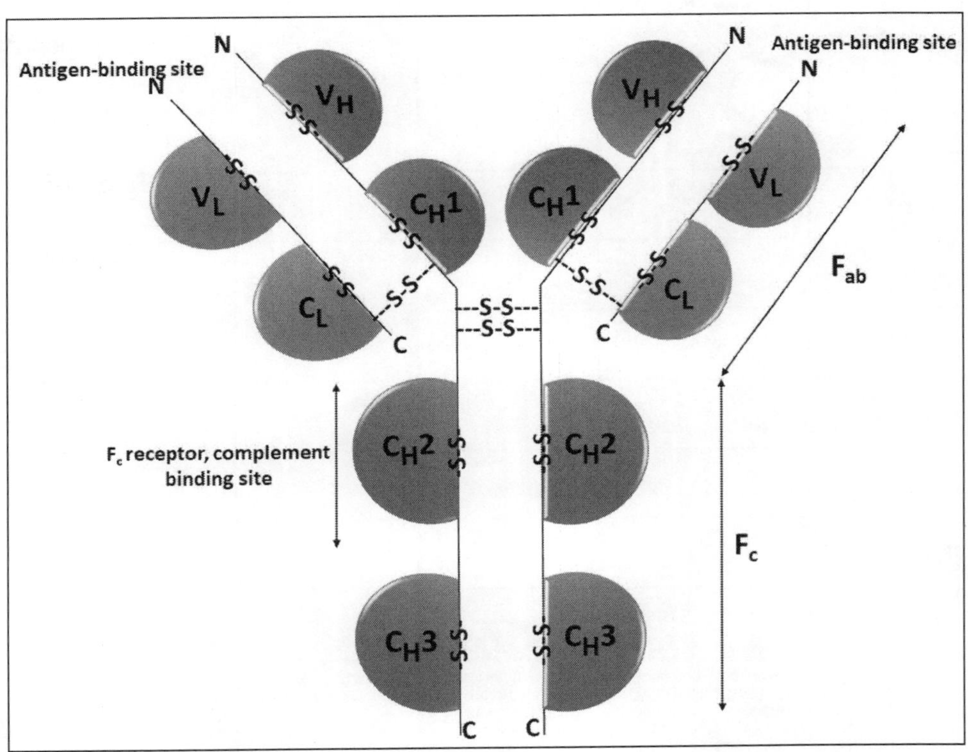

Figure 4.7: Structure of the Immunoglobulin.

Immunoglobulins

The design of the immunoglobulin particle is dictated by the Primary, secondary, tertiary, and quaternary association of the protein. Immunoglobulin structure comprises heavy and light chains. Both heavy and light chains are comprised of 110 amino acids long and each containing one intrachain disulfide bond. A light chain comprises one variable (V_L) and one constant (C_L) domain. Likewise, heavy chains contain one variable and three constant chains. (C_H1, C_H2, C_H3). The γ, δ, α- heavy chains contain an extended peptide sequence between the CH1 and CH2 domains that has no homology with other domains. This region is called the hinge region that is rich in proline and cysteine residues and is flexible [11-14].

Types of Immunoglobulins

The Five Immunoglobulin (Ig) Classes					
	IgM pentamer	IgG monomer	Secretory IgA dimer	IgE monomer	IgD monomer
			Secretory component		
Heavy chains	μ	γ	α	ε	δ
Number of antigen binding sites	10	2	4	2	2
Molecular weight (Daltons)	900,000	150,000	385,000	200,000	180,000
Percentage of total antibody in serum	6%	80%	13%	0.002%	1%
Crosses placenta	no	yes	no	no	no
Fixes complement	yes	yes	no	no	no
Fc binds to		phagocytes		mast cells and basophils	
Function	Main antibody of primary responses, best at fixing complement; the monomer form of IgM serves as the B cell receptor	Main blood antibody of secondary responses, neutralizes toxins, opsonization	Secreted into mucus, tears, saliva, colostrum	Antibody of allergy and antiparasitic activity	B cell receptor

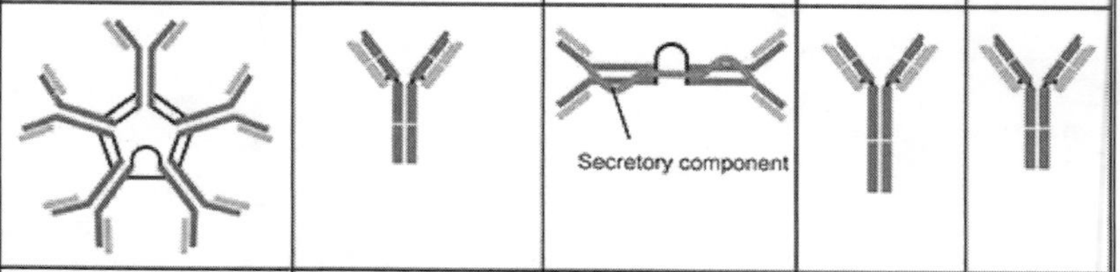

Figure 4.8: Types and Properties of different Immunoglobulins. (Ref: https://microbiologyinfo.com/antibody-structure-classes-and-functions/)

Effector Functions Generated by the Antibody

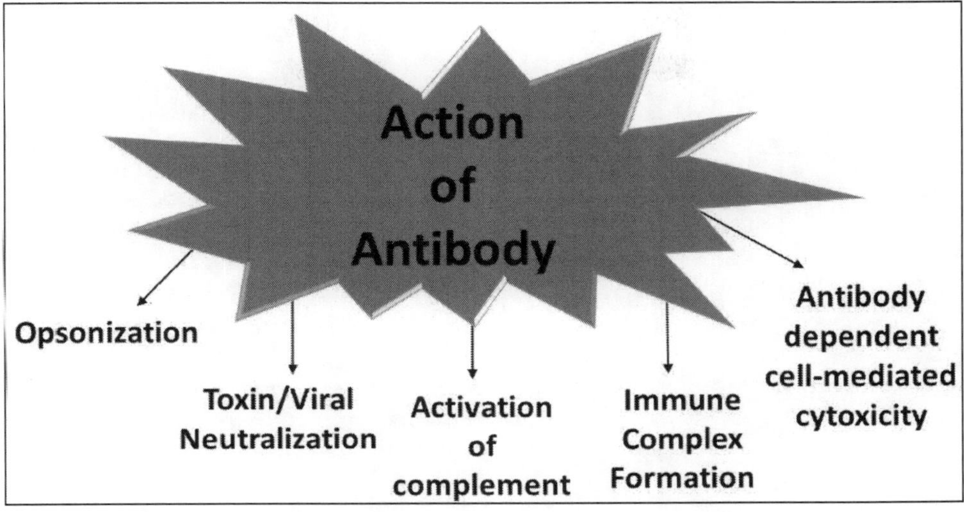

Figure 4.9: Different Effect or Functions Generated by the Antibody.

Antigen and Antibody (Ag-Ab) Interaction

Antigen-antibody interactions are very specific and weak non-covalent interactions are involved with this. The binding forces between the antigen and antibody are weak and reversible. The epitope present on the surface of the antigen is responsible for binding with the paratope of the antibodies. The number of epitopes present on the surface of antigens depends on the valence of the antigen. Valence is defined as the number of the antibody bind with the antigen at one time.

Different Factors Affect the Antigen-Antibody Interactions

- Affinity: For the stable interaction, there should be the presence of the higher affinity of the antibody with the antigen.
- Avidity: Avidity is defined as the overall binding of the antibodies with the multivalent antigen. So, for stable complexes to form reaction between multivalent antigens and multivalent antibodies are preferred.
- The physical form of the antigen plays a major role. Generally, particulate antigens when interacted with antibodies produce agglutination whereas soluble antigens upon interaction with antibodies give precipitation of the antigen to show the interactions.
- The antigen-Antibody ratio gives the size of the complex formed which is related to the concentration of antibody and antigen both.

Adjuvants

An adjuvant is a substance that is combined with the immunogen and then injected into the host for enhancing the immune response against the immunogen.

Aluminum potassium sulfate (alum) is the common adjuvant used for human vaccines as alum has the ability to prolong the persistence of the antigens.

Table 4.1: General difference between the MHC Class I and II

Features	MHC Class I	MHC Class II
Structure	MHC class I molecules composed of one membrane-spanning α chain (heavy chain), and one β chain (light chain or β2-microglobulin).	MHC class II molecules consist of two membrane-spanning chains, α and β, of similar size and both produced by MHC genes.
Types of APCs	MHC I glycoproteins are present in all nucleated cells.	MHC II glycoproteins are only present on specialised antigen-presenting cells (APCs), including macrophages, dendritic cells, B cells that produce antibodies.
Nature of Antigen Presentation	MHC class I glycoproteins present endogenous antigens that originate from the cytoplasm	MHC II proteins present exogenous antigens that originate extracellularly from foreign bodies such as bacteria.
Size of Peptide	MHC Class I present 8-10 amino acid peptides	MHC Class II presents 14-18 amino acid peptides.
T-cells Response	Present antigen to cytotoxic T cell lymphocytes (CD8+ T Cells)	Present antigen to helper T cell lymphocytes; (CD4+ T cells).
Sources of protein antigens	Cytosolic proteins	Endosomal/lysosomal proteins
Co-receptor	Binds with CD8 coreceptors molecules on cytotoxic T cells	Binds with CD4 co-receptors molecules on helper T cells
Enzymes for peptide generation	Cytosolic proteasome	Endosomal and lysosomal proteases
Site of peptide loading of MHC	Endoplasmic reticulum	Specialized vesicular compartment
Molecules involved in transport of peptides and loading of MHC molecules	• Chaperones • TAP in ER	• Chaperones in ER • invariant chain in ER • Golgi and MHC Class II compartment

Major Histocompatibility Complex

MHC is a complex composed of a cluster of genes that helps in the recognition of intracellular pathogens and differentiates between the self or non-self. MHC is localized in chromosome number 6 in humans and on 17 chromosomes in mice which is termed Human leukocyte antigen (HLA) complex and H-2 (histocompatibility-2) complex. MHC is highly polymorphic. MHC genes responsible for the polymorphism of the MHC are further divided into three classes; MHC class I, MHC class II, and MHC class III. The table below, **Table 4.1** highlights the important features of different types of MHC class and also distinguishes between MHC class I and MHC class II.

Facts About Major Histocompatibility Complex

- ☆ Each MHC molecule has only one binding site. Different peptides can bind with this site only at one time.
- ☆ MHC molecules especially, class I and class II are membrane-bound molecules and are mainly recognized by T-cells.
- ☆ Cytokines generally increase the level of MHC expression, mainly interferon-γ.
- ☆ Exogenous peptides coupled with class II MHC which are recognized by T_H cells whereas the endogenous peptides are coupled with class I MHC that is recognized by T_C cells.

Antigen Processing and Presentation

T-cell receptors detect the antigen molecules for further destruction. But T-cell receptors can recognize only the antigen that is bound to MHC molecules. Both the T_H and T_C cells can recognize the antigen when the antigen is being presented by a self-MHC molecule and it is termed a self-MHC restriction. Generally, CD4 T_H cells specifically recognize the antigen that is bound with the class II MHC molecule whereas CD8 T_C cells specifically recognize the antigen that is bound with the class I MHC molecule. The generation of the peptide antigens from proteins inside cells, the binding of the peptides to the respective MHC molecules, and formation of the peptide-MHC complexes for the recognition by the T-cell, all these accumulatively known as antigen processing and presentation.

Two different pathways are being followed by two types of antigens exogenous and endogenous for processing and presentation to cytotoxic T-cells and helper T-cells.

Endogenous Antigen Processing and Presentation: Cytosolic Pathway

- ☆ Endogenous antigens are secreted inside a cell, by different pathogens that have infected the cell.
- ☆ MHC I proteins represent peptide antigens that are synthesized by the endogenous protein antigen.

☆ The whole processing of the endogenous antigens takes place in the cytoplasm with the help of an enzyme proteasome. These proteins cleave them into peptides about 15 amino acids in length.

☆ The transporters associated with antigen processing (TAP) helps to transport the peptides into ER which take place by the energy-dependent reaction.

☆ After the peptides enter ER, they start binding with the MHC class I protein with the help of chaperon proteins such as calnexin, tapasin, calreticulin and ERp57.

☆ After the association with the MHC-I complex, a peptide with MHC goes to the Golgi apparatus.

☆ The chaperones release the MHC-I peptide complex and go to the cell surface where it amalgamates into the membrane and is then recognized by the T_C cells.

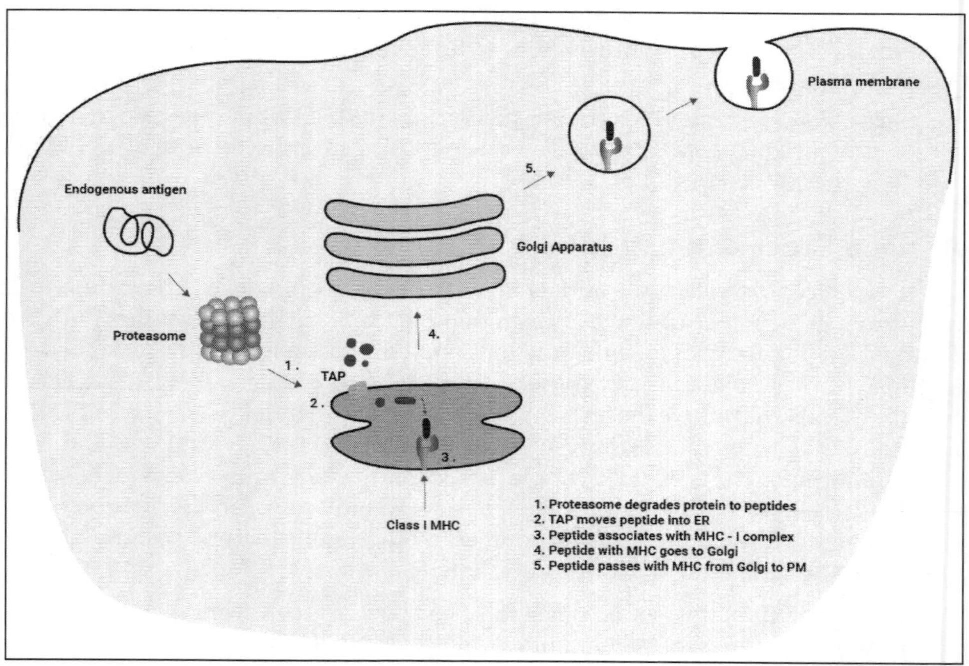

Figure 4.10: Cytosolic Pathway (Endogenous antigen processing and presentation).

Exogenous Antigen Processing and Presentation: Endocytic Pathway

☆ The foreign peptides are presented to helper T-cells from the endosomes.

☆ In a special endosomal compartment, the processed antigens bind to the pre-assembled class II heterodimers.

- ☆ After the binding of the peptide to the class II MHC protein, the MHC protein undergoes conformational changes to entrap the peptides in the groove for presentation on the cell surface to the T_H cells.
- ☆ An invariant chain, a special trimeric protein ensures the blocking of the binding capability of the class II MHC with endogenous antigen.
- ☆ MHC complex is then transported through the Golgi apparatus to the endocytic pathway compartments.
- ☆ The invariant chain is cleaved by the proteases in the late endosome and is further degraded, leaving the CLIP fragment.
- ☆ The exogenous antigen is taken up and the degraded fragments are transported to the endocytic pathway compartments.
- ☆ Further, the class II MHC peptide is transported to the plasma membrane.

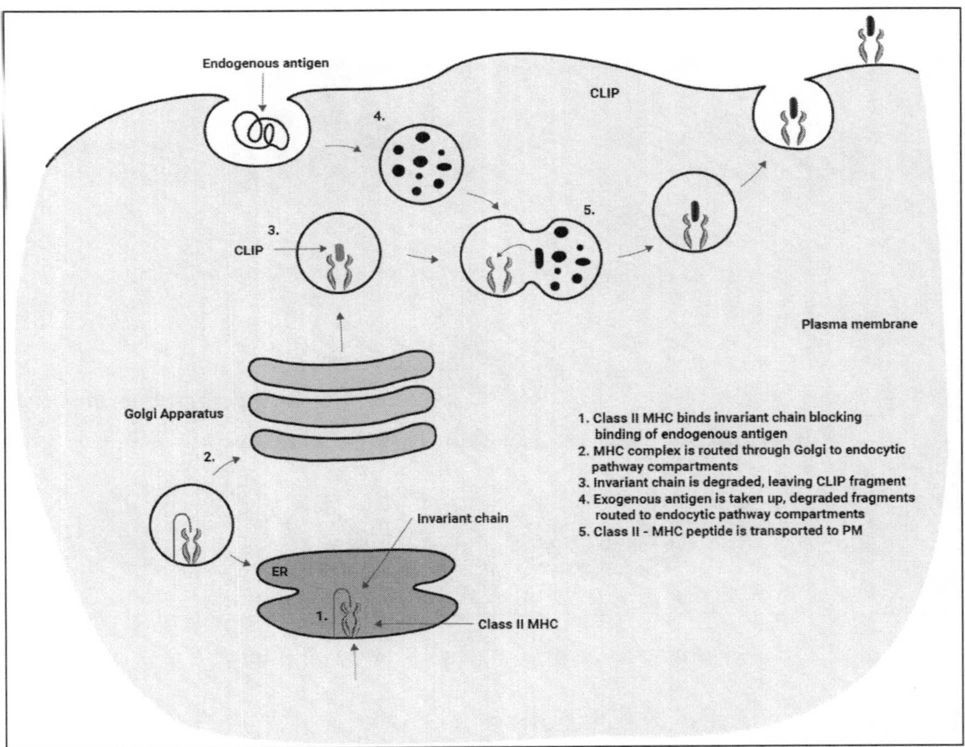

Figure 4.11: Endocytic Pathway (Endogenous antigen processing and presentation).

Clonal Selection Theory

In the clonal selection theory, clonal is explained from the fact that the adaptive immune system consists of a variety of families and clones of lymphocytes that contains T and B cells. Each of the ancestral cells that differentiates into the further cells are already committed to producing one specific antigen-specific receptor protein and due to the clone, it is understood that all the cells have the same specificity. The clonal selection theory was formulated by Sir Macfarlane Burnet.

Clonal selection theory states that an animal randomly generates lymphocytes and then those lymphocytes that can react against the foreign antigens that the animal was supposed to interact with are specifically chosen and proliferated. When the lymphocyte interacts with the antigen in the lymphoid organ, after binding with the receptors it activates the lymphocyte thereby initiating the proliferation and differentiation into the effector cells. An antigen further stimulates only those cells that can express the complementary antigen-specific receptors and that is how the adaptive immune response is termed antigen-specific.

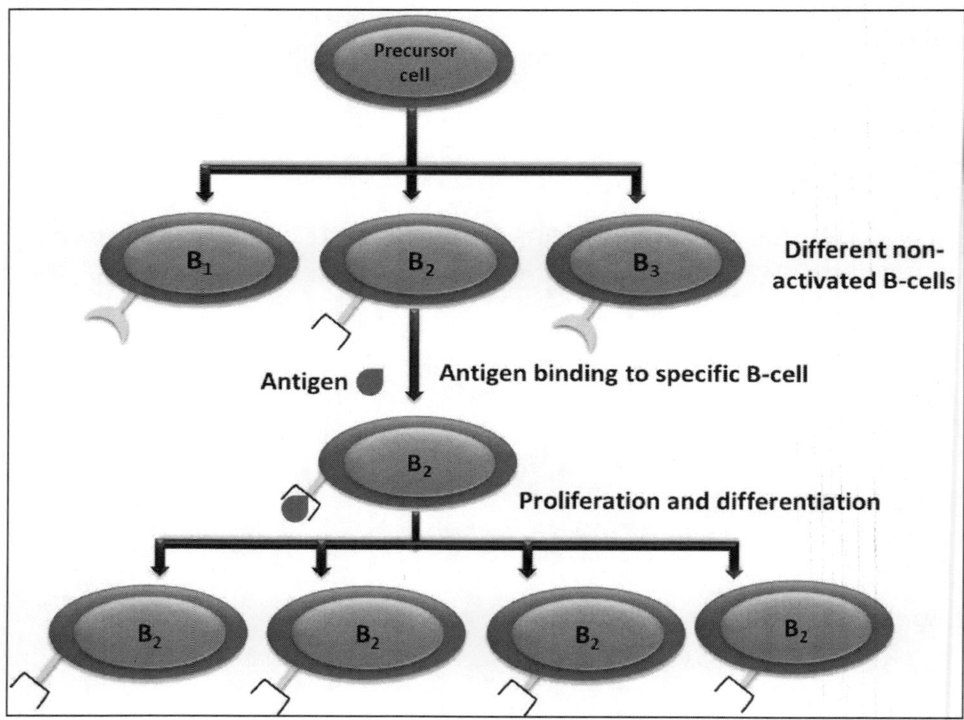

Figure 4.12: Clonal Selection Theory of B-cells.

Kinetics of Antibody Response

Antibody Response comes with two types of responses primary and secondary responses.

The primary response is the primary immunization that an individual develops when they are exposed to a first immunogen. Thus, the primary response generated by the host is further divided into four phases.

1. Lag Phase: It is the immediate phase that arises after the detection of the antigenic stimulus but no detectable amount of antibodies are found. The phase stays for one to two weeks.

2. Log or exponential Phase: In this state, there is a steady rise of the concentration of antibodies in the serum exponentially.
3. Steady-state or Plateau: The phase where there is an equilibrium maintained between antibody synthesis and degradation of antibodies.
4. Decline Phase: In this phase, there is a rapid decline in the concentration of antibodies.

In the primary response, the initial first-class antibody detected is IgM and IgG. But there is a sudden change or shift of the antibody detected in the case of secondary response. There is a shift of the class response termed class switching. In secondary response, IgG antibodies are appearing at much higher concentrations and with greater persistence than IgM. Along with this, IgA and IgE also start appearing, and collectively IgG, IgE and IgA are called secondary classes of antibodies. After a certain point in time of immunization, there is an increase in the affinity of the antibodies that are produced against the immunogen and this phenomenon is called affinity maturation that arises due to the point mutation occurring in the light and heavy chain of the V-region coding sequences.

On the other hand, the secondary response arises when the individual is exposed to the same immunogen. The secondary response is also called a memory response and memory cells participate in this.

Monoclonal Antibodies and Hybridoma Technology

Monoclonal antibodies are monospecific. These types of antibodies are secreted from a clone of a single lymphocyte that is directed against a single epitope. Therefore, monoclonal antibodies are directed against a single epitope.

When a specific antibody-producing B-cell is fused with a myeloma cell (cancerous B-cell) for synthesizing hybrid cell lines, the phenomenon is called Hybridoma Technology. The antibodies produced by this method are monoclonal antibodies.

Super Antigens

- Superantigens are the bacterial or viral proteins that generally bind with the variable domain of β of a T-cell receptor and to the α- chain of the MHC class II molecule.
- Superantigens can activate a large number of T-cells disregarding their antigenic specificity.
- Generally, superantigens can endogenous as well as exogenous. Endogenous superantigens are the cell membrane proteins that are encoded by the viruses that eventually infect the mammalian cells.
- Exogenous superantigens are the soluble proteins synthesized by bacteria.

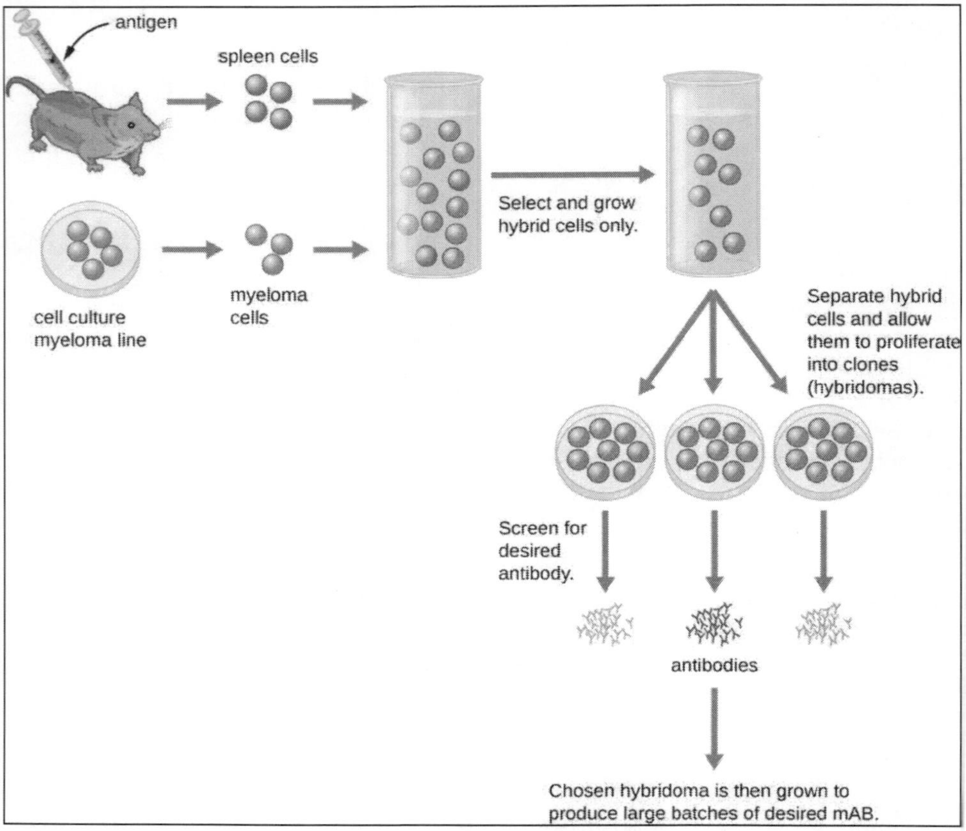

Figure 4.13: Monoclonal Antibodies Production (Ref: https://courses.lumenlearning.com/microbiology/chapter/polyclonal-and-monoclonal-antibody-production/)

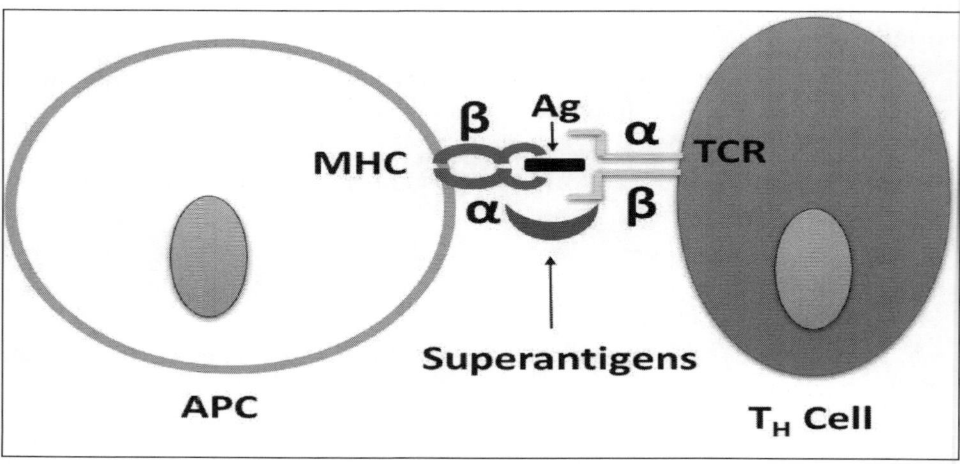

Figure 4.14: Superantigen.

Cytokines

Cytokines are a low molecular weight of less than 30kDa soluble glycoproteins. Cytokines have been playing a major role in the development of the cellular and humoral immune response, regulation of the hematopoiesis, control the cellular differentiation and proliferation, and elicitation of the inflammatory responses. Different biological activities exhibited by cytokines are pleiotropy, redundancy, synergy, and antagonism. Cytokines have been named by their origin, such as monokines (substances produced by macrophages or monocytes), lymphokines (synthesized by lymphocytes). Cytokines have been further grouped into the categories, such as interleukins, interferons, chemokines, hematopoietins, and tumor necrosis factors (TNF).

Role of Cytokines

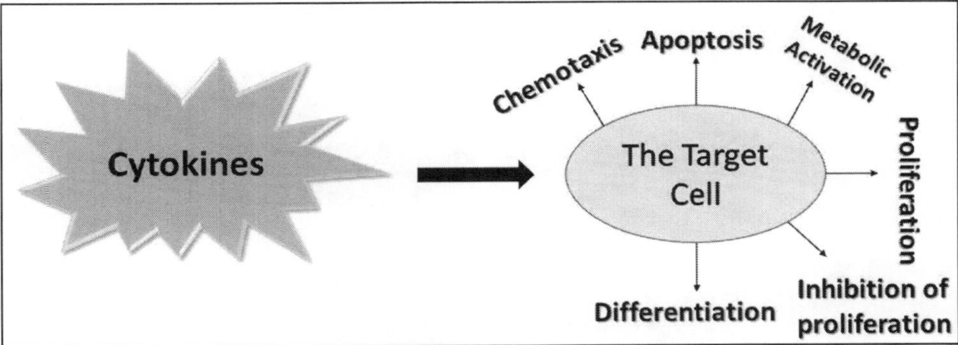

Figure 4.15: Role of Cytokines in the Immune System on the Target Cell.

Complement System

The complement system is composed of around 30 serum and cell surface proteins which together play a major role in inducing the immune responses. Various functions are performed by the complement systems. That includes:

1. Lysis of cells
2. Inflammatory Responses
3. Opsonization
4. Neutralization
5. Solubilization of immune complexes
6. Clearance of immune complexes

Also, different complement components are involved to run the complement systems. These complement components are again a group of glycoproteins. They are given names by numerals (C1-C9). Mainly, these complement components are produced by liver hepatocytes. Its been studied that normally the complement components are found in the serum in an inactivate state in the form of zymogens or proenzymes but once the components are activated one after the other, they start following complement activation pathways. Upon the activation of the components, they start splitting into small fragments denoted by small letters. They start splitting into larger, and smaller fragments. The smaller fragments get diffused and initiate the inflammatory response and on the other hand, the larger fragments bind with the target near to the site of activation. Three pathways are being followed, lectin, classical and alternative pathways.

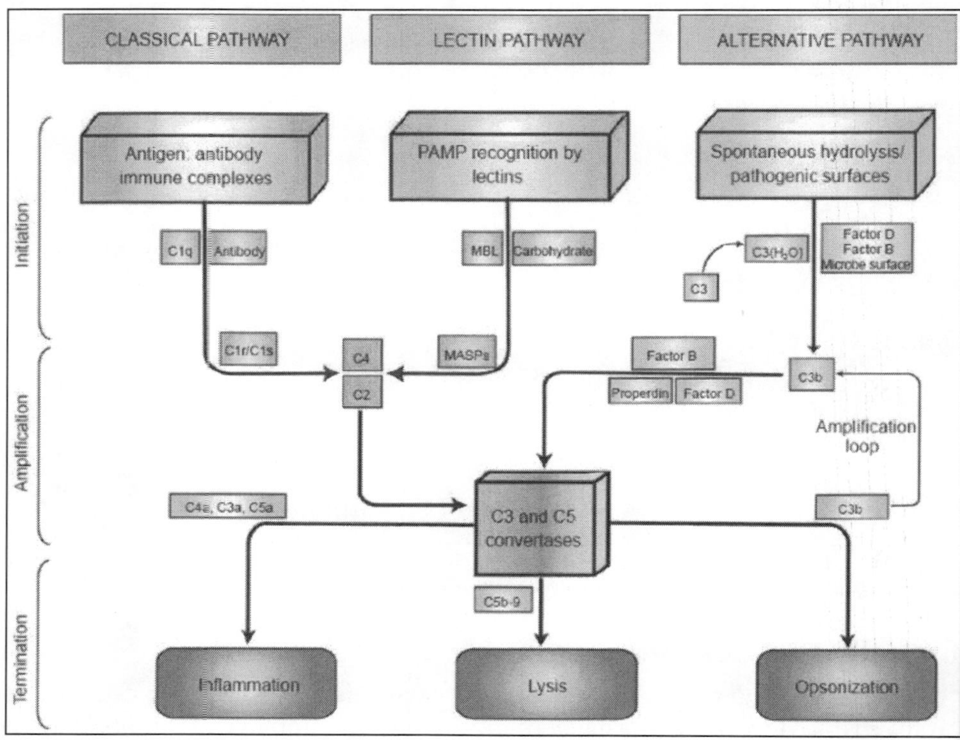

Figure 4.16: Complement System and their Types.
(Ref: https://www.nature.com/articles/cr2009139/ [15]).

Hypersensitivity

Hypersensitivity is an immune response that results in tissue damage and is divided into two types immediate and delayed ones completely on the basis of the time needed for the sensitized individual o develop the clinical reactions on the re-exposure of the antigen. They are typically divided into four types.

1. Type I Hypersensitivity (allergic reaction)
2. Type II Hypersensitivity (cytotoxic reaction)
3. Type III Hypersensitivity
4. Type IV Hypersensitivity (Delayed-Type Hypersensitivity)

Type I Hypersensitivity (Allergic reaction)

- This hypersensitivity is induced by allergens which act as antigens.
- Type I hypersensitive reactions are IgE-mediated humoral immune responses.
- IgE-specific F_C receptors present on the mast cells and basophils binds with the IgE.
- Upon crosslinking of IgE induced by the antigens, the IgE triggers the basophils and mast cells to secrete primary mediators (histamines, proteases, eosinophils, *etc.*)
- These mediators normally cause the consequences of an acute inflammatory reaction.
- It is said that Type I hypersensitivity can be anaphylaxis, which is rapid, causes a severe whole-body allergic reaction, and can be life-threatening.
- This can also atopic allergy which develops from hereditary to certain substances, such as pollen, insect venom, *etc.*

Type II Hypersensitivity (Cytotoxic reaction)

- This hypersensitivity is termed cytotoxic reaction because of the destruction caused to host cells by lysis or other toxic mediators.
- The antibodies that mediate the Type II hypersensitivity are IgM and IgG classes.
- Two different antibody-mediated mechanisms are followed by this.
- Complement-mediated hypersensitivity reactions trigger the synthesis of the antibodies that react with the cell membrane component, which leads to complement fixation by activating the complement cascade that either causes lysis or opsonization of the cell.
- Antibody-dependent cell-mediated cytotoxicity (ADCC) uses F_C receptors present on different cell types. ADCC causes the lysis of the targeted cells by releasing cytoplasmic granules perforin and granzymes that activate the cascade events to apoptosis

Type III Hypersensitivity

- Type III hypersensitivity is mediated by IgG antibodies.
- The immune complexes circulating resides at tissue sites from where they activate the complement system and further induce cell lysis.
- Generally, these complexes are phagocytosed but due to the presence of a larger number of soluble antigens, the antigen-antibody complexes can not remove the immune complexes, and accumulation of these arise the hypersensitivity reaction.

Type IV Hypersensitivity

- It is a delayed-type of hypersensitivity.

- This hypersensitive reaction is mediated or triggered by antigen-specific T cells. Mainly it is mediated by T_H cells or their subtypes T_H1 and in few cases T_C cells as well.
- There is no role of antibodies in this type of hypersensitivity.
- In this, there is an activation of T_H1 cells that release cytokines that accumulate and activate the macrophages and cause local damage.

Autoimmune Diseases

The individuals can recognize their self particles from foreign particles and accordingly raise the immune responses against it. When T and B-cells are activated against the self-proteins or antigens, there is a formation of the condition known as autoimmunity. The disease used by this condition is known as autoimmune disease. Autoimmune disease cause destruction to the self-proteins, organs by autoimmune antibodies (Hashimoto's thyroiditis) or self-reactive T-cells (Rheumatoid arthritis). Below, is the table of different types of autoimmune diseases, the organs they affect, and the mechanism they show.

Table 4.2: Autoimmune Diseases of Humans

Disease	Affected Area	Mechanism
Juvenile Diabetes	Pancreas	Cell-mediated immunity and autoantibodies against surface and cytoplasmic antigens of islets of Langerhans (II & IV)
Myasthenia gravis	Skeletal Muscle	Autoantibodies against acetylcholine receptors on skeletal muscle (II)
Goodpasture's Syndrome	Kidney	Autoantibodies against basement membrane of kidney glomeruli (II)
Rheumatoid arthritis	cartilage	Autoantibodies against the self IgG antibodies
Hashimoto's Disease	Thyroid	Autoantibodies produced to thyroid surface antigens (II)
Pernicious Anemia	Intrinsic factors	Autoantibodies prevent the absorption of vitamin B_{12} (III)
Addison's Disease	Adrenal Glands	Autoantibodies to the adrenal cell antigens (II)

Immunodeficiency Diseases

When there is a defect in the components of the immune system, it rises immunodeficiencies. Immunodeficiencies are again divided into two types primary and secondary immunodeficiency.

Primary Immunodeficiency: It is caused by a defect in more than one gene which takes part in the development and function of the immune system. Examples of primary immunodeficiency diseases are Severe combined immunodeficiency (SCID), Chediak-Higashi syndrome, DiGeorge Syndrome.

Secondary Immunodeficiency: It is caused when acquired after birth due to some infections which are not related to any genetic defect.

Vaccines

An individual is capable of inducing the production of antibodies on their own once exposed to foreign particle or antigens but another type of immunity called artificial immunity also play the similar role to induce the production of antibodies in the body. The component utilized for inducing this artificial immunity is the antigen itself or mixture of antigens and is known as vaccines. The process of creating such an immune response is known as immunization [16-17].

There are now several basic types of vaccine. Following are the different types of vaccines discussed.

Attenuated Whole-Agent Vaccines

In this living but attenuated (weakened) microbes are used. Live vaccines are capable to closely mimic an actual infection. Lifelong immunity is often achieved without booster immunizations and effectiveness. These vaccines do not require booster doses and can show immunogenicity in long run. But there is a disadvantage of these types of vaccines where it is mostly associated with the risk of taking the form of virulent strain.

The Sabin polio vaccine is an example of the attenuated vaccine, which consists of three attenuated strains of poliovirus. Sabin polio vaccine induces the production of IgA that acts against the defense of the naturally acquired poliovirus.

Inactivated (Killed) Vaccines

Inactivated vaccines are produced by inactivating or killing the microorganisms with the help of heat or chemical treatment so that they cannot replicate massively in the body. These vaccines require booster doses. They are generally more stable than attenuated whole-agent vaccines. The immunity induced by these vaccines is mainly humoral. The good part of these vaccines is they do not revert into the virulent form.

The Salk Polio Vaccine is an example of the inactivated vaccines.

Toxoids

Toxoids are also inactivated vaccines. There are many exotoxins that are modified chemically to retain their antigenicity but they are no longer toxic. This sort of modified exotoxin is called toxoids.

The Diptheria and Tetanus vaccines are being purified and made by the bacterial exotoxins, inactivating them with the formaldehyde treatment to produce toxoids.

Subunit Vaccines

Subunit vaccines use the antigenic fragments of the microorganisms which induce the immune response. These vaccines are produced with the help of genetic modifications, therefore, it is termed recombinant vaccines.

The first recombinant antigen vaccine used is the hepatitis B vaccine.

DNA Vaccines

DNA vaccines are known as genetic vaccines. These use the genetic material of the pathogens to raise the immunity of the individual. The antigenic proteins present on the fragments of the pathogen's genome are directly injected into the host cells where they get integrated into the chromosomal DNA thereby generating both humoral and cell-mediated immunity.

Recombinant Vector Vaccines

In these types of vaccines, the genes that specifically code for antigens are isolated from the pathogen and then inserted back into the non-virulent viruses or bacteria. These recombinant microorganisms are termed vectors that replicate within the host and express the gene product of the pathogen that are encoded with antigenic proteins.

Immunological Tests or Assays

Antigen-antibody interactions are very specific and with the help of these interactions, various immunological tests and assays are being performed. Three prime terms affinity, avidity, and cross-reactivity give the interaction mechanisms of the Ag-Ab complex.

1. Affinity: Affinity is the ability with which a monovalent ligand binds, generally non-covalent interactions between the epitope and paratope.
2. Avidity: Avidity is the ability of antigen-antibody binding when multiple epitopes on an antigen interact with multiple binding sites of an antibody.
3. Cross-reactivity: Cross-reactivity is the ability of the antibodies to bind with more than one antigenic determinant.

REFERENCES

1. Akira, S., K. Takeda, and T. Kaisho. 2001. Toll-like receptors: Critical proteins linking innate and acquired immunity. Nature Immunol. 2: 675.
2. Burnet, F. M. 1959. The Clonal Selection Theory of Acquired Immunity. Cambridge University Press, Cambridge.
3. Cohen, S. G., and M. Samter. 1992. Excerpts from Classics in Allergy. Symposia Foundation, Carlsbad, California.
4. Desour, L. 1922. Pasteur and His Work (translated by A. F. and B. H. Wedd). T. Fisher Unwin Ltd., London.

5. Fritig, B., T. Heitz, and M. Legrand. 1998. Antimicrobial proteins in induced plant defense. Curr. Opin. Immunol. 10: 12.

6. Appelbaum, F. R. 1996. Hematopoietic stem cell transplantation. In Scientific American Medicine. D. Dale and D. Federman, eds. Scientific American Publishers, New York.

7. Banchereau J., F. Briere, C. Caux, J. Davoust, S. Lebecque, Y. J. Liu, B. Pulendran, and K. Palucka. 2000. Immunobiology of dendritic cells. Annu. Rev. Immunology. 18: 767.

8. Bendelac, A., M. N. Rivera, S-H. Park, and J. H. Roark. 1997. Mouse CD1-specific NK1 T cells: Development, specificity and function. Annu. Rev. Immunol. 15: 535.

9. Clevers, H. C., and R. Grosschedl. 1996. Transcriptional control of lymphoid development: lessons from gene targeting. Immunol. Today 17: 336.

10. Cory, S. 1995. Regulation of lymphocyte survival by the BCL-2 gene family. Annu. Rev. Immunol. 12: 513.

11. Frazer, J. K., and J. D. Capra. 1999. Immunoglobulins: structure and function. In Fundamental Immunology, 4th ed. W. E. Paul, ed. Philadelphia, Lippincott-Raven.

12. Kohler, G., and C. Milstein. 1975. Continuous cultures of fused cells secreting antibody of predefined specificity. Nature 256: 495.

13. Kraehenbuhl, J. P., and M. R. Neutra. 1992. Transepithelial transport and mucosal defence II: secretion of IgA. Trends Cell Biol.2: 134.

14. Immunology Today, The Immune Receptor Supplement, 2nd ed.1997. Elsevier Trends Journals, Cambridge, UK (ISSN 1365-1218).

15. Dunkelberger JR, Song WC. Complement and its role in innate and adaptive immune responses. Cell Res. 2010 Jan;20(1): 34-50.

16. Afzal, M. F., *et al.*, 2000. Clinical safety issues of measles, mumps, and rubella vaccines. WHO Bull. 78: 199.

17. Bloom, B. R. 1998. The highest attainable standard: ethical issues in AIDS vaccines. Science 279: 186.

Chapter 5

Molecular Biology

Riya Mukherjee, Ramendra Pati Pandey*

Centre for Drug Design Discovery and Development (C4D), SRM University, Delhi-NCR, Rajiv Gandhi Education City, Sonepat – 131 029, Haryana, India

****e-mail: ramendra.pandey@gmail.com***

ABSTRACT

The area of molecular biology has a major influence in life science research. Over the last four decades, major developments in molecular biology have sparked study and development in almost every field of life science. This has revolutionized developments not only in molecular biology, but also in biochemistry, biophysics, biotechnology, cell biology, and genetics, by altering the logic and approach to scientific experiments. One major example is the development of high-throughput biology, next-generation sequencing, and recombinant DNA technology, which enabled scientists to reveal the genome's high complexity and elucidate the precise mechanisms for genetic information transmission. Gene expression, DNA replication, DNA repair, and sister chromatid segregation are now shown to be processes that are far more complex than previously thought. This complexity involves, but is not limited to, the presence of intertwined regulatory pathways involving previously unknown actors, such as non-coding RNAs; the importance of epigenetic mechanisms and post-transcriptional modifications; and the importance of epigenetic mechanisms and post-transcriptional modifications. Despite the fact that this module focuses on life sciences, it is important to note the biomedical significance of molecular biology-related research for drug discovery and the advancement of more personalized medicine. We focused on applied basic to advanced aspects of molecular biology in this chapter since molecular biology is a discipline that is continuously changing and evolving.

Keywords: *High-throughput biology, Next-generation sequencing, Recombinant DNA technology; Gene expression, DNA replication, DNA repair, Post-transcriptional modifications, Personalized medicine.*

Nucleic Acids: DNA and RNA Structure

Nucleic acids are nucleotide-based compounds that bear a cell's genetic blueprint. A pentose sugar, a nitrogenous base, and a phosphate group make up each nucleotide. DNA and RNA are the two types of nucleic acids. The genetic blueprint of a cell is borne by DNA, which is passed on from parents to offspring. The two strands of double-stranded DNA form a helical pattern with the two strands going in opposite directions. The two strands are chemically complementary to each other and are connected by hydrogen bonds. The double helix is also stabilized by "base piling" interactions. A pentose sugar (ribose), a nitrogenous base, and a phosphate group make up RNA, which can be single-stranded or double-stranded. Protein synthesis as a messenger, protein synthesis regulation, other regulatory mechanisms, and some catalytic action are all supported by RNA. Deoxyribonucleic acid (DNA) and ribonucleic acid (RNA) are the two primary groups of nucleic acids (RNA). The presence or lack of a hydroxyl group at the C2 site of the ribose, also known as the 2′ position, is the key distinction between these two groups of nucleic acids. The word "deoxy" ribonucleic acid derives from the lack of ribose and the presence of a hydrogen atom at that position, whereas RNA has a hydroxyl functional group at that site. Nucleotides are monomers that makeup DNA and RNA. To form a nucleic acid polymer, individual nucleotides condense with one another. A nitrogenous base, a pentose sugar, and a phosphate group are the three components of each nucleotide.

The Nitrogenous Base

The nitrogenous bases of nucleotides are organic compounds with carbon and nitrogen as constituents. They are bases because they contain an amino group that can bind additional hydrogen, allowing the hydrogen ion content in the local atmosphere to decrease. Adenine (A), guanine (G), cytosine (C), and thymine (T) are the four nitrogenous bases that can be found in DNA (T). Instead of thymine, RNA includes adenine (A), guanine (G), cytosine (C), and uracil (U). Adenine and guanine are classified as purines. Purines have a double carbon-nitrogen ring as their main identifying characteristic. Pyrimidines are the bases of cytosine, thymine, and uracil. A single carbon-nitrogen ring separates them structurally. Each of these ring structures has functional groups that can be used in many chemistries and interactions, and you should be able to recognize them.

The Pentose Sugar

There are 5 carbon atoms in the pentose sugar. The sugar molecule's carbon atoms are called 12 , 22 , 32 , 42 , and 52 (12 implies "one prime"). The two major functional groups attached to the sugar are often referred to by the carbon number to which they are bound. The phosphate residue, for example, is attached to the sugar's 52 carbon, while the hydroxyl group is attached to the sugar's 32 carbon. Be very familiar with the composition of the pentose sugar and we can often use the carbon number to refer to functional groups on nucleotides. The pentose sugar in DNA is called deoxyribose, and in RNA, the sugar is ribose. The difference between the sugars in the presence of the hydroxyl group on the 2′ carbon of the ribose and its absence on the 2′ carbon of the deoxyribose.

The Phosphate Group

The 5′ carbon of the sugar will have up or three phosphate groups bound to it. Nucleotide Monophosphate refers to a nucleotide that has only one phosphate bound to it (NMP). Nucleotide Diphosphate refers to a nucleotide that has two phosphates bound to it (NDP). A Nucleotide Triphosphate is formed when three phosphates are bound to a nucleotide (NTP). The phosphoanhydride bonds that bind the phosphate groups have chemical properties that make them useful for many biological functions. In biological conditions, the hydrolysis of the bonds between the phosphate groups is thermodynamically exergonic, and evolution has developed various pathways to couple this negative shift in free-energy to help accelerate much of the cell's reactions.

Double Helix Structure of DNA

DNA is made up of two helixes. The base of DNA is made up of sugar and phosphate, which are found on the outside of the helix. The nitrogenous bases are stacked in pairs in the interior, like steps on a staircase, and are linked by hydrogen bonds. Each base pair in the double helix is 0.34 nm away from the next base pair. The helix's two strands pass in opposite ways, so one strand's 52 carbon end will face the 32 carbon end of its corresponding strand.

Deoxyribonucleic acid (DNA) and ribonucleic acid (RNA) are the two primary groups of nucleic acids (RNA). From single-celled bacteria to multicellular animals, DNA is the genetic material present in all living organisms. It's found in eukaryotes' nuclei, as well as chloroplasts and mitochondria. DNA is not encased in a membranous shell in prokaryotes but rather floats naturally in the cytoplasm. The genome is a cell's whole genetic material, and genomics is the analysis of genomes. DNA forms a complex of histone proteins to form chromatin, the material of eukaryotic chromosomes, in eukaryotic cells but not in prokaryotes.

The instructions are not read immediately by the ribosomes until the mRNA has entered them. Instead, a different type of RNA known as transfer RNA (t-RNA) is needed to transform the information from the mRNA into a form that can be used. The t-RNA binds to the mRNA, but with base pairings that are reversed. The series is then read in codons, which are three-base groups. Every three-letter combination of A, C, U, and G (*e.g.*, AAA, AAU, GGC, and so on) is a distinct instruction, and the correspondence between these instructions and amino acids is known as the "genetic code." Though there are modifications or changes to the code, the basic genetic code remains true in the vast majority of species.

The ribosome serves as a giant clamp, locking all of the players in place and allowing base pairing between the messenger and transition RNAs as well as chemical bonding between amino acids. Since they function in the ribosome, ribosomal RNAs (r-RNA) are special subunits of the ribosome. These subunits are part of the ribosome machinery, which is used to produce proteins from mRNAs. They do not hold instructions for making particular proteins (*i.e.*, they are not messenger RNAs). The translation is the method of producing proteins by translating instructions from mRNA.

(a) DNA Replication

James Watson and Francis Crick's discovery of the structure of the double helix gave a clue as to how DNA is replicated during replication. Separating the double helix strands would provide two models for the synthesis of new complementary strands, but it was still uncertain how new DNA molecules were created. The two strands of the double helix divide during DNA replication in one model, semiconservative replication, and each strand acts as a template from which the new complementary strand is copied; after replication, each double-stranded DNA comprises one parental or "old" strand and one "new" strand.

Because of the small size of the genome and the proliferation of mutations, DNA replication in bacteria has been widely studied. A single circular chromosome in *E. coli* comprises 4.6 million base pairs (Mbp), and it is repeated in 42 minutes, beginning from a single replication origin and continuing around the circle bidirectionally (*i.e.*, in both directions). This translates to around 1000 nucleotides being added per second.

There are three types of DNA polymerases present in bacteria: DNA pol I, DNA pol II, and DNA pol III. DNA pol III is now recognized to be the enzyme necessary for DNA synthesis, while DNA pol I and DNA pol II are primarily needed for DNA repair. DNA pol III adds deoxyribonucleotides to the 3′-OH group of the growing DNA chain one by one, each complementary to a nucleotide on the template strand. The inclusion of these nucleotides necessitates the spending of resources. Similar to how energy is contained in the phosphate bonds of adenosine triphosphate, this energy is found in the bonds of three phosphate groups bound to each nucleotide (a triphosphate nucleotide) (ATP).

Initiation

The origin of replication is a particular nucleotide sequence where different proteins bind to initiate the replication process. On its single chromosome, *E. coli* (like most prokaryotes) has a single replication origin called oriC. The replication origin is about 245 base pairs long and includes a lot of adenine-thymine (AT) sequences. Any of the proteins that bind to the replication origin play a role in allowing single-stranded DNA regions to be replicated.

The DNA strands are then separated by an enzyme called helicase, which splits the hydrogen bonds between the nitrogenous base pairs. Note that AT sequences have fewer hydrogen bonds than guanine-cytosine (GC) sequences, which therefore have weaker interactions. ATP hydrolysis is necessary by these enzymes. Replication forks are Y-shaped structures that form when the DNA opens up. At the origin of replication, two replication forks form, allowing for bidirectional replication and the creation of a structure that resembles a bubble when seen through a transmission electron microscope; as a result, this structure is known as a replication bubble.

Elongation

The addition of nucleotides happens at a maximum rate of around 1000 nucleotides per second during the elongation of DNA replication. The replication fork is hindered by the fact that DNA polymerase III can only stretch in the 5′ to

3′ direction. The DNA double helix is antiparallel, meaning one strand is oriented 5′ to 3′ and the other is oriented 3′ to 5′. (see Structure and Function of DNA). Since polymerase can add nucleotides in this direction, one strand, which is complementary to the 3′ to 5′ parental DNA strand, is synthesized continuously toward the replication fork during replication. The leading strand is the one that is continually synthesized.

The leading strand can be expanded with only one primer, while each of the short Okazaki fragments includes a new primer. The lagging strand will be 3′ to 5′ in length, and the leading strand will be 5′ to 3′ in length. The DNA polymerase is held in place by a protein called the sliding clamp as it proceeds to incorporate nucleotides. A ring-shaped protein called the sliding clamp attaches to DNA and locks the polymerase in place. Topoisomerase also stops the over winding of the DNA double helix when the DNA opens up ahead of the replication fork by creating temporary nicks in the helix and then resealing it. The RNA primers are eventually replaced by DNA as the synthesis progresses. The primers are replaced by DNA polymerase I's exonuclease operation, and the holes are filled in. The enzyme DNA ligase seals the nicks that remain between the newly synthesized DNA (that replaced the RNA primer) and the previously synthesized DNA by catalyzing the formation of a covalent phosphodiester linkage between the 3′-OH end of one DNA fragment and the 5′ phosphate end of the other, stabilizing the sugar-phosphate backbone of the DNA molecule.

Termination: After the entire chromosome has been repeated, DNA replication must be halted. While much is known about replication initiation, little is known about replication termination. The full circular genomes of prokaryotes are concatenated after replication, which means that the circular DNA chromosomes are interlocked and must be removed. The action of bacterial topoisomerase IV accomplishes this by inserting double-stranded breaks into DNA molecules, causing them to differentiate from one another; the enzyme then reseals the circular chromosomes. Because of their circular chromosomes, concatemer resolution is a challenge unique to prokaryotic DNA replication. Since bacterial DNA gyrase and topoisomerase IV differ from their eukaryotic counterparts, these enzymes are used as targets for quinolone antimicrobial drugs.

(b) DNA Transcription

Transcription is the method of converting DNA into RNA, which involves the creation of an RNA strand on the DNA template. The unwinding of DNA is also involved in this process, and transcription begins at a certain stage. Only one of the two strands of DNA produces the necessary RNA in this situation. The enzyme RNA polymerase catalyzes the reaction, which necessitates the nucleotide forms of the building blocks A, U, G, and C. The base sequence in DNA specifies the base sequence in RNA in this manner. As a consequence, DNA details have been transcribed to RNA. The building blocks, which are free ribonucleotides (A, U, C, and G), align and shape complementary RNA according to the base paring law, with A pairing with U (U in RNA replaces T in DNA), G pairing with C, and so on. As a consequence, the information encoded in the sequence of bases in DNA is transmitted to RNA.

Initiation

Proteins that make an RNA copy of a particular piece of DNA (transcription) must first be able to identify the start of the entity being copied. A promoter is a DNA sequence that various proteins, collectively referred to as the transcription machinery, bind to and begin transcription.

Promoters are located upstream (5′ to the coding region) of the genes they control in the vast majority of cases. The sequence of a promoter is critical because it determines whether the gene's coding portion is transcribed all of the time, half of the time, or only rarely. While promoters differ between organisms, a few sequence elements are frequently conserved. There are two promoter consensus sequences, or regions that are identical over several promoters and organisms, at the -10 and -35 regions upstream of the initiation site. Some proponents will have a sequence that is very similar to the consensus sequence (which includes the most typical sequence elements), and others will have a very different sequence. The intensity in which the transcriptional machinery can bind to the promoter to start transcription is impaired by these sequence variations. This allows you to keep track of how many transcripts you're making and how long you're making them.

Elongation

The template strand, one of the two strands of double-stranded DNA, is often used to initiate transcription. Except for uracil (U) in place of the thymine (T) present in DNA, the RNA product is complementary to the template strand and virtually identical to the non-template strand, known as the coding strand. RNA polymerase travels around the DNA template during elongation, attaching nucleotides by base-pairing with the DNA template in a manner identical to DNA replication, with the exception that the synthesized RNA strand does not stay attached to the DNA template. The DNA is constantly unwound ahead of the central enzyme and rewound behind it as elongation progresses. Note that the direction of synthesis is identical to that of synthesis in DNA–5′ to 3′.

Termination

If a gene has been transcribed, the bacterial polymerase must be ordered to detach from the DNA template and release the newly formed mRNA. There are two types of termination signals, based on the gene being transcribed. The first is protein-based, while the second is RNA-based. Rho-dependent termination is regulated by the rho protein, which follows the polymerase along the mRNA chain as it grows. The polymerase stalls at the end of the gene as it comes across a run of G nucleotides on the DNA template. As a result, the rho protein and the polymerase collide.

The mRNA is released from the transcription bubble as it interacts with rho. Relevant sequences in the DNA template strand regulate Rho-independent termination. As the polymerase reaches the end of the transcribed gene, it comes across an area rich in CG nucleotides. The complementary CG nucleotides bind together as the mRNA folds down on it. As a result, the polymerase forms a stable hairpin that causes it to stall as soon as it starts transcribing an area rich in AT nucleotides. The complementary UA region of the mRNA transcript interacts with the template DNA very weakly. This, together with the stalled polymerase, allows the central enzyme to break free and liberate the new mRNA transcript.

(c) Post-transcriptional Processing

RNA is transcribed, but before translation can begin, it must be translated into a mature form.

Post-transcriptional modification is the sorting that happens after an RNA molecule has been transcribed just before it is converted into a protein. This post-transcriptional level, like the epigenetic and transcriptional stages of processing, can be regulated to control gene expression in the cell. There will be no protein synthesized if the RNA is not processed, shuttled, or translated.

Alternative RNA splicing genes were discovered for the first time in the 1970s. When various combinations of introns and exons are deleted from the transcript, alternate RNA splicing causes different protein products to be produced from the same gene. The frequency of different splicing alternatives is regulated by the cell as a means to regulate the output of different protein products in different cells or at different stages of growth. This alternative splicing may be haphazard, but it is most commonly controlled and serves as a method of gene regulation. Alternative splicing is now accepted as a widespread method of gene control in eukaryotes; according to one estimation, alternative splicing is responsible for the expression of 70 percent of human genes as multiple proteins. After transcription, post-transcriptional regulation can occur at any level, including RNA splicing, nuclear shuttling, and RNA stability. After RNA has been transcribed, it must be converted into mature RNA that can be translated. Introns that do not code for protein are omitted in this process. To detach the introns and ligate the exons together, spliceosomes bind to the signals that mark the exon/intron boundary. When this happens, the RNA can be translated. The nucleus generates and splices RNA, so it must be transferred to the cytoplasm to be translated. RNA is transported to the cytoplasm through the nuclear pore complex. The period that RNA spends in the cytoplasm before being degraded, known as RNA stability, can be modified to regulate the total amount of protein synthesized. The RNA stability can be improved, resulting in a longer cytoplasmic residence time, or reduced, resulting in a shorter time and less protein synthesis. RNA-binding proteins (RBPs) and microRNAs regulate RNA stability (miRNAs). These RPBs and miRNAs bind to the RNA's 5′ or 3′ UTRs, increasing or declining RNA stability. Stability may be substantially increased or decreased depending on the RBP; however, miRNAs often decrease stability and encourage decay.

(d) Translation of Genetic Code

The cellular mechanism of transcription produces messenger RNA (mRNA), which is a handheld molecular replica of one or more genes with the letters A, C, G, and uracil in its alphabet (U). The mRNA prototype is converted into a protein product, translating nucleotide-based genetic information. Protein sequences are made up of 20 amino acids that are usually present, so the protein alphabet is made up of 20 characters. The triplet codon is a three-nucleotide sequence that distinguishes each amino acid. The genetic code is the association between a nucleotide codon and its accompanying amino acid. Given the different numbers of "letters" in the mRNA and protein "alphabets," combinations of nucleotides corresponded to single amino acids. Using a three-nucleotide code means that there is a total of 64 (4 × 4 × 4) possible combinations; therefore, a given amino acid is encoded by more than one nucleotide triplet. Three of the 64 codons interrupt protein synthesis and allow the polypeptide out of the translation apparatus. Stop codons are the term for these triplets. AUG, another codon, has a specific feature. It also acts as the start codon for translation, in addition to defining the amino acid methionine. The AUG start codon near the 5′ end of the mRNA sets the reading frame for translation. The genetic code is the same for everybody. With a few exceptions, almost all animals use the same genetic code for protein synthesis, providing convincing proof that all organisms on Earth evolved from a single source. Protein synthesis can be divided into three stages, analogous to mRNA synthesis: initiation, elongation, and termination. Prokaryotes and eukaryotes both go through the same translation process. Here, we'll look at how translating functions in *E. coli*, a model prokaryote, and discern between prokaryotic and eukaryotic translation.

Since the fundamentals of polypeptide elongation are the same in prokaryotes and eukaryotes, we'll look at it from the perspective of *E. coli*. It has large ribosomal subunit is classified into three compartments: The A site is responsible for binding incoming charged t-RNAs (t-RNAs with their attached specific amino acids). Charged t-RNAs carrying amino acids that have formed bonds with the increasing polypeptide chain but have not yet dissociated from their corresponding t-RNA are bound by the P location. The E site dissociates t-RNAs, allowing them to be recharged with free amino acids.

The ribosome catalyzes each of the three processes by transferring one codon at a time. Each step adds a charged t-RNA to the complex, lengthens the polypeptide by one amino acid, and eliminates an uncharged t-RNA. GTP, a molecule similar to ATP, supplies the energy for each bond between amino acids. The *E. coli* translation apparatus adds each amino acid in less than 0.05 seconds, suggesting that a 200-amino-acid polypeptide could be converted in less than 10 seconds. When a stop codon (UAA, UAG, or UGA) is found, translation is terminated. The growing polypeptide is released and the ribosome subunits dissociate as the ribosome encounters the stop codon. The fundamental dogma explains how genetic material travels from genes to mRNA to proteins in the cell. The method of transcription is used to create mRNA, and the process of translation is used to synthesize proteins. The genetic code is the three-nucleotide mRNA codon of an amino acid correspondence. The t-RNA molecules "translate" the genetic code by associating a particular codon with a specific amino acid. Since 64 triplet codons in mRNA specify just 20 amino acids and three stop codons, the genetic code is degenerate. This implies that each amino acid is represented by several codons. Almost all of the world's animals have the same genetic code. Bonds are generated between consecutive amino acids specified by the mRNA template in conjunction with the genetic code. The ribosome recognizes charged t-RNAs and catalyzes bonding between the new amino acid and the growing polypeptide's end as it passes down the mRNA.

(e) Regulation of Gene Expression and Protein Synthesis Inhibitors of Protein Synthesis

Gene expression is the mechanism of using a gene to generate a protein. It involves the processes of DNA transcription and mRNA translation in protein synthesis. It may also require extra protein processing after synthesis. Gene expression is regulated to ensure that the right proteins are generated at the right time and in the right place. From the start of the transcription step of protein synthesis to the production of a protein after synthesis, regulation can occur at any point in the expression of a gene. This term focuses on the regulation of transcription, which is one of the most complex forms of gene regulation in eukaryotic cells.

Regulating proteins or transcription factors regulate transcription. These proteins bind to regulatory factor or promoter regions of DNA, which are found near promoters. The promoter is the section of a gene where RNA polymerase binds to commence mRNA transcription from DNA. Regulatory proteins may interact with RNA polymerase after binding to regulatory elements. The bulk of regulatory proteins are either activators or repressors. Activators are regulatory proteins that enable RNA polymerase to interact with the promoter to facilitate transcription. Enhancers are long strings of DNA that can loop back and interact with the promoter of a gene to increase transcription.

In the early stages of an organism's development, gene expression control is crucial. To grow natural organs and organ systems, regulatory proteins must turn on specific genes in specific cells at precisely the right time. A broad number of genes known as homeobox genes control growth during the embryonic period. There are an estimated 235 activated homeobox genes in humans. They can be found on any chromosome and are commonly found in groups. Homeobox genes contain instructions for shaping homeodomains, which are 60-amino-acid chains. Homeodomain-containing proteins function as transcription factors, binding to and regulating the activity of other genes. The homeodomain is the portion of the protein that binds to and regulates the expression of the target gene. Homeobox genes, which code for amino acid chains are known as homeodomains, are key regulators of growth. Mutations of genes that regulate the cell cycle affect certain forms of cancer. Tumor-suppressor genes and proto-oncogenes are two groups of regulatory genes where cancer-causing mutations are most common.

(f) DNA Repair Mechanisms

DNA in living cells is subject to many chemical modifications (a fact that is often ignored in the excitement of being able to sequence DNA on dried and/or frozen specimens). Some chemical modifications must be reversed if the genetic material contained in DNA is to remain uncorrupted. A failure to repair DNA produces a mutation.

There are several mechanisms of DNA repair

- ☆ Direct chemical reversal of the damage.
- ☆ Excision Repair, in which the damaged base or bases are removed and then replaced with the correct ones in a localized burst of DNA synthesis. There are three modes of excision repair, each of which employs specialized sets of enzymes.
    1. Base Excision Repair (BER)
    2. Nucleotide Excision Repair (NER)
    3. Mismatch Repair (MMR)

Direct Reversal of Base Damage

The random addition of a methyl group (CH3-) (an example of alkylation) to Cs accompanied by deamination to a T is perhaps the most common cause of point mutations in humans. Fortunately, enzymes called glycosylases to restore the bulk of these modifications by eliminating the mismatched T and restoring the right C. This is achieved without breaking the DNA backbone. Removal of the weakened base by a DNA glycosylase (estimated to occur 20,000 times per day in each cell in our body). There are at least eight genes that code for different DNA glycosylases, each of which is responsible for detecting and extracting a particular form of base damage. The deoxyribose phosphate in the backbone is eliminated, resulting in a void. In cells where genes are actively transcribed on the DNA strand that acts as the basis for transcription, nucleotide-excision repair happens most easily. Mismatch repair is concerned with fixing usual basis mismatches, or errors to preserve Watson-Crick base pairing (A•T, C•G). It may use enzymes that are active in both base-excision repair (BER) and nucleotide-excision repair (NER), as well as enzymes that are specially designed for this reason.

(g) Applied Aspects of Purine and Pyrimidine Metabolism

An antimetabolite is a compound that prohibits the use of a metabolite, which is a chemical that exists naturally in the body. Antifolates, which interfere with the use of folic acid, have a composition that is identical to that of the metabolite they interfere with. Antimetabolites may have harmful effects on cells, such as reducing or preventing cell growth or division. Antibiotics are made from antimetabolites. Antimetabolite antibiotics are classified into three groups. The first is that antifolates interact with folic acid's function, causing DNA and RNA output to be interrupted. Methotrexate, for example, is a folic acid analog that binds to and inhibits the enzyme dihydrofolate reductase, preventing the production of tetrahydrofolate, due to its structural resemblance to folic acid. Tetrahydrofolate deficiency can cause DNA, RNA, and protein production to be inhibited because it is necessary for purine and pyrimidine synthesis. Pyrimidine analogs, which resemble the structure of metabolic pyrimidines, are the second category of antimetabolite antibiotics. Cytosine (C), thymine (T), and uracil (U), three nucleobases present in nucleic acids, are pyrimidine derivatives, and pyrimidine analogs interrupt their production, blocking DNA and RNA synthesis. Purine analogues are the third category of antimetabolite antibiotics, and they resemble metabolic purines in structure. Adenine and guanine, two of the four bases of nucleic acids, are purines.

Purine analogues inhibit the development of nucleic acids. Azathioprine, for example, is the most frequently used immunosuppressive cytotoxic agent in transplants to regulate rejection reactions by inhibiting DNA synthesis in lymphocytes.

(h) Genetic Engineering: Recombinant DNA Technology

Biotechnology is the study of using living systems to support humans. Domestication of plants and animals by farming and breeding practices is scientifically a form of biotechnology. In today's world, though, we equate biotechnology with the overt modification of an organism's genetics to produce desired characteristics through the process of genetic engineering. Recombinant DNA technology, in which a DNA genome is manipulated in vitro to produce recombinant DNA molecules with new variations of genetic material, is used in genetic engineering. After that, the recombinant DNA is inserted into a host organism.

The bacterial strain that produces human insulin is an example of a transgenic microorganism. The human insulin gene was incorporated into a plasmid. The bacteria were then inoculated with the recombinant DNA plasmid. This transgenic microbe will now generate and secrete human insulin as a result. By "mating" with other cells (conjugation), viral infection (transduction), and sucking up DNA from the environment, certain prokaryotes can absorb foreign DNA and integrate usable genes into their genome (transformation). Note that horizontal gene transfer happens as genetic material is passed between cells of the same age. DNA molecules are manipulated using naturally occurring enzymes obtained predominantly from bacteria and viruses in recombinant DNA technology. The use of naturally occurring restriction endonucleases (restriction enzymes), bacterial enzymes developed as a defense mechanism to cut and break foreign cytoplasmic DNA, which is most commonly a product of bacteriophage infection, allows for the development of recombinant DNA molecules. In their 1960s studies on how E. coli limits bacteriophage replication during infection, Stewart Linn and Werner Arber discovered restriction enzymes. A palindrome is a letter series that reads the same in both directions. (For example, the word "stage" is a palindrome.)

Palindromic DNA sequences have the same base sequences on one strand as they do on the complementary strand in the 5 to 3 direction. When a restriction enzyme recognizes a DNA palindrome, it cuts each backbone in the palindrome at the same place. Such restriction enzymes cut to create molecules with complementary overhangs (sticky ends), while others cut to produce blunt ends without any overhangs.

At their sticky ends, molecules with complementary sticky ends will quickly anneal, or form hydrogen bonds between complementary bases. The single-stranded overhangs may be hybridized during the annealing process. The joining of two complementary single strands of DNA is referred to as hybridization. Blunt ends may still bind to each other, but not as well as sticky ends due to the lack of complementary overhangs to help the process. In any case, DNA ligase may use covalent bonding to connect the two sugar-phosphate backbones of the molecule, resulting in a continuous double strand.

(i) DNA and Diagnostics

The letters "DNA" has come to stand for crime-solving, paternity tests, human identity, and genetic testing. Skin, blood, and saliva can all be used to remove DNA. Each person's DNA is distinct, and these identifying characteristics can be used to identify variations between individuals within a species. Beyond forensics, DNA analysis has a wide variety of uses. In humans, DNA testing is used for several purposes, including paternity assessment, genealogy analysis, pathogen detection, and archaeological research, disease outbreak monitoring, and researching human migration patterns. DNA is used in diagnostics, vaccine production, and cancer treatment in medicine. Each human cell has 23 chromosome pairs, with one set inherited from the mother and the other from the parent. A mitochondrial genome, which is inherited solely from the mother and can play a role in inherited genetic diseases, is also present.

(j) DNA Repair Mechanisms and Related Disorders

Diseases, syndromes, and other diseases caused by mutations in one or more genes or chromosomal abnormalities are known as genetic disorders. Genetic diseases are most often found at birth, although they should not be confused with congenital disorders, which are all conditions present at birth, regardless of cause. Genetic mutations or chromosomal variations do not affect all congenital conditions. Rather, they are triggered by complications that occur during embryonic or fetal development, as well as during the birthing period. Fetal alcohol syndrome is an example of a nongenetic congenital condition. A genetic defect caused by a mutation may be passed on over the years. As a result, people who have a genetic disease in their families may be worried about raising children with it. A genetic counselor will assist them in assessing the probability that their children will be affected. If they want to have infants, they will be recommended to undergo prenatally ("before birth") tests to assess if the fetus has any genetic defects. Amniocentesis is one form of pregnancy examination. The fetal chromosomes are analyzed after a few fetal cells are removed from the fluid containing the fetus in utero. This approach can be used to identify Down syndrome and other chromosomal anomalies.

Symptoms of genetic defects may be treated or avoided in some cases. The amino acid phenylalanine, for example, builds up to unsafe levels in the body in the genetic disease phenylketonuria (PKU). PKU is caused by a mutation in a gene that usually codes for a phenylalanine-degrading enzyme. When a person with PKU eats phenylalanine-rich foods (which include many high-protein foods), PKU can build up and cause severe health problems. The accumulation of phenylalanine in babies and young children will lead to intellectual disability, delayed growth, and other serious issues.

(k) Telomers, Telomerases

Telomeres are essential, and their steady shrinking with each mitosis could result in cells having a finite life span. In truth, this is the case. When regular (non-cancerous) cells are cultured, they do not expand forever. Cells taken from a premature baby and grown in culture can multiply almost 100 times. However, their rate of mitosis continues to decrease long before the end (to less than once every two weeks). If my cells (I am 81 years old) were cultured, they would only be able to complete a few hundred mitoses until they started dividing and died out. Replicative senescence is the name for this phenomenon. Telomerase is a DNA strand-modifying enzyme that attaches telomere repeat sequences to the 3′ end. DNA polymerase can complete the synthesis of the "incomplete ends" of the opposite strand by lengthening this strand. Telomerase is a ribonucleoprotein that controls telomere lifespan. Its single snoRNA molecule, TERC ("Telomere RNA Component"), serves as a CCAAUC template for the insertion of GGTTAG in mammals. The catalytic activity is given by TERT ("Telomere Reverse Transcriptase"), a protein part.

(l) Inhibitors of DNA Replication, Apoptosis

A cell will die either deliberately (referred to as apoptosis or programmed cell death), or accidentally (referred to as "cellular suicide") (necrosis). The microscopic examination of these two systems indicates that they use very different mechanisms. As the cytoskeleton is degraded during apoptosis, the cell starts to shrink and lose structure, and the organelles, except the nucleus, start to bundle together. The chromatin condenses within the nucleus and binds to the nuclear envelope, which then loses its cohesion and continues to disintegrate. The cell membrane starts to exhibit abnormalities, which are referred to as blebs, and the cell gradually breaks up into vesicles, which are conveniently washed up by phagocytes attracted to the site by apoptotic signals released by the dying cell. Necrosis, on the other hand, is a total tragedy. The cell starts to expand, and the integrity of the plasma membrane continues to deteriorate. It starts to leak cytoplasm and leaves behind cell waste, which can collect and cause necrotic death in surrounding cells. A cascade of caspases, a class of proteolytic enzymes, is essentially responsible for activating apoptosis. The caspase family of enzymes is normally made up of proenzymes that are activated by other caspase members. After the initial trigger activates one group of caspases, they will cleave a number of proteins, including procaspases, which will then activate and hydrolyze many more proteins, including even another form of procaspase, and so on. Of necessity, other enzymes are activated as well, and they contribute to the reaction by stimulating other proteases and apoptotic enzymes. The apoptotic cascade is normally activated by one of two pathways: an internal stimulus, which is initiated by binding an extracellular signal molecule to activate a "death receptor," or an external trigger, which is initiated by binding an extracellular signal molecule to activate a "death receptor." While both stimuli have several differences, they follow identical pathways to the ones we'll use here.

REFERENCES

1. Brunstein J. DNA and RNA structure: nucleic acids as genetic material. MLO Med Lab Obs. 2013 Jan;45(1): 26, 28.
2. Durland J, Ahmadian-Moghadam H. Genetics, Mutagenesis. 2020 Sep 20. In: StatPearls [Internet.Treasure Island (FL): StatPearls Publishing; 2021 Jan–. PMID: 32809354.

3. Chatterjee S, Pathmasiri W, Plashkevych O, Honcharenko D, Varghese OP, Maiti M, Chattopadhyaya J. The chemical nature of the 2′-substituent in the pentose-sugar dictates the pseudoaromatic character of the nucleobase (pKa) in DNA/RNA. Org Biomol Chem. 2006 May 7;4(9): 1675-86.
4. Kim S. Structure of the DNA double helix. Preface. Top Curr Chem. 2014;344: v-viii. PMID: 25013884.
5. Ekundayo B, Bleichert F. Origins of DNA replication. PLoS Genet. 2019 Sep 12;15(9): e1008320.
6. Mercadante AA, Dimri M, Mohiuddin SS. Biochemistry, Replication and Transcription. 2020 Aug 28. In: StatPearls [Internet. Treasure Island (FL): StatPearls Publishing; 2021 Jan–. PMID: 30986011.
7. Bhattacharyya S, Go MF, Dunn BE, Phadnis SH. Transcription and Translation. In: Mobley HLT, Mendz GL, Hazell SL, editors. Helicobacter pylori: Physiology and Genetics. Washington (DC): ASM Press; 2001. Chapter 26. PMID: 21290729.
8. Dalhus B, Laerdahl JK, Backe PH, Bjorås M. DNA base repair—recognition and initiation of catalysis. FEMS Microbiol Rev. 2009 Nov;33(6): 1044-78.
9. Lanigan TM, Kopera HC, Saunders TL. Principles of Genetic Engineering. Genes (Basel). 2020 Mar 10;11(3): 291.
10. Miglani M, Rain M, Pasha Q, Raj VS, Thinlas T, Mohammad G, Gupta A, Pandey RP, Vibhuti A. Shorter telomere length, higher telomerase activity in association with tankyrase gene polymorphism contribute to high-altitude pulmonary edema. Hum Mol Genet. 2020 Nov 4;29(18): 3094-3106.

Chapter 6

Plant Physiology

Sangeeta Kumari

Amity Institute of Biotechnology, Amity University Haryana, Gurugram (Manesar) – 122 413, Haryana, India
e-mail skumari@ggn.amity.edu

ABSTRACT

Plant physiology is the first and most important way for plants to communicate with their surroundings and climate. A variety of cellular processes are involved in the control and regulation of physiological growth. The most important abiotic factors for plants are light, carbon dioxide, water, temperature, nutrients, and salinity biotic factors. Their actions are interrelated in a functional network involving all major processes of plant physiology in the ecological performance of plants. Plant physiology is the study of how plants function on a physiological level. It is a descriptive analysis of plant variation and structure at the molecular and cellular level that leads to ecological, physiological, and biochemistry-related aspects of plant exploration (Figure 6.1).

Keywords: *Plant physiology, Water movement, Translocation, Light and dark reactions, Respiration, Plant growth regulators, Plant defence mechanism, Photoperiodism, Vernalization.*

Introduction

In plant physiology, natural phenomena operating in the living plants and plant parts are studied. It is a discipline of botany where the structure of the cell, tissues and organs is associated with processes and functions. The different responses of organisms to environmental alternations and the resultant growth and development which are the outcome of such responses are also studied in plant physiology.

A process comprises a series of sequential events operating under natural conditions. Some of the most important processes operating in plants are stomatal

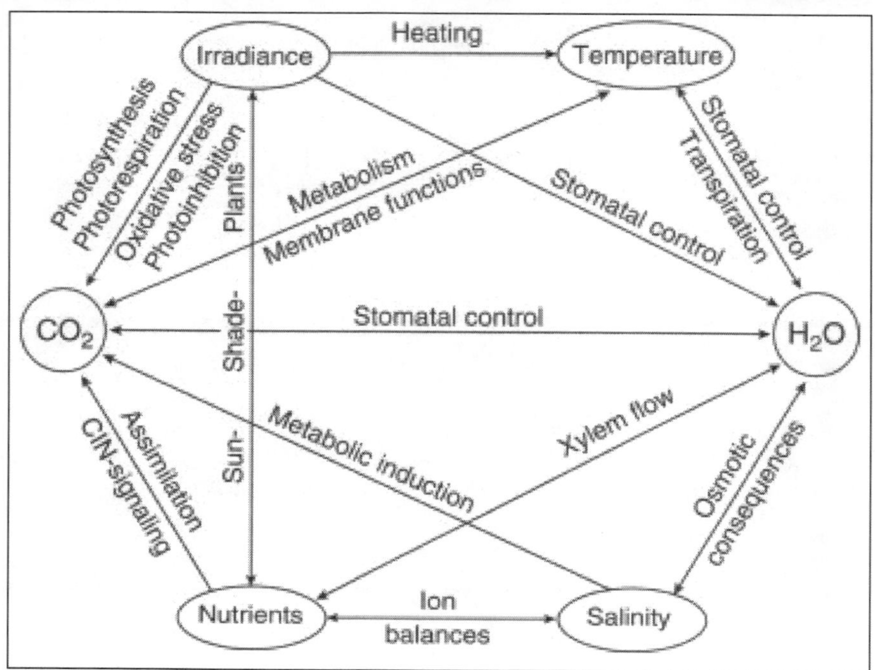

Figure 6.1: Function of Plant Physiology.
(Image Credit: Plant Physiology, U. Lüttge, in Encyclopedia of Ecology, 2008).

mechanism; water and mineral absorption; photosynthesis, respiration, *etc.* A plant physiologist tends to understand, describe and explain such processes.

The natural activity of the cells, tissues, organs and organisms is referred to as their function. A plant physiologist must understand, describe and explain these functions as well. These functions are explained at the cellular and molecular levels. In plant physiology, an attempt is also made to study the factors which modify growth and development.

In other words, a plant physiologist must understand and explain how external stimuli and factors modify plant responses. In brief, in plant physiology, comprehensive information on the structure, processes and functions operative at the cells, tissues, organs are desired in order to explain the processes of growth and development in an organism.

These days, a plant physiologist must have a sound knowledge of chemistry, biochemistry, physics, statistics and plant molecular biology. In fact, these sciences have contributed immensely in elucidating the functional and structural aspects of plants.

Plant physiology is evidently not a static discipline, and it will always change and be enriched by the discovery including the use of new methodologies and tools. This is also a reason why differential views exist with one process. The observations depend on the methods used, while the perspectives depend on the understanding of divergent chemical and physical phenomena.

Water Relation

The Spectrum of Soil, Plants, and Environment

The regulation of water movement through the soil, through roots, through the plant, and out into the air as a set of closely interrelated processes is an important contribution to plant water relations.The soil–plant–atmosphere continuum (SPAC) (Philip, 1966) is a useful term for stressing the importance of considering all aspects of water.

Water movement through soil, roots, stems, and leaves, as well as its evaporation into the air, can be studied in terms of the driving forces and resistances operating in each section, different plant and environmental influences water movement by affecting either the driving or the controlling factors.

Mostly plant absorb water from the soil and less than 2 per cent of all the water is available for the plant called chesard. Majority of water enter into water table but during percolation soil particles hold some water called capillary water. Root hair present in the absorption zone. The water enters the root hair by osmosis. The osmotic pressure of soil is always less than 1 atmosphere where as the osmotic pressure of cell-sap of root hairs is about 2.5 atmosphere or more.

The Diffusion Pressure created by diffusing molecules from one area of its greatest concentration to the lesser concentration. Pure water has maximum diffusion pressure. Diffusion pressure deficit is the reduction of diffusion pressure of the substance over its pure state due to the bonding of its molecule or pressure of other particles. DPD initially equivalent to its osmotic pressure. When cell under osmosis it increases its turgor, pressure forces the cytoplasm against the cell wall also exerts equal and opposite pressure called wall pressure.

Relationship expressed as

DPD (WATER POTENTIAL) *psi* = OP-TP

Water moves from region of high-water potential to one of low water potential, further addition of solutes causes lowering of water potential. Pure water at atmospheric pressure has zero water potential. Addition of solutes cause lowering of water potential.

Incipient plasmolysis condition in the plant cell in which the cell wall has reached its limit of contraction but protoplasm has not yet receded from the wall called incipient plasmolysis. In the point where the cell-sap attains smallest volume but keeps the protoplasm in contact with cell wall. At the point of incipient plasmolysis, the wall pressure and turgor pressure of the cell stands zero.

Ascent of Sap

The upward movement of water from base to top of the tree through mostly xylem. Godlewski(1884) proposed the vital theory of " relay pump hypothesis" according to which the pumping activity of the cells of wood parenchyma and medullary ray are responsible for ascent of sap. JC Bose (1923) Pulsation Theory.

He suggested that ascent of sap due pulsatory activity of inner most cell. Dixon and Jolly widely accepted theory transpiration pull/cohesion and adhesion theory. The magnitude of cohesion force of water molecules ranges upto 350 atmosphere. It is much in excess of the minimum required 20 atm in a tallest tree as 1 atm. Osmotic pressure can result in water upto 10 meters.

Transpiration

Its vital physiological process, there are three types of transpiration occur: cuticular (3 per cent),lenticular (.1 per cent), and stomatal (97 per cent).

The opening of stomata during day time occurs because the guard cells photosynthesize and produce osmotically active sugars. The osmotic value of guard cell sap greater than the other epidermal cells and it is highest when stomata are open is lowest when stomata is closed.

Significant Water-Translocation Theories

The following are the theories: 1. Capillarity 2. Root Tension 1. Theory of Cohesion.

Capillarity

Capillarity is a principle that allows water to move from one place to another.

The adhesion between water molecules and the tube wall through which the process is taking place causes such an increase in water in narrow tubes. Water appears to crawl up the side of the container due to this adhesion, which forms a meniscus. As the water flows upward along the wall, strong cohesive forces between water molecules begin to function and pull the water upward. This upward pull of water continues until the forces of adhesion and cohesion are balanced by downward force of gravity.

Root Tension

While root pressure produced in the xylem of the roots can lift water to a certain height, it does not appear to be a useful force in the ascent of sap for the following reasons:

1. Root pressure is relatively low in magnitude (about 2 bars).
2. Sap ascent continues even when there is no root tension.
3. Roots absorb mineral ions from the soil and deposit them in the xylem vessels. The lowering of osmotic potential is caused by the accumulation of ions in vessels.
4. In temperate regions, where transpiration is rapid during the summer, root pressures are normally negligible.

Cohesion and Adhesion

The presence of H-bonds between water molecules keeps them linked. While the H-bond is weak, when they are present in large quantities, as they are in water, a very strong reciprocal force of attraction or cohesive force forms between water molecules, causing them to stay in the xylem in the form of a continuous water column. Since the magnitude of this force is so great (around 350 atm or bars), the xylem's continuous water column cannot be easily broken by gravity or any other means of resistance. Evaporation of water from the leaf to the atmosphere, according to this theory, causes a decrease in the water potential of epidermal cells in direct contact with the atmosphere. Water from neighbouring cells replaces water lost by epidermal cells along a water potential gradient. Water passing from xylem elements in leaf veins replaces the water lost by leaf cells (*i.e.*, xylem elements). A tension is formed in the water in the xylem elements of the leaves as a result of this pattern of water movement. Ligno-cellulose, which makes up the walls of xylem vessels, has a high affinity for water molecules. Since the water potential of root cells is smaller than that of soil, water moves from the soil to the roots. Water uplift is also known as transpiration pull.

Translocation

Translocation mostly occur through phloem particularly through sieve tubes,in contrast to the unidirectional movement of water through xylem vessels, whereas translocation of food occurs both in directions *e.g.*, from leaves to roots downwardly and from roots to growing tips upwardly.

Diffusion, activated diffusion, protoplasmic streaming, interfacial flow, electro-osmosis, transcellular threads, contractile proteins, and mass flow are among the theories proposed to understand the mechanism of organic nutrient translocation through the phloem. The most critical are as follows:

De Vries (1885) proposed the Cytoplasmic Streaming Hypothesis, which Curtis later expanded on (1929-35). The transport is thought to occur by a combination of two forces, diffusion and cytoplasmic streaming, according to the hypothesis. Chemical solvents or food materials are carried by cytoplasmic streaming from one end of a sieve tube cell to the other, where they disperse according to their concentration. The theory explains how substances can move in both directions within the same sieve element. The hypothesis has many flaws: I the rate of cytoplasmic streaming is too slow to account for phloem transport (5 cm/hr vs. 50-150 cm/hr for phloem transport); (ii) the rate of cytoplasmic streaming is too slow to account for phloem transport; and (iii) the rate of cytoplasmic streaming is too slow to account for phloem.

Thaine proposed a theory called the Transcellular Streaming Hypothesis (1962, 1969). Sieve tubes are thought to have tubular threads that run from one tube cell to the next through sieve pores. Tubular or transcellular strands travel in a peristaltic motion that aids the passage of organic substances. The transcellular fibres, on the other hand, have not been observed in the sieve tube.

Munch made the suggestion (1927,1930) according to that the o rganic substances in a mass flow transfer from a region of high osmotic pressure to a region of low osmotic pressure, according to this theory, as a turgor pressure gradient develops. Two interconnected osmometers, one with a high solute concentration and the other with a low osmotic concentration, can be used to demonstrate thisexperiment. The apparatus' two osmometers are submerged in water. In comparison to the other, more water reaches the osmometer with high solute concentration. As a result, it will develop a high turgor strain, forcing the solution to flow into the second osmometer in a mass flow. The mass flow may be increased if the solutes are replenished in the donor osmometer and immobilised in the recipient osmometer. The sieve tube device is perfectly suited to solute mass movement. Due to the lack of tonoplast, the vacuoles are completely permeable. The source or supply area, such as mesophyll cells, has a constant high osmotic concentration (due to photosynthesis).

An active process passes the organic substances present in them into the sieve tubes through their companion cells. As a result, a high osmotic concentration forms in the source's sieve tubes. The sieve tubes collect water from the xylem around them and build up a lot of turgor strain. It allows the organic solution to flow towards the low turgor pressure field. The turgor pressure is mild.

Photosynthesis

Photosynthesis is the conversion of solar energy into chemical energy by plants, algae, and some bacteria. We'll go through the fundamentals of photosynthesis and how scientists are using what they've learned to grow sustainable fuels and renewable energy sources.

Photosynthesis Classifications

Photosynthetic processes can be divided into two categories: oxygenic and anoxygenic. Although the basic concepts of anoxygenic and oxygenic photosynthesis are somewhat similar, plants, algae, and cyanobacteria use oxygenic photosynthesis.

Light energy moves electrons from water (H_2O) to carbon dioxide (CO_2) during oxygenic photosynthesis, resulting in the production of carbohydrates. The CO_2 is "reduced," or receives electrons, while the water is "oxidised," or loses electrons, during this transfer. Finally, oxygen and carbohydrates are generated.

Oxidative photosynthesis serves as a counterbalance to respiration by removing carbon dioxide released by all breathing organisms and reintroducing oxygen to the atmosphere. Anoxygenic photosynthesis, on the other hand, does not use water as an electron donor. Purple bacteria and green sulphur bacteria, which are found in a variety of aquatic environments, are the most common bacteria that undergo this process.Despite the fact that both forms of photosynthesis are multistep processes, the overall process can be neatly summarised as a chemical equation.

The following is a formula for oxygenic photosynthesis:

$$6CO_2 + 12H_2O + \text{Light Energy} \rightarrow C_6H_{12}O_6 + 6O_2 + 6H_2O$$

Using light energy, six carbon dioxide (CO_2) molecules combine with 12 water (H_2O) molecules. The end result is a single carbohydrate molecule ($C_6H_{12}O_6$, or glucose), as well as six breathable oxygen and water molecules each.

Similarly, the various anoxygenic photosynthesis reactions can be represented as a single generalized formula:

$$CO_2 + 2H_2A + \text{Light Energy} \rightarrow [CH_2O] + 2A + H_2O$$

In the equation, the letter A stands for a variable, and H2A stands for a potential electron donor.

The Photosynthetic System

The following are photosynthesis-critical cellular components.Pigments are molecules that give plants, algae, and bacteria colour while also effectively trapping sunlight. Different colours absorb light at different wavelengths. The three key classes are mentioned below.

Chlorophylls are green pigments that can absorb blue and red light. Chlorophylls are classified into three types: chlorophyll a, chlorophyll b, and chlorophyll c. Chlorophyll an is present in all photosynthesizing plants, according to Eugene Rabinowitch and Govindjee in their book "Photosynthesis" (Wiley, 1969). This pigment is mainly seen in purple and green bacteria, which perform anoxygenic photosynthesis. Carotenoids are pigments that are red, orange, or yellow in colour and absorb bluish-green light. Carotenoids include xanthophyll (yellow) and carotene (orange), which are responsible for the colour of carrots.

Phycobilins: These red or blue pigments absorb light wavelengths that chlorophylls and carotenoids do not. Cyanobacteria and red algae all contain them.

Plastids typically contain pigments or have the ability to store nutrients. According to Geoffrey Cooper's book "The Cell: A Molecular Approach," colourless and nonpigmented leucoplasts store fats and starch, chromoplasts produce carotenoids, and chloroplasts contain chlorophyll (Sinauer *et al.*, 2000).

The grana and stroma regions of the chloroplasts are where photosynthesis takes place. The grana is the organelle's innermost part, consisting of a series of disc-shaped membranes stacked like plates in columns. Specific discs are referred to as thylakoids. The movement of electrons takes place right here. The stroma is made up of the empty spaces between grana columns.

Chloroplasts, like mitochondria, the cells' energy centres, have their own genome, or array of genes, found within circular DNA. These genes code for proteins that are needed for the organelle's function as well as photosynthesis. Chloroplasts, like mitochondria, are thought to have evolved from primitive bacterial cells through endosymbiosis.

Antennae are antennas that are used to transmit information.

Pigment molecules are linked to proteins, allowing them to travel freely toward light and toward one another. According to an article by Wim Vermaas, a professor at Arizona State University, "antennae" are a wide array of 100 to 5,000 pigment molecules. These structures effectively absorb photons, which are the sun's light energy.

Light energy must eventually be passed to a pigment-protein complex capable of converting it to chemical energy in the form of electrons. Light energy is passed to chlorophyll pigments in plants, for example. When a chlorophyll pigment expels an electron, the energy is converted to chemical energy, which can then be transferred to another recipient.

Centre of Reaction

Reaction centres are pigments and proteins that convert light energy to chemical energy and initiate the electron transfer process.

The photosynthetic process is a biological process that takes place in the presence of sunlight

Plant photosynthesis reactions are classified as either requiring or not requiring sunlight. Light-dependent reactions in the thylakoid and light-independent reactions in the stroma take place in chloroplasts. Light-dependent reactions (also known as light reactions) occur when a photon of light strikes the reaction core, releasing an electron from a pigment molecule such as chlorophyll.

The released electron travels through an electron transport chain, generating the energy required to produce ATP (adenosine triphosphate, a chemical energy source for cells) and NADPH. A water electron is used to fill the "electron hole" in the original chlorophyll pigment. Oxygen is emitted into the environment as a result of this process. The Calvin cycle is made up of light-independent reactions (also known as dark reactions): The rich energy sources that drive dark reactions are ATP and NADPH, which are generated by light reactions. The Calvin cycle is made up of three chemical reaction steps: carbon fixation, reduction, and regeneration. Water and catalysts are used in these reactions. When carbon dioxide atoms are constructed, they are "fixed."

Photosynthesis Process

In terrestrial–land–ecosystems, plants are the most prevalent autotrophs. While all green plant tissues can photosynthesize, photosynthesis takes place primarily in the leaves in most plants. The primary site of photosynthesis is the mesophyll, which is a layer of cells in the middle layer of leaf tissue. Chloroplasts are specialised organelles found in mesophyll cells that carry out photosynthesis reactions. Most plants have small pores on the surface of their leaves called stomata–singular, stoma.

Thylakoids, disc-like structures found inside chloroplasts, are organised in grana–singular, granum–piles that look like stacks of pancakes. Chlorophylls, which are green pigments that absorb light, are found in the membrane of each thylakoid.

The Calvin Cycle and Light-Dependent Reactions

Many steps are involved in photosynthesis in plant leaves, but they can be divided into two stages: light-dependent reactions and the Calvin cycle.

Light-dependent reactions occur in the thylakoid membrane and necessitate a constant supply of light energy. Chlorophylls absorb light energy, which is then converted into chemical energy by the creation of two compounds. ATP an energy storage molecule–and NADPH a reduced (electron-bearing) electron carrier. Water molecules are converted to oxygen gas, which is what we breathe, during this process.

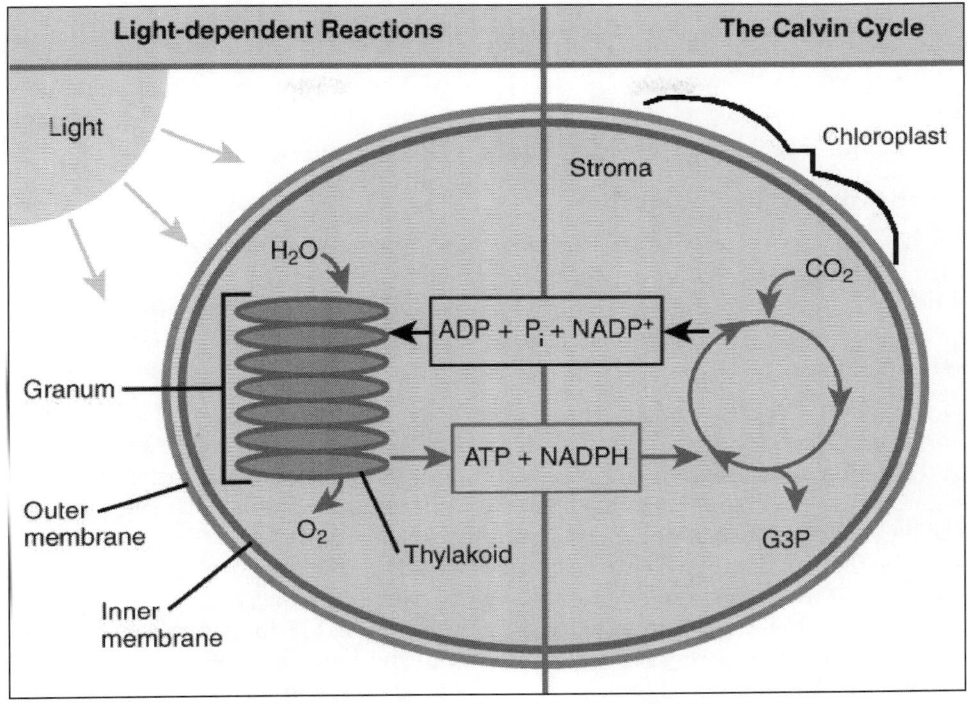

Figure 6.2: Image credit: Modified from "Overview of photosynthesis: Figure 6" by OpenStax College, Biology.

Photophosphorylation (Light Dependent Reaction)

The method of transferring energy from a light-excited electron into the pyrophosphate bond of an ADP molecule is known as photophosphorylation. As light excites the electrons in water in the presence of P680, this happens. The energy transfer resembles the chemiosmotic electron transport that takes place in the mitochondria. A molecule of P680 that is part of Photosystem II loses an electron when it is exposed to light energy. The P680 requires an electron, which is obtained from a water molecule, resulting in the formation of H^+ and O-2 ions. The diatomic O_2 that is produced is made up of these O-2 ions. The electron is "boosted" to a higher energy state and bound to a primary electron acceptor, kicking off a sequence of reactions. As light strikes a P700 molecule in Photosystem I, an electron is "boosted" to a higher potential. A separate primary electron acceptor is attached to the electron (that is a different molecule from the one associated with Photosystem II). After passing through a series of redox reactions, the electron is bound to $NADP^+$ and H^+ to form NADPH, an energy carrier. As a result, electrons from water flow continuously to NADPH. Carbon Fixation uses this electricity. Some eukaryotes and primitive photosynthetic bacteria have cyclic electron flow. Only ATP is made, no NADPH. This happens when cells need more ATP or when there isn't enough $NADP^+$ to convert to NADPH. Electron gradients formed in the thylakoid membrane drive the pumping of H ions into the thylakoid and the conversion of ADP + P into ATP in Photosystem II.

This produces electrons, which power an ADP-ATP pump, which generates ATP from sunlight without the use of chlorophyll. This lends credence to the idea that chemiosmotic processes can produce ATP in any environment.

Light Independent Reaction

The Calvin cycle, also known as light-independent reactions, occurs in the stroma and does not involve light directly. Instead, light-dependent reactions produce Calvin ATP and NADPH, which fix carbon dioxide and produce three-carbon sugars (glyceraldehyde-3-phosphate, or G3P) molecules, which combine to form glucose.

The light-dependent reactions, in general, absorb light energy and temporarily store it in chemical forms ATP and NADPH. ATP broken down to release energy and NADPH donates electrons to the process of converting carbon dioxide molecules into sugars in the end, the energy that began as light becomes stuck in the sugar bonds. The light-dependent reactions, in general, absorb light energy and temporarily store it in chemical forms. Photosynthesis and cellular respiration are almost opposite processes at the stage of overall reactions. As seen in the diagram below, the only difference is the type of energy consumed or released. Photosynthesis isn't just cellular respiration in reverse at the stage of individual steps. Photosynthesis, on the other hand, follows its own set of steps, as we'll see in the rest of this section. Photosynthesis and cellular respiration, on the other hand, have several striking similarities. Photosynthesis and cellular respiration, for example, both require a sequence of redox reactions (reactions involving electron transfers). Electrons flow from glucose to oxygen in cellular respiration, forming water and releasing energy. They go in the opposite direction in photosynthesis, beginning with water and ending with glucose–an energy-intensive process driven by light. Photosynthesis, like cellular respiration, uses an electron transport chain to produce a product. By chemiosmosis, a concentration gradient causes ATP to begin synthesis.

Dark Reaction

The molecule ribulose biphosphate absorbs carbon dioxide (RuBP). RuBP is a chemical that has five carbon atoms in it. The Calvin Cycle takes six molecules of carbon dioxide and produces one molecule of glucose in the end. Melvin Calvin determined the reactions involved in this process.

Phosphoglycerate (PGA), a 3-carbon compound, is the Calvin Cycle's first stable product. The photosystems' energy is used to bind phosphates to (phosphorylate) the PGA using ATP and NADPH energy carriers. Two of the 12 molecules of glyceraldehyde phosphate (also known as phosphoglyceraldehyde or PGAL, a 3-C) are extracted from the cycle to produce glucose.

The cycle is reactivated when the remaining PGAL molecules are converted to 6 RuBP molecules by ATP energy. Remembering the complexities of life, each reaction in this process is catalysed by a different reaction-specific enzyme, just as in Kreb's Cycle.

C-4 Cycle

The Calvin Cycle (also known as a C-3 pathway) has a preamble step that some plants have established. This preamble step is referred to as C-4. While most C-fixation starts with RuBP, C-4 starts with phosphoenolpyruvate (PEP), a 3-carbon molecule that is converted to oxaloacetic acid (OAA, a 4-carbon molecule) when carbon dioxide is incorporated. OAA is converted to Malic Acid, which is then transferred from the mesophyll cell to the bundle-sheath cell, where it is broken down into PEP and carbon dioxide. PEP returns to the mesophyll cell after the carbon dioxide reaches the Calvin Cycle. The sugars that result is now near the leaf veins and can be easily transported across the plant. The enzyme PEP carboxylase, which has a higher affinity for carbon dioxide than RuBP carboxylase, is responsible for PEP's carbon dioxide capture. RuBP is catalysed with oxygen instead of carbon dioxide when carbon dioxide levels fall below the threshold for RuBP carboxylase. The reaction produces glycolic acid, which cannot be broken down by photorespiration and thus dismantles the Calvin Cycle by producing neither NADH nor ATP. To avoid photorespiration, C-4 plants, which also grow close together, have had to adapt to lower levels of carbon dioxide by artificially raising the carbon dioxide concentration in specific cells. Plants that developed in the tropics and are adapted to higher temperatures than those that evolved at higher latitudes are known as TC-4 plants. C-4 plants include crabgrass, corn, and sugar cane, among others. Since OAA and Malic Acid are involved in other processes, scientists believe that the chemicals must have been present in all plants, leading them to believe that C-4 pathways evolved several times independently (Figure 6.3).

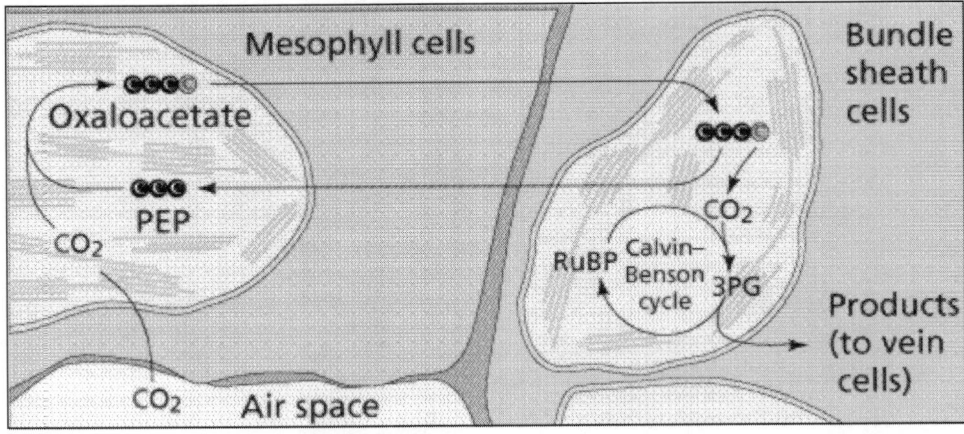

Figure 6.3: C-4 Photosynthsis Involves the Separation of Carbon Fixation and Carbohydrate Systhesis in Space and Time. (Image from Purves *et al.*, Life: The Science of Biology, 4th Edition, by Sinauer and WH Freeman).

Future Photosynthesis

Photosynthetic species can be a viable source of clean-burning fuels like hydrogen and even methane. Green algae's ability to generate hydrogen was recently exploited by a research team at the University of Turku in Finland. If green algae are first exposed to dark, anaerobic (oxygen-free) conditions and then exposed to light, they will emit hydrogen for a few seconds.

In the field of artificial photosynthesis, scientists have also made significant progress. For example, a team of researchers from the University of California, Berkeley, created a synthetic method to trap carbon dioxide using nanowires, which are wires with a diameter of a few billionths of a metre. The wires feed into a system of microbes that use energy to convert carbon dioxide into fuels or polymers.

Few researchers identified another artificial photosynthetic device that used specially engineered bacteria to produce liquid fuels from sunlight, water, and carbon dioxide. During photosynthesis, plants can only capture about 1 per cent of solar energy and use it to create organic compounds.

The researchers' artificial machine, on the other hand, was able to harness 10 per cent of solar energy to generate organic compounds.Scientists will find new ways to use renewable energy sources by continuing to study natural processes such as photosynthesis. Given the prevalence of sunlight, plants, and bacteria, harnessing the power of photosynthesis is a reasonable next step.

Plant Respiration

Plant respiration is a vital biochemical process in which different substrates are oxidised and carbon dioxide is released in most cases (CO_2). Adenosine triphosphate (ATP) formed by plant respiration (as well as photosynthesis) is known as adenosine triphosphate (ATP).

In plant cells, it's used to move things around the cell, make new molecules for growth, and power active transport (the pumping of ions or other substances across a cell membrane against an osmotic gradient). Most plant respiration is aerobic (that is, it requires oxygen and is often referred to as aerobic or cellular respiration) and involves the conversion of sugars to carbon dioxide. Anaerobic respiration, or fermentation, occurs when oxygen is not present, allowing some ATP synthesis. Fermentation is much less effective than aerobic respiration at extracting energy from organic molecules, and most plants cannot withstand prolonged anaerobiosis. Glycolysis, the Krebs cycle (also known as the citric acid cycle or the tricarboxylic acid cycle), and oxidative electron transfer are all part of plant respiration. With a few notable exceptions, it occurs in all plant cells and is essentially similar to animal respiration (such as a cyanide-insensitive respiration mechanism lacking in animals).

Glycolysis

The first step in the breakdown of glucose to extract energy for cellular metabolism is glycolysis. Glycolysis is a part of the metabolism of almost all living organisms. Since the mechanism does not use oxygen, it is classified as anaerobic. Both prokaryotic and eukaryotic cells undergo glycolysis in their cytoplasm. Glycolysis starts with a single glucose molecule's six carbon ring-shaped structure and ends with two molecules of pyruvate, a three-carbon sugar. Glycolysis is divided into two distinct stages. The first step in the glycolysis process traps the glucose molecule in the cell and uses energy to shift it so that the six-carbon sugar molecule can be equally divided into two three-carbon molecules. The second stage of glycolysis removes energy from molecules and stores it as ATP and NADH, a reduced form of NAD. Pyruvate Oxidation and the Citric Acid Cycle

Aerobic respiration can continue if oxygen is sufficient. Pyruvate molecules formed at the end of glycolysis are transported into mitochondria, which are the sites of cellular respiration in eukaryotic cells. Pyruvate is converted to an acetyl group, which is picked up and activated by a carrier compound called coenzyme A (CoA).

Acetyl CoA primary role is to transport the acetyl group from pyruvate to the next step in the glucose catabolism pathway. Pyruvate, a glycolysis product, must go through a series of transformations before it can join the next pathway. There are three stages to the conversion. A multi-enzyme complex transforms pyruvate to acetyl CoA once it enters the mitochondrial matrix. Carbon dioxide is released in the process, and one molecule of NADH is formed.

CO_2 is Generated by Converting Acetyl CoA

In the presence of oxygen, acetyl CoA transfers its acetyl group to oxaloacetate, a four-carbon molecule, to form citrate, a six-carbon molecule with three carboxyl groups; this process would harvest the remaining energy from what started as a glucose molecule. The citric acid cycle (for the first intermediate formed–citric acid, or citrate–when acetate joins to the oxaloacetate), the TCA cycle (because citric acid, citrate, and isocitrate are tricarboxylic acids), and the Krebs cycle (named after Hans Krebs, who first described the steps in the process in the 1930s). The citric acid cycle happens in the matrix of mitochondria, much like the conversion of pyruvate to acetyl CoA. Except for succinate dehydrogenase, which is embedded in the mitochondrion's inner membrane. The citric acid cycle, unlike glycolysis, is a closed loop: the last step regenerates the compound used in the first. The cycle's eight steps are a sequence of redox, dehydration, hydration, and decarboxylation reactions that result in two carbon dioxide molecules, one GTP/ATP molecule, and reduced NADH and FADH2. Since NADH and FADH2 are present, this is an aerobic pathway. Since the NADH and FADH2 formed must transfer their electrons to the next pathway in the system, which uses oxygen, this is called an aerobic pathway. The citric acid cycle's oxidation steps will not take place if this transition does not take place. It's important to remember that the citric acid cycle contains very little ATP and does not absorb oxygen directly.

The Citric Acid Cycle's By-products

Each acetyl group contributes two carbon atoms to the citric acid cycle, accounting for four of the six carbons in a single glucose molecule. On each cycle turn, two carbon dioxide molecules are released; however, these often do not contain the most recently added carbon atoms. Later turns of the cycle will release the two acetyl carbon atoms, resulting in the incorporation of all six carbon atoms from the initial glucose molecule into carbon dioxide. Three NADH molecules and one FADH2 molecule are formed with each cycle switch. To generate ATP molecules, these carriers can interact with the last portion of aerobic respiration. In addition, one GTP or ATP is produced in one cycle.

Oxidative Phosphorylation

As the two ATP-generating pathways in glucose catabolism: glycolysis and the citric acid cycle. However, most of the ATP generated during the aerobic catabolism of glucose does not come from these pathways. Rather, it is derived from a mechanism that starts with electrons being transported via a series of electron transporters that undergo redox reaction. Hydrogen ions accumulate in the matrix space as a result of this. As a result of passing through ATP synthase, a concentration gradient forms in which hydrogen ions disperse out of the matrix space. The catalytic action of ATP synthase, which phosphorylates ADP to produce ATP, is driven by hydrogen ions.

Electron Transport Chain

The electron transport chain is the final step in aerobic respiration and the only part of glucose metabolism that uses ambient oxygen. Electron transport is a sequence of redox reactions that mimic a relay race or bucket brigade in which electrons are quickly transferred from one link to the next until they reach the end of the chain, where they reduce molecular oxygen and produce water. The electron transport chain is made up of four protein and it is made up of the aggregation of these four complexes, as well as related mobile, accessory electron carrier. Eukaryotes' inner mitochondrial membrane and prokaryotes' plasma membrane both have several copies of the electron transport chain (Figure 6.4).

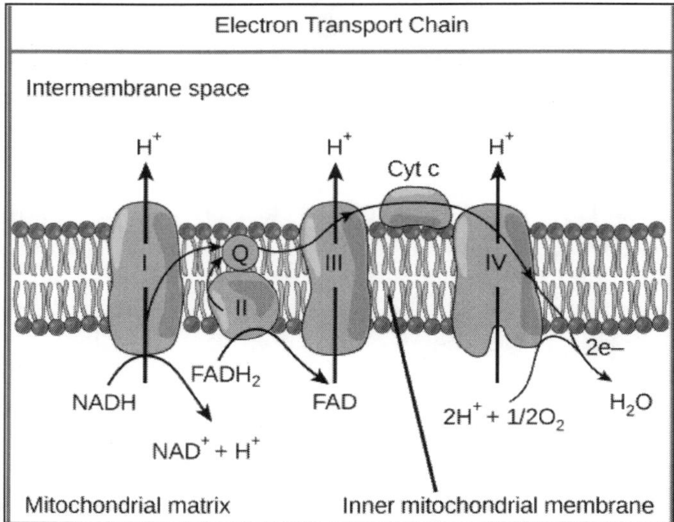

Figure 6.4: The Electron Transport Chain is a Network of Electron Transporters Embedded in the Inner Mitochondrial Membrane that Transports Electrons from NADH and FADH2 to Molecule Oxygen. Protons are pumped from the mitochondrial matrix to the intermembrane space, and oxygen is reduced to form water.

Chemiosmosis

The free energy produced by the redox reactions just described is used to pump hydrogen ions (protons) across the membrane in chemiosmosis. Due to the positive charge of hydrogen ions and their aggregation on one side of the membrane, the unequal distribution of H+ ions across the membrane creates both concentration and electrical gradients (thus, an electrochemical gradient). The ions would begin to diffuse back across the membrane into the matrix if the membrane was open to diffusion by hydrogen ions, guided by their electrochemical gradient. Many ions need the assistance of ion channels to diffuse through the nonpolar regions of phospholipid membranes. The force of the hydrogen ions diffusing through it, down their electrochemical gradient, turns this complex protein into a tiny generator. Using the potential energy of the hydrogen ion gradient, the turning of sections of this molecular machine allows the addition of a phosphate to ADP, creating ATP. Chemiosmosis is the method used in the light reactions of photosynthesis to harness the energy of sunlight in the process of photophosphorylation. It also generates 90 per cent of the ATP generated during aerobic glucose catabolism. Remember that oxidative phosphorylation is the method of producing ATP in mitochondria by chemiosmosis. The energy of the electrons extracted from hydrogen atoms is used to produce ATP, which is the end result of these reactions. Originally, these atoms were a part of a glucose molecule. The electrons are then used to reduce an oxygen molecule to oxygen ions at the end of the pathway. Water is produced when extra electrons on oxygen attract hydrogen ions (protons) from the surrounding medium.

Take a way points : Water and ATP are the end products of the electron transport chain. As low-energy electrons reduce oxygen molecules and form water, electrons travelling through the electron transport chain gradually lose energy. High-energy electrons donated to the chain by either NADH or FADH2 complete the chain. In NADH or FADH2, the amount of free energy of the electrons decreases from about 60 kcal/mol to about 0 kcal/mol in water. The anabolism of other biochemical substances, such as nonessential amino acids, carbohydrates, and lipids, may be diverted from the citric acid cycle's intermediate compounds. The glucose pathways will use the same molecules as energy sources.

Photorespiration

The light-dependent evolution of CO_2 is known as photorespiration. The oxygenation of RuBP by RUBISCO, accompanied by photorespiratory glycolate metabolism, is known as photorespiration. The rate of carbon assimilation, the energetic efficiency of photosynthesis, and the photosynthetic quotient (PQ = O_2 produced/CO_2 assimilated) are all affected by the competition between O_2 and CO_2. Rubisco produces a 3carbon compound, 3phosphoglycerate, and a 2carbon compound, phosphoglycolate, by oxidising ribulose1,5bisphosphate. While photorespiration appears to be a wasteful operation, it can serve as an essential energy sink by consuming ATP and NADPH and thus preventing the over-reduction of the PQ pool when leaf intercellular CO_2 concentrations are restricted. Photorespiration's protective function may be particularly significant in stressful situations like drought. Photorespiration decreases photosynthesis efficiency for a variety of reasons. First, carbon is given an oxygen boost. In other words, the carbon is oxidised, as opposed to photosynthesis, which involves the conversion of carbon to carbohydrate. Second, the ribulose bisphosphate must be resynthesised and the phosphoglycolate must be reduced. The CalvinBenson pathway can accept 3phosphoglycerate from photorespiration, but the phosphoglycolate must be recycled in order to produce a useful compound. The peroxisome, a specialised organelle, is responsible for this recycling. Peroxisomes are found in the plant cell between the chloroplasts and mitochondria, and they are responsible for passing on the 2 carbon products of oxygenation for further metabolism. Phosphoglycolate is dephosphorylated in the chloroplast. Glycolate is transported to the peroxisome, where it is further oxidised to glyoxylate by the presence of molecular oxygen. Peroxisomes are located between the chloroplasts and the mitochondria in the plant cell, and they are in charge of passing on the two carbon products of oxygenation for further metabolism. In the chloroplast, phosphoglycolate undergoes dephosphorylation. Glycolate is transported to the peroxisome, where molecular oxygen further oxidises it to glyoxylate. In the peroxisome, the glyoxylate is amidated to the amino acid glycine. Glycine is then transferred to the mitochondrial matrix, where two glycines are converted to one serine with the loss of CO_2 and NH 3 from the fixed molecule pool. The serine is carried to the peroxisome, where it is deaminated and converted to glycerate. The glycerate is returned to the chloroplast, where it is recycled, where it is phosphorylated to 3 phosphoglycerate for the Calvin Benson cycle (Figure 6.5).

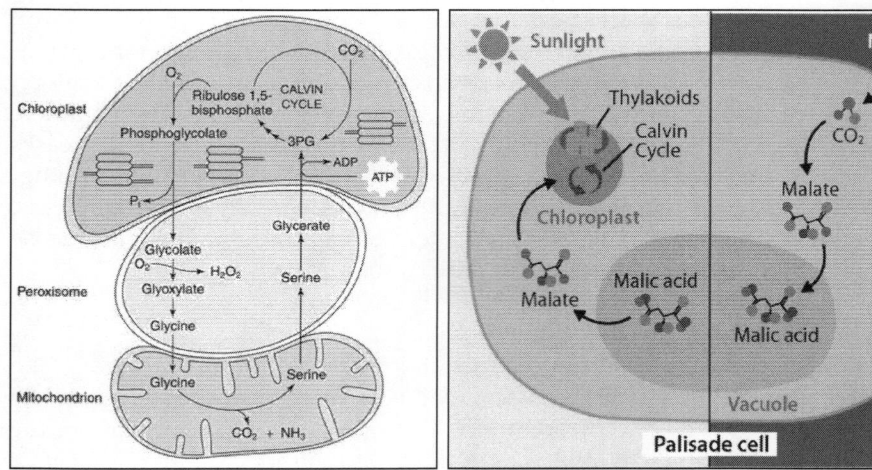

Figure 6.5: C3 Cycle/CAM Cycle.

C_4 Cycle

In land plants, two mechanisms have evolved to suppress photorespiration rates. First mechanism is C_4 Cycle. If Rubisco could receive CO_2 more efficiently than by diffusion through the leaves, photorespiration could be avoided. A bypass mechanism for the transmission of CO_2 to Rubisco has developed in a variety of

C_4 plants, including grasses including maize (corn) and bamboo. The enzyme phosphoenolpyruvate carboxylase transforms CO_2 to oxaloacetate first in these C_4 plants. Rubisco has a lower K m for CO_2 than PEP carboxylase. In addition, oxygen is a weak substrate for this enzyme. This means that, at low CO_2 concentrations, carbon is delivered more efficiently into photosynthesis products than in C_3 plants, and oxygenation does not occur. PEP carboxylase is concentrated in the leaf's outermost mesophyll cells. This ensures that the cells that are the most exposed to the environment are the most effective at transforming CO_2 into organic products. Rubisco photosynthesis is more prevalent in the bundle sheath cells, which are located in the inner part of the leaf and transported to various part of the plant. The oxaloacetate generated by PEP carboxylase is transported to the bundle sheath cells. NADPH converts it to malate before transporting it to the bundle sheath cells. Since this also produces NADPH, the C_4 cycle absorbs no reducing equivalents. Pyruvate is transferred back to the mesophyll cells, where it is rephosphorylated to phosphoenolpyruvate, using the equivalent of two ATP "high energy phosphates." Malic enzyme breaks down malate into pyruvate and CO_2 for Rubisco in bundle sheath cells. To deliver CO_2 to Rubisco, the C_4 cycle needs two ATP equivalents. This is not a concern during active photosynthesis since Photosystems I and II generate plenty of ATP. Why aren't C_4 plants sweeping the globe? Because of the higher energy demands, these plants are less effective in low-light situations. This hypothesis is supported by the fact that C_4 plants are often found in tropical climates, while C_3 plants are found in more temperate climates. Photorespiration is more expensive at high temperatures because high temperatures promote the oxygenation reaction more than the carboxylation reaction. If stomata near, causing a low CO_2 partial pressure in the leaf, photorespiration is particularly costly in water-limited environments (oxygenation and carboxylation compete so low CO_2 leads to a high rate of oxygenation).

CAM Cycle

Second is Crassulacean Acid Metabolism, or CAM, is the first. This is a highly adaptable metabolism in which some or all CO_2 absorption takes place at night (Black and Osmond, 2003). CO_2 is processed as a carboxylic acid, often malate, during the night. During the day, stomata close and CO_2 is released into the now-relaxed atmosphere. CAM plants have identical biochemistry to C4 plants, but the two carboxylations are now isolated in time rather than space. Malic acid is made from carbohydrates by PEP carboxylase and processed in the vacuole at night. Malate is decarboxylated in the cytosol during the day by PEP carboxykinase or NAD(P)-malic enzymes, and CO_2 is re-fixed by the Calvin-Benson cycle and carbohydrate reformed. Water or salt stress will then trigger CAM, causing gene expression to turn on for the synthesis of component enzymes.

Plant Growth Regulators

Mighty Massengers

Thimann coined the word phytohormones to describe growth hormones (1948). It is characterised as "organic substances synthesised in minute amounts in one part of the plant body and transported to another part of the plant body where they influence specific physiological processes."

Auxin

Auxins (Gk. auxein = to grow) are weakly acidic growth hormones with an unsaturated ring structure that promote cell elongation, especially in shoots (more pronounced in decapitated shoots and shoot segments) at concentrations less than 100 ppm, but are inhibitory to roots. Auxins were the first growth regulators to be discovered among the growth regulators.

Natural auxins: These are auxins that occur naturally in plants and are thus classified as phytohormones. The most well-known and ubiquitous auxin is indole 3-acetic acid (IAA). It can be present in all types of plants and fungi.

Synthetic auxins: are synthetic substances that elicit the same physiological responses as IAA. 2, 4-D auxin is one of the most effective synthetic auxins (2, 4-dichlorophenoxy acetic acid). IBA is a form of auxin that is both natural and synthetic (Figure 6.6).

Auxins have a variety of functions in plants. They regulate a variety of growth processes. The following are some of them: Auxins stimulate cell elongation in all directions, which promotes the elongation and development of stems and roots, as well as the enlargement of many fruits. Apical dominance occurs when the apical bud develops while the lower axillary buds are suppressed in many plants (Figure 6.6).

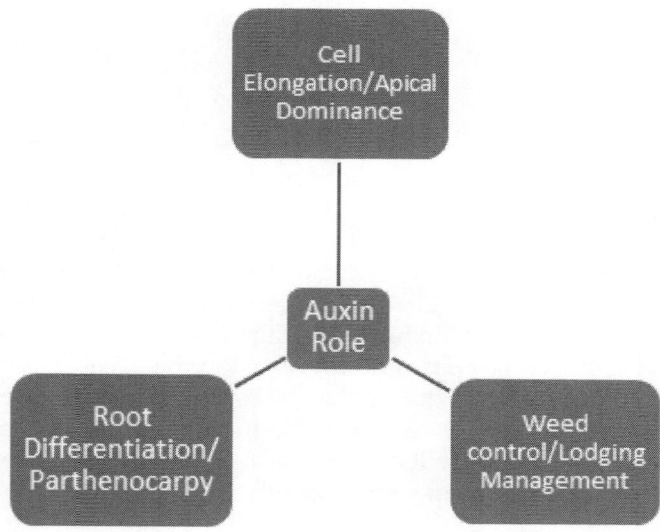

Figure 6.6: Showing Role of Auxin as Growth Regulator.

Chemical compounds with an aromatic ring and a carboxylic acid group are known as auxins. In plants, tryptophan is a precursor to auxin biosynthesis. Auxin causes signal responses to be triggered by stimulating or inhibiting gene expression.

It activates glutathione S-transferases, auxin homeostasis proteins including GH3, and the Aux/IAA repressor, among other primary response genes. Auxin signalling pathway: Auxin sensitive factors initiate ARE-mediated transcription of auxin genes (ARF). The binding of the AUX/IAA protein complex inhibits transcription. In the absence of auxin, the AUX/IAA protein complex binds to ARFs and inhibits their transcriptional activity. When auxin is present, a molecular complex form between T1R1 protein and AUX/IAA, resulting in ubiquitone-mediated AUX/IAA proteolysis. ARF will then bind to the promoter and begin transcription (Figure 6.7).

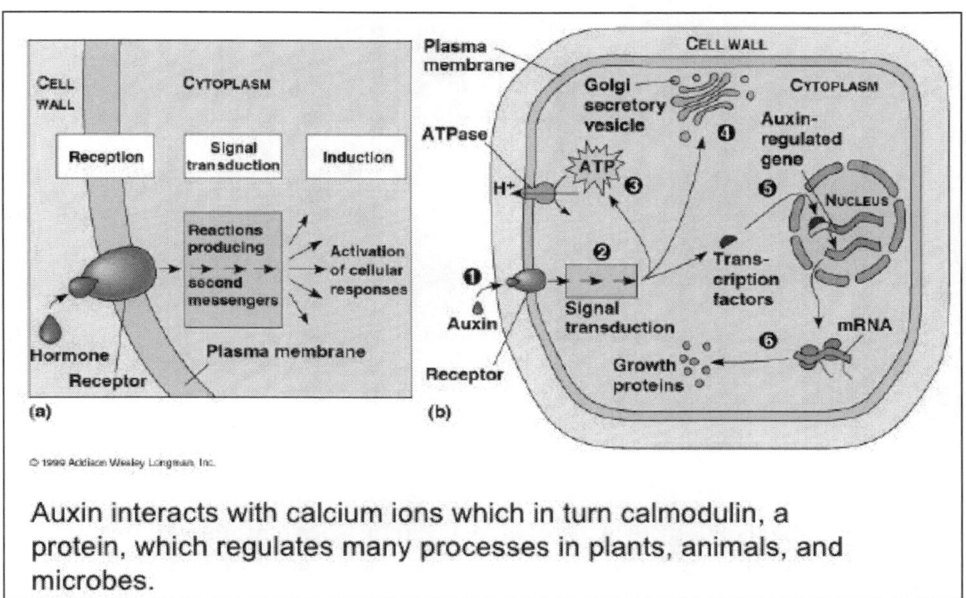

Auxin interacts with calcium ions which in turn calmodulin, a protein, which regulates many processes in plants, animals, and microbes.

Figure 6.7: Diagrammatic Representation of Signal Transduction in Plant.

Cytokinin

Cytokinin is a hormone that is produced by the body. PGRs derived from adenine are known as cytokinins. It encourages cell division in the roots and shoots of plants. Zeatin is the most common form of naturally occurring cytokinin. 6-Benzyl amino purine and 6-phenyl amino purine are two examples of synthetic cytokinin. The precursor to cytokinin biosynthesis is 5′-AMP. A plant protein known as a cytokinin signalling and response regulator protein is involved in the two-step cytokinin signalling and response regulation pathway (Figure 6.8). Cytokinin sensor kinases (CRE1/AHK4, AHK2, and AHK3) are activated in the presence of cytokinin and then auto-phosphorylate themselves by moving a phosphate from the kinase domain to the receiver domain. The phosphate is then moved to a protein called histidine phosphotransferase (AHPs). A reaction regulator is then phosphorylated by histidine phosphotransfer protein. Response regulators regulate gene expression in either a positive or negative way.

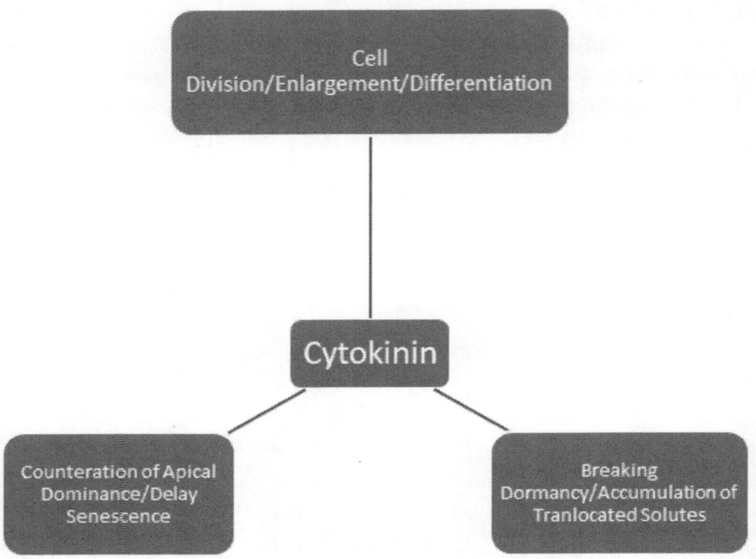

Figure 6.8: Showing Role of Cytokinins.

Gibberellins

Gibberellins are a form of gibberellin that is found Gibberellins (GAs) are a tetracyclic diterpenoid family of plant growth substance. It plays a role in seed germination as well as cell elongation (Figure 6.9). Ent-kaurene is a tetracyclic hydrocarbon that is a GA precursor. Three different types of transcriptional factors are involved in GA-induced signal transduction: Spindly or slender mutants,

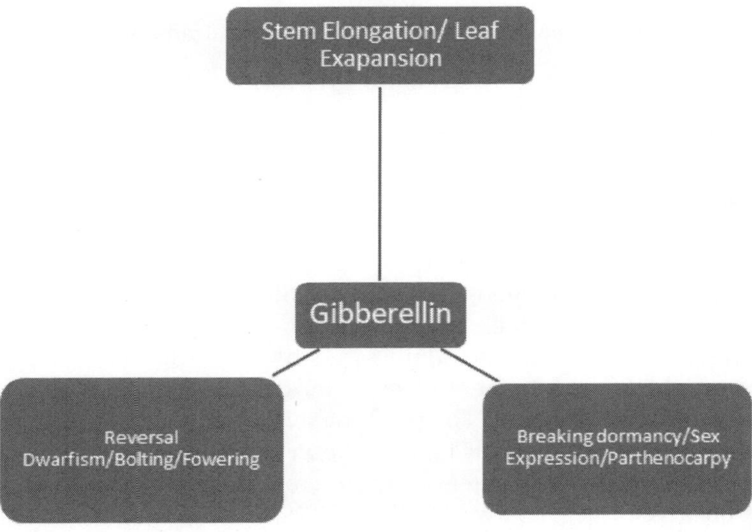

Figure 6.9: Showing Role of Gibberellin.

Gibberellin insensitive dwarf mutants (GAI), Gibberellin deficiency reversion mutants (RGA), and Gibberellin deficiency reversion mutants (RGA) (SPY). GAI and RGA (DELLA repressors) have a conserved region for DELLA proteins in the Gibberellin signalling pathway. GAI and RGA act as growth repressors. SPY is also a repressor that acts upstream of GAI and RGA, both of which inhibit or enhance the effect of GAI and RGA. These repressors are degraded in the presence of GA, allowing transcription of genes that lead to stem elongation.

Ethylene

Ethylene is a chemical that can be found in several different Plants produce ethylene, a PGR that aids in the ripening and ageing process (Figure 6.10). Ethylene is formed from the amino acid methionine. The ethylene signalling pathway begins when ethylene is detected by a family of endoplasmic membrane receptors following its biosynthesis. Protein kinases, GTPases, and transcription factors are all involved in signalling (EIN2, EIN3). Ethylene signalling pathway: Copper cofactor receptor mediates ethylene signal perception and transmission. After that, protein kinases like CTR1 interact with the receptors. As ethylene binds to receptors, it inactivates both receptors and CTR1, resulting in the depression of the positive regulatory molecule EIN2. It is then transmitted from EIN2 to EIN3/EIL1, causing EIN3 factors to accumulate in the nucleus. It causes ethylene gene expression by inducing transcription of ethylene-regulated genes such as ERF1, EBF1, 2, 3, and 4.

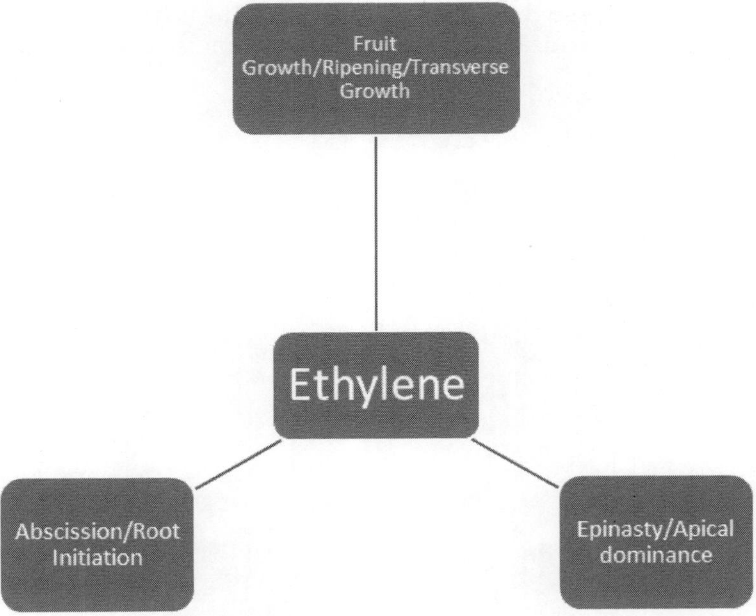

Figure 6.10: Showing Role of Ethylene.

SPY is also a repressor that acts upstream of GAI and RGA, both of which inhibit or enhance the effect of GAI and RGA. These repressors are degraded in the presence of GA, allowing transcription of genes that lead to stem elongation.

Abscisic Acid

Abscisic acid is a plant growth regulator involved in seed and bud dormancy, organ size regulation, and stomatal closure. It's an inhibitory hormone found in plants that aids in stress adaptation. Xanthoxin is a more advanced ABA biosynthetic precursor. ABA is essential in the response to various stress signals such as drought, cold, and salinity. The presence of cis acting elements known as ABRE is required for ABA-induced gene expression (ABA responsive element). ABA gene expression in plants is regulated by transcriptional factors such as AREB, DREB2A, DREB2B, MYC/MYB, RD22BP1, and AtMyB2, which are responsible for regulating ABA gene expression in plants during environmental stress. The ABA-dependent stress signalling pathway activates AREB, which binds to the ABRE factor and induces the stress-responsive gene. A protein similar to LEA is encoded by the stress sensitive gene (RD29B) (Late Embryogenesis Abundant Protein). DREB2A, DREB2B, and DRE cis-element transcription factors aid in maintaining osmotic balance in plant cells during stress. The MYC/MYB transcription factors bind to the MYBRS and MYCRS cis-elements and aid in the activation of the RD22 gene. Overall, these transcription factors interact with one another to achieve the best stress tolerance response.

Plant growth regulators have an effect on the growth and production of plants. In plants, the function of these regulators can be individualistic or synergistic, resulting in a promoting or inhibiting response (Figure 6.11). Plant growth regulators are affected by factors such as temperature and light, which influence plant growth events (vernalisation). As a result, studying the signalling behaviour of plant growth regulators in plants is critical for understanding the molecular processes at work in plants.

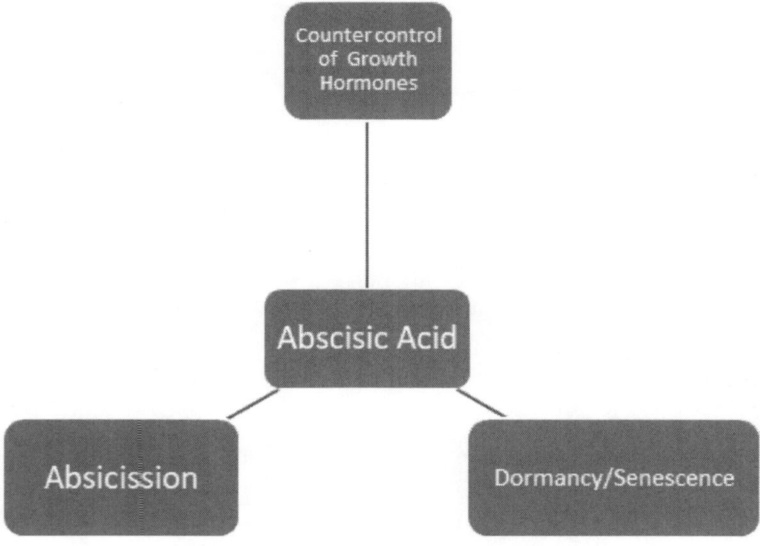

Figure 6.11: Showing Role of Abscisic Acid.

Plant Defence Mechanism

Plants have evolved multiple layers of sophisticated surveillance mechanisms that detect potentially harmful pathogens and react quickly before they cause serious damage. These surveillance systems are connected to complex defensive responses that are pre-programmed.

Innate immunity, also known as **basal resistance**, is the first line of protection that protects plants against whole classes of pathogens. When plant cells identify microbe-associated molecular patterns (MAMPs), such as unique proteins, lipopolysaccharides, and cell wall components found in microbes, basal resistance is activated. As a result, living plant cells become more resistant to attack. Owing to the widespread existence of these molecular components in plant cells, both non-pathogens and pathogens are capable of triggering basal resistance. Pathogens have evolved countermeasures to inhibit basal resistance in a variety of plant species. If a pathogen suppresses basal defence, plants can retaliate with a new line of defence: the **hypersensitive response (HR)**. At the infection site, the HR is characterised by deliberate plant cell suicide. The HR can restrict pathogen access to water and nutrients by sacrificing a few cells in order to save the rest of the plant, which is drastic compared to basal resistance. HR is more pathogen-specific than basal resistance, and it is often activated when gene products in the plant cell recognise the presence of specific disease-causing effector molecules introduced into the host by the pathogen. Plant tissues can become highly resistant to a wide range of pathogens for an extended period of time once the hypersensitive response has been activated. This phenomenon is known as **systemic acquired resistance (SAR)**, and it refers to a state of readiness in which plant resources are mobilised in the event of another attack.

Researchers have discovered that spraying plants with chemicals known as plant activators can artificially cause SAR. These chemicals are gaining popularity in agriculture because they are much less harmful to humans and animals than fungicides or antibiotics, and their protective effects can last much longer. Plants can protect themselves against viruses through a variety of mechanisms, including a sophisticated genetic defence system known as **RNA silencing**, in addition to the hypersensitive response. During replication in a host cell, several viruses generate double-stranded RNA or DNA. Plants can detect these foreign molecules and react by breaking down the genetic strands into useless fragments, effectively stopping the infection. Chlorosis and mottling are common symptoms of virus infection in plants, but if RNA silencing is active, disease symptoms can eventually disappear. Furthermore, the plant can retain a template of the digested genetic strand that can be used to quickly respond to future attacks by similar viruses, similar to how vertebrate immune systems remember.

While plants have evolved surveillance systems to identify insect pests and react with specific defence mechanisms, mechanical damage caused by insects is not commonly considered a "real" plant disease. The presence of elicitors found in the saliva of chewing insects allows plants to differentiate between general wounding and insect feeding. Plants can produce volatile organic compounds (VOCs), such as monoterpenoids, sesquiterpenoids, and homoterpenoids, in response. These chemicals can repel harmful insects while also attracting beneficial predators that eat the pests. Wheat seedlings infested with aphids, for example, can produce VOCs that repel other aphids.

Stress Resistance

The ability to adapt or acclimate to stress is needed for stress resistance.

A sudden change in environmental condition is normally the cause of plant stress. Exposure to a specific stress in stress-tolerant plant species, on the other hand, leads to a time-dependent acclimation to that specific stress. As a result, plant stress and acclimation are closely related. The signal for the plant to activate processes necessary for the establishment of a new homeostasis associated with the acclimated state can be thought of as the stress-induced modulation of homeostasis. Because of their genetic capacity to adapt or acclimate to stress and develop a new homeostatic state over time, plants exhibit stress resistance or stress tolerance.

The attainment of the acclimated state can be thought of as a dynamic, time-nested response to a stress, according to a hierarchy of short- and long-term responses. Differential expression of specific sets of genes associated with exposure to a specific stress is commonly associated with acclimation. The amazing ability to regulate gene expression in a timed manner in response to environmental change.

Photoperiodism

Photoperiodism is a plant's reaction to the relative lengths of light and dark cycles. The initiation of flowering is the most important photoperiodic response in plants. Flowering in plants necessitates a brief light-dark phase. The time period is referred to as the critical period. It was first discovered in the tobacco variety Maryland Mammoth (*Nicotiana tabacum*). All plants do not take the same duration of light and dark cycles for flowering, according to Garner and Allard's observations. Butler *et al.*, discovered phytochromes, which are photoreceptor flower stimulating pigments found in plants, in 1959. All green plants are thought to contain it. Phytochrome is a bili-protein that comes in two different forms chemically. The Pr form absorbs red light with a wavelength of 660 nm, while the Pfr form absorbs far red light with a wavelength of 730 nm. The two types of phytochrome can be converted into each other, as shown below:

Pr is also known as P 660 and Pfr is P 730 based on their absorption spectra. Pr encourages flowering in short-day plants while Pfr suppresses it, and vice versa in long-day plants.

Vernalization

T.D. Lysenko, a Russian physicist, coined the word vernalization in 1920. Many species, especially biennials and perennials, are induced to flower at temperatures ranging from 1 to 10 degrees Celsius. This is referred to as vernalization. The response of all plants to the cold temperature stimulation is not the same. The measures for inducing vernalization are as follows: Depending on the plant, seeds are allowed to germinate before being exposed to cold treatment for a period of time. After this treatment, the germinated seeds are allowed to dry before being sown. Vernalization has been used by Russian scientists to reduce the time it takes for a crop to mature by hastening the flowering processes caused by cold treatment. Vernalization allows crops to be processed sooner. They can be grown in areas where they don't grow naturally. Plant breeding can be sped up by using vernalization.

Summary

It also provides a quick overview of how physiological processes affect the environment. The chapter on plant physiology discusses various plant structures as well as how they function. It aims to describe plant processes such as photosynthesis, mineral nutrition, respiration, transportation, and, ultimately, plant production and growth.

REFERENCES

1. L. W. Roberts, P. B. Gahan, and R. Aloni (2012). Plant growth regulators and vascular differentiation Springer Science and Business Media is a publisher of science and business books.
2. S. C. Minocha (1987). Plant growth regulators and morphogenesis in forest tree cell and tissue culture. In Forestry Cell and Tissue Culture (pp. 50-66). Dordrecht: Springer.
3. Salisbury, F.B. and ROSS, C.W. 1992: Plant Physiology. Wadsworth Publishing Company, Belmont - California.
4. Strasburger, E. 2008: Lehrbuch der Botanik für Hochschulen. 36. Auflage, G. Fischer Verlag, Stuttgart-Jena-New York.
5. Hopkins, W.G., Huner, N.P.A. 2009: Introduction to Plant Physiology, 4th Edition. John Wiley and Sons, Inc., Hoboken, USA.
6. Taiz, L. and Zeiger, E. 2002 and 2010: Plant Physiology, 3rd and 5th Edition. The Benjamin Cummings Publishing Company, Redwood City - California.
7. Luttge, U.2008: Plant Physiology, Encyclopaedia of Ecology.Pages 2837-2845.
8. Rabinowitch and Govindjee 1969 : Photosynthesis (Wiley).

Chapter 7

Genetics

Anand K. Singh

Interdisciplinary School of Life Sciences,
Banaras Hindu University, Varanasi – 221 005, Uttar Pradesh, India
e-mail: anandksingh@bhu.ac.in

ABSTRACT

Genetics is the branch of biology that defines the mechanism of similarities and differences in the characters among the organisms from the same family. Studies on the inheritance of such characters from one generation to next generation started from thousands of years but significant progress has been made in 1865 by an Austrian monk Gregor Johann Mendel who defined the fundamental laws of character inheritance. In this introductory chapter "Genetics" the fundamental understanding of chromosome-based inheritance and variation in organisms has been discussed. Deviation in Mendelian genetics due to epigenetic interactions or linkage of genes present on the same chromosome suggest that character transmission is a highly regulated and complex process. Inheritance of genes associated with sex chromosomes, the chromosomal basis of sex determination and phenomenon of dosage compensation to equalize the expression of sex-linked and autosomal genes has also been discussed. In brief, this chapter covers most of the fundamental understanding of genetics.

Keywords: *Allele, Chromosome, DNA, Epigenetics, Gene, Mutation.*

Introduction

The term "genetics" was given by British biologist *William Bateson* in 1905, which was derived from the Greek word "genesis" that means "origin". Genetics is the branch of biology that defines the transmission of characters from one generation to the next generation with two contradictory aspects of character transmission-heredity and variation. *Heredity* is the transmission of characters from parents to their offspring and thus acts as the basis of similarities while *Variation* is the cause of differences in individuals.

Studies on the transmission of characters from one generation to the next generation have been started long back and different theories have been proposed by various scientists before the rediscovery of Mendelian laws of genetics.

- *Theory of Preformation:* This theory was proposed by two Dutch biologists, *Swammerdam* and *Bunnet* (1720-1793). According to this theory, a miniature human called *homunculus* already used to be present in egg and sperm and the development of a zygote resulted only in the growth of that miniature human.
- *Theory of Epigenesis:* This theory was supported by German biologist *Wolff* (1738-1794). According to this theory, egg and sperm are undifferentiated cells and differentiation in various organ takes place only after fertilization from the zygote that results in the development of various organs.
- *Theory of acquired characters*: This theory was proposed by French biologist *Lamarck* (1744-1829). This theory states that a newly acquired character by an individual shall pass on to its progeny. This theory was disproved by *Weismann* who demonstrated that by cutting the tail of mice for 22 successive generations the newly born baby mice has the tail.
- *Theory of Pangenesis*: This theory was proposed by an English naturalist *Charles Darwin* (1809-1882). This theory states that invisible copies of each body organ and component called *gemmules* are transported by the bloodstream to the sex organs. These *gemmules* are assembled in the gametes and after fertilization, they move out to the different part of the body resulting in the development of the respective organ.
- *Theory of Germplasm*: This theory was supported by German biologist *August Weismann* (1889). According to this theory body tissues are of two types, *viz.*, germplasm and somatoplasm. The germplasm refers to reproductive tissues while somatoplasm includes all other body tissues. Thus, the transmission of characters from one generation to another generation takes place only through germplasm. Any change in germplasm will lead to a change in the next generation.

Mendelian Genetics

- The most accepted and scientifically proven theory of character transmission from one generation to the next generation was proposed by Austrian monk, *Gregor Johann Mendel*.
- Mendel (1822-1884) published his famous pea plant experiments in *Proceedings of Natural History Society* in 1865, but unfortunately, his findings were ignored until 1900.
- Mendel's finding received recognition when it was independently rediscovered by three scientists- *Hugo de Vries* in Holland, *Carl Correns* in Germany, and *Eric von Tschermark*-Seysenegg in Austria.
- Mendel used the garden pea (*Pisum sativum*) plant which is a good model system for hybridization experiments as it has very distinct variation in

phenotypes, high reproduction, controlled mating, short life span, and convenience in handling.

- Mendel set the crosses between plants from the contrasting characters and proposed that in heterozygous condition, the expression of one character dominates over the other.
- The character that appears in F1 heterozygous condition is called the *dominant character* while the one with suppressed expression is called the *recessive character*. Dominant characters are represented with capital letters while recessive characters are shown in small letters.

Mendel started with 34 pairs but finally consider only 7 pairs of such contrasting characters among its different variants.

Table 7.1: Seven Pairs of Dominant and Recessive Traits that Mendel Monitored in the Pea Plant Crosses

Characters	*Traits (Dominant)*	*Traits (Recessive)*
Plant height	Tall (T)	Dwarf (t)
Pod colour	Green (G)	Yellow (g)
Flower/Pod Position	Axial (A)	Terminal (a)
Flower colour	Violet (V)	White (v)
Seed colour	Yellow (Y)	Green (y)
Seed shape	Round (R)	Wrinkled (r)
Pod shape	Inflated (I)	Constricted (i)

- Plants obtained from parent "P" to their first generation of cross termed first filial or "F1" generation and likewise, subsequent generations are called second filial "F2" generation, third filial "F3" generation and so on.
- The factors that represent the characters and responsible for their production are called *genes*.
- The alternative forms of a gene are called *alleles*.
- When diploid organisms have the same set of alleles from a particular gene, they are called *homozygous* while if they have a different form of a gene, the organism is called *heterozygous*.
- The allelic constitution of a strain is called *genotype* while the phenotypic appearance of that strain is called the *phenotype*.

Mendel's Law of Inheritance

1. Law of Segregation

Mendel's first law of inheritance is called the *law of segregation* which is also known as the *law of purity of gametes*. This law states that alleles of the same genes with contrasting characters in heterozygotes though remain together for a long time, but they do not contaminate or mix and segregate at the time of gametogenesis with each gamete receives only one allele having either dominant or recessive character. In brief, during gametogenesis alleles of a character segregates in each gamete. Mendel's law of segregation is based on the monohybrid cross where only one character has been monitored and F2 has the phenotypic ratio of 3:1.

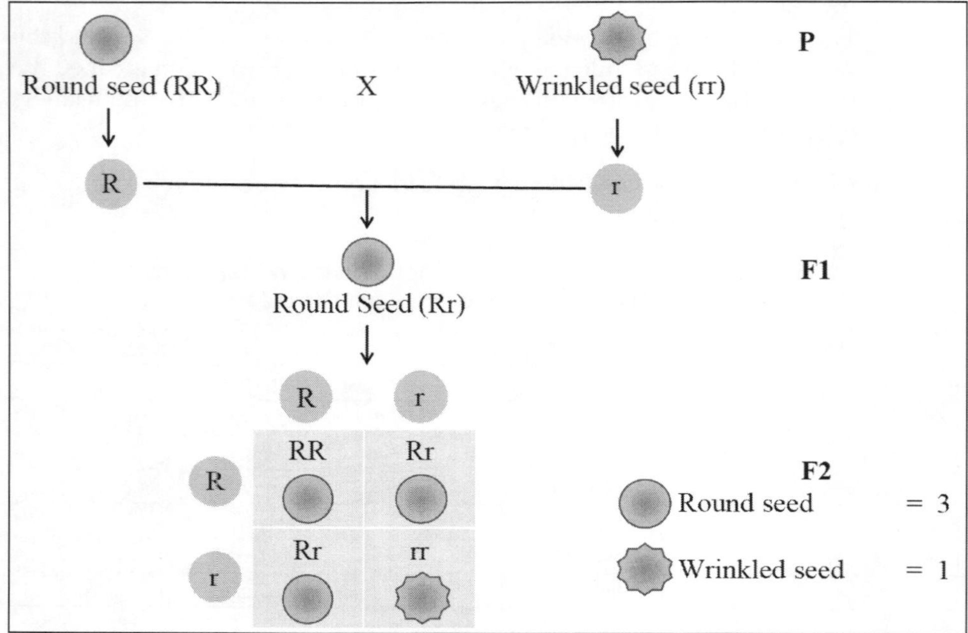

Figure 7.1: Diagrammatic Representation of Monohybrid Cross to Explain Mendel's Law of Segregation.

2. Law of Independent Assortment

Mendel's second law of inheritance is known as the *law of independent assortment*. This law states that alleles of different genes segregate independently of each other, which is based on the observations that the parents with two or more pairs of contrasting characters have the inheritance of one character independent from other pairs of character. Mendel's law of independent assortment is based on the dihybrid cross where two different characters have been considered simultaneously and F2 has the phenotypic ratio of 9:3:3:1.

Ratio of phenotypes in offspring from crosses of heterozygous parents:

- ☆ Monohybrid cross $(3:)^1$ = 3:1
- ☆ Dihybrid cross $(3:1)^2$ = 9:3:3:1
- ☆ Trihybrid cross $(3:1)^3$ = 27:9:9:9:9:3:3:3:1
- ☆ Multihybrid crosss $(3:1)^n$ where n is number of hybrids

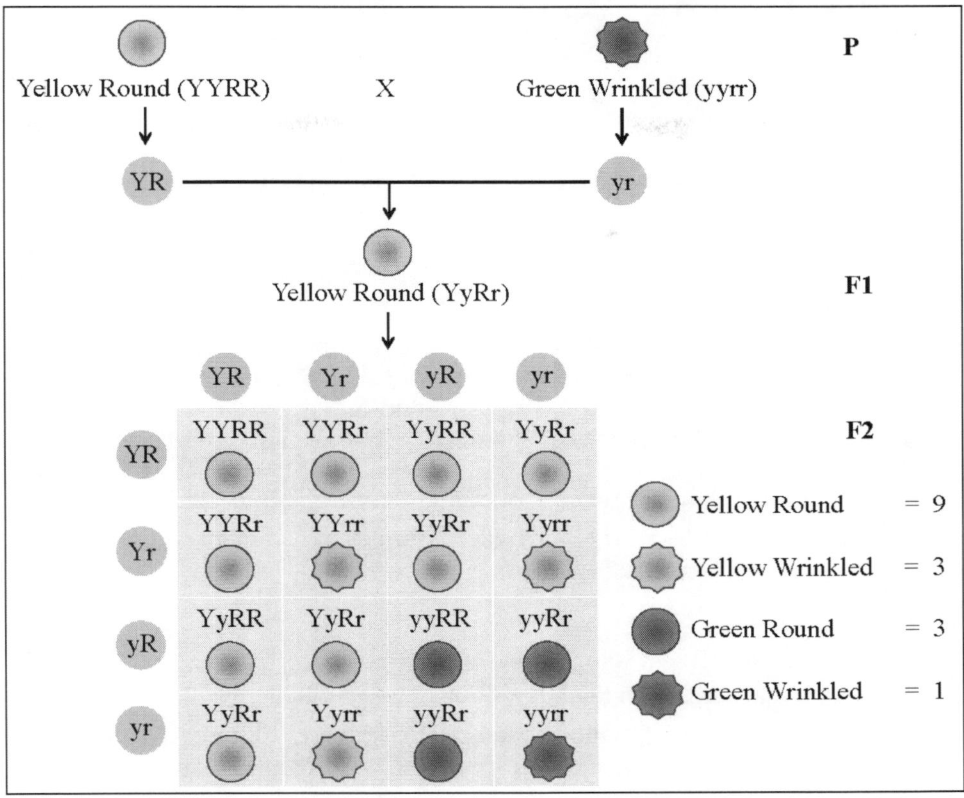

Figure 7.2: Diagrammatic Representation of Dihybrid Cross to Explain Mendel's Law of Independent Assortment.

Back Cross and Test Cross

- Crosses between an F1 individual with one of its parents is called *back cross* while if the individual is backcrossed specifically with recessive parents, then it is called *test cross*.
- Test cross tests whether an F1 individual is homozygous or heterozygous. If only one phenotype appears in progeny that means the organism is homozygous while if both dominant and recessive phenotype appears that means the organism is heterozygous.
- One of the main reasons for Mendel's success was that he always used pure homozygous plants to start his experiments which he generates by selfing for several generations.

Incomplete Dominance and Codominance

- A completely dominant allele has the same phenotypic effect in both homozygous as well as the heterozygous condition that means both RR and Rr individuals would be phenotypically identical. However, there are a few exceptions where heterozygotes are phenotypically different from homozygotes.

- If the heterozygotes generate an intermediate phenotype of both the parents, then it is called *incomplete* or *partial dominance*. For example, the flower colour of snapdragon, *Antirrhinum majus* are white or red in the homozygous condition of colour determining alleles while in the heterozygous condition they become pink in colour. The allele for red colour (W) is therefore called incomplete dominant over allele of white colour (w).
- Likewise, if two alleles of a gene expressed independently of each other and thus both factors express without affecting each other, then it is called *codominance*. For example, M and N antigen producing alleles in human blood express M or N antigen in homozygous condition, while in the heterozygous condition they express both M and N antigen and that behaves differently from M or N antigen-expressing cells.
- The phenotypic ratio of F2 in both incompletely dominant and codominant allele condition is 1:2:1.

Multiple Allele

- Alleles are an alternative mutant form of a gene and basically, they are named according to the phenotype of that mutant.
- Mendel proposed that one gene can exist in form of only two alleles but later many genes have been reported that have more than two alleles.
- A classic example of a gene with multiple alleles is the one that controls human blood type A, B, AB, and O. The allele I^A produces antigen A, I^B produces antigen B and I^O produces no antigen.
- Another example of a gene with multiple alleles is the one that controls rabbit coat colour. The coat colour determining gene in rabbit has four alleles c^+ (wild type), c (*albino*), c^h (*himalayan*), and c^{ch} (*chinchilla*) with a dominance relation $c^+ > c^{ch} > c^h > c$.
- The allele that has no function and thus has no phenotypic effect is called a *null* or *amorphic allele* while partially functional alleles that are recessive to a more functional allele is called a *hypomorphic allele*.
- The mutation that alters the morphology of the organism is called *visible mutation* while mutation that affects the reproduction capacity are called a *sterile mutation*.
- The mutation that alters the essential function and thus leads to organismal death in homozygous condition is called a *lethal mutation*.
- Lethal allele could be both dominant and recessive.
- *Dominant lethal allele* kills the organism in both homozygous as well as the heterozygous condition and therefore, eliminates from the population in the same generation in which it arose.

- *Recessive lethal allele* kills the organism only when in homozygous condition. Heterozygous condition of recessive lethal allele survives with or without any distinct phenotypes.
- Mutations that have phenotypic effect in both heterozygotes, as well as homozygotes, are called *dominant mutation* while mutation that has phenotypic effect only in homozygotes are called a *recessive mutation*.
- Recessive mutations typically generate *loss-of-function* allele.
- Some dominant mutations that interfere with the wild type allele function in heterozygous condition are called *dominant-negative* mutations.
- Some dominant mutations that generate a novel function for that gene product are called *gain-of-function* mutations.
- The phenomenon of multiple effects of a single gene is called pleiotropism and such genes are called *pleiotropic genes*.

Penetrance and Expressivity

- The ability of a given gene or gene combination to be expressed phenotypically to any degree is called *penetrance*. A trait through penetrance may be quite variable in its phenotypic expression.
- The degree of the effect produced by a penetrant genotype is called *expressivity*.
- Penetrance depends on genotype while expressivity depends on environmental condition. For example, polydactyly in feet or hand only is penetrance while its variation at different temperature is expressivity.

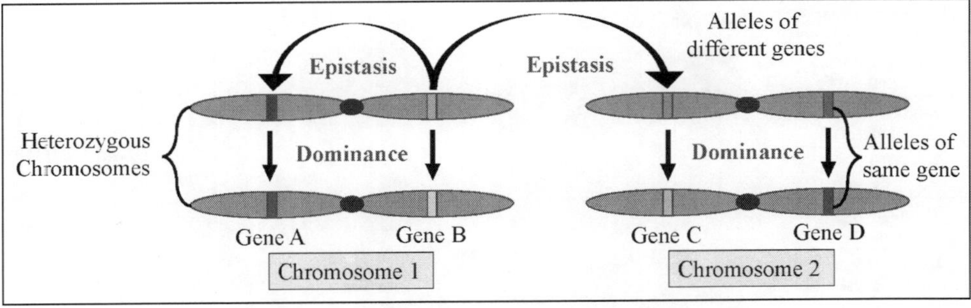

Figure 7.3: Diagrammatic Representation of Inter-allelic (Epistasis) and Intra-allelic (Dominance) Gene Interaction.

Epistatic Gene Interaction

- The gene or locus that has an overriding effect on another gene present at a different locus is called an *epistatic gene* while the gene that gets suppressed by the epistatic gene is called a *hypostatic gene* and this phenomenon is called *epistasis*.

☆ Dominance is intra-allelic gene suppression which means the allele of a gene suppresses the expression of an allele of the same gene while epistasis is inter-allelic gene suppression where the allele of a gene suppresses the expression of an allele from another gene.

Kinds of Epistasis

1. Dominant Epistasis

When out of two genes, the dominant allele (X) of one gene masked the activity of the allele of another gene (Y) and expressed itself phenotypically, then gene X is called epistatic to the gene Y. Because the dominant allele X can express itself both in the presence of either Y or y allele, therefore such type of epistasis is called *dominant epistasis*. The phenotypic ratio of dihybrid cross in dominant epistasis modifies from 9:3:3:1 to 12:3:1.

2. Recessive Epistasis

When recessive alleles of one gene (aa) mask the expression of alleles of another gene locus (BB, Bb, bb), the phenomenon is called *recessive epistasis*. The phenotypic ratio of dihybrid cross in recessive epistasis modifies to 9:3:4.

3. Duplicate Recessive Genes or Complementary Genes

In this case, both gene loci have homozygous recessive allele, and both produce an identical phenotype. Both dominant alleles when present together, complement each other, and called *complementary genes* and produce a different phenotype. The phenotypic ratio of dihybrid cross in complimentary genes modifies to 9:7.

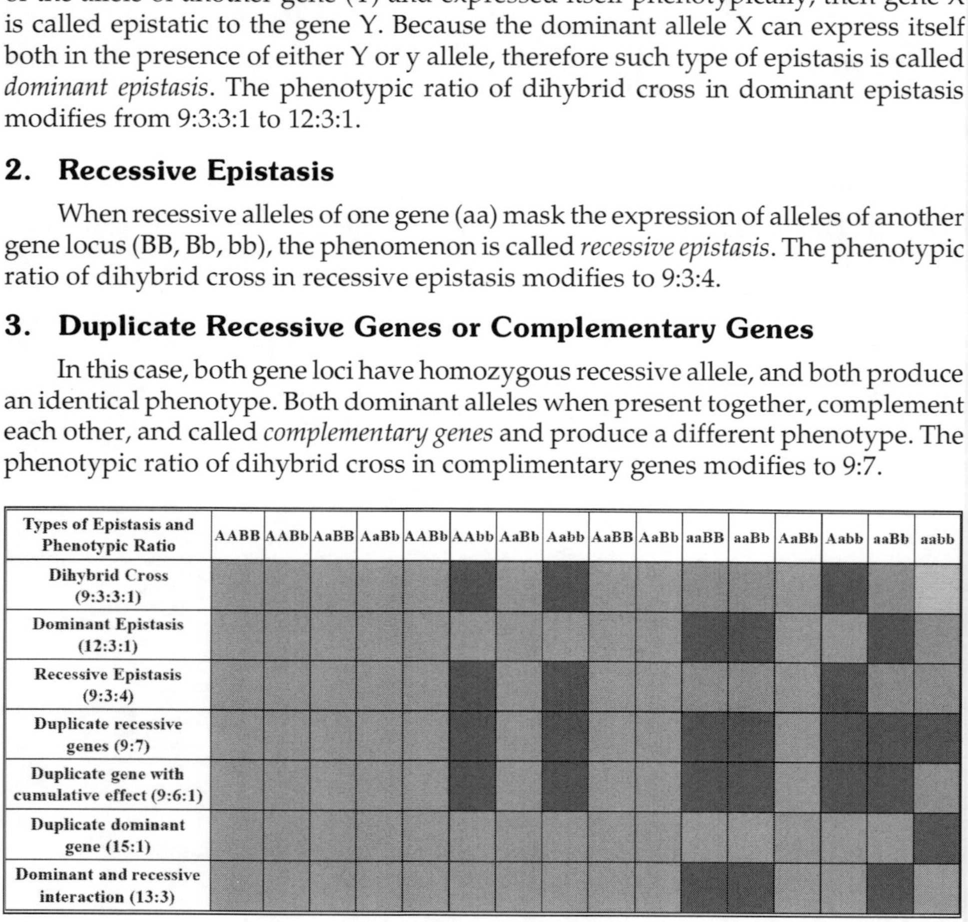

Types of Epistasis and Phenotypic Ratio	AABB	AABb	AaBB	AaBb	AABb	AAbb	AaBb	Aabb	AaBB	AaBb	aaBB	aaBb	AaBb	Aabb	aaBb	aabb
Dihybrid Cross (9:3:3:1)																
Dominant Epistasis (12:3:1)																
Recessive Epistasis (9:3:4)																
Duplicate recessive genes (9:7)																
Duplicate gene with cumulative effect (9:6:1)																
Duplicate dominant gene (15:1)																
Dominant and recessive interaction (13:3)																

Figure 7.4: Graphical Representation of Phenotypic Ratios from different Types of Epistatic Gene Interactions.

4. Duplicate Genes with the Cumulative Effect

In this case, dominant condition at either locus, but not both, produces the same phenotype because those phenotypic traits depend on the dominant allele of two gene loci. Here the phenotypic ratio of dihybrid cross modifies to 9:6:1.

5. Duplicate Dominant Genes

In this case, the dominant allele of both genes produces the same phenotype without cumulative effect. Here the phenotypic ratio of dihybrid cross modifies to 15:1.

6. Dominant and Recessive Interactions

In this case, the dominant allele of one gene locus, in homo or heterozygous condition, and homozygous recessive allele (bb) of another gene locus produce the same phenotype. Here the phenotypic ratio of dihybrid cross modifies to 13:3.

Linkage

- ☆ The tendency of two or more genes that are present on the same chromosome and inherit together is known as linkage.
- ☆ These genes do not follow Mendel's law of independent assortment and tend to stay together in the same combination of their parents.
- ☆ Since heredity unit number is much larger than the number of chromosomes, therefore each chromosome must contain many genes.
- ☆ *T.H. Morgan* proposed the theory of linkage by using the strong genetic tools of the *Drosophila* model system.

There are three key points in the theory of linkage.

- ☆ The genes are present in a linear fashion on chromosomes.
- ☆ The genes showing linkage are situated on the same chromosomes and remain bound by chromosomal material during the process of inheritance.
- ☆ The distance between the linked genes determines the strength of linkage as closely located genes have strong linkage while widely located genes have weak linkage.

Types of Linkage

- ☆ *Complete linkage*- If the parental combination of characters appears together for two or more generations continuously and regularly. Here genes are in very close proximity.
- ☆ *Incomplete linkage*: Here homologous non-sister chromatids may exchange segments of varying length with one another during the meiotic prophase. This phenomenon is called *crossing over*.
- ☆ The linked genes which are widely located on chromosomes and have chances of separation by crossing over are called incomplete linkage genes and the phenomenon is called *incomplete linkage*.

☆ *Linkage group*: All the linked genes of a chromosome form a linkage group. Thus, the number of haploid chromosomes = Number of linkage groups.

Female human = 22 pairs autosomes + 1 pair sex chromosome
= 22 autosomal linkage groups + 1 X chromosome linkage group
= 23 linkage groups

Male human = 22 pairs autosomes + 2 heteromorphic sex chromosomes
= 22 autosomal linkage groups + 1 X chromosome linkage group + 1 Y chromosome linkage group
= 24 linkage groups

Crossing Over

☆ Crossing over is a process that produces new combinations of genes by interchanging corresponding segments between non-sister chromatids of homologous chromosomes.

☆ The crossing over could be single, double, or multiple times on the same chromosome.

☆ Crossing over can happen in somatic cells during mitotic cell division while in germinal cells it happens during meiotic cell division.

☆ *Somatic crossing over*- Crossing over that occurs in somatic cells of the body during mitotic cell division is known as somatic or mitotic crossing over. This is a very rare incidence and reported to happen in *Drosophila* and *Aspergillus nidulans*.

☆ *Germinal crossing over*- Crossing over that occurs in the germinal cell during meiotic cell division is known as germinal or meiotic crossing over. This is a universal phenomenon with great genetic importance. However, male *Drosophila* and female *Bombyx mori* has no crossing over. The four major steps in germline crossing over are homologous chromosome condensation, Synapsis, crossing over and terminalization.

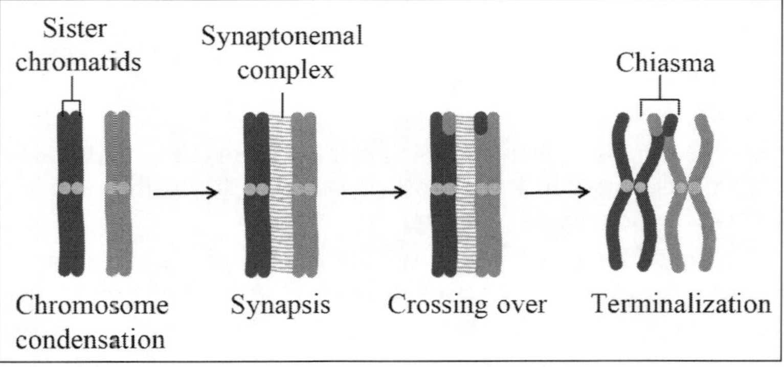

Figure 7.5: Diagrammatic Representation of Chromosomal Arrangement at different Stages of Crossing Over.

DNA as the Genetic Material

- Several attempts have been made to characterize the molecular nature of genes. Initially, it was thought that the proteins associated with chromosomes have genetic information because nucleic acids are too simple to carry genetic information, the *tetranucleotide hypothesis*.
- The first conclusive evidence that supports the DNA is genetic material was from transformation experiments by *Fredrick Griffith* in 1928.
- In his experiment, *Griffith* transfected the mice with virulent and avirulent *Diplococcus Pneumoniae* and found that mice suffered and died only with the virulent strain. When he infected mice with heat-killed virulent form, they did not suffer but when he infects with the mixture of the heat-killed virulent strain and live nonvirulent strain the mice suffered from pneumonia and died. These mice have both virulent and avirulent strains in their body which suggests that heat-killed strain transforms the avirulent strain into virulent strain.
- Latter three scientists *Oswald Avery*, *Colin MacLeod* and *Maclyn McCarty* in 1944 purified the DNA and then demonstrated that the transformation of nonvirulent strain to virulent strain occurs due to DNA transfection.
- Later in 1952, two scientist *Alfred Hershey* and *Martha Chase* demonstrated that DNA injected by phage particle into a bacterium contains all the information required to synthesize progeny phage particle. They radioactively labelled both DNA and protein with $^{32}PO_4$ and $^{35}SO_4$, respectively and examined the phage progeny after infection. They found that phage progeny carried only labelled ^{32}P and not ^{35}S. This experiment confirms that only DNA and not protein carries all the genetic information and hence DNA is the sole genetic material.
- The term gene was given by Danish botanist *Wilhelm Johannsen* in 1911 to define the mendelian hereditary factor.
- The gene is the conceptual hereditary unit that transmits characters from one generation to the next generation.
- The place where a gene is present on the chromosome is called the *locus*.
- Morgan proposed that genes are just like beads and chromosomes acts as a string for those beads.
- Muller classified the mutant genes based on their comparison to wild type genes. Genes with relatively less effective phenotypic expression are called *hypomorphs* while genes with very less effect are called *amorphs*.

Sex Chromosomes and Sex Determination

Sex-linked Inheritance

- Mendel's law of genetics equally applies to both males and females because all the genes he analysed were present on autosomes.

- However, genes that are present on sex chromosomes do not follow Mendel's law of inheritance.
- The recessive genes present on the X chromosome in males express phenotypically because the Y chromosome has no dominant allele of that gene to rescue its phenotype.
- The genes that are present on the X chromosome are called *X-linked genes* while genes that are exclusively present on the Y chromosomes are called *Y-linked genes* or holandric genes.
- Inheritance of genes present on these sex chromosomes is called *sex-linked inheritance*.

1. X-linked Inheritance

- X-linked genes show their phenotype in males irrespective of whether they are dominant or recessive.
- They show the criss-cross pattern of inheritance *i.e.*, X-linked recessive genes transmitted from P1 male parent to F2 male progeny, through its F1 heterozygous female progeny which acts as a carrier.
- There are several examples of X-linked recessive genes like Eye colour in *Drosophila*, Red-green colour blindness (Daltonism), Haemophilia, and Duchenne muscular dystrophy in human *etc.*
- In birds, moth and butterflies, females are heterozygotic ZW while males are homozygotic ZZ. Here also the sex-linked genes follow the criss-cross pattern. A typical example of Z-linked recessive gene inheritance is wing colour in Plymouth rock hen.

2. Y-linked Inheritance

- Genes in the nonhomologous region of the Y chromosomes pass directly from male to male.
- A typical example of Y-linked gene inheritance in human is hypertrichosis that has excessive development of hairs on ear pinna.

Sex-limited Genes

- These are autosomal genes, but their phenotypic expression is determined by the presence or absence of one of the sex hormones.
- This phenotypic effect is limited to individuals of one sex. For example, beard development and male voice in male human and cock feathering in male chicken.

Sex-Influenced Genes

- The expression of sex-influenced genes is manipulated by the sex of the bearer. In this case, both male and female individuals may be similar for a particular trait but give a different phenotypic expression of the same trait.

☆ A typical example of sex influenced gene inheritance is baldness in human.

Table 7.2: Table Showing Male- and Female-Specific Phenotypes of Sex Influenced Genes Responsible for Baldness in Human

Genotype	*Male*	*Female*
BB	Bald	Bald
Bb	Bald	Normal
bb	Normal	Normal

Chromosome Mapping

Linkage Mapping

☆ The first linkage map has been constructed for *Drosophila* by *Sturtevant* and *C. B. Bridges*. Linkage mapping in maize has been done by *Barbara McClintock*.

☆ A diagrammatic graphical presentation of relative distances between linked genes of a chromosome is called *linkage map* or *genetic map* and this method is called *genetic mapping*.

☆ Linkage group can be determined by defining the traits that always remain together.

☆ An arbitrary unit called a *map unit* has been assigned to describe the distance between genes from the linkage group.

1 per cent crossing over = 1 map unit

100 per cent crossing over = 100 map unit = 1 Morgan

1 per cent crossing over = 1 centimorgan (cM)

10 per cent crossing over = 1 decimorgan (dM)

Cytological Mapping and Gene Structure

☆ Polytene chromosomes are the giant interphase stage of chromosomes that are formed by multiple rounds of endoreplication without chromosomal segregation.

☆ Polytene chromosomes of *Drosophila melanogaster* was sketched by *C. B. Bridges* in 1935.

☆ *Bridges* divide the arms of salivary gland polythene chromosomes into 102 *divisions* designated by a number from 1 to 102.

☆ Each of the five main arms X, 2L, 2R, 3L, and 3R contains 20 divisions while the short chromosome 4 contains only two divisions.

☆ The divisions are divided further into 6 subdivisions, each designated with capital letters from A to F.

☆ Thus, each band of salivary gland chromosomes can be identified by giving the division number, subdivision, and the number of the band starting from the beginning of the subdivision.

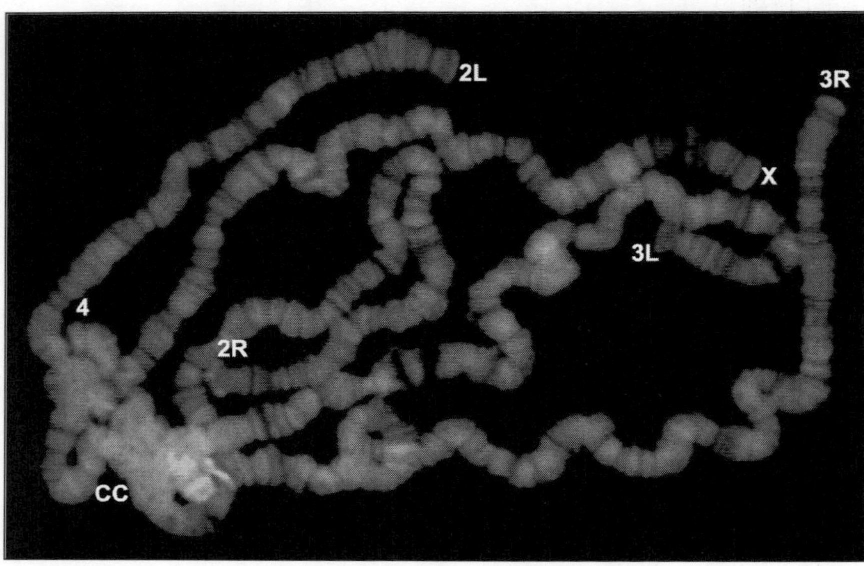

Figure 7.6: Polytene Chromosomes from 3rd Instar Larval Salivary Gland of *Drosophila melanogaster*. The chromosomes were stained with DAPI and image was captured under fluorescent microscope. Different chromosomal arms are labelled with X, 2L, 2R, 3L, 3R and 4. Chromocenter is labelled as CC.

Sex Determination

1. Chromosomal Basis of Sex Determination

☆ The X-chromosome was first observed by a German biologist, *Hermann Henking* in 1891 during the spermatogenesis in male bug and was described as X-body.

☆ The chromosomal theory of sex determination was proposed by *Edmund Wilson* and *Nettie Stevens* (1902-1905). They named the X and Y chromosomes as sex-chromosomes or allosomes and other chromosomes of the cell as autosomes.

☆ Sex chromosomes carry genes that are responsible for the determination of sex. X-chromosomes carries female determining genes and Y-chromosomes has male determining genes.

☆ The number of X and Y chromosomes determines the female or male sex of the individual while autosomes carry genes for the somatic characters.

A. Heterogametic Males

- **XX–XY type:** In most insects including *Drosophila* and human beings the females possess two homomorphic sex chromosomes XX, while males contain two heteromorphic sex chromosomes XY. Hence the males produce two types of gametes/sperms, either with X-chromosome or with Y-chromosome and therefore they are called Heterogametic.
- **XX–XO type:** In roundworms and some insects, the females have two sex chromosomes XX, while males have only one sex chromosomes X. There is no second sex chromosome. Therefore, the males are designated as XO. The females are homogametic because they produce only one type of eggs. The males are heterogametic with half the male gametes carrying X-chromosome while the other half are without X-chromosome.

B. Heterogametic Females

- **ZW-ZZ type:** In birds and some reptiles, the males are represented as ZZ and the females are ZW. Here males are homogametic while females are heterogametic.
- **ZO-ZZ type:** Here females have only one sex chromosome ZO while the males have two homomorphic sex chromosomes ZZ. In this case, also females are heterogametic while males are homogametic.

2. Genetic Basis of Sex Determination

- The gene-based sex determination was defined in *Drosophila* by *C. B. Bridges* in 1921.
- He suggests that the sex of an individual depends on the ratio of the number of X chromosomes and autosomes.
- If the ratio of the number of X chromosomes to the number of sets of autosomes is 1 then that would be *female* and if the ratio is 0.5 the organism would be *male*. If the ratio is more than one the fly would become *super female* while if the ratio is less than 0.5 then flies would become *supermale*. If the ratio is between 0.5 to 1.0 the organism would become the *intersex*.

Table 7.3: Table Showing Genotype (Left), the Ratio of Number of X Chromosomes to Sets of Autosome (Middle) and their Corresponding Phenotype (Right) in *Drosophila melanogaster*

Chromosomes	Ratio	Phenotypes
XXXAA	1.5	Super female
XXAA	1	Normal female
XXAAA	0.67	Intersex
XAA	0.5	Normal male
XAAA	0.33	Super male

- *Gynandromorphs* are individuals with a mosaic of male and female genotype in which a part of the body express male characters whereas another part of the body express female characters.
- These individuals in *Drosophila* are formed due to the permanent loss of one X chromosome during early embryonic stage of the cell division.
- The portion of the body that has AAXX chromosomes will make female while AAXO will make male. The presence of the Y chromosome has no role in determining the sex of *Drosophila* and it only requires during spermatogenesis and thus fertility.
- Human have XX-XY type of sex determination but here Y chromosome contains most of the sex-determining gene and thus acts as the determiner of sex and fertility of males.
- Any alteration in human chromosomal pattern induces multiple abnormalities called "Syndrome". For instance, Turner's syndrome with XO chromosome is sterile female while Klinefelter's syndrome with XXY chromosomes is sterile male.

Dosage Compensation

- The term dosage compensation was coined by *Muller* in 1932.
- This is a process to equalize the expression of sex-linked and autosomal genes in the heterogametic sex.
- Dosage compensation in different organism occurs either due to hyperactivation or hypoactivation of the X chromosome.
- In mammals, including human, the homogametic females with XX chromosomes have one X chromosome characteristically inactivated. These condensed chromosomes are called *Barr body* after the name of their discoverer *Murray Barr* in 1949.
- *Lyon* in 1972 proposed that the number of Barr bodies are one less than the total number of X chromosomes and this inactivation is a very random phenomenon between maternal and paternal X chromosomes. This is popularly known as *Lyon's hypothesis*.
- Lyon reported that the presence of one Barr body in normal female (XX) and male (XXY), two Barr bodies in male (XXXY) and metafemale (XXX). Thus, in any case, only one X chromosome is active in such organism.
- Dosage compensation in *Drosophila* happens with hyperactivation of one X chromosome in male while female has normal expression of both X chromosomes.

REFERENCES

1. B. Alberts; A. Johnson; J. Lewis; M. Raff; K. Roberts and P. Walter. 2015. *Molecular Biology of the cell*, 6th ed., Garland, New York, USA.

2. D. P. Snustad and M. J. Simmons. 2003. *Principles of Genetics*, 3rd ed., John Wiley and Sons, Inc., New Jersey, USA.

3. P. S. Verma and V. K. Agarwal. 2012. *Cell Biology, Genetics, Molecular Biology, Evolution and Ecology*, Multicolour ed., S. Chand and Company Ltd., New Delhi, India.

4. R. H. Tamarin. 2014. *Principles of Genetics*, 7th edition, Tata McGraw-Hill Education, Uttar Pradesh, India

5. W. S. Klug; M. R. Cummings; C. A. Spencer and M. A. Palladino. 2012. *Concepts of Genetics*, 10th ed., Pearson Education, Inc., California, USA.

Chapter 8

Recombinant DNA Technology

Bhuvnesh Yadav* and Manish Shandilya

Department of Chemistry,
Biochemistry and Forensic Science, Amity School of Applied Sciences,
Amity University Haryana, Gurugram, Haryana, India
****email: bhuvneshyadav@gmail.com***

ABSTRACT

This book chapter will provide the basic knowledge of gene, their types, structure and expression in eukaryotes and prokaryotes to the students. The students will be able to explain the concept of genetic engineering and the essentials for recombinant DNA production including DNA modifying enzymes (types and utility), vectors (for both prokaryotes and eukaryotes), host etc. They will understand the procedure of genetic engineering (selection, modification, and screening), the construction of gene and cDNA libraries, techniques involved in genetic modification like sequencing methods, PCR, NGS, mutagenesis etc.

Keywords: *Gene, Genetic engineering, Enzymes, PCR, Vectors, DNA sequencing, Mapping.*

1. Concept of Gene

1.1 Gene

- ☆ The **gene** is the basic unit of genetic information. Gene usually represents the genetic information transcribed into a single RNA molecule, which is in turn translated into a single protein.
- ☆ Genes are located on **chromosomes**, and the region of the chromosome where a particular gene is found is called the **locus** of that gene.
- ☆ Genes can be classified into two functional categories: structural genes and regulatory genes.

1. ***Structural genes*** (*Protein coding genes*) code for polypeptides or RNAs needed for the normal metabolic activities of the cell, *e.g.*, enzymes, structural proteins, transporters, and receptors, among others.
2. ***Regulatory genes*** code for proteins whose function is to control the expression of structural genes. Regarding molecular composition both classes of genes are similar.

Regulatory Sequences Associated with Genes

a. **Promoter** (P): Site for starting transcription, binds RNA polymerase, and a specific start point for transcription.
b. **Transcriptional unit** (TC): The DNA region that is copied into RNA. Within the transcriptional unit, there may be regulatory sites for translation From T_L (start site) to t_C (stop signal).
c. **Upstream and downstream sequences**: Involved in the control of gene expression.

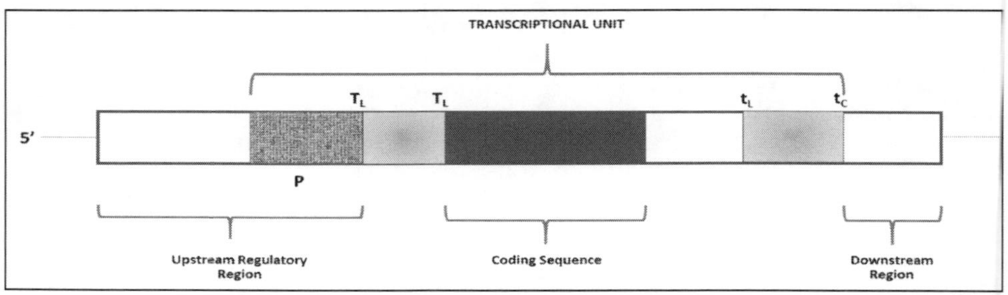

- ✰ The exact chromosomal gene location is defined by specific sequences for the start and termination of its transcription.
- ✰ The human genome contains approximately 25, 000 protein coding genes, which represents the **phenotype**.
- ✰ **Alleles:** Different forms of the same gene are known as alleles. Different varieties of the same gene, resulting in different phenotypic characteristics, are called **alleles.**

1.2 Gene Structure

1.2.1 Prokaryotes

Genes are found in groups called operons. The **operon** is a cluster of genes that are related and under the control of a single promoter/regulatory region, *e.g.*, the *lac* operon.

Lac operon: in lac operon, there are **three structural** genes within an operon that code for proteins, an upstream control region which has the **promoter** and a regulatory site called the **operator**.

The lac operon consists of:

- ✰ **Regulatory gene *i*** –codes for the repressor protein.

- *z* **gene** –codes for beta-galactosidase which catalyzes the hydrolysis of lactose into glucose and galactose.
- *y* **gene** –codes for permease which regulates the lactose permeability in the cell.
- *a* **gene** –codes for transacetylase which assists the enzyme beta-galactosidase.

These genes help in **lactose metabolism** and lactose acts as an inducer. When lactose is provided to bacteria, the regulatory gene gets activated. The inducer binds to the repressor protein and renders it inactive which allows transcription of the operon.

1.2.2 Eukaryotes

Gene regulation in eukaryotes is regulated by **transcriptional activators and repressors**. The repressors bind to specific DNA sequences and inhibit transcription. In eukaryotes, transcription involves several steps. It occurs in both, nucleus (transcription) and cytoplasm (translation).

- Lac operon contains genes involved in metabolism.
- The genes are expressed only when lactose is present, and glucose is absent.
- The operon is turned on and off in response to the glucose and lactose levels: catabolite activator protein and lac repressor.
- The lac repressor blocks the transcription of the operon. In the presence of lactose, it stops acting as a repressor.
- Catabolite activator protein activates the transcription of the operon, only when glucose levels are low.

2. DNA Modifying Enzymes

The **enzymes** present in eukaryotic and prokaryotic cells, which help in the maintenance of the integrity of their genome by repairing and controlling the damage caused by internal and external factors. Following are the DNA modifying enzymes:

1. Nuclease
2. Restriction enzymes
3. DNA polymerase
4. Ligase
5. Alkaline phosphatase

2.1 Nucleases

- Nuclease enzyme *hydrolyses the phosphodiester bond* on DNA strand and creates 3′-OH group and 5′-P group.
- Nuclease cut DNA on either side of distortion caused by thymine dimers or intercalating agents.

☆ The gap is filled by DNA polymerase and the strand is joined by DNA ligase.

Nucleases are of two types:

1. **Endonuclease** recognizes specific base sequences (restriction sites) within DNA or RNA molecule and cleaves internal phosphodiester bonds within a DNA molecule (*e.g.*, EcoRI, Hind III, Bam HI, *etc.*).
2. **Exonuclease** catalyzes the hydrolysis of terminal nucleotides from the end of DNA or RNA molecule either 5′to 3′ direction or 3′ to 5′ direction (*e.g.*, exonuclease I, exonuclease II, *etc.*).

2.2 Restriction Enzymes

☆ A restriction enzyme is a nuclease enzyme that **cleaves DNA sequence** at random or specific recognition sites known as restriction sites.

☆ In bacteria, restriction enzymes form a combined system **(restriction + modification system**) with modification enzymes that methylate the bacterial DNA.

☆ **Methylation of bacterial DNA** at the recognition sequence typically protects the own DNA of the bacteria from being cleaved by the restriction enzyme.

2.2.1 Classification of Restriction Endonucleases

There are three major classes of restriction endonucleases based on the types of sequences recognized, the nature of the cut made in the DNA, and the enzyme structure:

a. Type I restriction enzymes
b. Type II restriction enzymes
c. Type III restriction enzymes

a. Type I Restriction Enzymes

☆ These enzymes have both *restriction and modification activities.*

☆ Cleavage occurs approximately *1000 bp away* from the recognition site and the recognition site is *asymmetrical*.

☆ Restriction depends upon the methylation status of the target DNA.

☆ These enzymes require *S-adenosylmethionine* (*SAM*), *ATP*, and *magnesium ions* (Mg^{2+}) for activity.

☆ These enzymes are composed of mainly **three subunits**, a specificity subunit that determines the DNA recognition site, a restriction subunit, and a modification subunit.

b. Type II Restriction Enzymes

☆ *Restriction and modification are mediated by separate enzymes*, so it is possible to cleave DNA in the absence of modification.

- ☆ Cleavage of nucleotide sequence *occurs at the restriction site.*
- ☆ These enzymes recognize rotationally *symmetrical sequences* (palindromic sequence).
- ☆ They require Mg^{2+} as a cofactor and *ATP* is not needed for their activity.
- ☆ These enzymes are widely used for *mapping and reconstructing DNA* in vitro.

c. *Type III Restriction Enzymes*

- ☆ These enzymes *recognize and methylate* the same DNA sequence but cleave 24–26 bp away.
- ☆ *Cleave only one strand*. Two recognition sites in opposite orientation are needed for cleavage of double-strand.
- ☆ They have *two subunits;* one subunit is responsible for the recognition and modification of DNA sequence and the second subunit has nuclease action.
- ☆ They require Mg^{2+} *ions and ATP* for DNA cleavage.

2.3 DNA Polymerase

- ☆ DNA polymerase enzyme synthesizes nucleotide complementary to the template strand.
- ☆ It adds nucleotide to the free 32 OH end and helps in the elongation of the strand.
- ☆ It also helps to fill the gap in double-stranded DNA.
- ☆ Most commonly used DNA polymerases: for gene cloning- DNA polymerase-I (isolated from E. coli), for PCR amplification- Taq polymerase (isolated from *Thermus aquaticus*).

2.4 Ligase

- ☆ Ligase enzyme catalyzes the joining of two large molecules of DNA by forming a new chemical bond.
- ☆ It joins two DNA strands to generate the chimeric DNA and incorporate of foreign DNA in the vector.
- ☆ The enzyme requires *ATP or* NAD^+ as a cofactor to catalyze ligation reaction.
- ☆ *Ligase-AMP complex* is generated with ATP and this complex binds with 3′ and 5′ end of DNA having nick and brings them together.
- ☆ AMP is released and phosphodiester linkage is formed between 3′ and 5′ end to seal the cleavage.

2.5 Alkaline Phosphatase

- ✰ The enzyme that removes the phosphate group from the 5′ ends of the DNA molecule.
- ✰ Alkaline phosphatase digests linear plasmid containing cohesive ends on both sites with phosphate tends to re-circularize.
- ✰ Alkaline phosphatase is used to remove the 5′ terminal phosphate group to prevent circularization.

2.6 End Modification Enzymes

- ✰ The enzymes that change the end of a DNA molecule, *e.g.* Terminal Deoxynucleotidyl Transferase (Tdt).
- ✰ This enzyme is involved in homopolymer tailing by making cohesive ends.
- ✰ It adds nucleotides on the 3′-OH termini of a ds DNA molecule. It is called homopolymer because of the presence of only one type of deoxyribonucleotide.

2.7 Polynucleotide Kinase

- ✰ Its action is opposite to alkaline phosphatase, it adds phosphate at 5′ ends, so it is mostly used in the end-labeling of DNA molecule.

3. Concept of Vectors

3.1 Vector

Vector can be defined as a DNA molecule in which a fragment of foreign DNA can be introduced, and which can replicate in the desired host organism.

It can be classified into cloning vectors and expression vectors.

Cloning vectors- these are the vectors that are used for cloning of foreign DNA, whereas.

Expression vectors- are made so that the DNA is transcribed into RNA and then it is translated into protein.

Properties of a good vector are

a. Must have an **origin of replication (ori),** which makes vector capable of autonomous replication independent of the host genome.

b. The vector should be small DNA molecules, to facilitate isolation and handling.

c. It should have some **selectable marker** that helps in the detection of vectors in a host cell.

d. It should have at least one **unique restriction endonuclease recognition site** to enable DNA to be inserted during the production of recombinants.

3.2 Types of Cloning Vectors

1. Plasmids
2. Bacteriophages: bacteriophage λ (Lambda), M13
3. Cosmids
4. Yeast artificial chromosomes (YAC)
5. Bacterial artificial chromosomes (BAC)
6. P1 Artificial Chromosomes (PAC)
7. Mammalian Artificial Chromosomes (MAC)
8. Vectors for plants

3.2.1 Plasmids

- Plasmids are extrachromosomal circular, double-stranded DNA molecules.
- Plasmids occur naturally in bacteria, nuclei of yeast, and some higher eukaryotic cells, existing in a parasitic or symbiotic relationship with their host cell.
- These encode enzymes that provide antibiotic resistance.
- The size of the plasmid genome ranges from a few thousand bps to more than 100 kilobases (kb).
- *E. coli*-based plasmids are most frequently used in recombinant DNA technology.

  Plasmids can be classified into two groups:

  1. **Conjugative** plasmids (mediate their own transfer between bacteria by the process of conjugation, have *tra* (transfer) and *mob* (mobilizing) regions).
  2. **Non-conjugative** plasmids (not self-transmissible, mobilized by a conjugation-proficient plasmid if their *mob* region is functional).
- Plasmids can be modified by a reduction in size (~3 kb), inserting multiple cloning sites and restriction enzyme sites, to optimize their use as vectors in DNA cloning.
- *Examples:* pBR322, pAT153.

3.2.2 Bacteriophages

- Bacteriophages/phages are viruses that infect bacteria (bacteria eaters).
- Bacteriophages are classified into three main groups based on their structure: **(1) tailless, (2) head with a tail, (3) filamentous**.
- These may contain single or double-stranded DNA/RNA as genetic material which is enclosed in a protein head called **capsid.**
- Depending on their life cycles phages can be classified as **virulent** or **temperate.**

- ❒ **Lytic growth cycle**: When a phage enters a bacterial cell, produces more phages, and kills the host cell (**virulent).**
- ❒ **Lysogenic cycle**: When a phage integrates into the chromosome forming a prophage and remains in a quiescent state without killing the cell (**temperate**).

✫ Most used bacteriophages as cloning vectors: λ (Lambda), M13.

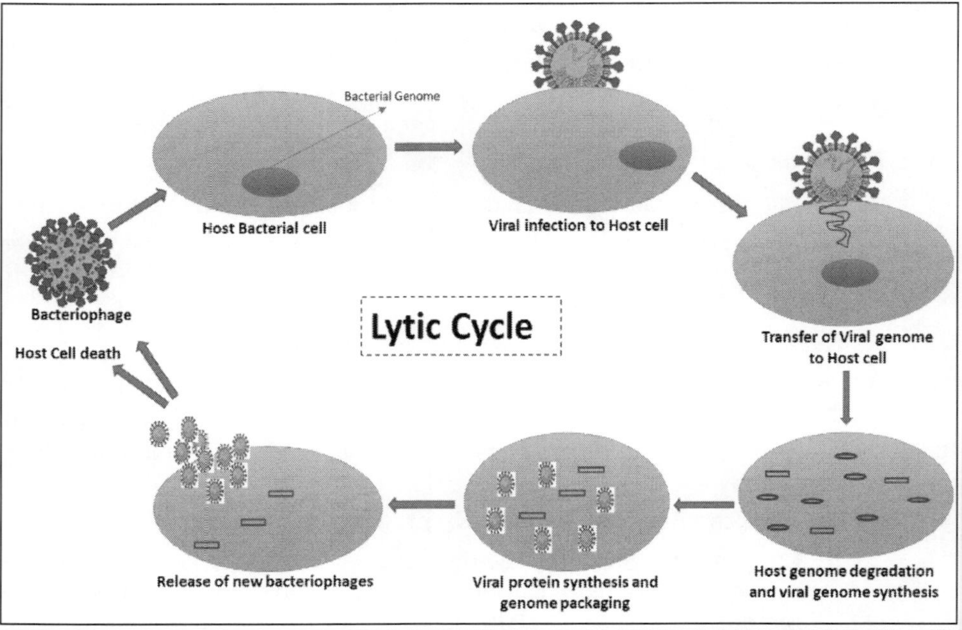

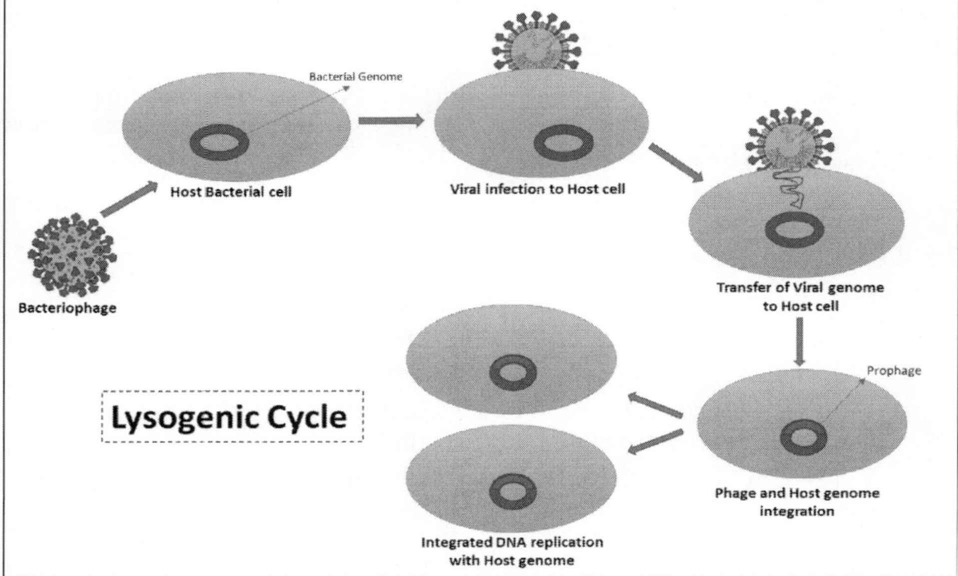

3.2.2.1 Bacteriophage λ (Lambda)

- ☆ Phage λ consists of a head (containing 48.5 kb double-stranded DNA linear genome and single-stranded *cos*) and a long flexible tail.
- ☆ The cos site helps in the circularization of linear DNA inside a cell and acts as a recognition site for endonucleases.
- ☆ It can incorporate 20 kb size of foreign DNA fragments, which is significantly larger than fragments suitable for plasmids (~10 kb).
- ☆ The infection process is about a thousand times more efficient than a transformation of bacterial cells with plasmid vectors.
- ☆ Such vectors have two main classes: (1) **insertion vectors** and (2) **replacement/substitution vectors.**

Insertional Lambda Vectors

The non-essential part that is present is deleted and the fragments are ligated, at least one unique restriction site is present which accommodates the new inserted DNA. The insert size of DNA can be 8-12 kb, it also depends upon the non-essential part deleted.

Replacement Vector

A stuffer fragment is contained by two identical restriction sites, the foreign DNA is inserted by deleting the stuffer fragment. DNA up to 23kb of length can be cloned. It is mainly used in making genomic libraries.

3.2.2.2 Bacteriophage M13

- ☆ The Restriction fragment is like a plasmid and can be isolated and manipulated using the same techniques.
- ☆ It is a filamentous bacteriophage that has 6407 nucleotide long single-stranded DNA.
- ☆ Unlike phage λ, M13 does not have any non-essential genes.
- ☆ Phage M13 particles are released out without lysing cell membrane.

3.2.3 Cosmids

- ☆ A cosmid vector is produced by inserting the cos sequence from λ-phage DNA into a small *E. coli* plasmid vector.
- ☆ Cosmid vectors contain all the essential components found in plasmids.
- ☆ Recombinant plasmids containing inserted fragments up to 45 kb can be introduced into host cells.
- ☆ The injected DNA does not encode any λ-phage proteins, no viral particles form in infected cells.

3.2.4 Yeast Artificial Chromosomes (YAC)

- ☆ YACs are constructed by ligating the components required for replication and segregation of natural yeast chromosomes to very large fragments of target DNA, which may be more than one Mb in length.

- YAC vectors contain *two telomeric sequences, one centromere, one autonomously replicating sequence,* and genes that act as *selectable markers* in yeast.
- YAC selectable markers usually do not confer resistance to antibiotic substances.
- YACs have a limitation that these can accommodate very large DNA fragments they may be unstable, *i.e.,* they often lose parts of the fragments during propagation in yeast.
- Based on replication mode yeast vectors are grouped into 4 classes :
  - Yeast Episomal Plasmids (YEP)
  - Yeast Integrative Plasmids(YIP)
  - Yeast Centromeric Plasmids (YCP)
  - Yeast Replicating Plasmids (YRP)
- Also called shuttle vectors as these can replicate in both *E.coli* and *S. cerevisiae.*

3.2.5 Bacterial Artificial Chromosomes (BAC)

- BAC vectors are developed to prevent problems encountered with YACs and are based on the fertility factor (F factor) of *E. coli.*
- The F plasmid, ~ 100 kb circular double-stranded DNA is present in *E. coli* with only 1-2 copies.
- The synthetic BAC vectors have ~7.5 kb double-stranded DNA circles with replication origin (oriS) and the gene repE of the F plasmid, which provide proper initiation and orientation of replication of the BAC vector. Also contain a selectable marker gene and a cloning site for the insertion of target fragment DNA.
- These vectors contain up to 300–350 kb of insert sequence.
- These can be stably propagated and replicated in *E. coli,* are easily introduced into their host cell by transformation.
- A large number of vectors can be produced in a short time due to the fast growth of *E. coli* and are simple to purify.

3.2.6 P1 Artificial Chromosome (PAC)

- PAC vectors permit the cloning of larger DNA fragments.
- The basic elements of PAC vectors are derived from P1 (temperate phage with ~100 kb long genome).
- PACs are circular molecules that are replicated in bacteria, and their preparation is easy as that of plasmids.

3.2.7 Mammalian Artificial Chromosomes (MAC)

- MACs are the potential artificial chromosome for gene therapy of humans.
- For gene therapy, a gene including its promoters and all the control elements is needed in human DNA fragments.

- This gene should be introduced into the target cells efficiently and must be stably maintained inside the nucleus.
- The DNA introduced in the genome should be expressed properly without interfering with the function of other genes.
- Such a large artificial human chromosome, if (1-10 Mb) is stable upto 100 generations.

3.2.8 TOPO Cloning

- A technique in which DNA fragments can be cloned into specific vectors without DNA Ligase.
- Taq polymerase has a non-template-dependent terminal transferase activity that adds a single deoxyadenosine (A) to the 3′-end of the PCR products.
- The technique utilizes the inherent biological activity of DNA topoisomerase I.
- Topoisomerase I specifically recognizes DNA sequence 5′-(C/T)CCTT-3′. During replication, the enzyme digests DNA specifically at this sequence, unwinds the DNA, and re-ligates it again at the 3′ phosphate group of the thymidine base.
- TOPO vectors are designed in such a way that they carry this specific sequence 5′-(C/T) CCTT-3′ at the two linear ends.
- The linear vector DNA already has the topoisomerase enzyme covalently attached to both of its strands' free 3′ ends.
- The TA TOPO cloning technique relies on the ability of adenine (A) and thymine (T) (complementary base pairs) on different DNA fragments to hybridize and, in the presence of ligase or topoisomerase, become ligated together.
- Polymerases or restriction enzymes that produce blunt ends can also be used for TOPO cloning.

3.2.9 Vectors for Plants

- Plasmids which are present in Agrobacterium species (Ti plasmid- *Agrobacterium tumefaciens* and Ri plasmid - *Agrobacterium rhizogenes*).
- Ti plasmid contains ori site, T DNA segment, vir genes region (helps in transferring T DNA) and opine catabolism region (acts as nitrogen source).

4. Gene Library

Gene sequences are randomly arranged in the genome and selecting or isolating a gene is a big task especially when the genomic sequences are not known. A small portion of the genome is transcribed to give mRNA whereas a major portion remained untranscribed. There are two ways to represent genomic sequence information into the multiple small fragments in the form of a library:

1. Genomic library
2. cDNA library

4.1 Preparation of Genomic Library

A genomic library represents a complete genome in multiple clones containing small DNA fragments. Depending upon the organism and size of the genome, this library can be prepared in a bacterial vector or yeast artificial chromosome. Genomic library can be prepared by following steps:

1. Isolation of genomic DNA
2. Generation of suitable size DNA fragments
3. Cloning in a suitable vector system (depending on size)
4. Transformation in a suitable host

1. Isolation of Genomic DNA

- ☆ Cells are lysed with lysis buffer containing detergent.
- ☆ Incubate and lyse the cells with digestion buffer containing protease-K, SDS to release genomic DNA from DNA-protein complex.
- ☆ Isolate aqueous phase containing DNA with phenol: chloroform mixture. Chloroform: phenol mixture has two phases, aqueous phase, and organic phase. Phenol denatures the remaining proteins and keeps the protein in the organic phase.
- ☆ Genomic DNA present in aqueous phase is precipitated with alcohol.
- ☆ DNA is analyzed on an agarose gel.

2. Generation of Suitable Size Fragments

- ☆ Genomic DNA can be digested with restriction enzymes (*e.g.*, EcoRI, BamHI) to generate the random sizes of DNA fragments.
- ☆ The size of the DNA fragments is large enough to contain a complete genome in very few numbers of clones.

3. Cloning into the Suitable Vector

- ☆ The suitable vector can be selected based on the size of the fragment of genomic DNA and the carrying capacity of the vector.
- ☆ Vector can be digested with the same restriction enzyme and put for ligation to get a clone.

4. Transformation to get Colonies

- ☆ Post ligation, clones are transformed into a suitable host to get colonies.
- ☆ A suitable host can be a bacterial strain or yeast.

4.2 Construction of cDNA Library

A cDNA library represents mRNA population present at a particular stage in an organism into multiple clones containing small DNA fragments. It has the following steps:

1. Isolation of mRNA
2. Preparation of complementary DNA fragments
3. Cloning in a suitable vector system
4. Transformation in a suitable host

1. Isolation of mRNA

- ☆ Release of total RNA by lysis buffer or by homogenization.
- ☆ Mixing of poly-T containing beads with the total RNA preparation. Due to mutual exclusive affinity, mRNA binds to the poly-T beads.
- ☆ Wash the beads with washing buffer to remove non-specific cross contaminating species.
- ☆ Elute the mRNA from beads; its purity can be checked on a polyacrylamide gel.

2. Preparation of Complementary DNA (cDNA)

- ☆ *First-strand synthesis with a reverse transcriptase*: An oligo dT primer and reverse transcriptase are used to amplify the first strand of DNA from mRNA. Terminal transferase is used to add C nucleotides on 3 of both mRNA and the newly synthesized DNA strand.
- ☆ *Removal of RNA template:* DNA-RNA hybrid is loaded on an alkaline sucrose gradient to hydrolyze RNA.
- ☆ *Second strand synthesis*: cDNA is used as a template and oligo dG primer, reverse transcriptase, and dNTPs are used to prepare the second strand of DNA.

Differences between Genomic Library and cDNA Library

- ☆ The genomic library has both coding and non-coding regions whereas the cDNA library has only coding regions.
- ☆ The introns have been removed in the cDNA library, but the genomic library has both introns and

3. Cloning of cDNA into the Vector

- ☆ The cDNA is ligated into a suitable vector to generate clones.

4. Transformation to get Colonies

- ☆ Post ligation, clones are transformed into a suitable host to get colonies.
- ☆ A suitable host can be a bacterial strain or yeast.

4.3 Screening for Cloned DNA

There are *three criteria* to identify a particular gene from an organism:

- **DNA Hybridization-**This properties can be used to search both genomic library and cDNA library to identify the gene.
- **Expression of a particular protein with immunogenic epitope-**This property can be partially useful to screen genomic libraries due to truncation of a full gene or no expression of a gene fragment. But this approach suits well to screen cDNA clones.
- **Enzymatic-based screening-** This property exploits the ability of a protein fragment to exhibits enzymatic activity. It is useful for the screening of the cDNA library but not much for the genomic library.

4.3.1 DNA Hybridization Method

In this method desired DNA sequence can be identified by a complementary single-stranded DNA sequence called **Probe**. The steps followed for this process are given below:

1. Suitable radioactive probe preparation	
Random primer method- random primer →anneal to the template→PCR reaction→ labeling with radioactive nucleotide	***Terminal transferease***-terminal transferase enzyme will label the probe at the ends to the last nucleotide → incubated with the labeled nucleotide→ partial purification with gel filtration column will give labeled primer.

2. Replica plate preparation and blotting	
Replica plate containing clones is prepared from original genomic or cDNA library	Blotting-The clone is transferred on a nitrocellulose membrane. Cells are lysed and released DNA is denatured

3. Hybridization with a specific probe	
A labeled probe is added	Probe binds to the target DNA due to base pairing. Unbound probes are removed by washing the membrane

4. Aautoradiography
The position of labeled probe is detected by autoradiogram. The position of signal on membrane can be matched with the master plate to get location of corresponding colony.

4.3.2 Immunological Method

In this method, the specificity of the antibody towards its antigenic epitope present on the protein expressed in a particular clone is utilized for desired sequence identification. Steps for immunological screening:

1. Replica plate preparation

Replica plate containing clones is prepared from original genomic or cDNA library

2. Blotting

The clone is transferred on a nitrocellulose membrane to get similar pattern of colonies on master plate. Cells are lysed and released DNA is denatured

3. Binding with primary antibody

Nitrocellulose (NC) membrane is incubated with antibody having immunoreactivity towards a Specific protein. The primary antibody will binds to the target protein and unbound antibodies are removed by washing

4. Treatment with secondary antibody

NC membrane is incubated with primary antobody specific enzyme labelled secondary antibody. Excessive secondary antibody is washed off after binding

5. Blot development

The secondary antibody is detected by performing enzymatic activity by analysing and matching the signal on membrane with master plate

4.3.3 Enzymatic-based Screening

Based on the ability of a protein to exhibit an enzymatic activity. However, this method not specific but helps us in the identification of proteins with known enzymatic activity.

Transformed cell selection could be done by two ways-

a. Integrate selectable marker.
b. Integrate screenable marker.

a. Integrate Selectable Marker

produces the product that allows artificial selection of transformed cells. Based on selection, they can be divided into two categories-

1. *Positive selectable marker*- which promotes the growth of cells by providing resistance to transformed cells.
2. *Negative selectable marker*- which promotes the cell death by increasing sensitivity of transformed cells.

b. Screenable Marker

Generates the product which is detectable using the quantitative assay. Mostly reporter genes, *e.g.* lac z gene, GFP, chloramphenicol acetyltransferase (CAT), are used which measure the expression of genes and help in localization of intracellular proteins.

5. DNA Sequencing

☆ Method of determining the sequence of the nucleotide's bases (A, T, G, C) in DNA segment.

- ☆ DNA is sequenced by a chemical procedure that breaks a terminally labeled DNA.
- ☆ The length of the labeled fragments calculated by identifying the position of bases.

5.1 Methods of DNA Sequencing

1. Maxam – Gilbert method
2. Chain-termination method (Sanger method)
3. Dye-terminator method

5.1.1 Maxam-Gilbert Sequencing Method

Based on chemical modification of DNA and subsequent cleavage at specific bases. Radioactive labeling at one end is done and purification of the DNA fragment to be sequenced. Small proportions of one or two of the four nucleotide-based in each of four reactions (G, A+G, C, C+T) are generated by the chemical treatments. The fragments in the four reactions are arranged side by side in gel DNA.

5.1.2 Chain-termination Method

Sanger method is more efficient and uses fewer toxic chemicals and radioactive substances and uses di-deoxynucleotide triphosphates (ddNTPs) as DNA chain terminators. Four separate sequencing reactions with nucleotides (with standard dATP, dGTP, dCTP, dTTP and only one of the four di-deoxynucleotide ddATP, ddGTP, ddCTP, ddTTP), DNA polymerase and primers are set. ddNTPs are the chain-terminating nucleotides as they lack a 3′-OH group and result in amplification of DNA fragments of varying length. The relative position of bands and fluorescence enables easy DNA sequencing.

5.1.3 Dye-terminator Sequencing

This sequencing technique utilizes labeling of the chain terminator ddNTPs, which helps in sequencing in a single reaction. Each labeled ddNTPs emit fluorescence with different wavelengths.

5.2 Applications of Genome Sequencing

- ☆ Analysis of protein structure and function by DNA sequence.
- ☆ Determination of function of a specific sequence
- ☆ Detect mutation by comparison of sequences.
- ☆ Kinship study
- ☆ DNA fingerprinting

6. Gene Mapping

- ☆ Method to identify the locus of a gene and the distances between genes.
- ☆ A widely applicable approach to scanning the genetic information of an organism for genes that are responsible for a specific trait.
- ☆ Gene mapping is helpful in the understanding of genetic diseases.

6.1 Gene Mapping can be of two types

6.1.1 Genetic Mapping

- ☆ Based on recombination of chromosomes to determine the relative positions of DNA landmarks to one another.
- ☆ It uses linkage analysis to determine the relative position between two genes on a chromosome.

6.1.2 Physical Mapping

- ☆ Involves determination of the positions of DNA landmarks by measurement of the physical quantity of DNA. Involves artificial breakage of DNA molecules using radiation, DNA-modifying enzymes, or shear forces.
- ☆ Determines the frequency at which DNA landmarks co-occur on the same chromosome segment.

7. High Throughput Sequencing (HTS)

- ☆ Sequencing multiple DNA molecules in parallel, producing hundreds of millions of DNA molecules to be sequenced at a time.
- ☆ Helpful in the creation of large data sets generate more comprehensive insights of cellular genomic and transcriptomic modifications in various disease conditions and developmental stages.

7.1 HTS can be of the following Types

- ☆ Whole-genome sequencing (WGS) provides the sequence of DNA bases across the genome.
- ☆ Whole exome sequencing can be used to identify novel variants and other mutations.
- ☆ Targeted sequencing covers a relatively small set of genes or targeted regions.

7.2 HTS is Useful in

- ☆ De novo sequencing.
- ☆ Metagenomics
- ☆ Epigenetics
- ☆ Whole-genome, targeted resequencing, and Exome sequencing
- ☆ RNA sequencing (Whole transcriptome)

8. Next-Generation Sequencing (NGS)

- ☆ Technology to determine the sequence of DNA or RNA to study genetic variation associated with diseases or other biological phenomena.
- ☆ Also known as "high-throughput sequencing" but initially named as "massively parallel sequencing", as it enabled the sequencing of many DNA strands at the same time.

- NGS enables the analysis of hundreds to thousands of genes at one time in multiple samples.
- It also helps in the diagnosis and analysis of different types of genomic features in a single sequencing run, from single nucleotide variants, RNA fusions, copy numbers, and structural variants.

8.1 NGS-based Approaches have the Following Advantages

- Prior knowledge of the genome or genomic features is not required.
- Provides the ideal throughput per run.
- Studies can be performed quickly and cost-effectively.
- Requires lower sample input.
- Has higher accuracy, and ability to detect variants at lower allele frequencies than Sanger sequencing.

9. Polymerase Chain Reaction (PCR)

It is an enzymatic process of in-vitro amplification of the desired DNA fragments in a temperature regulating instrument called Thermocycler. It is also called 'Molecular Xeroxing'.

Components for Polymerase Chain Reaction

1. DNA template (1-10ng genomic/cytoplasmic DNA depending upon type of amplification)
2. Primers (Forward and reverse)
3. Polymerase enzyme (Taq Polymerase)
4. dNTPs (dATP, dGTP, dCTP, dTTP)
5. Tris-HCl, pH 8.3 (25°C)
6. Magnesium chlorid
7. Potassium chloride
8. Bovine serum albumin (BSA)

(Items 5–7: For optimal pH, interaction, salt conditions, and enzyme activity)

9.1 PCR Protocol

Three main steps:

1. Denaturation
2. Annealing
3. Elongation

1. Denaturation

The reaction mixture is heated to 94 °C which causes denaturation of hydrogen bonds of double-stranded DNA molecule leading to form two single-stranded molecules.

2. Annealing

Temperature is lowered (50-65°C) and primers bind to template DNA, the annealing time is 15-30 secs, and it depends on the length and bases of the primers.

3. Extension

New DNA strands are synthesized in the 5 to 3 direction using primer and deoxyribonucleoside triphosphates (dNTPs). The reaction is held at 70-72°C for the final extension of the DNA strand. Finally, amplified DNA is held at 4°C until analysis.

9.2 Applications of PCR

- Genotyping
- Genomic cloning
- Drug discovery
- DNA Fingerprinting
- Pre-natal diagnosis
- Disease diagnosis
- Site-directed mutagenesis
- Gene therapy
- Gene expression studies
- Epidemiological studies

9.3 Types of PCR

1. Real-time PCR (quantitative PCR)
2. RT PCR (Reverse Transcriptase PCR)
3. Multiplex PCR
4. Hot Start PCR
5. Nested PCR
6. Asymmetric PCR

Quantitative and Reverse transcriptase PCR is most used in biological experiments and are explained below:

9.3.1 Real-Time PCR (Quantitative PCR)

- Technique to monitor the real-time progress of a PCR reaction.
- The technique is based on the detection of the fluorescence produced by a reporter molecule which increases, as the reaction proceeds.
- Faster than normal PCR, a relatively small amount of PCR product can be quantified, and the efficiency of reaction can be precisely calculated.
- Can be used in gene expression analysis, disease diagnosis, food testing, and animal and plant breeding.

- The principle of amplification is the same as that of PCR (*i.e.*, Denaturation, Annealing, Extension).
- The reaction can be analyzed in real-time with the camera/detector placed into a real-time PCR.
- With an increase in the number of gene copies during the reaction, fluorescence increases, indicating the progress of the reaction.
- Different types of markers are used in Real-time PCR but most used are:
  - **TaqMan probe**: based on quencher tetramethylrhodamine (TAMRA) on 3′ and fluorescein (FAM) 5′ combination. Once quencher is digested by nuclease activity, fluorescein is free to emit signals and the fluorescence released corresponds to the number of newly synthesized DNA strands.
  - **SYBR Green**: based on dye that emits a prominent fluorescent signal when it binds at the minor groove of DNA. It also provides information about cycles of amplification but lack specificity.

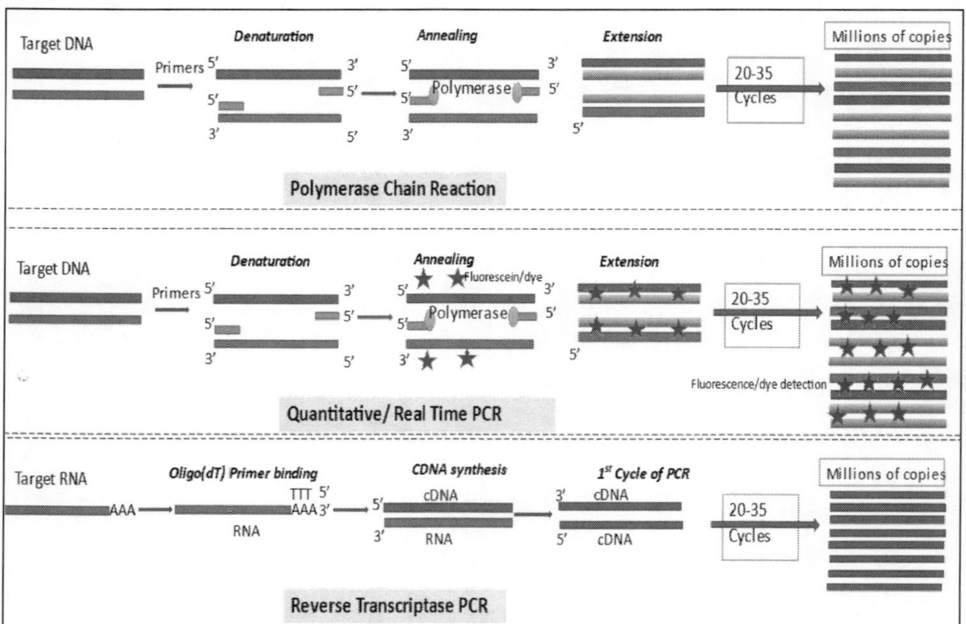

9.3.2 RT PCR (Reverse Transcriptase PCR)

- The process involves amplification of mRNA using reverse transcriptase.
- This technique is used for low levels of gene expression by analyzing the PCR product of cDNA prepared from the mRNA transcript.
- RNA extracted from the cells, target specific oligo primers, and reverse transcriptase enzymes are used for the synthesis of complementary DNA (cDNA) from the extracted RNA.

- The RNA and cDNA strands are denatured and then DNA-specific primers and Taq polymerase enzyme are used for DNA strand synthesis.
- The denaturation, annealing, and extension cycles are used repeatedly to get multiple copies of desired DNA.

9.3.3 Multiplex PCR

- For amplification of several different DNA sequences simultaneously in a single reaction volume.
- Multiple site-specific primers are used for amplification of more than one DNA location.
- The reaction is optimized in such a way that all primer pairs can work at the same annealing temperature.

9.3.4 Hot Start PCR

- A preferred method to minimize nonspecific primer binding and amplification.
- Taq polymerase in this case is in an inactive state until temperature increases above 70°C.
- Inactivation of Taq polymerase can be done by binding it with enzyme-linked antibodies or its enclosure in wax beads.
- Once there is an increase in temperature, Taq polymerase gets activated and amplification starts.

9.3.5 Nested PCR

- Involves the use of two primer sets and two successive PCR reactions to improve sensitivity and specificity.

9.3.6 Asymmetric PCR

- Preferentially amplify one strand of the original DNA more than the other.
- The technique has applications in some types of sequencing and hybridization probing where having only one of the two complementary strands is required.

10. Analysis of Gene Expression

Involves the isolation or capture of transcribed RNA within a sample, followed by amplification and subsequent detection and quantitation.

Different techniques are used to analyze gene expression:

- Northern blotting
- Real-time PCR (qPCR)
- Microarray analysis

10.1 Northern Blotting

- ✰ A technique that is used to study gene expression by detection of RNA. This technique was developed in 1977 by James Alwine, David Kemp, and George Stark at Stanford University.
- ✰ Procedure for northern blotting

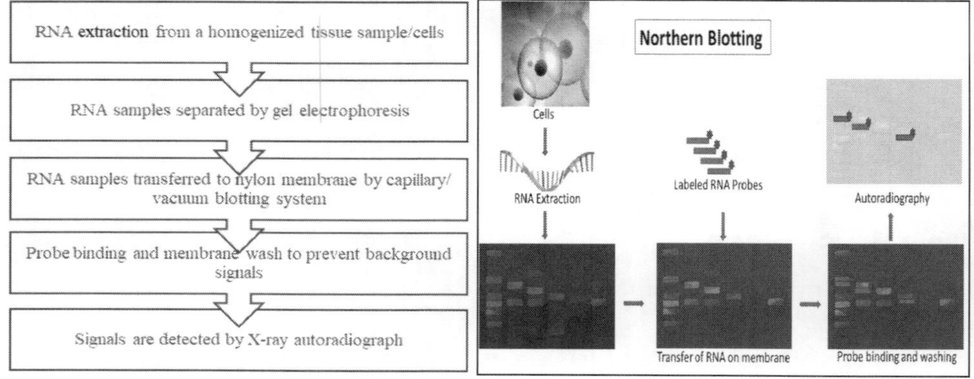

10.2 Real-time PCR

- ✰ (Explained in detail in PCR section).

10.3 Microarray Analysis

- ✰ The method uses microchips containing anchored arrays of probes (short DNA elements) for the large-scale interrogation of gene expression.
- ✰ Can detect the expression of thousands of genes at the same time.
- ✰ Microscope slides that contain DNA sequences or genes on thousands of tiny spots at defined positions.
- ✰ Unknown DNA molecules are digested with restriction enzymes, fluorescent markers are attached to these DNA fragments and put on the microarray plate.
- ✰ Applicable for tests for intellectual disability, developmental delay, autism spectrum disorders, *etc.*

11. Introduction of Recombinant DNA in Host Clone

Gene delivery is the necessary step for gene recombination. There are many methods of introducing foreign DNA into a eukaryotic host:

- ✰ Physical methods
- ✰ Chemical methods
- ✰ Biological methods

11.1 Physical Methods

- *Electroporation:* Permeability of the cell membrane increased with the application of the electrical field, allowing DNA to be introduced into the cell.
- *Microinjection:* Glass micropipette is used to inject a desired substance into the target living cells
- *Gene gun*: Mechanical force is used to deliver exogenous DNA/RNA to cells. Gene of interest is coated on heavy metal and fired these micro-projectiles into cells.
- *Magnetofection*: DNA delivery mediated by a magnetic force acting on associations of magnetic particles.
- *Impalefection*: Nanostructures are synthesized and Plasmid DNA containing the gene is attached to the nanostructure surface.
- **Continuous infusion, cell squeezing,** and **sonication** are other physical methods.

11.2 Chemical Methods

- Liposome mediated gene transfer.
- Calcium phosphate mediated gene transfer.
- DEAE- Dextran mediated gene transfer.
- Polyethylene glycol mediated gene transfer.

11.3 Biological Methods

- *Transfection:* Process of introducing DNA molecule by non-viral means in eukaryotic cells. Recombinant proteins can be produced by transfection as it enhances or inhibits gene expression in transfected cells. It is applied to study the function and regulation of genes or gene products, to produce transgenic organisms, and for gene therapy.

  Types of transfection: *Transient transfection and Stable transfection*
- *Transformation*: Uptake of DNA from the environment. In this process, recombinant DNA fragments are produced which are transferred into the cell by increasing membrane permeability. The transferred DNA is integrated into the chromosomal DNA where it is maintained and replicated.
- **Transduction:** Transfer of DNA by bacteria-specific viruses called bacteriophage.

12. Knockout Mice

- Are modified mice in which existing gene is inactivated (knocked out) by replacing/disrupting it with an external DNA.

- These mice are used to study the impact of the absence of specific genes. The functions of knocked-out genes (biochemical, developmental, physical, and behavioral) are studied.
- The knockout technique involves the construction of DNA containing the desired mutation. The knockout gene is replaced by a drug resistance marker.
- The cell's repair mechanism recombines the foreign DNA into the existing DNA.

13. Cloning

- Process for creating an exact copy of the genetic, or inherited, traits of a donor.
- The species that have been successfully cloned are cattle, swine, sheep, mice, rats, rabbits, cats, mules, horses and goats, *etc.*
- Artificial cloning is of three types:
    1. ***Gene cloning***: produces copies of genes or segments of DNA.
    2. ***Reproductive cloning***: produces copies of whole animals.
    3. ***Therapeutic cloning:*** useful in studying the structure and function of genes. Helps in the synthesis of vitamins, hormones, and antibiotics.

14. Mutagenesis

- Mutagenesis is a process in which genetic information of an organism is changed, causing interruption/modification in the function of an existing gene on the chromosome, resulting in a mutation.
- Mutagenesis can be achieved either by natural processes, chemicals, or biological procedures.

14.1 Transposon Mutagenesis

First studied by Barbara McClintock. Transposon mutagenesis is a biological process that allows genes to be transferred to a host chromosome. This procedure more effective than chemical and natural methods as it incorporates selective markers that induce single hit mutations and the chances of host cell death are less.

14.1.1 Tn5 transposon system

It is a model system in which a bacterial composite transposon Tn5 is used, in which genes are flanked by two nearly identical insertion sequences, IS50R and IS50L.

14.1.2 Sleeping Beauty Transposon System

It is non-viral vector for incorporation of a gene cassette into a vertebrate genome.

14.2 Site-directed Mutagenesis

- One of the most important laboratory techniques for the generation of DNA libraries by introducing mutations into DNA sequences.
- Also called 'Oligonucleotide-directed mutagenesis' and is used to make specific and intentional changes to the DNA sequence of a desired gene/ gene product.
- Short DNA primers complementary to the template DNA with the desired mutation are synthesized. These primers hybridize with the DNA of the gene of interest. DNA is amplified and introduced in the host cell. Mutants are selected by DNA sequencing.
- There are different methods for site-directed mutagenesis:
  - PCR site-directed mutagenesis
  - Whole plasmid mutagenesis
  - *In vivo* site-directed mutagenesis method
  - CRISPR

14.3 Applications of Mutagenesis

- Improvement of quality of the protein.
- Production of genetically modified proteins that have high commercial values.
- In gene synthesis and gene-editing technology.
- For the study of gene characteristics.
- Used in cloning.
- Screening of SNP.
- Construction of the map of the regulatory elements of a gene.

15. Transgenic Organisms

These are the genetically modified organisms that have inserted DNA (transgene) of different species origin.

15.1 Transgenic Plants

- Transgenic plants are genetically engineered plants with new characteristics.
- Recombinant DNA techniques are used for the insertion of foreign genes.
- The new traits which are naturally not available in plants are inserted (transgene).
- The transgene can be from unrelated plants or species.

The purpose of the development of transgenic plants is to:

i. Improve shelf life and quality of the crop.

ii. Increase yield and tolerance to heat, cold, drought, and biotic and abiotic stress.

iii. Provide resistance against pests, insects, viruses, *etc.*

iv. Increases expression of foreign proteins with industrial and pharmaceutical value.

15.2 Transgenic Animals

- ☆ Animals that have a foreign gene deliberately inserted into their genome.
- ☆ The insertion of the transgene into the pronuclei of a fertilized egg is usually done by microinjection. This egg is subsequently implanted into the oviduct of a surrogate mother.
- ☆ Transgenic livestock has been used to increase animal welfare, decrease livestock disease, enhance nutrition, protect the environment, and subsequently improve human health.

16. RNA Interference (RNAi)

- ☆ Also called 'Post-Transcriptional Gene Silencing'.
- ☆ It is the RNA-dependent gene silencing process and is controlled by the RNA-induced silencing complex.
- ☆ The silencing of a gene is a consequence of the degradation of RNA into short RNAs that activate ribonucleases to target homologous mRNA.
- ☆ dsRNA degraded in small interfering RNAs (siRNAs) by an RNase III-like activity and then these siRNAs join an RNase complex, RISC (RNA-induced silencing complex), which acts on the cognate mRNA and degrades it.
- ☆ RNAi has applications in functional genomics, therapeutic intervention, agriculture, and other areas.

REFERENCES

1. Sandy B. Primrose, Richard Twyman. Principles of Gene Manipulation and Genomics, 7th Edition, 2006. ISBN: 978-1-405-13544-3.

2. Desmond S. T. Nicholl. An Introduction to Genetic Engineering, 3rd Edition, Cambridge University Press 2008, ISBN-13 978-0-511-39858-2.

3. Daniel L. Hartl, Elizabeth W. Jones. Genetics: Principles and Analysis, 4th Edition, Jones and Bartlett Publishers, Harvard University.

4. Cornel Mülhardt. Molecular Biology and Genomics, The Experimenter series Translated by E.W. Beese, Academic Press, Copyright © 2007, Elsevier Inc ISBN-13: 978-0-12-088546-6.

Chapter 9

Plant Biotechnology

Kusuma Kumari Panda

Amity Institute of Biotechnology, Amity University Uttar Pradesh
Noida – 201 313, Uttar Pradesh
e-mail: pkkumari@amity.edu

ABSTRACT

Plant biotechnology offers powerful tools and technologies for the development of new plant varieties with improved traits and enable us to improve crop yield and food quality in agriculture and to produce a large variety of products in industries. Plant biotechnology is having a significant impact on agriculture, horticulture and forestry. It can be regarded as a new age technology for large scale production of plants through micropropagation, transgenics, artificial seeds, secondary metabolites, biopharmaceuticals etc. Development of tissue culture methods along with genetic engineering techniques allowed us to produce improved plant varieties and novel agricultural products in large scale and would contribute significantly towards achieving global food security. Micropropagation and in vitro conservation proved especially useful in producing high quality, disease-free planting material of a wide range of crops. Many transgenic cultivars of major food crops have been produced with resistance to herbicides, insects and pathogens.

In this chapter, various plant tissue culture-based techniques and genetic engineering aspects for the improvement of plant varieties and agro products are discussed. Plant tissue culture-based industries equipped with recent technologies are expanding fast and the future can hold great promise with exciting possibilities.

Keywords: *Tissue culture, Callus, Micropropagation, Haploids, Somatic hybrid, Agrobacterium, Transgenics.*

Biotechnology is an assemblage of different technologies that enable us to improve agricultural produce qualitatively and quantitatively and to produce a wide range of products in industries.

Plant biotechnology/Agricultural biotechnology aims at manipulation of plants for the benefit of mankind. Various technologies applied in plant biotechnology includes:

1. Tissue culture
2. Genetic engineering/recombinant DNA technology
3. Molecular breeding – MAS

By using these biotechnological tools, crop improvement can be achieved faster by facilitating transfer of genes from unrelated species.

Plant tissue culture involves in vitro cultivation of all plant parts under aseptic conditions. Plant tissue culture has enabled mass clonal propagation, production of virus-free plants, secondary metabolite production, preservation of germplasm and serves as an indispensable tool for regenerating transgenic plants. All this has been possible due to the formulation of different types of media and plant hormone combinations. Plant tissue culture is one of the most dynamic and promising experimental biology techniques and its various applications include:

- ☆ **Crop Improvement**: Plants with built in resistance to pest and diseases, tolerance to abiotic stresses, improved qualitative characters
- ☆ **Pharmaceuticals/Industrial:** Plants for production of edible vaccines, secondary metabolites, plastics, fuels, having Improved taste and nutrition, and other products
- ☆ **Plant breeding:** For creating genetic diversity and manipulating genetic variability, that biotechnology including tissue-culture techniques is having its most significant impact.
- ☆ **Wide hybridization**: in vitro fertilization can be used to overcome pre-zygotic barriers, such as the failure of pollen to germinate or inhibition of pollen-tube growth. Post-zygotic barriers (poor endosperm development) may be overcome by embryo, ovule or pod culture. Embryo culture has also been successful in overcoming problems of slow seed germination, low seed set, seed dormancy, inducing embryo growth in the absence of a symbiotic partner, and in the production of monoploids of barley.
- ☆ **Somatic hybridization:** Somatic hybrids were produced by fusing protoplasts which can be used for developing unique hybrid plants which cannot be produced by conventional sexual hybridization.
- ☆ **Haploid plant production:** Haploids are of special interest to plant breeders as doubled haploid plants can be used immediately as homozygous breeding lines for the immediate expression of recessive/ mutated genetic traits
- ☆ **Micropropagation**: Large scale propagation of plants from explants and/ or callus has been made possible for large number of species using in vitro vegetative propagation. Laboratory-scale micropropagation is the widest use of plant tissue-culture technology.

- ☆ **Synthetic seeds:** Somatic embryos produced through tissue culture can be encapsulated with gelly like coating resembling a zygotic seed are called as synthetic seeds/artificial seed. These can be exported anywhere for vegetative propagation analogous to a zygotic seed.
- ☆ **Pathogen free plants**: Apical meristems are found to be having low incidence of virus or are virus-free. Culturing of apical meristems, combined with chemo- or thermo-therapy, has been successfully employed to produce virus-free and generally pathogen-free material for micropropagation.
- ☆ **Germplasm preservation:** in vitro conditions can be employed for storage of plant tissues/propagules under slow-growth conditions (at low temperature and/or with growth-retarding compounds) or cryopreservation or as desiccated synthetic seed. It serves as an alternative to seed banks

Types of Culture

Callus Culture

Callus represents an undifferentiated or unorganized mass of cells. Culturing of any excised tissue or plant parts such as leaf, stem parts, root parts, cotyledon, hypocotyls *etc.*, under suitable culture/media conditions produces callus. It is generally composed of parenchymatous cells in division phase. Callus can be continuously proliferated using plant growth hormones or can be directed to form organs (organogenesis) or somatic embryos (embryogenesis).

Somaclonal variations can be induced into callus through which desired variants can be selected.

Cell-suspension Cultures

Callus cultures can be used to establish Single-cell cultures and suspension cultures by transferring a piece of friable callus tissue into liquid growth medium and subjecting it to continuous shaking. They can be maintained as batch cultures grown in flasks or as bioreactors employed for the production of valuable secondary metabolites or recombinant proteins. Some important secondary metabolites present in plants are flavonoids, alkaloids, steroids, tannins, and terpenes but are produced in very small quantities under normal conditions. The production process can be scaled up and automated using bioreactors for commercial production. Many strategies such as biotransformation, cell permeabilization, elicitation, and immobilization have been used to make cell suspension cultures more efficient in the production of secondary metabolites. Transgenic plant cell cultures are gaining popularity in the large-scale production of recombinant proteins, thus making them integral parts of molecular farming. Pharmaceutical compounds include antibodies, interleukins, erythropoietin, human granulocyte–macrophage colony-stimulating factor (hGM-CSF), and hepatitis B antigen have been produced by suspension cultures.

Organ Cultures

Isolated organs or tissues such as stem, leaf, or roots, can be cultured under in vitro conditions for its specific purpose:

Seed Culture

Seed germination efficiency can be improved of seeds that are difficult to germinate in vivo

Embryo Culture

It is a technique in which isolated embryos from immature ovules or seeds are cultured in vitro and is a useful tool for direct regeneration in species where seeds are dormant, recalcitrant, or abort at early stages of development. Embryo culture is specifically employed in the production of interspecific hybrids between incompatible crosses, where seeds are discarded because of their inability to germinate. Embryo culture enables embryo rescue in distant (interspecific or intergeneric) hybridization by overcoming embryo abortion due to incompatibility barriers. In addition, immature embryos can be used to produce embryogenic callus and somatic embryos.

Ovary or Ovule Culture

A common explant for the initiation of somatic embryogenic cultures, for the production of haploid plants, overcoming abortion of embryos of wide hybrids

Anther and Microspore Culture

Anthers or isolated microspores can be used to produce haploid plants. These haploids are used for production of homozygous diploid lines through chromosome doubling. It is a powerful toon in plant breeding.

Protoplast Cultures

Protoplasts are plant cells without cell walls. They can be isolated and used in somatic hybrid production. Protoplasts enable efficient and direct gene transfer to plant cells and are now increasingly used in cell culture studies mostly to study transient transgene assays and localization of proteins.

Meristem Culture

Apical meristem tips (roots, shoots) can be used to produce disease-free plants. This technique is used for elimination of viruses, also for bacterium- or fungus-free plants. Apical meristems in plants are suitable explants for the production of virus-free plants since the meristems typically devoid of viruses. Meristem culture in combination with thermos or chemotherapy has resulted in successful production of virus-free plants.

Media and Culture Conditions

Basal Media

The growth medium is comprised of all the minerals, vitamins, sugar and all other components that are essential for a plant's growth and development, in sterile or axenic conditions. The minerals consist of macronutrients such as nitrogen, potassium, phosphorus, calcium, magnesium, sulphur and micronutrients such as manganese, zinc, iron, boron, cobalt, molybdenum, and copper. The vitamins used are thiamine (vitamin B1), pyridoxine (B6), nicotinic acid (niacin), and thiamine. In addition, biotin, folic acid, ascorbic acid (vitamin C), and vitamin E (tocopherol) are also sometimes added to some specific media formulations. Myoinositol, a sugar alcohol, is included in most plant culture media to improve the growth of cultures. Plants require an external supply of carbon source as sugar as cultures grown in vitro cannot photosynthesize sufficiently to support the carbon needs of the growing tissues. Maltose, and sorbitol are also used as carbon source in some cultures. The pH of the medium plays important role in the uptake of various components of the medium as well as regulating a wide range of biochemical reactions of plant tissue cultures. Most media are adjusted to a pH of 5.2 – 5.8. Both liquid or semi-solid medium can be used for growing the cultures. The Semi-solid media are easy to handle and provide a support system for the explants. Solidification is achieved using agar derived from seaweed or agar substitutes such as GelriteTM or PhytagelTM.

Table 9.1: Most Frequently Used Media and their Composition

Medium Components (mg.l^{1-})	*MS*	*G_5*	*W*	*LM*	*NN*
Macronutrients					
NH_4NO_3	1650.0			400.0	720.0
KNO_3	1900.0	2500.0	80.0		950.0
$CaCl_2.2H_2O$	440.0	150.0		96.0	166.0
$MgSO_4.7H_2O$	370.0	250.0	720.0	370.0	185.0
KH_2PO_4	170.0			170.0	68.0
$(NH4)_2SO4$		134.0			
$NaH_2PO_4.H_2O$		150.0	16.5		
$CaNO_3.4H_2O$			300.0	556.0	
Na_2SO_4			200.0		
KCl			65.0		
K_2SO_4				990.0	
Micronutrients					
KI	0.83	0.75	0.75		
H_3BO_3	6.20	3.0	1.5	6.2	10.0
$MnSO_4.4H_2O$	22.30		7.0		25.0
$MnSO_4.H_2O$		10.0		29.43	
$ZnSO_4.7H_2O$	8.6	2.0	2.6	8.6	10.0
$Na_2MoO_4.2H_2O$	0.25	0.25		0.25	0.25
$CuSO_4.5H_2O$	0.025	0.025		0.25	0.025
$CoCl_2.6H_2O$	0.025	0.025			
Na_2EDTA	37.3	37.3		37.3	37.3
$FeSO_4.7H_2O$	27.8	27.8		27.8	27.8

Medium Components (mg.l⁻¹)	MS	G_5	W	LM	NN
Vitamins and other supplements					
Inositol	100.0	100.0		100.0	100.0
Glycine	2.0	2.0	3.0	2.0	2.0
Thiamine HCl	0.1	10.0	0.1	1.0	0.5
Pyridoxine HCl	0.5		0.1	0.5	0.5
Nicotinic acid	0.5		0.5	0.5	5.0
Ca-panthothenate			1.0		
Cysteine HCl			1.0		
Biotin					0.05
Folic acid					0.5

A variety of media formulations are available for plant tissue culture. The basal medium is designed to keep plant tissues alive and thriving. The composition of nutrients varies from medium to medium. Majority of tissue cultures of plants use MS media as the choice medium, other than MS are also used. The following are the media used for specific culture systems.

1. Knudson's medium- For orchid tissue culture and is also used for fern tissue culture.
2. Murashige and Skoog- To induce organogenesis, and regeneration of plants in cultured tissues
3. White- Initially developed for root culture, can be used for the purpose of shoot culture and callus culture. It is suitable for culture Musa and Daucus species
4. Linsmaier and Skoog- Used for the purpose of organogenesis, callus culture, cell suspension, and micropropagation
5. Gamborg (B5)- Used for the purpose of protoplast culture
6. Nitsch and Nitsch (1969): To establish the anther culture.

The composition of nutrients varies from medium to medium. For example, MS medium has higher macronutrients than does WPM, which is suitable for most plant species, but woody plants respond better in WPM than MS medium. It is important to select the right medium for culture and is determined empirically for optimal response of the plant species in tissue culture condition.

The success of tissue culture lies in the selection and composition of the growth medium with combinations of growth regulators(hormones) and culture conditions such as temperature, pH, light, and humidity.

Growth Regulators

Hormones or plant growth regulators are added to in basal media as discussed above to direct the developmental program of tissues in desired way as to produce callus or callus tissue to proliferate, or produce roots or shoots. Auxins, cytokinins, and gibberellins are the important growth regulators used. Auxins promote cell growth and root growth. The most commonly used auxins are IAA (indole acetic acid), NAA (naphthalene acetic acid), 2,4-D (2,4-dichlorophenoxyacetic acid), IBA (indole butyric acid). Cytokinins promote cell division and shoot growth, BAP (benzylaminopurine), zeatin, and kinetin are the most commonly used cytokinins. Sometimes an auxin-like compound TDZ (thidiazuron) has been used to improve the success rate of plant regeneration in many species. Other hormones such as abscisic acid and jasmonic acid have also been used in plant cell culture for specific growth requirements.

In addition to these hormones, compounds like adjuvants such as spermidine, spermine, and putrescene can also be added to the growth media to have an enhanced and positive effect on morphogenesis. By manipulating the quantity and combination of growth hormones, whole plants regeneration under in vitro conditions can be established.

It is important to transfer the tissues to fresh medium regularly (every week to monthly, as per species and experiment). This is known as sub culturing.

Sterile Conditions

All tissue culture operations are done in sterile environmental conditions and use laminar flow cabinet for this purpose. The laminar flow cabinets are equipped with a high-efficiency particulate air (HEPA) filter to maintain sterile environment as they filter and do not allow the microorganisms to enter inside the cabinet. The hood is also cleaned and sterilized by wiping it with 70 per cent alcohol. All the instruments used should kept dipped in 70 per cent ethanol and sterilized using flame or glass beads just before use. Hands should be disinfected with ethanol before handling cultures. Maintenance of sterile/axenic conditions is essential throughout the all phases of cultures: from explant stage to the regeneration of whole plants.

All the tissues/explants should be sterilized prior to tissue culture as they may inherently have various bacteria and fungi on their surfaces. These pathogens can grow fast and compete with the plant tissue for nutrition, thus depriving the plant tissues of nutrients. Surface sterilants like 10 per cent Sodium hypochlorite or 70 per cent ethanol or 0.2 per cent mercuric chloride, or 0.1 per cent silver nitrate and fungicides are the common chemicals used for surface sterilization of the explants when using field-grown tissues. The concentration of sterilants and time of sterilization is dependent on the type of tissue; for example, a tough seed coat will require a longer sterilization time with higher concentration time than the softer leaf tissues. Biological detergents like Tween added to the sterilants can improve surface contact with the tissue for efficient sterilization. In addition to surface contamination, internal contamination of tissues or systemic contamination can be controlled to a certain extent by use of a low concentration of antibiotics in the medium with frequent transfer to fresh medium.

Culture Conditions and Vessels

Culture rooms or chambers must be maintained as sterile as possible to control any airborne contaminants Cultures are grown in growth rooms or growth chambers. Controlled temperature, light and humidity conditions are also important for proper growth of cultures. An optimum temperature of 22 – 25°C is used in most of the cultures, with 16-h light photoperiod. A relative humidity of 50 – 90 per cent is maintained in the growth chambers. Some cultures are also incubated in the dark. Cultures can be grown in various kinds of sterile vessels such as petri plates, test tubes, "Magenta boxes," bottles and flasks.

In vitro Regeneration Methods of Plants

Genesis of whole plant from cultured explants directly through multiple shoots or indirectly via callus phase is called regeneration. This process is exploited in tissue culture due to the totipotent nature of plant cells. Totipotency is the inherent ability of a plant cell to give rise to a whole plant under defined conditions.

A differentiated cell, to express its totipotency, it first undergoes dedifferentiation (mature cell reverting to the meristematic state and forming undifferentiated callus tissue) followed by redifferentiation (Individual cells of callus tissue to develop whole plant or plant organs). The is termed 'dedifferentiation'. This capacity of cell to form organs or embryos can be exploited to regenerate plants This process of in vitro regeneration is very important for transgenic plants production from single transformed cells.

Morphogenesis

Origin of form is termed as morphogenesis. Under in vitro conditions this can be achieved by two routes: **de novo origin of organs**, either shoots or roots from the cultured tissues precisely termed as organogenesis and **de novo origin of embryos** with distinct root and shoot poles on opposite ends from the somatic cells called as somatic embryogenesis

Organogenesis

A process by which cells are directed to produce unipolar structures in the form of root or shoot primordia with vascular connection to the parental tissue finally leading to the production of roots or shoots. This depends on the balance of auxin and cytokinin and the ability of the tissue to respond to phytohormones during culture. Under the influence of phytohormones, cells initially become competent to dedifferentiate and morphogenesis. It can be achieved by two ways: direct and indirect.

Indirect Organogenesis

In this mode organs are formed via a callus phase. This route does not ensure clonal fidelity, but variations can be exploited in the form of somaclonal variants for desired characters and also for mass multiplication. The callus phase has been used for the production of transgenic plants in which (i) the callus cells may be transformed and plants regenerated or (ii) the explant is transformed initially and callus is formed, then shoots are developed from the explant.

Direct Organogenesis

The production of direct buds or shoots from explant with no intermediate callus phase is termed direct organogenesis. Direct organogenesis is the method for clonal propagation and production of transgenic plants. Indirect organogenesis better method for transgenic plant production.

Axillary Bud Induction/Multiple-bud Initiation

Axillary shoots are formed directly from preformed meristems at nodes and mutation rates of the shoot meristem are relatively low. This technique is often referred to as multiple-bud induction. This technique ensures the production of uniform planting material without genetic variation and is the most common method employed for micropropagation. Many economically important plants have been propagated using this method.

Somatic Embryogenesis

Production of a bipolar embryo with a closed vascular system from somatic tissues of a plant is known as Somatic embryogenesis. It is a nonsexual developmental process and has become one of the most powerful techniques in plant tissue culture for mass clonal propagation. These somatic embryos can be produced directly or via a callus phase. Direct somatic embryogenesis is always preferable for clonal propagation as there is less possibility of somaclonal variations. Indirect somatic embryogenesis may be used when we want to select desired somaclonal variants and for the production of transgenic plants. Main advantage of somatic embryogenesis is that somatic embryos can be directly germinated into viable plants thus mimicking the natural germination process.

Synthetic Seeds

These somatic embryos can be used as seed material for the production of viable plants.

Somatic embryos when encapsulated in an alginate matrix are known as synthetic seeds. Alginate matrix serves as an artificial seed coat. Synthetic seeds are easy to handle, they can be cryopreserved and stored for a long time, and there is potential for scaleup and low cost of production. Large-scale production of synthetic seeds using bioreactors and germination of these seeds to plantlets has been accomplished in bamboo, coffee, sandalwood, and many other plant species.

Micropropagation

Multiplication of genetically identical copies of a cultivar by asexual reproduction is called clonal propagation. Large scale in vitro clonal propagation is called as Micropropagation and has the advantage of large number of true-to-type plantlets production in relatively short time and space from a single individual.

Types of explants used in micropropagation: shoot tip, axillary bud, lateral bud, shoot tip, root tip, nodal segments, floral parts *etc.*

Various Stages of Micropropagation

Stage 0 - Preparative stage: Preparation of mother plants to provide quality explants for better establishment of aseptic cultures

Stage 1: In this period, exposing the stock plants to suitable light, temperature and growth regulator treatments to improve the quality of explants. Contamination problem is reduced in the subsequent stages, mother plant is grown in a glasshouse and watered regularly.

Stage 2

Multiplication

Following approaches have been followed to achieve in vitro multiplication.

Callusing: Cultured cells may be induced to develop into plant. Differentiation may occur via organogenesis or somatic embryogenesis. Somatic embryogenesis is most preferred form of differentiation from a commercial point of view.

Somatic embryos being small, uniform and bipolar are more amenable to automation at the multiplication stage and as seeds for field planting with cost advantages. Synthetic seeds can also be stored through cold storage, cryopreservation or desiccation for prolonged periods.

On the other side callus cultures for shoot multiplication may be disadvantageous due to the genetic instability of their cells.

Adventitious buds: Development of buds from any place other than leaf axil or the shoot apex are termed adventitious buds. Culture conditions can be optimized to enhance adventitious bud formation.

Enhanced axillary branching: With optimized concentrations of cytokinin to auxin in the medium I of shoot multiplication can be increased by axillary branching.

Stage 3

Rooting of regenerated shoots (Manual shoot separation from culture medium and rooting)

Efficient rooting of in vitro grown shoots is very important for the success of micropropagation. A pre-formed radical is already present in somatic embryo and may develop directly into plantlet. However, conversion rate into plantlets is very low. Shoots developed from axillary and adventitious buds in the presence of a cytokinin generally lack roots. For rooting, Individual shoots measuring around 2 cm in length are excised and transferred to the rooting medium from shoot multiplication medium with different combinations of hormones and salts.

Stage 4

Transplantation, Hardening under greenhouse environment.: The plants grown in vitro as above are exposed to a unique set of controlled growth conditions (high levels of sucrose, growth regulators, inorganic and organic nutrients, high humidity, low light, poor gaseous exchange). These conditions may induce high growth rate and multiplication but may also induce structural and physiological abnormalities. The ability to transfer plants out of culture to the field on a large scale with high survival rates is the key factor for the successful micropropagation industry commercially.

This requires that the plants be hardened-off before transfer to the field. This gradual transition from laboratory conditions to harsh field conditions is termed as acclimatization. During this acclimation process, plants are first transferred to a growth chamber or greenhouse and covered by domes to minimize the loss of water. This process is essential to survive transition from culture/laboratory conditions to the greenhouse and finally to field. Plantlets or shoots are transferred to potting mix and slowly and gradually conditions are adjusted from low concentration of inorganic nutrients, gradual reduction of relative humidity and high light intensity of light for initiation of photosynthesis by plantlets. The success of acclimatization of a plantlet greatly depends on root system production. Rooting of trees and woody species is difficult as compared to herbaceous species. Several factors are known to affect rooting. Exogenous application of auxins and compounds like phloroglucinol, Catechol *etc.* have a positive effect on rooting. During acclimatization, contamination, high transpiration rates, browning, hyperhydration are the common problems we encounter. These problems can be addressed by application of antitranspirants (1 per cent acropol), frequent subculturing with medium containing compounds like ascorbic acid, citric acid, PVP *etc.* low cytokinins in the medium and usage of $CaSO_4$ to reduce hyperhydration.

Advantages of Micropropagation

- ☆ Clonal mass propagation – exponential multiplication of plants in short time. We can obtain more than 1,000,000 plants per year from one initial explant in place of may be 10000 plants in an year from an initial cutting through vegetative propagation.
- ☆ Clonal multiplication of woody species (Mango, Banana, Pineapple, Rubber, Coffee, Tea, Quercus, Eucalyptus, Tectona, Santalum sps. *etc.*)
- ☆ Culture is initialized from small parts of plants – Large number of plants can be produced in small space initially and once established, they can be distributed to nurseries.
- ☆ One of the rapid methods for cloning of disease free trees. Production of disease free new cultivars and virus free plantlet through micropropagation leads to simplification of international exchange of plants and no phytosanitary certification required
- ☆ Micropropagation enables growers to increase the production of plants that normally propagate very slowly such as Narcissus and other bulbous crops.
- ☆ Vegetative propagation of sterile hybrids can be used as parent plants for seed production. *e.g.* Cabbage
- ☆ Breeding cycle can be shortened.
- ☆ Long-time storage of these in vitro cultures is possible through cryopreservation.

Disadvantages of Micropropagation

1. Initial lab set up with laboratory equipment and services can be expensive
2. Acclimatization to the field is a common problem (hyperhydricity)
3. More problems in inducing rooting
4. Risk of genetic changes in the form of somaclonal variation.
5. May not get uniform growth of original plant in culture conditions. Each explant has different in vitro growth rates and maturation. Thus cannot be used for floriculture crop production where uniformity is critical

Haploid Production

Haploids are defined as saprophytes with gametophytic chromosome constitution and production of haploids become an important component of biotechnology programmes with applications in genetics and plant breeding. Haploids are produced in a variety of plant species using a variety of methods following delayed pollination, irradiation of pollen, temperature shocks, colchicine treatment and distant hybridization (bulbosum technique), however they are not dependable always. Currently following in vitro methods are being utilized to produce haploids

Anther or pollen culture (in *Datura innoxia* by Guha and Maheswari 1968)

Ovule culture (in *Hordeum vulgare* 1976)

This technique of haploid production through anther culture has been extended to numerous plant species including cereals, vegetables, oil and tree species.

Methodology Followed

- ☆ Flower buds of the appropriate developmental stage (uni-nucleate anthers) are collected, surface sterilized and their anthers are excised and placed horizontally culture medium.
- ☆ Avoid injury to anthers otherwise it may induce callus formation from injured anther walls.
- ☆ Alternatively, pollen grains can be isolated from anthers either mechanically or by 'float culture method' and cultured on a suitable medium.
- ☆ Density gradient centrifugation can be also used which allows the separation of embryogenic grains from a mixture of embryogenic and non-embryogenic grains with 30 per cent sucrose solution, centrifuged at 1200 g for 5 min. The androgenic, vacuolated pollen grains formed a band at the top of the sucrose solution.

Factors Influencing Androgenesis

- ☆ Genotype of the donor plant: This controlled by many genes.
- ☆ Pre-treatment of anthers: Cold and heat shock treatment or with chemicals like etherel (2-chloroethylphosphonic acid), sucrose, agar and other

nutrients specific to certain genotype found to improve the success rate.

- Physiological status of the donor plant: Exposures of donor plants to nutrient and water stresses shown to promote androgenesis
- Anther wall factors: Extracts from anthers stimulates embryo production
- Culture medium and culture density: Nitsch and MS medium along with coconut milk, yeast extract, high sucrose Fe, activated charcoal have shown positive effect.

Development of Pollen Embryo

Pollen grains exhibit pollen dimorphism. Most of them are bigger, stain deeply with acetocarmine and contain plenty of starch. But small portions of the pollen grains are smaller and stain light with acetocarmine; these are called S-grains. These S-grains only respond during anther culture. The responsive pollen grains become multicellular and ultimately burst open to release the cell mass. This cell mass may either assume the shape of a globular embryo and undergo the developmental stages of embryogeny or it may develop into callus depending on the species. Regeneration of plants from pollen callus or pollen embryos may occur on the original medium or it may require transfer to a different medium. The pollen embryos exhibit considerable similarity with zygotic embryos in their morphology and certain biochemical features. To raise full plantlets from pollen embryos it is necessary to excise a cluster of the secondary embryos along with a part of the parent embryo and plant them on fresh medium.

Haploids: Applications

- As gene action is immediately manifested in haploid condition, even recessive alleles also get expressed.
- Production of homozygous lines will make fast release of new varieties.
- Very important advantage of haploids is that they display mutations with successive effects in single dose.
- Double haploid plants can be immediately produced using colchicine
- Very effective in mutagenesis studies
- Development of virus free and disease resistant lines from pure lines
- Production of 100 per cent High yielding male plants in asparagus
- Production of homozygous transgenic lines

Ovule Culture

Haploid production can be done using immature ovules in cases of incompatibility where pollination is successful but for certain reason the seeds do not develop beyond a certain stage. Before the embryo aborts, the ovules can be excised soon after fertilization and cultured on suitable medium. The components of the culture medium include inorganic nutrients that are essential for the plant to complete its life cycle, such as sugar, vitamins, amino acid, organic supplement such coconut water, growth regulators, agar as a gelling agent, and other supplements that are deemed necessary. In the case of orchids, the Knudson medium is being utilized as it is specially formulated for orchids.

The medium may need to be supplemented with some fruit/vegetable juice to accelerate initial growth. Ovules have been successfully cultured after fertilization to obtain mature embryos/seeds in a number of species of Malvaceae, Fabaceae, Cruciferae, Solanaceae, *etc.*, involving difficult interspecific/intergeneric crosses. Nevertheless, ovule culture is mainly useful in those conditions, where embryo aborts very early, and embryo culture is not possible due to difficulty of its excision at a very early stage.

Gynogenic Haploids: Advantages

- Valuable substitute for the production of homozygous lines in cases where cytoplasmic male sterility prevents the use of microspores.
- Reduction in the frequency of albino plants especially cereals.

Limitations

- Successful only in few species
- The frequency of responding ovaries (1-5 per cent) and the number of plantlets/ovary (1-2) is quite low.
- Therefore, anther culture is preferred over ovary culture.
- ovary culture assumes significance only in those cases where anther culture fails. *e.g.* sugar beet and for male sterile lines

Production of Virus Free Plants

The viral diseases cause lot of losses in yield and reduce the quality of the produce of agricultural crops. It is very difficult to eradicate virus infection in plants therefore developing and growing virus free plants is the only viable option for the plant breeders. Virus free plants can be produced through tissue culture in some ornamental plants at the commercial level. Among the culture techniques, meristem-tip culture is the most reliable method for virus and other pathogen elimination. Meristem can be cultured under in vitro conditions as these tissues are free of infection. The size of the meristem used in cultures play a very critical role in regeneration potential of the plant. Meristems are initially treated with heat shock (34-36°C) to inactivate the virus. The culture medium can also be treated with chemicals *e.g.* addition of cytokinins suppressed the multiplication of certain viruses leading to the production of virus free plants. These techniques eliminated viruses from a number of economically important plant species *e.g.* potato virus X from potato, mosaic virus from cassava *etc.*, led to significant improvement in the yield and production.

Somaclonal Variation

Plants regenerated from tissue and cell cultures show heritable variation for both qualitative and quantitative traits; such a variation is known as somaclonal variation. Variations can be induced into regenerated plantlets during in vitro culture and can be detected as genetic or phenotypic traits. in addition to the variants/ mutants (cell lines and plants) obtained as a result of the application of a selective agent, transient physiological and developmental disturbances may be caused by culture environments. They can be either calliclones (somaclones from callus cultures) and protoclones (somaclones from protoplast cultures) They may be genetic or epigenetic. When the variations are genetically controlled, they are passed to the next generation which is known as somaclonal variation. Somaclonal variation are considered as both a boon and a bane in tissue culture. It may adversely affect clonal propagation, but can also generate desirable variants that can be selected for the development of agronomically useful and novel cell lines viz Salt-tolerant heavy-metal-tolerant, disease-resistant, and herbicide-resistant, *etc.*

Causes of Somaclonal Variations

Genetic (Heritable Variations)

- ☆ Occur at high frequency
- ☆ Pre-existing variations in the explant
- ☆ Caused by mutations and other DNA changes due to methylation of DNA
- ☆ Change in chromosome number and structure
- ☆ Gene Mutation like Tansition, Transversion, Insertion, Deletion
- ☆ Transposable element activation

Epigenetic (Non-heritable Variations)

- ☆ Occur at low frequency
- ☆ Variations generated during tissue culture for short period
- ☆ Caused by temporary phenotypic changes

Physiological Cause

- ☆ Exposure of culture to plant growth regulators
- ☆ Culture conditions like culture media, type of explant, successive transfer of culture, temperature, pH *etc.*
- ☆ Lack of photosynthetic ability due to alteration in carbon metabolism Genetic Cause

Detection and Isolation of Somaclonal Variants

- ☆ Analysis of morphological characters
- ☆ Detection by karyotypic studies using the root tip, leaf tip
- ☆ Variations can be detected by molecular markers like RAPD, RFLP, AFLP, SSR *etc.*

Advantages of Somaclonal Variations

- ☆ Help in crop improvement
- ☆ Creation of additional novel genetic variations
- ☆ Improved production of secondary metabolites

- Selection of plants resistant to various toxins, herbicides, high salt concentration and mineral toxicity
- Suitable for breeding of tree species

Following are the ex. of some of the crops with trait specific improvement

- Sugarcane: variants showing resistance to downy mildew (*Sclerospora sacchari*), eye spot disease (*Helminthosporium sacchari*) and Fiji disease (Virus) were isolated.
- Potato: Soma clones having resistance to late blight (*Phytophthora infestans*) and early blight (*Alternaria solani*).
- Maize: Somaclones were produced with the characters of male fertility and *Drechslera maydis* toxin resistance due to alterations in mtDNA which is responsible for toxin tolerance.
- Rice: Somaclones of dihaploids cultivar Norin 10 showed improved chlorophyll development, plant height, heading date, maturity and grain yield.
- Mutants with abiotic stress resistance *e.g.* salt tolerance in tobacco and maize, aluminium tolerance in carrot,
- Somaclonal variants with herbicide resistance *e.g.* tobacco resistant to sulfonylurea.
- Improved variety of *Lathyrus sativa* (Lathyrus Bio L 212) with reduced levels of neurotoxin.
- Somaclonal variant of Citronella java (with 37 per cent more oil and 39 per cent more citronellon), a medicinal plant as Bio-13 for commercial cultivation.

Disadvantages of Somaclonal Variations

- Selected variants are random and genetically unstable
- It is a serious problem where clonal uniformity is essential, as in the horticulture and forestry industries where clonal propagation through tissue culture is employed for rapid propagation of elite genotypes.
- Can lead to undesirable results
- Require extensive and extended field trials for many generations
- Not suitable for complex agronomic traits like yield, quality *etc.*

Protoplast Fusion/Somatic Hybridization

Protoplast are single cells without cell wall exposing the plasmalemma. Isolation of protoplast by mechanical method was done initially by Klercker in 1892. Later large scale isolation of protoplasts was demonstrated by Cocking (1960) through enzymatic degradation method. Isolated protoplast from two genetically distant taxa or species or genera can be made to fuse experimentally to obtain parasexual hybrid protoplasts. The process of fusion of isolated protoplasts from somatic cells hybrid plants regeneration from the fusion products is called somatic Hybridization. First somatic hybrid production in the genus tobacco was achieved. Later it has been applied to various crop species with improved characters. Through Somatic hybridization both nuclear and cytoplasmic genes can be fused simultaneously unlike sexual hybridization or genetic engineering.

Somatic hybridization technique includes the following essential steps:

Isolation of Protoplasts

Any plant part *i.e.* root, leaf, fruit, tuber, endosperm, pollen mother cell *etc.* can be used for isolation of protoplasts. Isolation can be achieved by Mechanical method and Enzymatic method. In mechanical method plant cells are incubated in plasmolyzing solution and then cut with a sharp knife. This method yields very less protoplasts and is very tedious and can be applicable only to vacuolated cells. In Enzymatic method, cell wall degrading enzymes (cellulase, hemicellulase and pectinase) are used for the isolation of protoplast. And yield good percentage of viable protoplasts.

Protoplasts Fusion

During the enzyme treatment, protoplast can fuse spontaneously from adjoining cells through their plasmodesmata to form multinucleate protoplasts. More efficient fusion can also be achieved by using fusion inducing chemical or physical agents which reduce the electronegativity of the isolated protoplast and allow them to fuse with each other. Chemicals such as polyethylene glycol (PEG), Calcium ions (Ca2+), sodium nitrate *etc.* are used for fusion. Freshly isolated protoplasts from the two selected parents mixed in appropriate proportions and are treated with 15–45 per cent PEG (1,500–6,000 MW) solution. After 20-30 min, the protoplasts are gradually washed with the culture medium containing a high level of Ca^{2+} ions (50 mM $CaCl_2.2H_2O$) and the pH is adjusted to 9–10.

Alternatively, Electrofusion technique can be used where an electric field of low strength (10Kv/m) for some milliseconds or a high strength of electric field (100Kv/m) for some micro seconds are applied which leads to fusion.

Culture of Protoplasts and Regeneration of Somatic Hybrid Plants

This can be achieved by using either Semi solid medium or liquid medium in the form of suspension cultures with specific organic and inorganic nutrient composition and culture conditions.

Selection of Hybrid Cells and Hybridity Verification

- Can be done by cytological analysis
- Use of molecular techniques such as isozyme analysis and DNA analysis by RFLP, RAPD, SSR, AFLP *etc.*
- Use of GISH (Genomic *In situ* Hybridization) 3. FISH (Fluorescence In Situ Hybridization)

Fusion Products

The mixture of two protoplasts may or may not contain fused protoplasts and the fusion can be in variety of forms. The fused binucleate cells are known as heterokaryon or heterocyte. When nuclei and cytoplasm both are fused, the cells are known as somatic hybrid or synkaryocyte. When only cytoplasms fuse and one of the two nuclei is lost, it is known as cybrid *i.e.* cytoplasmic hybrid or heteroplast.

Application of Somatic hybridization

- ☆ Protoplast fusion overcomes sexual incompatibility barriers. In some cases somatic hybrids between two incompatible plants have also found application in industry or agriculture.
- ☆ Protoplasts of sexually sterile (haploid, triploid, and aneuploid) plants can be fused to produce fertile diploids and polyploids.
- ☆ Very useful for transgenic plant production
- ☆ Somatic cell fusion is useful in the study of cytoplasmic genes and their activities and this information can be applied in plant-breeding experiments.
- ☆ Cybridization has been successfully used to make intergeneric and interspecific transfer of cytoplasmic traits, such as male sterility and disease and herbicide resistance.

Trasngenic Plants Production

Molecular biology and genetic engineering offer new tools and are source of genetic variability that can be used in crop improvement and fulfilling agricultural needs. Production of transgenic plants is a multi-step process and includes the major following steps:

- ☆ **Identification of gene of interest**: Identification of required gene is driven by the aim and for the resultant organism and is based on earlier research. Genetic screening is done to determine potential genes and best candidate genes are identified using molecular and genomic approaches.
- ☆ **isolation and cloning of genes:** The chosen gene can be accessible from a genetic library or If the DNA sequence is known, it can also be artificially synthesised. Once the gene is isolated it is ligated into a plasmid that is then inserted into a bacterium. After transformation of the bacterium with the plasmid/vector, large number of copies of the inserted gene can be cloned by allowing the transformed bacterium to divide.
- ☆ **Insertion of cloned DNA or gene of interest into the host genome:** There are a variety of direct and indirect methods are available to insert required gene or gene of interest into the host genome.

Indirect or Vector-mediated Gene Transfer

The most common indirect method used to introduce the gene package into plant cells is through Ti plasmid of Agrobacterium tumefaciens. The gene transfer method is based on tumour inducing mechanism of the soil bacterium *Agrobacterium tumefaciens*, causal organism for crown gall disease and another closely related species *Agrobacterium rhizogenes* causing hairy root disease. This bacterium *Agrobacterium* is known as "natural genetic engineer" of plants because of its natural way of infecting the plants at wound site and subsequent insertion of the T- DNA of its Ti plasmid into plant cell genome. This infection causes unorganized growth of a cell mass under the influence of T DNA of Ti plasmid and results in the crown gall disease in plants. The gene of interest or foreign gene is cloned in to Ti-plasmid in place of the T-DNA region. Ti plasmids are used as vectors for carrying and delivering useful foreign genes into target plant tissues.

Structure and Functions of Ti Plasmid

Ti plasmids have four regions:

- Region A: There are two special sites on this region i) An 'Onc' region hosts T-DNA responsible for tumour induction, and mutations in this region lead to the production of tumours with altered morphology (shooty or rooty mutant galls). T-DNA consists of three genes "tms1 and tms2" representing 'shooty locus' and one gene "tmr" representing 'rooty locus'. Once inserted, these genes encode the enzymes responsible for the synthesis of indole acetic acid (an auxin) and isopentyladenosine 5′-monophosphate (a cytokinin). These phytohormones alter the developmental programme of the plant leading to the uncontrolled cell division and formation of crown gall. Ii) The second site is an 'os' region responsible for the synthesis of special types of amino acid or sugar derivatives, which are known as opines. Two most common types of opines are octopine and nopaline and the corresponding enzymes octopine synthase and nopaline synthase are coded by os region of T- DNA.
- Region B: Responsible for replication.
- Region C: Required for conjugation.
- Region D: Responsible for infection mechanism or virulence and plays a crucial role in the transfer of T-DNA into the plant nuclear genome.

Most of the higher plants cannot utilize opines, but can be metabolized by Agrobacterium and the products are utilized as a source of carbon and nitrogen. Ti plasmid carries the opine catabolizing genes, outside the T-DNA region. The T-DNA region is flanked by 25bp cis acting direct repeat sequences, essential for T-DNA transfer. Any DNA sequence, flanked by these 25bp repeat sequences in the correct orientation, can be transferred to plant cells. This characteristic property has been successfully utilized for Agrobacterium mediated gene transfer in higher plants for the production of transgenic plants.

Besides 25bp flanking border sequences (with T DNA), vir region is also essential for T-DNA transfer. vir region is capable of functioning even in trans orientation. T-DNA and vir region can be separated onto two different plasmids and still can affect T-DNA transfer, provided both the plasmids are present in the same Agrobacterium cell. This property played an important role in designing the well-established vector systems for gene transfer in higher plants. The vir region (approx 35 kbp) is organized into six operons, namely vir A, vir B, vir C, vir D, vir E, and vir G. The vir A and vir G gene products regulate the expression of other vir loci. Genes vir A, B, D, and G are absolutely required for virulence; the remaining two genes vir C and E are required for tumour formation. The vir A locus is expressed constitutively under all conditions.

The product of Vir A is a chemoreceptor located on the inner membrane of Agrobacterium cells senses the presence of phenolic compounds (found in the vicinity of wounded plant tissue), such as acetosyringone and β-hydroxyacetosyringone. Signal transduction proceeds via activation (possibly phosphorylation) of Vir G and its product in turn induces expression of other vir genes.

For transformation of plants, embryogenic callus (in case of monocots) or leaf discs (in case of dicots) are infected with Agrobacterium carrying recombinant disarmed Ti-plasmid vector in suitable culture medium. This way co-cultivation allows the transfer of foreign genes into plant cells. The transformed plant tissues (leaf discs/calli) are then placed on plant regeneration medium supplemented with optimized concentration of an antibiotic for selection of transformed cells and also to selectively eliminate non-transformed tissues. After 3-5 weeks, the regenerated shoots are transferred to root-inducing medium. Once roots are initiated, complete plants are transferred to soil followed by acclimatization process to obtain regenerated plants. The regenerated plants are checked for the transferred new gene using the molecular techniques like PCR and southern hybridization and presence of foreign genes can be confirmed in the transgenic plants. techniques Agrobacterium mediated transformation infection (utilizing its plasmids as vectors) has been extensively utilized for transfer of foreign genes into a number of plant species for improvement of a variety of characters.

Direct or Vectorless Gene Transfer

the foreign gene of interest can be delivered into the host plant cell without the help of a vector in some case where engineered vectors do not work out well particularly in monocot species.

Some of the direct transfer methods are as following:

Chemical Mediated Gene Transfer

Chemicals like polyethylene glycol (PEG) can induce direct foreign DNA uptake by protoplasts. PEG at 15-25 per cent) concentration can precipitate ionic macromolecules such as DNA and stimulate their uptake by protoplasts through the process of endocytosis. This is followed by cell wall formation and initiation of cell division. These cells can now be plated at low density on selection medium. Initially this method has been applied to Nicotiana and Petunia and has been used in other plant systems. PEG is also used to stimulate the uptake of liposomes and to improve the efficiency of electroporation.

Calcium phosphate precipitation method for gene transfer

Foreign DNA can also be carried with the Ca^{2+} ions, and is released inside the cell due to the precipitation of calcium in the form of calcium phosphate.

Electroporation

introduced by Fromm and his coworkers in 1986. Mixture of plant protoplasts and external foreign DNA mixed in buffer and are exposed to short electrical impulses of high field strength. The electric pulse is generated by discharging a capacitor across the electrodes in a specially designed electroporation chamber. Either a high voltage (1.5 kV) wave pulse of short duration or a low voltage (350V) pulse of long duration is used. These impulses increase the permeability of protoplast membrane and facilitate entry of DNA molecules into the cells. Using linear instead of circular DNA and addition of PEG after adding DNA improves the transformation frequency. Successful transfer of genes was achieved with the protoplasts of tobacco, petunia, maize, rice, wheat and sorghum using electroporation method.

Microinjection

Glass micropipettes with 0.5-10μm diameter tip are used for transfer of macromolecules like DNA into the cytoplasm or the nucleus of a recipient cell or protoplast. The recipient cells are immobilized on a solid support (cover slip or slide, *etc.*) or held by a pipette under suction Specially designed micromanipulator is used for microinjecting the foreign DNA. Although, this technique gives high rate of success, the process is slow, expensive and requires highly skilled and experienced personnel.

Particle Gun or Gene Gun or Microprojectiles or Biolistics for Gene Transfer

Projectile Bombardment method is demonstrated by Klein and his colleagues in 1987. The micro-projectiles (small high density particles of tungsten or gold) are accelerated to high velocity by a particle gun apparatus. When these particles coated with foreign DNA penetrate the cells and membranes also carry foreign DNA inside of the bombarded cells. These microprojectiles of 1-3pm in diameter, are carried by a 'macroprojectile' or the 'bullet' and are accelerated into target living plant cells (protoplasts, cultured cells, cells in differentiated tissues and meristems) The acceleration is achieved either by an explosive charge (cordite explosion) or by using shock waves initiated by a high voltage electric discharge. This method is otherwise called as "Biolistics Method". Transformation has been achieved using this technique in many plant species including soybean, tobacco, maize, rice, wheat, *etc.*

Liposome Mediated Gene Transfer (Lipofection)

Engineered plasmids carrying foreign DNA can be enclosed in small lipid bags known as Liposomes. They can be induced to fuse with protoplasts in presence of PEG, and therefore have been used for gene transfer. The technique is found to be advantageous because of low cell toxicity and stability and protection of nucleic acids from nuclease digestion due to encapsulation in liposomes, the technique has been successfully used to deliver DNA into the protoplasts of a number of plant species (*e.g.* tobacco, petunia, carrot, *etc.*)

Sonication Method

The explant tissue is excised and cut into segments, immersed in sonication buffer containing plasmid DNA and Carrier DNA in a sterile glass culture vessel.

Samples were sonicated with an ultrasonic pulse generator at 0.5 c/cm^2 acoustic intensity for 30 minutes. After 30 minutes, the explants were rinsed with buffer solution and transferred to the culture medium.

Transgenic Plants and their Applications

Some success stories related to the production of transgenic plants are described below.

The major successes have been achieved in the transfer of: 1. Genes for herbicide tolerance. 2. Insect tolerant genes. 3. Virus resistance through Coat protein genes for cross protection. 4. Genes responsible for certain antisense RNA and 5. Molecular farming

1. Transgenics for Herbicide Tolerance

The transgenic plants thus produced show expression of foreign genes resulting in a higher level of herbicide tolerance. In 1986, Shah and his co-workers isolated a cDNA clone encoding an enzyme 5-enolpyruvyl-shikimate phosphate (EPSP) synthase from a glyphosate tolerant Petunia hybrida cell line. This cell line over produced the enzyme upto 20 times more. The chimeric EPSP synthase gene was constructed using cauliflower mosaic virus 35 promoter and introduced into the non-tolerant Petunia cell lines. The calli from transformed cell lines showed tolerance to glyphosate and the plants regenerated from them were tolerance to the herbicide whereas the control plants died after spraying the herbicide.

De Block and his co-workers transferred a gene conferring resistance to bialaphos and phosphinothricin called bar gene isolated from *Streptomyces hygroscopicus,* into tobacco, tomato and potato in 1987. This gene encodes for an enzyme, phosphinothricin acetyltransferase which prevents toxicity due to phosphinothricin. This gene has been transferred to tobacco, tomato and potato with the help of 35 S promoter of CaMV. The transformed plants showed high levels of resistance against field dose applications of the bialaphos and phosphinothricin. This technique can also be extended to engineer resistance to various herbicides into other important crops.

2. Transgenic Plants for Insect Tolerance

Bacillus thuringiensis is a bacterium that produces proteinaceous crystals during sporulation. These crystal proteins have insecticidal properties especially to Lepidopteran insects. The use of *Bacillus thuringiensis* as a microbial insecticide offers advantages over chemical control agents in that the species-specific action of its insecticidal crystal proteins (ICPs) makes it harmless to non-target insects, to vertebrates, to the environment and the user. The chimeric genes containing the CaMV 35 S promoter and the *B. thuringiensis* crystal protein coding sequences constructed Fischhoff and his colleagues in 1987. The engineered *B. thuringiensis* gene has been introduced into tomato and tobacco and the level of resistance to Lepidopteran insects had increased in transgenic plants. The larvae fed on transgenic plants were killed within 48 hours and there was little evidence of feeding damage to leaves of transformed plants. Thus the introduction of toxin genes into plants seems to be a practical approach for providing protection against certain insect pests.

3. Use of Coat Protein Genes Expression for Virus Protection

Cross-protection is a common practice to protect the plants from viruses and the coat protein of viruses have an important role in systemic cross protection. A chimeric gene containing a cloned cDNA of the coat protein (CP) gene of TMV was introduced into tobacco cells on a Ti plasmid of *A. tumefaciens* from which tumour inducing genes have been removed. Plants regenerated from transformed cells expressed TMV mRNA and CP as a nuclear trait. Seedlings from self-fertilized transgenic plants were inoculated with TMV and observed for development of disease symptoms. The seedlings that expressed the CP gene showed delayed symptom development and 10-60 per cent of the transgenic plants failed to develop symptoms. This strategy would be useful to develop varieties with resistance to viruses where resistance to viruses have been difficult to develop through conventional plant breeding.

4. Molecular Farming

Plants have been engineered to produce materials they do not normally make. Plants are source of many high value compounds, owing ease of plants for large scale propagation, availability of natural organ systems for storage, possibility of scale up, plants have been employed for the production of high value products through transgenic technology. This ability to produce and isolate compounds from transgenic systems is popularly known as molecular farming. Various products like proteins of industrial and pharmaceutical value *e.g.*, monoantibodies, edible vaccines, human serum albumin, blood factors, antigenic proteins (hepatitis-B surface antigen), protein products like trypsin, collagen, aprotinin, human lactoferin, oligosaccharides like cyclodextrins have been in the process of successful production phase using plant systems as bioreactors. The useful product is purified from the harvest and then used in the standard pharmaceutical production process.

REFERENCES

1. Ainsley, P. and Aryan, A. 1998. Efficient plant regeneration system for immature embryos of triticale (xTriticosecale Wittmack). Plant Growth Regulation 24, 23–30.
2. Augustine, A.C. and D'Souza, L. 1997. Somatic embryogenesis in *Gnetum ula* Brongn. (*Gnetum edule*) (Willd) Blume. Plant Cell Rep., 16: 354-357.
3. Bhojwani S.S.and Dantu P.K. (2013) Somaclonal Variation. In: Plant Tissue Culture: An Introductory Text. Springer, India. https: / /doi.org/10.1007/978-81-322-1026-9_12
4. Carlson, P. S., Smith H. H. and Dearing, R. D. 1972. Parasexual interspecific plant hybridization. Proc. Nat. Acad. Sci. (U. S. A.) 69: 2292-2294.
5. Cocking, E. 1960.A Method for the Isolation of Plant Protoplasts and Vacuoles. *Nature* **187,** 962–963. https: / /doi.org/10.1038/187962a0
6. Cardoza, V and D'Souza, L. 2000. Direct somatic embryogenesis from immature zygtoic embryo of cashew. *Phytomorphology* 50(2): 201–204.

7. Cardoza, V. and D'Souza, L. 2002. Induction development and germination of somatic embryos from nucellar tissues of cashew (*Anacardium occidentale* L.). Sci. Hortic., 93: 367-372.

8. Fiona, S. and Shadwick, Pauline Doran. 2005. Foreign Protein Expression Using Plant Cell Suspension and Hairy Root Cultures. In book: Molecular Farming: Plant-Made Pharmaceuticals and Technical Proteins. DOI: 10.1002/3527603638. ch2

9. Fromm, M. E., Taylor, L. P., and Walbot, V., 1986, Stable transformation of maize after gene transfer by electroporation, *Nature* **319**: 791–793

10. Gamborg, O.L., Miller, R.A. and Ojima, K. 1968 Nutrient requirements of suspension cultures of soybean root cells. Exp. Cell Res. 50, 151-158.

11. Kartha, K.K. 1986. Production and indexing of disease-free plaints. In: Withers LA, Alderson PG (eds) Plant tissue culture and its agricultural applications. Butterworths, London, pp 219–238

12. Krens, F. A., Molendijk, L., Wullems, G. J., and Schilperoort, R. A. 1982, In vitro transformation of plant protoplasts with Ti-plasmid. DNA, *Nature* **296**: 72–74.

13. Larkin, P.J., Scowcroft, W.R. 1981. Somaclonal variation - a novel source of variability from cell cultures for plant improvement. Theor Appl Genet. Oct;60(4): 197-214. doi: 10.1007/BF02342540. PMID: 24276737.

14. Linsmaier E.M.and Skoog F. 1965 Organic growth factor requirements of tobacco tissue cultures. Physiol. Plant. 18, 100- 127.

15. Lloyd, G. and McCown, B. 1981. Commercially-feasible micropropagation of mountain laurel, *Kalmia latifolia*, by use of shoot-tip culture. Proc. Intl. Plant Prop. Soc. 30: 421–427

16. Migue,l A. Blázquez, David C. Nelson, and Dolf Weijers. 2020. Evolution of Plant Hormone Response Pathways. Annu. Rev. Plant Biol. 71: 4.1–4.27

17. Murashige, T. and Skoog, F. 1962. A revised medium for rapid growth and bioassays with tobacco tissue cultures. Physiol. Plant. 15: 473-97

18. Schenk, R.U. and Hildebrandt, A.C. 1972 Medium and techniques for induction and growth of monocotyledonous and dicotyledonous plant cell cultures. Can. J. Bot. 50, 199-204.

19. Ochatt, S.J., Marconi, P.L., Radice, S., Arnozis, P.A.and Caso, O.H. 1999. In vitro recurrent selection of potato: production and characterization ofsalt tolerant cell lines and plants. Plant Cell, Tissue and Organ Culture55: 1–8.

20. Wang, Q.C., Panis, B. Engelmann, F., Lambardi, M., and. Valkonen J.P.T. 2009. Cryotherapy of shoot tips: a technique for pathogen eradication to produce healthy planting materials and prepare healthy plant genetic resources for cryopreservation. Ann Appl Biol 154 351–363

21. White P.R. 1963 The Cultivation of Animal and Plant Cells. 2nd edition. Ronald Press, New York.

Chapter 10

Animal Biotechnology

Anil Kumar[1], Sunil Kumar[2] and Sneh Shalini[3]

[1]School of Engineering and Sciences, GD Goenka University, Gurgaon – 122 103, Haryana, India
[2]Department of Biological Sciences, Science Research Center (SRC) for Immune Research on Non-lymphoid Organ (CIRNO), Sungkyunkwan University, Jangan-gu, Suwon, Gyeonggi-do 16419, South Korea
[3]Molecular Oncology Laboratory, National Institute of Cancer Prevention and Research, Noida – 201 301, Haryana, India
**e-mail: anil.stem@gmail.com*

ABSTRACT

Animal biotechnology aims to promote an understanding and knowledge of animal cell structure and function with particular emphasis on in vitro proliferation and differentiation. Cell culture is the foundation to understand many biological processes. That is why it has attracted the attention of people working in the area of stem cells, gene therapy, drug discovery, pharmacy to name a few. The potential of this animal cell culture is enormous with lots of promises to make for future. The advancements in the methods of transfection techniques are giving us more possibility in the area of gene transfer. This is also giving us further hope in terms of the management of the disease burden. With advancement in the technology we do have many ethical concerns to address and with increasing awareness and acceptance of the science we are getting more and more avenues to serve the society.

Keywords: *Animal cell culture, Transfection, Gene therapy, Ethics.*

Tissue Culture: The Beginning

Tissue culture as the name implies, was developed first with culture of small tissue fragments with migration of cells from the tissue fragment and subsequent division and growth of the cells. Tissue culture with explants of tissue dominated the field for more than 50 years and that is why this term is used as a generic term for cell culture, tissue culture and even for organ culture.

Study of cells in isolation has always been a matter of great curiosity since very beginning. A stimulus to this was given when Rudolf Virchow postulated that pathological characteristics may be detected on a cellular level.

Culture of animal cells started with fragments from a tissue or an organ of animals which had natural capacity to regenerate lost tissue, for example, amphibians, which can regenerate some of their lost organs.

Initially many challenges were there the first and foremost challenge was of a tissue culture media which can support the growth and survival of the tissue and cells in isolation. People started with various salt broths initially. Wilhelm Roux, in the year 1885 isolated nerve fibers of chicken embryos can be kept them alive in a warm salt-broth.

In 1895 Paul Ehrlich successfully cultivated and propagated mouse tumor cells within mice by intra-peritoneal injection of the tumor cells. This in-vivo cultivation was a direct evidence that that the fluids from the living animals is the ideal mix to maintain and support cell proliferation. A major breakthrough in this regard was achieved in 1907 by Ross Harrison who cultivated spinal cords of frogs in a hanging drop of coagulated frog's lymph and studied the proliferation of nerve fibers in this *in-vitro* cultivation and propagation system.

This inference and observation that biological fluids will support the growth of tissue and cells were quite obvious as we see most of the organs thereby tissue and cells are bathed in the fluid. Scientists in the beginning of the twentieth century used various components of the biological fluids from the living organism to study the behavior of animal cells in an environment free of systemic variations.

This was the beginning of the tissue culture and very little was known about the behavior of these tissue or cells in culture. Especially about their life span in culture condition. In 1912 Alexis Carrel reported on the Permanent Life of Tissues outside the organism when he cultivated embryonic chicken cells in an extract of chicken embryos. He introduced aseptic methods and cultivated the cells as monolayers in glass flasks. He was of the opinion that cells can be maintained in culture for decades. He was of the view that if one is well trained cell culture scientist then the cells can be cultured for decades in an in-vitro condition, which is certainly not true as we know today, unless until the cells are tumorous in nature or are transformed. Generally for non-transformed cells or for non-tumorous cells that means for normal cells the in *vitro* proliferation is limited to about 50 divisions. This was shown in culture conditions by the investigations of Hayflick and Moorhead (Hayflick Limit).

Life Span of Cells in Culture: Hayflick Limit

The life span of cells in culture was a subjected which attracted the attention of leading cell culture scientists. The scientists in the beginning were divided in their opinion on the life span of primary cells (nontransformed/nonmalignant) in tissue culture. The history of this phenomenon starts way back in 1881 when the German biologist August Weismann speculated that "death takes place because a worn-out tissue cannot forever renew itself, and because a capacity for increase by means of cell division is not ever- lasting but finite". Alexis Carrel in 1912 suggested that all cells explanted in culture are immortal. Carrel was further of the view that the lack of continuous cell replication was due to ignorance on how best to cultivate the cells. However, reports were beginning to emerge of difficulties in long-term cell culture when Leonard Hayflick and Paul Moorhead entered the field.

In 1961, Hayflick and Moorhead published on the serial cultivation of human diploid cell strains. Hayflick discovered that cultured normal human cells have limited capacity to divide, after which they become senescent.

This work and subsequent studies changed the tenor of research, eventually leading Sir Macfarlane Burnett, Nobel laureate from Australia, to coin the phrase "the Hayflick limit" for the first time in his book Intrinsic Mutagenesis.

The concept of the Hayflick Limit helped scientists study the effects of cellular aging on human populations from embryonic development to death, including the discovery of the effects of shortening repetitive sequences of DNA, called telomeres, on the ends of chromosomes.

Now we understand the Hayflick limit in view of several scientific theories such as Telomere Shortening (Nobel Prize in Physiology or Medicine in 2009), Genomic Damage, Mitogens and Proliferation-Associated Signals, Epigenomic Damage and Activation of Tumor Suppressors.

The downstream signals responding to different kind of cellular stress determine the consequences of cell fate. These signals function primarily to protect ageing tissues from cancer formation. However, the same pathways can promote tissue dysfunction and selection of malignant clones during ageing, involving both cell-intrinsic and cell-extrinsic alterations that are activated in response to genome damage. Lot of insight has accumulated and research is still continuing, it will take a long way to understand the ageing of cells. Understanding the process of cellular ageing will give us many insights in understanding the developmental biology to uncontrolled cell growth.

Primary Culture, Cell Lines and Continuous Cell Lines

Cells in culture can be of three types depending upon their life span and homogeneity during tissue culture.

The cells derived from a tissue explant *i.e.,* isolated and raised directly from a tissue biopsy are called primary culture. When we passage the cells they attain homogeneity and the cells are now called secondary culture or cell line. The cell line may be characterized, and the characteristics will apply for most of its finite life span in culture condition. The derivation of *continuous cell* lines usually implies a phenotypic change, or *transformation -when* a particular type of cells are selected from a culture, by cloning or by some other method, the subline is known as a *cell strain. Monolayer culture signifies that, given* the opportunity, the cells will attach to the substrate and that normally the cells will be propagated in this mode. *Anchorage dependence means that attachment to and usually,* some degree of spreading onto the substrate is a prerequisite for cell proliferation.

Monolayer culture is the mode of culture common to most normal cells, with the exception of hematopoietic cells. *Suspension cultures are derived from cells* that can survive and proliferate without attachment (*anchorage independent*); (*hematopoietic cells,* transformed cell lines, and cells from malignant tumors).

Cultured cell lines are more representative of precursor cell compartments *in vivo than of fully differentiated cells, as, normally, most* differentiated cells do not divide.

First continuous human cell line, HeLa, named after the donor of the cells Henrietta Lacks, was established during middle of the 20th century. This was the period when the tissue culture was growing at a very rapid pace because of the very rapid developments in the tissue culture and introduction of antibiotics into culture to curb the culture contamination, although a large fraction of the scientific group was already against continuous use of the antibiotic because of the associated risk of harboring cryptic, or antibiotic-resistant, contaminations.

The 1950s were also the years of the development of defined media which led ultimately to the development of serum-free media.

Regardless of the method employed, primary culture is the first in a series of selective processes that may ultimately give rise to a relatively uniform cell line.

In primary explantation, *selection occurs by virtue of the cells'* capacity to migrate from the explant, whereas with dispersed cells, only those cells that both survive the disaggregation technique and adhere to the substrate or survive in suspension will form the basis of a primary culture.

If the primary culture is maintained for more than a few hours, a further selection step will occur. Cells that are capable of proliferation will increase, some cell types will survive but not increase, and yet others will be unable to survive under the particular conditions of the culture.

Hence, the relative proportion of each cell type will change and will continue to do so until, in the case of monolayer cultures, all the available culture substrate is occupied.

It should be realized that primary cultures, although suitable for some studies such as cytogenetic analysis, may be unsuitable for other studies because of their instability. Both cell population changes and adaptive modifications within the cells are occurring continuously throughout the culture, making it difficult to select a period when the culture may be regarded as homogeneous or stable.

After *confluence is reached* (*i.e., all the available growth* area is utilized and the cells make close contact with one another), cells whose growth is sensitive to contact inhibition and density limitation of cell proliferation will stop dividing, while any transformed cells, which are insensitive to density limitation, will tend to overgrow.

Keeping the cell density low (*e.g.,* by frequent subculture) helps to preserve the normal phenotype in cultures such as mouse fibroblasts, in which spontaneous transformants tend to overgrow at high cell densities [Todaro and Green, 1963].

Some aspects of specialized function are expressed more strongly in primary culture, particularly when the culture becomes confluent. At this stage, the culture will show its closest morphological resemblance to the parent tissue and retain some diversity in cell type.

Generation of Continuous Cell Line from Cell Line

The primary culture after the first subculture, or passage is known as a *cell line and may* be propagated and subcultured several times before it reaches senescence. With each successive subculture, the component of the population with the ability to proliferate most rapidly will gradually predominate, and nonproliferating or slowly proliferating cells will be diluted out, this will lead to the homogeneity of the cell culture population

This is very much obvious from the first subculture, in which differences in proliferative capacity are compounded with differential abilities of the different cell populations to withstand the trauma of trypsinization and grow after each successive transfer. Although some selection and phenotypic drift will continue, by the third passage the culture becomes more stable and is typified by a rather hardy, rapidly proliferating cell.

The steps involved in the formation of a cell line from a primary culture implies

1. The increase in the total number of cells over generations or increasing passage number. The cells are of heterogeneous in nature in the beginning.
2. As the no of generation or passage number increases the cells of a particular type or cell lineages with the capacity for high growth dominate in terms of number, resulting in
3. A degree of uniformity or homogeneity in the cell population at later passages or over generations

Methods of Cell Culture

To begin with a culture of cells from the primary tissue, there are mainly three cell culture methods are employed. Depending upon the type of tissue and handling aspects. Though establishing a culture from a unknown tissue type is a hit and trial method. We can always refer to the work of the previous people and the available literature to start with. Here a brief methodology of different types of culture techniques employed in listed below.

Suspension Culture

Suspension culture is when we dissociate the tissue into single cell suspension and then we plate them in to culture flask where they may grow suspended in the media or adhered to the cell culture vessel. We can understand this by taking an example of suspension culture of skin tissue cells. The skin tissue has to be made into single cell suspension by enzymatic treatment, we rely on trypsin for most of the tissue dissociation into single cell suspension. After adding trypsin into the culture flask, we may incubate the culture flask at 37°C to provide an optimum temperature for the enzyme to act. We keep observing the cells under an inverted microscope to see their dislodgement from the surface. We may also tap the culture flask gently to provide mechanical force for their dislodgement.

After the cells have fully dissociated form the culture vessel we add trypsin inhibitor to avoid the damage to the cells further once they have dislodged from the parent tissue.

After making the tissue into single cells, we count the number of viable cells and the total cell population; after viability count, the cells are seeded onto a culture dish at a density which is optimum for their growth for example we may say 10,000 cells/cm^2 area of the culture flask (Figure 10.1). We may coat the plate before seeding the cells with fibronectin, which helps the cells to adhere, it is only advisable, if we are working on the adherent cell population. The culture vessel is then incubate into an animal cell culture CO_2 incubator. Normally we keep the cells at 37°C with 5 per cent CO_2 supply.

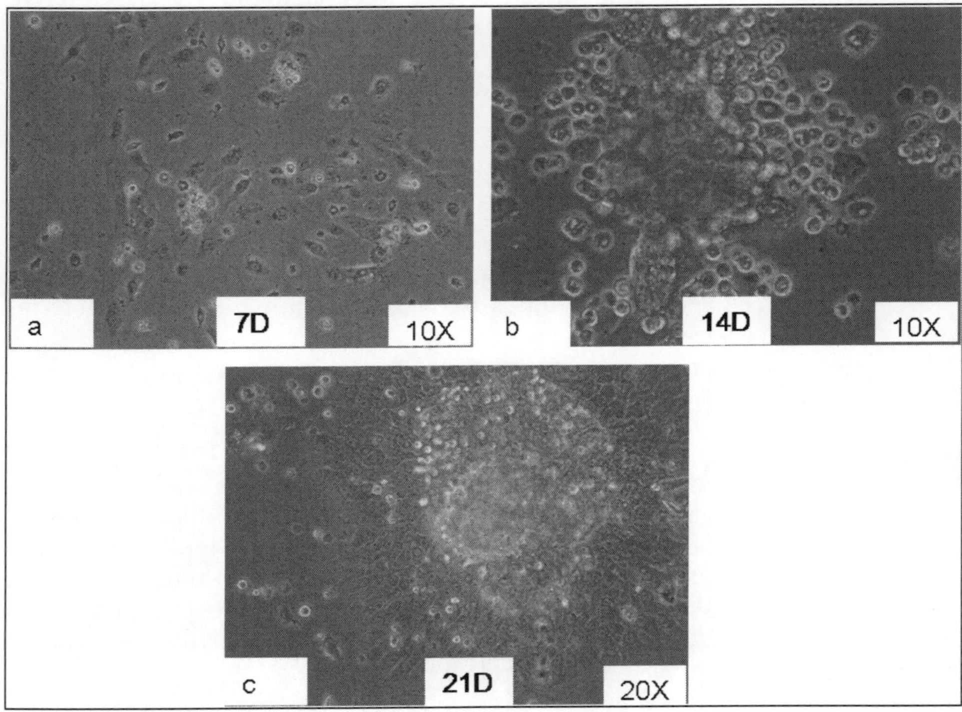

Figure 10.1: Photomicrograph Showing the Skin Stem Cell Colony Obtained by Cell Suspension Culture Method over Fibronectin Coated Culture Dish. The 80- 90 percent confluent culture was achieved after 35-40 days from day of seeding. The cell seeding density was 5000 cells/sq. cm. area of the culture dish. The photomicrographs a, b and c represent the culture at day 7, 14 and 21 respectively.

Explant Culture

In explant culture tissue is not made into single cells but it is chopped into small pieces. These chopped pieces and placed into a culture flask separated by an optimum distance and allowed to grow by adding the media and proper incubation.

We can use fibronectin coated flasks for culture as they provide additional anchorage to the tissue and help them in adherence over the culture flask.

If for example we have to do explant culture of the skin tissue, we first of all make the skin biopsy into small chopped pieces.

The sizes of the explants used for the culture should be kept optimum which has to standardized for different tissue types but mostly it works good with a size of of 2mm x 2 mm. One explants/sq. cm. area of the culture dish may generally be placed. So if for example we are using a 35mm culture dish approximately 9 explants can be placed. Initially, a small volume of media is added to avoid the floating of the explants. After approximately 6-8 hrs, approximately some more media is added very carefully to avoid the floating of the explants. The culture dish can be incubated in a 5 per cent CO_2 incubator at 37°C (Figure 10.2). The media was changed generally every 3rd day or by looking at the media nutrient consumption. This we can infer by looking at the media colour, which changes due to physiological activity of the cells.

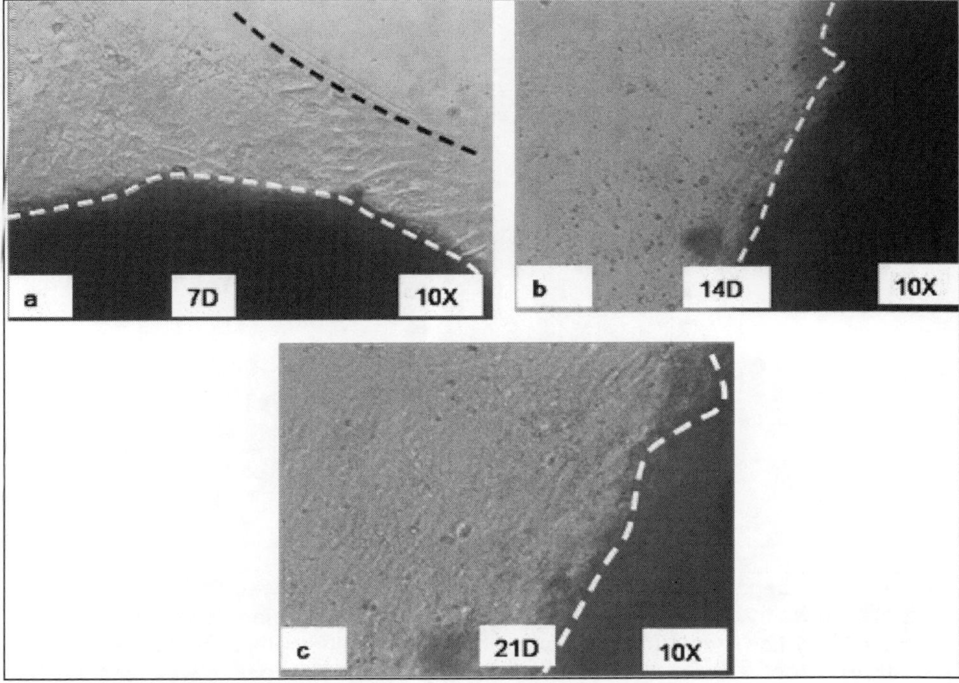

Figure 10.2: Photomicrograph Showing the Explant Culture of Skin Tissue Over Fibronectin Coated Culture Dish. The cells started coming out from the explant periphery after a week in culture media. White dashed line shows the explant boundary and the black dashed line shows the boundary of cells expanded from the tissue explant. The photomicrographs a, b and c represent the culture at day 7, 14 and 21 respectively.

Feeder Layer Culture

Feeder layer cultures are done over the a layer of cells which is treated in such a way that the cells no longer can divide and grow, however the cells are physiologically active.

3T3 mouse fibroblast cell line is a cell line of choice which is used to make feeder layer. To make a feeder layer a confluent culture of mouse fibroblast cell line 3T3 is incubated with mitomycin C or irradiated with gamma rays to convert it into feeder layer. The cells to interest to be cultured are cells are seeded onto the culture dish with feeder layer at an optimum density. The culture dish is incubated in a 5 per cent CO_2 incubator at 37°C (Figure 10.3). The media is changed every 3rd day.

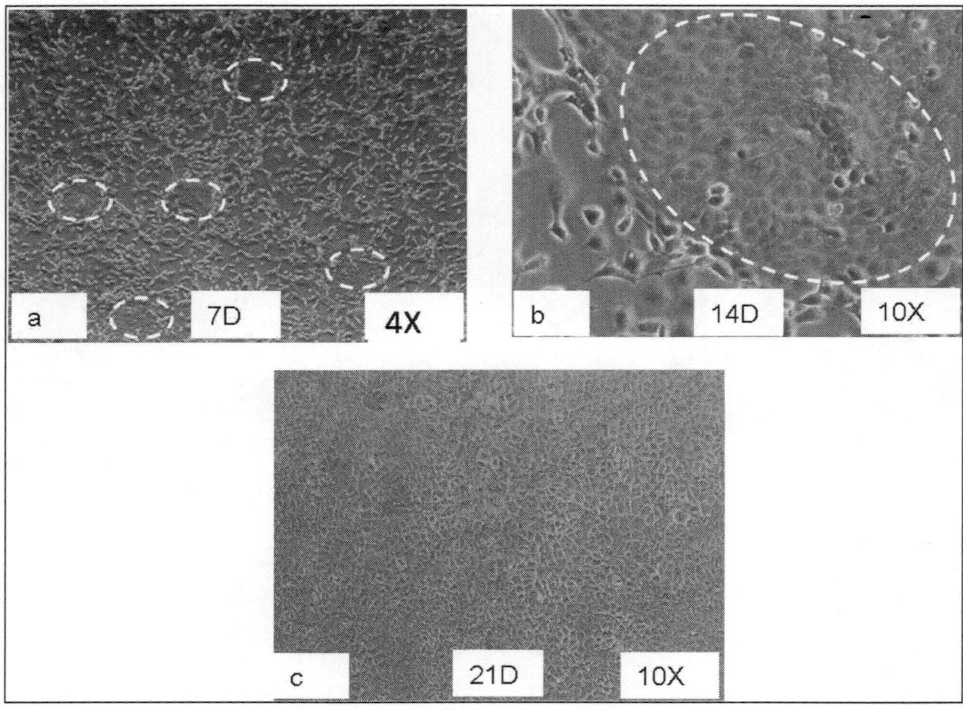

Figure 10.3: Expansion of Skin Stem Cells Over Feeder Layer. The white dashed circle shows the colony of cells expanded over the fibroblast feeder layer. The cell colony has dynamically replaced the feeder cells (cells outside the white boundary). It took around 21 days when 80-90 per cent confluence was reached. The photomicrographs a, b and c represent the culture at day 7, 14 and 21 respectively.

Subculturing and Split Ration

The rate of cell proliferation in culture as we initiate the culture, starts from the lag phase as the cells establish themselves over the new surface area of culture they proliferate rapidly and enter into a log phase. As the cells start growing as per their growth kinetics they start acquiring the space which is available for them to acquire and when the cells in adherent cultures occupy all the available substrate and have no room left for expansion, or when the cells in suspension cultures exceed the capacity of the medium to support further growth, cell proliferation is greatly reduced or stops at all. Generally however we should not wait for the growth to cease, if we are interested in the propagation of the cells through subculture. Mostly one should do the passage (divide the cells into new culture flasks) when the cells have acquired about 80 per cent of the space available for them to grow (Figure 10.4). To keep the culture at an optimal density for continued cell growth and to stimulate further proliferation, the culture has to be divided and fresh medium supplied.

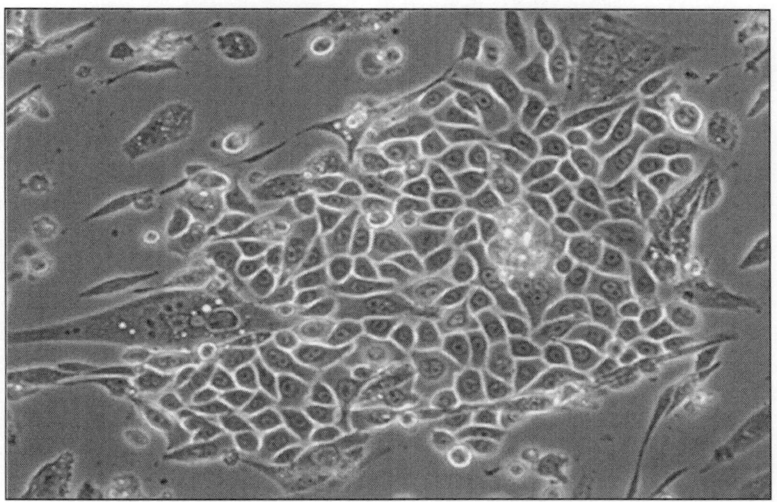

Figure 10.4.: Keratinocytes in Culture Viewed with a Phase Contrast Microscope Showing almost 70-80 Confluence.

Cells keep on growing till there is space for them to grow and nutrition is available. Once all the space and some key nutrients or all the nutrients have exhausted the cells enter into a stationary phase of and we observe a plateau phase in a growth curve. This plateau shows that the growth of cells has almost ceased.

To start with the passaging or sub culturing especially for the cells which are adherent we have to dislodge the cells from the surface. Different ways are there by which we can dislodge the cells from the surface like mechanical for example cell scrapers and tapping the culture vessel or by enzymatic methods such as trypsin EDTA where generally we can use 0.25 per cent Trypsin and 0.05 per cent EDTA solution. Trypsinization has proved to be very useful as it has got a very quick action and ease of handling.

While sub-culturing we trypsinize the cells if it is an adherent culture or simply spin down the cells if it is in suspension culture. After centrifugation we count the number of cells in the pellet and culture them on to new culture vessels by keeping an optimum seeding density. We may split the cells into for example 2 or 3 new flasks by keeping a seeding density for example 10,000 cells/cm^2 surface area of the culture vessel. If we are splitting the cells of one flask into two new flasks the split ration will be 1: 2 or 1:3, if we are splitting it into 3 new flasks.

Senescence

Cell culture derived from a healthy normal tissue can divide a limited number of times; hence, cell lines derived from normal tissue have finite life span in culture *i.e.*, fixed number of population doublings. This is a genetically programmed event involving several different types of genes and is known as *senescence.*

Senescence is a multifactorial process. Partly, it is thought to be determined by the inability of terminal sequences of the DNA in the telomeres to replicate at each cell division. This results in a progressive shortening of the telomeres until, finally, the cell is unable to divide further.

Exceptions to this rule are germ cells, stem cells, and transformed cells, which often express the enzyme telomerase, which is capable of replicating the terminal sequences of DNA in the telomere and extending the life span of the cells, infinitely in the case of germ cells and some tumor cells.

Cell Culture Media

The variety of cell culture media are available today. If we look back at the history of the cell culture media. It was the natural media which was utilized by the scientists for decades before scientists tried for the artificial media. The table below (Table 10.1) shows the basic categorization of the media, its examples and uses.

Table 10.1: Types of Natural and Artificial Media

	Media Type	*Example*	*Uses*
Natural media	Biological Fluids	plasma, serum, lymph, human placental cord serum, amniotic fluid	
	Tissue Extracts	Extract of liver, spleen, tumors, leucocytes and bone marrow, extract of the bovine embryo and chick embryo	
	Clots	coagulants or plasma clots	
	Balanced salt solutions	PBS, DPBS, HBSS, EBSS	
Artificial media	Balanced salt solutions	PBS, DPBS, HBSS, EBSS	Form the basis of complex media
	Basal media	MEM DMEM	Primary and diploid culture
	Complex media	RPMI-1640, IMDM	Supports a wide range of mammalian cells

Source: Labome (www.labome.com).

Table 10.2: Common Cell Lines and Recommended Growth Media

Cell Line	Morphology	Species	Medium	Applications
HeLa B	Epithelial	Human	MEM+ 2mM Glutamine+ 10 per cent FBS + 1 per cent Non Essential Amino Acids (NEAA)	Tumourigenicity and virus studies
HL60	Lymphoblast	Human	RPMI 1640 + 2mM Glutamine + 10-20 per cent FBS	Differentiation studies
3T3 clone A31	Fibroblast	Mouse	DMEM + 2mM Glutamine +5 per cent New Born Calf Serum (NBCS) + 5 per cent FBS	Tumourigenicity and virus studies
COS-7	Fibroblast	Monkey	DMEM+ 2mM Glutamine + 10 per cent FBS	Gene expression and virus replication studies
CHO	Epithelial	Hamster	Ham2 s F12 + 2mM Glutamine + 10 per cent FBS	Nutritional and gene expression studies
HEK 293	Epithelial	Human	EMEM (EBSS) + 2mM Glutamine + 1 per cent Non Essential Amino Acids (NEAA) + 10 per cent FBS	Transformation studies
HUVEC	Endothelial	Human	F-12 K + 10 per cent FBS + 100 μg/ml Heparin	Angiogenesis studies
Jurkat	Lymphoblast	Human	RPMI-1640 + 10 per cent FBS	Signaling studies

Source: Labome (www.labome.com).

Regrettably, the choice of medium is still often empirical. What was used previously by others for the same cells, or what is currently being used in the laboratory for different cells, often dictates the choice of medium and serum. For continuous cell lines it may not matter as long as the conditions are consistent, but for specialized cell types, primary cultures, and growth in the absence of serum, the choice is more critical (Table2)

There are two major advantages of using more sophisticated media in the absence of serum: they may be selective for particular types of cell, and the isolation of purified products is easier in the absence of serum. Nevertheless, culture in the presence of serum is still easier and often no more expensive, though less controlled.

Two major factors why serum media is more popular over serum free media

(a) Cost. Most people do not have the time, facilities, or inclination to make up their own media, and serum-free formulations, with their various additives, tend to be much more expensive than conventional media.

(b) Requirements for serum-free media are more cell type specific. Serum will cover many inadequacies revealed in its absence. Furthermore, because of their selectivity, a different medium may be required for each type of cell line.

(c) Initial attempts to culture cells were performed in natural media based on tissue extracts and body fluids, such as chick embryo extract, serum, lymph, *etc.*

(d) With the propagation of cell lines, the demand for larger amounts of a medium of more consistent quality led to the introduction of chemically defined media based on analyses of body fluids and nutritional biochemistry.

(e) Eagle's Basal Medium and, subsequently, Eagle's Minimal Essential Medium (MEM) became widely adopted, variously supplemented with calf, human, or horse serum, protein hydrolysates, and embryo extract.

However, many industrial-scale production techniques now use serum-free media, to facilitate downstream processing and reduce the risk of adventitious infectious agents.

A popular compromise for many laboratories is a mixture of a complex medium, such as Ham's F12, with one with higher amino acid and vitamin concentrations, such as DMEM.

Decontaminating Cultures with Antibiotics and Antimycotics

When an important culture which is irreplaceable becomes contaminated, we apply methods to eliminate the contamination from the culture.

First of all we need to figure out the type of organism responsible for the contamination *i.e.*, bacteria, fungus, mycoplasma, or yeast. First of all, isolate the contaminated culture from other cell lines so to minimize the chances of contamination to other culture flasks. Clean incubators and laminar flow hoods with a laboratory disinfectant, and check HEPA filters. Antibiotics and antimycotics at high concentrations can be toxic to some cell lines; therefore, we need to perform a dose response test to determine the level at which an antibiotic or antimycotic becomes toxic.

Application of Cell Culture

The cell culture has application in the alomost all disciplines across Biotechnology, Microbiology, Pharmacy, Drug discovery and many more. Some of the areas, but not limited to this where the cell culture find its applications are listed below.

1. Model Systems for Drug Screening/Drug Toxicity/Cancer Resarrch/ Developmental Biology
2. Cell based manufacturing: Large Scale production of viruses for developing vaccines. Large scale production of modified cells designed to produce proteins, hormoes; Large scale production of cells for various cell therapy clinical trials and therapeutics.

3. Genetic Engineering: Programming the cultured cells for the production of desired type of traits. Study of the effect of deletion or introduction of genes inside the cells and other types of transformation studies.
4. Gene Therapy: Production: Take out the cells from the affected person correcting them in *in-vitro* and introducing back the corrected cells into the patients having genetic defects for the gene corrections.
5. Study of Intracellular activity: Studies related to the translocation of hormone receptor complexes and resultant signal transduction processes, and membrane trafficking
6. Environmental interaction: Study of nutrition, infection, cytotoxicity, carcinogenesis, drug action, and ligand–receptor interactions.

Cryopreservation and Thawing

Cryopreservation of Cultured Cells

During the process of cell culture we need to store the cell lines in continuous culture for future use. This we do because cell cultures are prone to genetic drift, are fated for senescence, are susceptible to microbial contamination and we may lose our cells because of the failure in the working instrument, which can spoil the whole experiment.

After characterization, the expanded cultures of are cryopreserved for further experimental uses. For this, the cell monolayer is trypsinized using Trypsin EDTA (0.25 per cent Trypsin, 1mM EDTA). The cells are washed once with cell expansion media and centrifuged at 1500 rpm for 5 min at 25°C. The cell pellet was suspended in cold cryopreservation media containing 10 per cent dimethyl sulfoxide (DMSO) (Sigma-Aldrich, USA), 70 per cent FBS and 20 per cent 1X DMEM-LG, in a drop wise manner with regular tapping of the cells at a concentration of 1×10^6 cells/ml. An aliquot (20 ul) is used to check the viability and cell count. The cells with the cryopreservation media are put in pre labeled (name, date, cell concentration) cryovials (1.8ml) and shifted to rate controlled freezer for gradual drop in temperature at an average rate of 1°C/minute. Later, the vials are shifted to liquid nitrogen storage container (-196°C) for long term storage.

Thawing of Cryopreserved cells

Thawing is a revival process of the cryopreserved cells. As and when we require we can take the cryopreserved cells and revive them and keep multiplying the cells.

To start with the thawing process, cryovials are removed from liquid nitrogen storage container and thawed in a water bath set at 37°C. The vials are disinfected by soaking in 70 per cent ethanol and dried with a paper towel. Cells are transferred to a 15ml tube and appropriate cell culture media is added drop wise over 5 min. Cells are centrifuged at 1200 rpm for 5 min and the pellet is re-suspended in fresh media and viability counts is assessed by trypan blue exclusion. Cells are transferred to a T-25 culture flask and incubated overnight at 37°C, 5 per cent CO_2 and > 95 per cent humidity. Culture flasks are observed for the revival and growth of cells and protocol is followed to maintain them in culture.

Methods of Gene Transfer

There are various methods which are utilized for gene transfer which span from physical, chemical to viral vector methods. For example; in plants (cells) the genes are delivered via gene gun, electroporation, retroviral and lentiviral systems. In animal cells (cell lines), by electroporation, nucleofection, retroviral and lentiviral mediated transfer. In insects, microinjection electroporation, nucleofection, retroviral and lentiviral mediated transfer. We briefly write about some of these chemical, physical and viral vector methods of gene transfer techniques.

Transfection with Diethylaminoethyl dextran

Diethylaminoethyl (DEAE)-dextran is a polycationic derivative of the carbohydrate polymer dextran, and it is one of the first chemical reagents used to transfer nucleic acids into cultured mammalian cells by Vaheri and Pagano in 1965. It is a soluble polycationic carbohydrate that forms aggregates with DNA through electrostatic interactions. It provides the entire complex with a net positive charge, which allows it to interact with the negatively charged cell membrane and promotes uptake by endocytosis. The complexes are very small compared to the particles formed during calcium phosphate transfection. Also much less DNA can be used in each transfection experiment. Like the calcium phosphate method, the reagents are inexpensive and the procedure is simple and efficient. DEAE-dextran is suitable for transient transfections, and is not suitable for generating stable cell lines the efficiency of the transfection around 10 per cent.

Calcium Phosphate Transfection

The procedure was developed in 1973 by Frank L Graham and Alex J. van der Eb, for introducing DNA into mammalian cells. It was the first chemical transfection method to be used with animal cells. Calcium phosphate is probably the most widely used transfection method. This is a simple, reliable method applicable to many cultured cell lines, and the reagents are inexpensive. It can be used both for transient and stable transformation. The principle of the technique is that DNA in a buffered phosphate solution is mixed gently with calcium chloride, which causes the formation of a fine DNA-calcium phosphate coprecipitate. The precipitate settles onto the cells and some of the particles are taken up by endocytosis.

Lipofection

Gene transfer mediated by liposomes was first described by Fengler in 1980. Liposomes are used to form a fusogenic particle with DNA. They are hydrophobic, unilaminar phospholipid vesicles. Such vesicles when mixed with cells in culture, fuse with the cell membrane and deliver DNA directly into the cytoplasm. Lipofection technology uses tiny vesicular structures called **liposomes** that have the same composition as the cell membrane. A scientist performs a simple reaction that forms a liposome around the DNA sequence to be transfected. Depending on the liposome and cell type, the liposome can be endocytosed or directly fuse with the cell membrane to release the DNA construct into cells.

Physical Transfection

In physical methods the DNA is delivered directly into either the cytoplasm or the nucleus using some kind of physical force. There is no requirement for interaction with the plasma membrane. This avoids involvement with the endosomal pathway and thus limits the amount of damage sustained by the exogenous DNA. The physical transfection methods are usually expensive s they employ some sort of apparatus, which is required to administer the physical force. The DNA may be introduced free in solution, but it may be beneficial to protect it by forming chemical complexes (*e.g.* with polyamines) to reduce the damaging effects of shear forces during the transfer process.

Microinjection: Several Physical methods for introduction of DNA and RNA into cells have been developed over the years. Of these, microinjection is the most direct approach and is used currently for a number of applications. Using very small bore glass needles (outer diameter of usually less than 0.2 µm), DNA or other material is injected into the cell for subsequent integration and/or expression. The direct nature of the microinjection ensures delivery in almost every cell treated. Further, the exact copy number or number of DNA molecules delivered into each cell can be precisely controlled. Current applications include the delivery of genes into isolated cells for research purposes, generation of transgenic animals, and *in vitro* fertilization.

Electroporation

Electroporation is a biophysical phenomenon in which cell membrane permeability is increased through externally applied pulsed electric fields. The applied electric field generates small pores in the plasma membrane. These pores, called 'electropores', allow molecules, ions and water to pass from one side of the membrane to the other. If a suitable electric field pulse is applied, then the electroporated cells can recover, with the electropores resealing spontaneously, and the cells can continue to grow. Pore formation is extremely rapid (approximately 1 µs), while pore resealing is much slower, and is measured in the order of minutes.

Gene-gun delivery, a handheld form of biolistic system used for DNA vaccination consists of propelling DNA-coated colloidal gold or tungsten microprojectiles toward the tissue surface. Gas-accelerated particles penetrate into deeper layers based on adjustment of the discharge pressure. Some of the beads pass through the cell wall and into the cytoplasm of the target cells. Here, the bead and the DNA dissociate and the cells become transformed. The gene gun is particularly useful for transforming cells that are difficult to transform by other methods, *e.g.* plant cells. It is also gaining in use as a method for transferring DNA constructs into whole animals.

Retroviral Vectors

Retroviruses are the animal viruses that integrate into the host cell genome during the normal growth cycle. They are enveloped particles (approximately 100 nm in diameter), where the envelope takes the form of a lipid bilayer extracted from the host cell as the virus buds away from it. The envelope also contains some virally encoded proteins. Infection occurs as a result of the interaction of the envelope proteins with specific receptors on the surface of the host cell. Receptor binding results in the internalization of the viral particle (Figure 10.5).

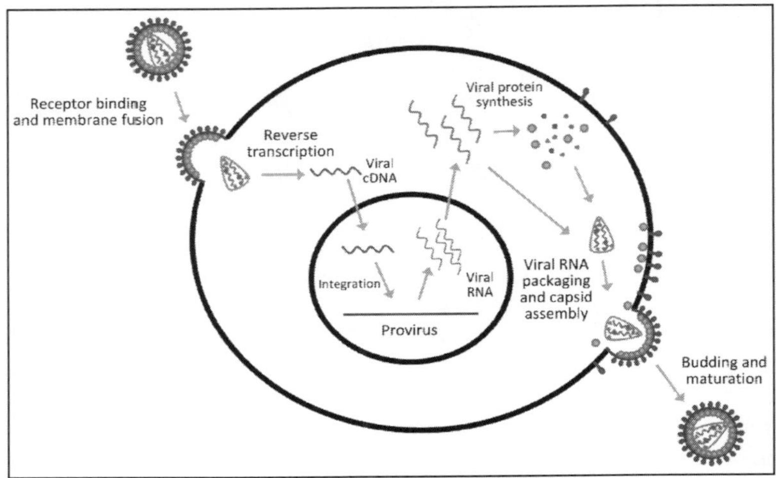

Figure 10.5: Retroviral Replication. Infection begins when the viral Env protein interacts with the cellular receptor and enters the cell. The RNA genome is reverse-transcribed by reverse trnacriptase into dsDNA which then enters the nucleus and is integrated into the host genome through the activity of integrase. After the accumulation of newly synthesized viral proteins and viral genomic RNA, the components are packaged and bud from the cell, acquiring a cellularly-derived membrane. Source credit: Labome (www.labome.com)

All The genetic material in retroviruses is in the form of RNA molecules, while the genetic material of their hosts is in the form of DNA. When a retrovirus infects a host cell, it will introduce its RNA together with some enzymes into the cell. This RNA molecule from the retrovirus must produce a DNA copy from its RNA molecule before it can be considered part of the genetic material of the host cell.

Retrovirus genomes commonly contain these three open reading frames that encode for proteins that can be found in the mature virus (Figure 10.6).

Group-specific antigen (gag) codes for core and structural proteins of the virus, polymerase (pol) codes for reverse transcriptase, protease and integrase, and envelope (env) codes for the retroviral coat proteins.

The process of producing a DNA copy from an RNA molecule is termed reverse transcription. It is carried out by one of the enzymes carried in the virus, called reverse transcriptase. After this DNA copy is produced and is free in the nucleus of the host cell, it must be incorporated into the genome of the host cell. That is, it must be inserted into the large DNA molecules in the cell (the chromosomes). This process is done by another enzyme carried in the virus called integrase. Now that the genetic material of the virus is incorporated and has become part of the genetic material of the host cell, we can say that the host cell is now modified to contain a new gene. If this host cell divides later, its descendants will all contain the new genes. Sometimes the genes of the retrovirus do not express their information immediately. Retroviral vectors are created by removal of the retroviral gag, pol, and env genes. These are replaced by the therapeutic gene. In order to produce vector particles a packaging cell is essential. Packaging cell lines provide all the viral proteins required for capsid production and the virion maturation of the vector. These packaging cell lines have been made so that they contain the gag, pol and env genes.

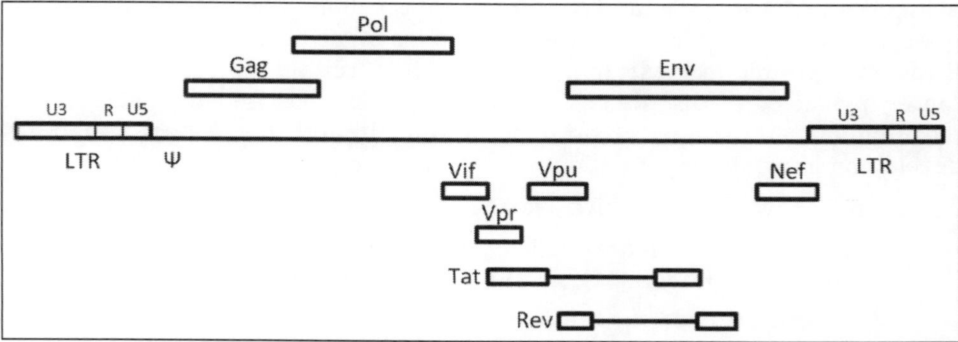

Figure 10.6: Complex Retrovirus Genome Structure.

The linear, nonsegmented, single-stranded RNA of retroviruses is 7-12 kb in length and encode the genes gag, pol, and env. The gag gene encodes a polyprotein that is translated from an unspliced mRNA which is then cleaved by the viral protease (PR) into the MA, CA, and NC proteins. the env gene also encodes a polyprotein precursor which is cleaved into the surface envelope glycoprotein gp120 and the transmembrane glycoprotein gp41. The pol gene is expressed as a Gag-Pol polyprotein and encodes the enzymatic proteins reverse transcriptase, protease and integrase. These three proteins are associated with the viral genome within the virion. Unlike simple retroviruses, complex retroviruses encode a series of accessory proteins including Vpu, Vif, Vpr, and Nef. The integrated provirus genome has 5' and 3' long terminal repeats (LTR) which consist of U3, R, and U5 regions. Finally, the psi (Ψ) sequence serves as the packaging signal for the RNA genome. Source credit: Labome (www.labome.com)

Complex Retrovirus (lentivirus)

The main feature of complex retroviral genomes distinguishing them from those of simple retroviruses is the presence of a set of accessory genes whose products are involved in the regulation of transcription, RNA transport, gene expression, and assembly. These include the Rev and Tat proteins as well as the accessory proteins Vpu, Vif, Vpr, and Nef. Rev is an RNA-binding protein that promotes late phase gene expression. It is also important for the transport of the unspliced or singly-spliced mRNAs, which encode viral structural proteins, from the nucleus to the cytoplasm. Tat is an RNA-binding protein that enhances transcription. The Nef protein inhibits T-cell activation. Vpu enhances the release of the virus from the cell surface to the cytoplasm during entry. The Vif protein is necessary for replication of lentiviruses due to its ability to downregulate the host's antiviral response

Viral Vectors in Gene Therapy

Gene therapy is a branch of science where genetic manipulations are done by recombinant DNA technology (genetic engineering) for the purpose to improve the desired needs. It is applied in plants, animals, insects, medical and pharmacological areas. In plants, it is basically used to improve vegetable, fruits and flowering qualities, including, to create drought and disease resistant. In animals, it is used to increase milk production in cows, goats and wool production in sheep's. In insects, to improve honey qualities and wax productions in honey bees (*Apis malifera*). The most widely used application of gene therapy is in medical and pharmacological fields, for example in medical, it is used to treat certain disease like: diabetes, cancer, hematological disorders *etc.* In pharmacological, it is used in drug discovery, recombinant bio-therapeutic proteins production and monoclonal antibodies developments against several immune and non-immune associated disorders.

There are two ways in which a genetic disorder is corrected.

1. *ex vivo gene correction*- cells of the diseased host removed, genetically modified with viral vector and transplanted back into a patient
2. *in vivo gene correction*- it is direct transfer of corrected genetic material inside the vector into patient

The Ideal Vector for Gene Transfer should have following features

- ✰ High concentration of virus allowing many cells to be infected or transduced
- ✰ Convenience and reproducibility of production
- ✰ Ability to transduce dividing and non-dividing cells
- ✰ Ability to integrate into a site-specific location in the host chromosome
- ✰ A transcriptional unit that can respond to manipulation of its regulatory elements
- ✰ Ability to target the desired type of cell

Lentiviral and retroviral gene delivery systems exploit aspects of retrovirus replication to provide stable integration of the desired nucleic acid sequence. Whereas transfection of nucleic acids results only in transient transgene expression, the activity of the viral integrase in retroviral and lentiviral-based systems allows for stable integration of the transgene which is then inherited and continuously expressed over repeated cell divisions. A key feature of both lentiviral and retroviral vectors is that they produce replication-defective, or self-inactivating, particles. This allows for delivery of the desired sequence, without continued viral replication in the target cells. More importantly, since some of these are developed from a human virus, it eliminates the dangers associated with the use of a live pathogen. The production of replication defective virus is accomplished through trans-complementation (Figure 10.7) in which the packaging cells are cotransfected with three separate plasmids (Figure 10.8) that together express all of the viral proteins necessary to generate infectious particles, as well as the nucleic acid sequence of interest that will be packaged within them for delivery. While many lentiviral vector systems are based on transduction of two helper plasmids (second generation) with the transfer plasmid, some newer systems (third generation) have the packaging and envelope constructs on three plasmids which are combined with the transfer plasmid. The typical transfer and two helper plasmids used in replication-defective retroviral or lentiviral production are:If genetic material happens to be inserted in the middle of one of the original genes of the host cell, this gene will be disrupted (insertional mutagenesis).

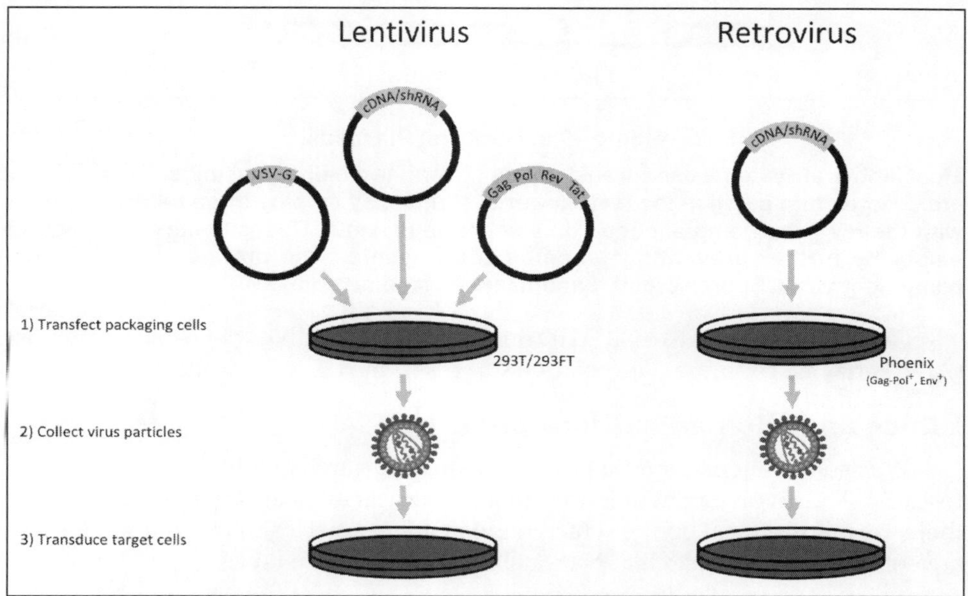

Figure 10.7: Making Lentiviral and Retroviral Vectors.

Lentiviral vectors (left) are created by cotransfection of a packaging cell line (293T/293FT) with the cDNA/shRNA expressing transfer plasmid along with two helper/ packaging plasmids which encode the structural and envelope (typically VSV-G) proteins. The packaging cells produce infectious particles, whose genome only encodes sequences from the transfer plasmid, which can be used to transduce the target cells. Retroviral vector production (right) occurs in a similar manner to lentivirus production, with the main difference being that the initial step is transfection with a single plasmid. The transfer plasmid alone is transfected into a packaging cell line (Phoenix) that already contains the helper constructs. adapted from AddGene. Source credit: Labome (www.labome.com)

If the gene happens to be one regulating cell division, uncontrolled cell division (*i.e.*, cancer) can occur. This problem has recently begun to be addressed by site directed integration for integration at specific chromosomal sites.

Gene therapy trials to treat severe combined immunodeficiency (SCID) were halted or restricted in the USA when leukemia was reported in three of eleven patients treated in the X-linked SCID (X-SCID) gene therapy trial.

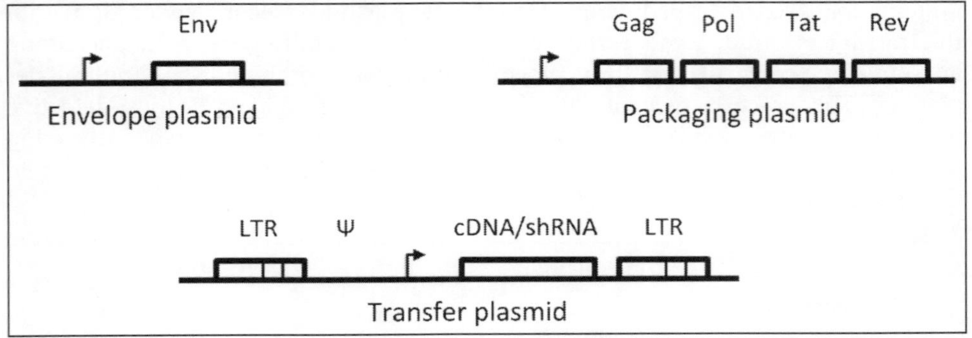

Figure 10.8: Lentiviral Plasmids.

Most lentiviral systems use a transfer plasmid and two helper plasmids. Their features are described in detail in the text. Newer systems may employ three helper plasmids with the rev gene being encoded on a separate plasmid. This is believed to improve safety by further preventing recombination events from producing replication-competent virus. Source credit: Labome (www.labome.com)

Gene therapy trials to treat SCID due to deficiency of the Adenosine Deaminase (ADA) enzyme continue with relative success in the USA, Italy and Japan.

Ethics and Biomedical Research

We need to understand that the biomedical research involves living entities in research. The involvement of living subjects attracts lot of ethical issues. Therefore there are many ethical bodies which regulate the research and development in the area of biomedical research at National and International levels.

Some of the prominent area of research which require to be regulated by the ethics committee are:

1. Preclinical Research – Research on Animals
2. Recombinant DNA research
3. Clinical Research-Research on Human Subjects
4. Stem Cell Research
5. Research on embryo (Destruction of Life/Rights of an Individual)

Ethics is not something related to personal beliefs, what polls and surveys reveal, the law and the religious beliefs.

Ethics is something which relies on justified principles and values, convincing argument, pragmatic payoff, values that have appeal outside your own group or nation and character and virtues that produce trust.

Ethics matters because ethics leads to the law. Ethics is what people care about when it comes to medicine and biotechnology. Ethics is required to protect patients and public health.

Therefore the institutions working on the biomedical research require ethics committees. We shall briefly mention some of the ethics committees.

Institutional Animal Ethics Committee (IAEC): Animal ethics committee clearance is required for the R and D projects which involve research on animal subjects. This is regulated by Animal Welfare Division of the Ministry of Environment, Forest and Climate Change, Govt. of India. (http://cpcsea.nic.in/Auth/index.aspx).

Institutional Biosafety Committee (IBC): IBC is required to be constituted by institutions working on Recombinant DNA research and Bio-containment. This is regulated by Department of Biotechnology, Ministry of Science and Technology, Govt of India. (https://ibkp.dbtindia.gov.in/Content/FlashPDF/IBSC per cent 20Handbook.pdf)

Institutional Ethics Committee for Stem Cell Research (IEC-SCR): IEC-SCR is necessary to be constituted by the Institutions which work on stem cell research (http://dbtindia.gov.in/regulations-guidelines/guidelines/national-guidelines-stem-cell-research- per cent E2 per cent 80 per cent 93-2017).

Hospitals and Institutions where human subjects are enrolled for different type of clinical trials are required to take the permission of Institutional Human Ethics Committee before they start the clinical trials.

IEC-SCR operates and follows the guidelines formulated by jointly by Indian Council of Medical Research and Department of Biotechnology, Govt of India.

REFERENCES

1. Freshney, R. Ian. *Culture of Animal Cells: A Manual of Basic Technique*. Hoboken, N.J.: Wiley-Liss, 2005.
2. S B Primrose; Richard M Twyman. Principles of gene manipulation and genomics. Malden, MA; Oxford : Blackwell Pub., 2006

Chapter 11

Environment Biotechnology

Ravneet Chug[1]* *and Babita Khosla*[2]

[1]*Amity Institute of Biotechnology, Amity University Rajasthan, Jaipur, Rajasthan, India*
[2]*Department of Environmental Sciences, Maharshi Dayanand University, Rohtak, Haryana, India*
**e-mail: rchug@jpr.amity.edu*

ABSTRACT

Onset of the 21st century, has seen environment biotechnology evolving as an emerging field for sustainable environmental protection. It provides ecofriendly solutions for developing clean processes and products which are less hazardous and have minimal adverse environmental impacts. Environment biotechnology not only focus on pollution control but also emphasizes on pollution prevention, judicial utilization of available resources and sustainable future development. Integration of innovative new technologies comprising the use of latest molecular biological and genetic engineering techniques in solving the environmental problems may offer an added advantage. This chapter describes the state-of-the-art and contribution of environmental biotechnology for the development and progression of a more sustainable society.

Keywords: *Bioremediation, Biofuels, Bioethanol, Heavy metal sequestration, Biodiesel, Biofertilizers, Biogas, IPM.*

1. Renewable and Non-renewable Energy Resources

A natural resource is the gift provided to us by nature which can be utilized as an energy source.

A renewable natural resource is the one which can be renewed, in a substantial amount of time (usually years or a human-life span), once it has been used. It is categorized as infinite resource.

Main advantage of using renewable energy resource is that since it is replenished from natural sources like sun, wind, rain, tides, and vegetation, so anytime we may regenerate it according to the requirement. For example, trees may be considered as a renewable resource because once a tree is removed, a new tree can be grown at its place.

Types of Renewable Energy Resources

1. **Solar Energy**: The sun's light contains energy which can be harnessed in the form of electromagnetic waves because when sunlight falls on an object, heat is generated. Similarly, when light hits certain objects like silicon, solar energy converts into an electrical current due to the photoelectric effect and it can be harnessed for power generation.
2. **Hydroelectric Energy**: Water falling from dams is used to turn the turbine of a generator in hydroelectric plants. Electricity production is then regulated using this generator.
3. **Geothermal energy**: It is the form of heat present beneath the sub-surface of the earth. The word **geothermal** is derived from the Greek words' geo (meaning earth) and therme (meaning heat).

   It is a renewable energy resource, since heat is constantly produced inside the earth which can be efficiently used to generate the electricity.
4. **Wind Energy**: Winds are generated due to rotation of earth, earth's surface irregularities and also due to heating effect of sun. Wind turbines can change the kinetic energy of the wind into mechanical power.

   As the wind blows and sun shines, the energy is produced which can be harnessed for power generation.
5. **Biomass Energy**: It is a sustainable and renewable resource of energy where animal or plant material including left over crops, leaves, tree branches, wood wastes from forests, animal manure, *etc.* are used to create heat or generate electricity.

2. Non-renewable Energy Resources

A nonrenewable resource is the one that is not replenished with the speed at which it is consumed. It is considered as a finite resource as it may eventually run out.

Most of the fossil fuels like coal, gas, and oil, minerals and metal ores are non-renewable.

These resources are formed from dead organic material of plant and animal remains which was into existence millions of years ago. It took millions of years to form, so it will also require millions of years to replenish.

Human beings extract non-renewable resources in the form of gas, liquid, or solids, and then these are converted into the forms which can be used commercially. Although, these are the main source of power supply for many industries, factories, vehicles, homes but there are numerous growing concerns over their negative environmental consequences as these are the notable contributors to global warming.

Types of Non-Renewable Natural Resource

1. **Coal Energy**: Coal is produced by putting pressure for millions of years on organic matter from trees, plants and ferns which are buried underground. It is extracted by excavating the ground and then taking out the coal solids for processing into energy.
2. **Oil Energy**: Crude Oil is referred to as Liquid Petroleum. Excessive pressure on small organisms like zooplankton and algae decomposes them leading to oil production. This oil may be utilized for gasoline, heating oil, and diesel fuel.
3. **Natural Gas**: Like oil reserves, decomposition is a longer process as high amount of heat and pressure are required. It is used as cooking fuel, vehicle fuel. It would take many generations, perhaps millions of years, to replenish natural gas.
4. **Nuclear Energy**: Nuclear energy uses radioactive material as a fuel. It generally relies on using Uranium-235, a radioactive chemical naturally found in the earth. It undergoes decay and, in this process, releases a large amount of heat. The heat produces the steam which is used to turn a turbine in a generator. Eventually, electricity production can be carried out. Although, no greenhouse gas emission takes place in this process, however, radioactive byproducts being produced must be stored safely, because they are environmental hazard.

Advantages of Non-renewable Energy

- It is easily accessible and more compatible.
- It is easy to store.

Disadvantages of Non-renewable Energy

- Non-renewable energy cannot be replaced/replenished easily
- Emission of greenhouse gases causes environmental hazard.
- Transportation of fossil fuels, excavation and mining activities, oil spills, pipeline leaks may result in nuclear accidents and which may cause harmful effects on the environment

Biofuels

Since many decades, energy requirements of human beings have been met by fossil fuels (coal, oil, gas). Fossil fuels account for over 80.3 per cent of the main energy consumed in the world, out of which 57.7 per cent is used in the transport sector. Even though, such fuels provide good cost/benefit ratio; but at the same time, they are causing harm to the environment.

Burning of conventional fuels aids to global warming due to the harmful release of greenhouse gases including carbon dioxide (CO_2), nitrogen oxide (NOx), volatile organic compounds (VOC) and hydrocarbons (HC).

These limitations compel the scientists and researchers for finding alternative substitutes. Biofuel has emerged as a novel, reliable and ecofriendly energy resource since last two decades. Production of biodiesel, biogas and bioethanol from variety of feedstock, various kinds of wastes, many types of biomass and agricultural residues, is economically feasible and sustainable option.

The term "bio" in biofuel refers to crop, plant, algae or wood-based raw materials like rice husk, molasses, corn and wood waste, which are converted into fuel. In short, biofuel is any fuel derived from biomass conversion.

Biofuel production from biomass is the result of thermochemical and biochemical processes. These processes include pyrolysis, gasification, liquefaction, supercritical fluid extraction, *etc.* which results into production of energetic exploitable liquid and gaseous products.

Biofuels include bioethanol, biodiesel and biogas which are produced by biochemical path ways, for *e.g.* alcoholic fermentation, anaerobic fermentation and trans-esterification.

Generations of Biofuels

These are categorized into three: First, second and third generation biofuels. These are characterized by the type of biomass, their limitation as a renewable energy resource, and their technological advancement. The main disadvantage of first-generation biofuels is that they come directly from the biomass which is also a food source. This leads to shortage of food item and presents a problem. Second generation biofuels are derived from non-food biomass, but still compete with food production for land use.

Third generation biofuels are the best possible alternative for fuel as they don't compete with food. However, still there are challenges in making them economically feasible.

First generation biofuels are made from sugar, starch or vegetable oil. These are also known as conventional biofuels. These are produced through known technologies and processes, like fermentation, distillation and transesterification. These processes are in existence since hundreds of years and use to make alcohol. Sugars and starches are fermented to produce mainly ethanol, although butanol and propanol are also produced in lesser quantities.

These biofuels are a step towards gaining energy independence and reducing off fossil fuels for energy demands. These biofuels also support agricultural industries as crop demand increases. These first-generation biofuels also offer many disadvantages as they pose a threat to increase in the food prices since the biomass used are food crops such as corn and sugar beet. They also pose adverse impact on biodiversity, additionally, biomass production requires lots of space for crop production.

Second generation biofuels are derived from organic waste, food waste, wood and specific biomass crops. The lignocellulose biomass derived from above sources is available in much higher quantities as compare to starch and sucrose containing substrates. It undergoes pretreatment process which involves thermochemical or biochemical reactions that unlock the sugars embedded in fibers of the plant. After this step, the process to generate plant ethanol resembles that of first-generation ethanol production.

These overcome many disadvantages of first-generation biofuels as no competition for production of fuel and food crops. Also, energy production is more per acre land. Less fertile lands may be used where food crops may not be able to grow. However, some biomasses for second-generation biofuels requires same climatic conditions as of food crops. Additionally, production of second-generation biofuels requires more energy and raw materials for pretreatment of biomass.

Third generation biofuels use algae as the energy source which is grown and harvested for oil extraction. The oil can then be converted into biodiesel through a similar process as first-generation biofuels, or it can be refined into other fuels as replacements to petroleum-based fuels. Algae are advantageous in that it can grow in areas unsuitable for first and second-generation crops. It is considered as low-cost, high-energy yield, and completely renewable sources of energy. Although, third generation biofuels are considered to be most advantageous, but still lot of scientific studies need be done to minimize cost of production and make this type of fuel production commercially viable.

Fourth-generation biofuels are similar to third-generation biofuels, fourth-generation biofuels are made using non-arable land. However, unlike third generation biofuels, they do not require the destruction of biomass. This class of biofuels includes electro fuels and photo biological solar fuels. Some of these fuels are carbon-neutral.

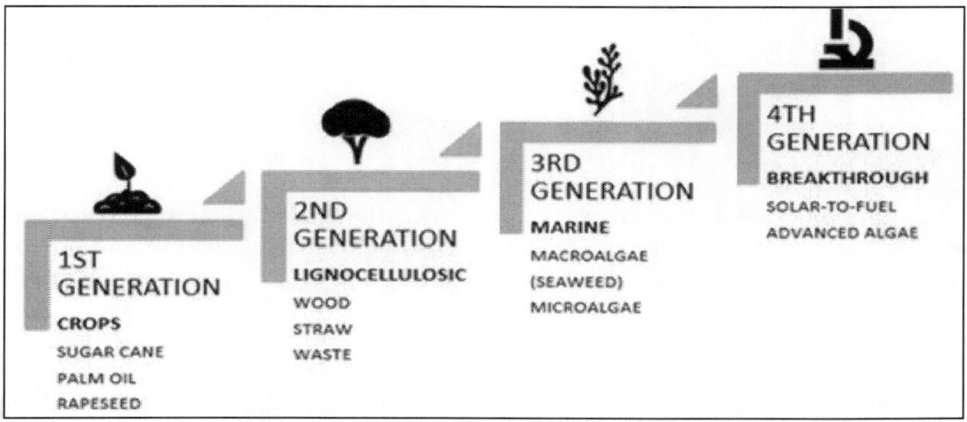

Figure 11.1: Generations of Biofuels.

Bioethanol

Bioethanol is an alcohol produced by fermentation, derived from carbohydrates sources such as sugar, starch, and cellulose.

Ethanol fermentation of the glucose is the oldest method being employed for producing alcoholic beverages. Agriculture based stuffs containing sugar, starch, and cellulose are employed as raw material. Normally, the fermentation process by the yeasts occurs at room temperature, anaerobically. Ethanol fuel is the most common biofuel worldwide, particularly as an alternative to gasoline used by flex-fuel vehicles in Brazil and as an oxygenate to gasoline in USA.

Alcohol fuels unlike petroleum is a renewable resource, that can be produced by fermentation of sugars derived from wheat, corn, sugar beets, sugar cane, molasses, potato and fruit waste or any sugar or starch.

Bioethanol is usually concentrated by distillation of aqueous solutions, but the composition of the vapor from aqueous ethanol is 96 per cent ethanol and 4 per cent water. Commercial ethanol contains 95 per cent by volume of ethanol and 5 per cent of water. Dehydrating agents can be used to remove the remaining water and produce absolute ethanol. Dehydrated alcohol contains not less than 99.0 percent v/v or 99.0 per cent w/w, which is not more than 100.0 per cent v/v or 100.0 per cent t w/w of ethanol. Anhydrous ethanol can be used as a fuel in petrol engines as a replacement for gasoline; but usually blended with gasoline in proportions varying from 5 to 85 per cent. The lower blends are compatible with conventional gasoline engines. Blends above 10 per cent ethanol content are only suitable for use in modified engines. Most of the vehicles on the road today can run on blends up to 10 per cent ethanol and the use of 10 per cent ethanol gasoline is mandated in many cities.

The ethanol can be produced by fermentation of sugar or by hydration of ethane ($CH_2=CH_2$) from petroleum or other sources.

The production of bioethanol by fermentation includes the following steps:

1. Biomass Pretreatment
2. Enzyme digestion/Hydrolysis (to release sugars from stored starches)
3. Fermentation of the sugars by Yeast
4. Distillation and drying

The simplest way to produce ethanol is to use biomass that contains six-carbon sugars that can be fermented directly to ethanol. If producing ethanol from starch-based crops another processing step is required. The two conversion routes are described below:

Bioethanol from Sugars

The process starts by grinding up the feedstock to extract the sugar, which is then added to yeast for the fermentation process. In a closed anaerobic chamber, the yeast secretes enzymes that digest the sugar, yielding several products, including lactic acid, hydrogen, carbon dioxide and ethanol. The most common feed stocks include sugarcane, sugar beet, sweet sorghum and other plants containing a large proportion of simple sugars. A gram of glucose can be converted to 0.511 grams of ethanol.

Bioethanol from Starches

Producing ethanol from starch-based crops requires another step in the process called saccharification, which entails breaking the large starch molecules into simpler sugars. There are two main methods for refining starches into sugars, primarily differing in the pre-treatment of feedstock. In the "wet milling" process the grains are soaked in water, usually with a sulphurous acid, to separate the starch-rich endosperm from the high-protein germ and high-fiber husks. In addition to ethanol, the process results in a number of high-value co-products, such as grain oil, gluten feed, germ meal, starches, dextrin and sweeteners. The simpler "dry milling process" entails grinding the unprocessed heterogeneous seed into granules. Compared to wet mills, dry mills are less capital intensive and produce fewer co-products; however, a very important co-product is the dried distiller's grains with solubles (DDGS), a high quality, nutritious livestock feed. "Both wet and dry mills also sometimes sell the CO_2 released during fermentation to the carbonating soft beverage industry".

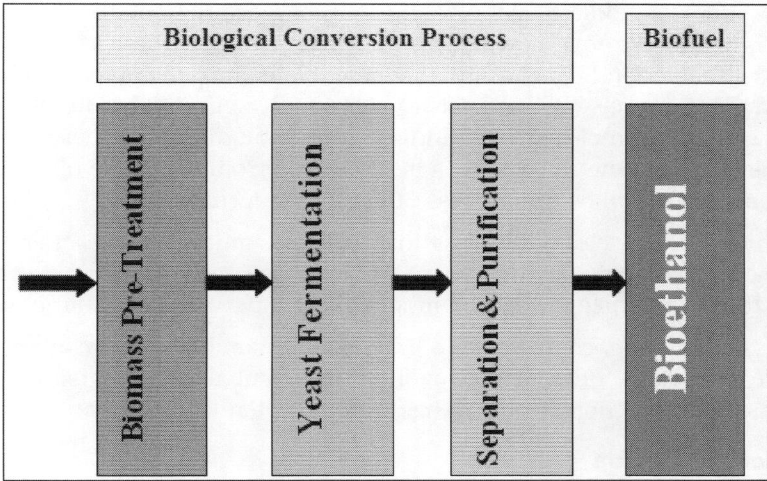

Figure 11.2: Bioethanol Production.

Advantages of Bioethanol as Fuel

1. Most existing car petrol engines can run on blends of up to 15 per cent bioethanol with petroleum/gasoline.
2. In high-altitude locations, some states mandate a mix of gasoline and ethanol as a winter oxidizer to reduce atmospheric pollution emissions.
3. Ethanol has a smaller energy density than that of gasoline; this means it takes more fuel (volume and mass) to produce the same amount of work.
4. Ethanol or ethanol blended gasoline has a higher-octane rating than ethanol-free gasoline, which allows an increase of an engine's compression ratio for increased thermal efficiency. Ethanol is also used to fuel fireplaces. As they do not require a chimney and are "flueless", bioethanol fires are

extremely useful for newly built homes and apartments without a flue. The downsides to these fireplaces are that their heat output is slightly less than electric heat or gas fires, and precautions must be taken to avoid carbon monoxide poisoning.

Bioethanol replaces gasoline, because when the gasoline is burned, it produces carbon dioxide, water, carbon monoxide and other impurities like sulfur oxides and nitrogen oxides at higher levels than bioethanol. Therefore, rapidly growing industrialization needed ecofriendly sustainable energy sources like bioethanol

Biodiesel

Mono-alkyl esters of long chain fatty acids such as plant oils, animal fats or algal sources are chemically processed for use in compression ignition (diesel) engines" are called as biodiesel. It can be replaced by conventional diesel as it is based on esters of long chain fatty acids.

ASTM International (originally known as the American Society for Testing and Materials) defines biodiesel as "A mixture of long-chain monoalkylic esters from fatty acids obtained from renewable resources, to be used in diesel engines". Blends with diesel fuel are indicated as "Bx", where "x" is the percentage of biodiesel in the blend. For instance, "B5" indicates a blend with 5 per cent biodiesel and 95 per cent mineral diesel fuel and B100 indicates pure biodiesel. Biodiesel chemically known as fatty acid methyl ester can be produced from vegetable oil, animal oil/fats, waste cooking oil by the process called transesterification.

Biodiesel is biodegradable, less toxic and its ignition in diesel engines can extract the total unburned hydrocarbons (HC) and polycyclic aromatic hydrocarbons (PAHs). It can minimize the carbon monoxide and particulate matter emission.

Across the globe, countries like Brazil, Malaysia, USA, Germany and many other European states are utilizing it owing to its potential for minimizing hazardous emissions and protection of human health from potential or probable threats.

Biodiesel Production

The feedstock for bioethanol production is dependent upon climatic conditions, soil conditions and agricultural practices being followed in an area. Across the globe, more than 350 oil crops have been shortlisted as sources of biodiesel production.

Feedstock required for biodiesel production is classified into following:

A. Edible plant oils

B. Non-edible plant oils

C. Waste or recycled oils

D. Animal and poultry fats

Some edible and non-edible oil sources used for biodiesel production are summarized in Table 1. Applications of edible oils may be detrimental to environment as it leads to soil destruction, deforestation and consumption of arable land/water.

Non-edible oils can replace the edible oil for biodiesel production. These are economical and are readily available in many parts of the world like the wastelands that are unsuitable for food crops, this eliminates competition for food, declines deforestation rate, are more ecofriendly, produce useful by-products.

Microalgae are photosynthetic microbes which have emerged as third generation biodiesel feedstock capable of converting sunlight, water and CO_2 to algal biomass, more proficiently when compared to conventional crops. High oil content and better productivity promotes the use of microalgae as better feedstock as compared to edible and non-edible oil.

Table 11.1: Some Non-edible and Edible Oil Sources Used for Biodiesel Production

Sl.No.	Non Edible Oil	Edible Oil
1	Jatropha	Palm
2	Rubber seed	Soyabean
3	Castor	Rapeseed

Biofuel production techniques widely vary, depending on the type of raw material, efficiency level, production volume, surrounding situation and end-user's requirement *etc.*

As mentioned above biodiesel can be produced from vegetable oil, animal oil/ fats, and waste oils, there are three basic routes to biodiesel production:

1. Base catalyzed transesterification of the oil.
2. Direct acid catalyzed transesterification of the oil.
3. Conversion of the oil to its fatty acids and then to biodiesel.

Almost all biodiesel is produced using base catalyzed transesterification as it is the most economical process requiring only low temperatures and pressures and producing a 98 per cent conversion yield.

The transesterification process is the reaction of a triglyceride (fat/oil) with an alcohol to form esters and glycerol. The nature of the fatty acids can in turn affect the characteristics of the biodiesel. During the esterification process, the triglyceride is reacted with alcohol in the presence of a catalyst, usually a strong alkaline like sodium hydroxide. The alcohol reacts with the fatty acids to form the mono-alkyl ester, or biodiesel and crude glycerol. In most productions, methanol or ethanol is the alcohol used (methanol produces methyl esters, ethanol produces ethyl esters) and is base catalyzed by either potassium or sodium hydroxide. Potassium hydroxide has been found to be more suitable for the ethyl ester biodiesel production; either base can be used for the methyl ester. The figure below shows the chemical process for methyl ester biodiesel. The reaction between the fat or oil and the alcohol is a reversible reaction and so the alcohol must be added in excess to drive the reaction towards the right and ensure complete conversion.

$$
\begin{array}{l}
CH_2-OCOR^1 \\
| \\
CH-OCOR^2 \\
| \\
CH_2-OCOR^3
\end{array}
\; + \; 3CH_3OH \; \xrightleftharpoons{\text{catalysts}} \;
\begin{array}{l}
R^1COOCH_3 \\
\\
R^2COOCH_3 \\
\\
R^3COOCH_3
\end{array}
\; + \;
\begin{array}{l}
CH_2-OH \\
| \\
CH-OH \\
| \\
CH_2-OH
\end{array}
$$

Plant Oil (Triglyceride) (Rapeseed, Soybean, etc) — Methanol — (Methyl ester compounds) — Glycerin

A successful transesterification reaction is signified by the separation of the ester and glycerol layers after the reaction time. The heavier, co-product, glycerol settles out and may be sold as it is or it may be purified for use in other industries, *e.g.* the pharmaceutical, cosmetics *etc.*

Straight vegetable oil can be used directly as a fossil diesel substitute however using this fuel can lead to some fairly serious engine problems. Due to its relatively high viscosity vegetable oil leads to poor atomization of the fuel, incomplete combustion, coking of the fuel injectors, ring carbonization, and accumulation of fuel in the lubricating oil. The best method for solving these problems is the transesterification of the oil.

Advantages of Biodiesel

1. **Produced from Renewable Resources**: Biodiesel is a renewable energy source unlike other petroleum products that will vanish in years to come.
2. **In- line with current engine technology**: Biodiesel can be used directly in any existing, unmodified diesel engines. Biodiesel can be used alone or mixed in any ratio ranging between 5-20 per cent with diesel made from fossil fuels.
3. **Energy Independence:** The total energy production is higher than which is invested throughout its manufacturing process.
4. **Environmental benefits**: Biodiesel substantially reduces unburned hydrocarbons, carbon monoxide and particulate matter in exhaust fumes. Sulphur dioxide emissions are totally eliminated as biodiesel contains 11 per cent oxygen by weight and does not contain sulphur. It can be described as 'carbon neutral fuel' that produces no net output of carbon. This effect occurs because when the oil crop grows it absorbs the same amount of CO_2 as is released when the fuel is combusted.
5. **Biodegradable, Safe and Non-toxic**: Biodiesel is rapidly biodegradable and completely non-toxic, meaning spillages represent far less of a risk than fossil diesel spillages. Biodiesel is safe to handle and transport.
6. **Grown, Produced and Distributed Locally:** Fossil fuels are limited and may not be able to fulfil our demand for coal, oil and natural gas after a certain period. Biodiesel can work as an alternative form of fuel and can reduce our dependence on foreign suppliers of oil as it is produced from

domestic energy crops. It is produced in local refineries which reduce the need to import expensive finished product from other countries.

Disadvantages of using Biodiesel

The main features to be considered in the use of methyl esters of vegetable oils in diesel engines are:

1. **Performance**: There is a slight loss of power and a slight increase in consumption due to a calorific value lower than that of gas oils, although the efficiency of combustion is somewhat higher.
2. **Limitations due to low temperatures**: The clouding points of the esters, in some cases superior to those of diesel, can cause problems in cold climates. These difficulties would be obviated with the use of additives.
3. **Incompatibility with materials**: Esters are more aggressive than diesel and can attack rubber and common types of paints. To avoid the risk of these attacks, it is convenient to use acrylic paints and replace the rubber pipes with Teflon or fluorinated rubber.
4. **Less stability and formation of carbonaceous deposits**: Due to the unsaturated bonds that these molecules carry, they have a lower stability in prolonged storage and are more easily decomposed in pre-reactions that occur before combustion.
5. **Delay of the injection point of the engine**: This solution, although effective, would involve the modification of the engine, which would reduce the advantages of biodiesel.
6. **Slight Increase in Nitrogen Oxide Emissions**: Biodiesel has about 10 per cent higher Nitrogen Oxide (NO_X) than other petroleum products. Nitrogen Oxide is the one gas that is used in the formation of smog and Ozone. Once it gets dissolved in atmospheric moisture, can cause acid rain.

Biogas

Microorganisms convert organic matter into biogas by anaerobic digestion. This process occurs in marshes, landfills, wetlands, and also in the digestive tract of ruminants. Biogas can be easily collected and used as an energy resource.

Substrates for Biogas Production

Generally, biomass of any kind containing carbohydrates (Starch, cellulose and hemicellulose), proteins and fats as major components can be used for biogas production.

Following points are to be considered for the choosing the biomass for biogas production:

- Composition of organic matter has to carefully selected for fermentation process.
- Organic matter should have high potential for biogas production

- Selected substrate must be pathogen free as it can harm fermentation process
- Biogas composition has to be examined proper for further use.

Biogas formation from plant fibers is generally a three-stage process:

A. Hydrolysis of biomolecules
B. Acetogenesis: acetic acid and carbon dioxide production
C. Methanogenesis: Formation of approximately 70 per cent CH_4 and 30 per cent CO_2 and the by-products NH_3 and H_2S by slow-growing archaea,

Anaerobic and facultative anaerobic bacteria are involved in these three stages, resembling to those in cow's rumen or wastewater treatment plants.

Composition of Biogas

Methane (CH_4) and carbon dioxide (CO_2) are major constituents of biogas with several impurities. Biogas containing methane ratio above 45 per cent is flammable. The content of hydrogen sulfide (H_2S) in biogas depends on the type of waste used. Without a desulfurizing step, the concentration of H_2S would often exceeds 0.2 per cent by volume.

Advantages of Biogas Production

1. **Biogas is Eco-Friendly:** Biogas is a renewable and clean source of energy. It actually reduces greenhouse emissions (*i.e.*, reduces the greenhouse effect).
2. **Biogas Generation Reduces Soil and Water Pollution:** Anaerobic digestion carried by bacteria deactivates pathogens and parasites; thus, effectively minimizing the incidence of waterborne diseases.
3. **Biogas Generation Produces Organic/Biofertilizer:** Biofertilizers are the by-product of the biogas generation process which is a perfect substitute for chemical fertilizers which have toxicity effects and can result in food poisoning
4. **Biogas production is a simple and low-cost Technology:** Left over agricultural residues which are no longer required can be utilized for bioenergy generation which is quite cheap and it can also be used directly for cooking and generation of electricity.

Disadvantages of Biogas Production

1. **Less efficient:** Less costly, new technologies are yet to be explored as the current technologies are less efficient. This means large scale production is yet not feasible.
2. **Contains Impurities:** Even after refinement and compression, biogas still contains impurities. This impure biogas if used to power automobiles, can corrode the metal parts of the engine.

3. **Effect of Temperature on Biogas Production:** Bacteria needs optimal temperature of around 37°C for digesting the waste which is difficult to maintain in cold climates. So, digesters require heat energy for constant biogas supply.

Bioremediation

Bioremediation is a branch of biotechnology in which chemical reactions mediated by (micro)biological organisms are used to degrade or transform contaminants, pollutants, toxins, to less toxic or nontoxic forms, thereby reducing or eliminating environmental contamination. The bioremediation process stimulates the growth of specific microorganisms that use the discharged chemical contaminants as a source of food and energy

Bioremediation can be performed in situ, where the contaminated material remains in its original location, or *ex situ*, after removal of the contaminated material from the original location for treatment, long-term storage, or permanent disposal.

Bioremediation of Heavy Metals

Heavy metals are generally considered to be those whose density exceeds 5g/ cm^3. Various industries like electroplating, mining, batteries, fertilizers, oil refineries and nuclear power plants release effluents enriched with toxic heavy metals. These toxic pollutants can affect the biological systems leading to many health hazards and causing detrimental diseases.

Although various physicochemical methods are available for combating heavy metal pollution but modern researchers and scientists are focusing more towards biological weapons for bioremediation of heavy metals owing to their low cost, eco- friendly nature and reduction in the discharged biological or chemical sludge.

Mechanism of Microbial Detoxification

In response to survive in the harsh environment including metal toxicity, microorganisms have developed their own unique mechanisms of heavy metal resistance and detoxification. These include electrostatic interaction, ion exchange, precipitation, redox process, and surface complexation.

The anionic groups present on the surface of microorganisms are hydroxyl, alcohol, phosphoryl, amine, carboxyl, ester, sulfydryl, sulfonate, thioether, and thiol groups. These negatively charged functional groups endow the microorganism with the potential to bind metal cation and enable its detoxification. In addition, microorganisms can detoxify metal ions by valence conversion, volatilization, or extracellular chemical precipitation.

Additionally, various factors including redox potential, chemical form of the metal ion and total metal ion concentration are some of the deciding factors which affect the metal removal potential of the microorganism. Environmental factors like temperature, pH, low molecular weight organic acids, and humic acids can also affect the bioavailability of heavy metals towards microorganisms.

Due to the increased hydrogen ion concentrations at acidic pH, more protons are available to saturate metal binding site which reduces attraction between biosorbent and metal ion and in turn increases its toxicity.

Temperature is an important parameter affecting heavy metal adsorption on the surface of adsorbent as increased temperature increases the bioavailability of metal ions. Also, the increase in temperature till a suitable range, accelerates metabolic and enzymatic activity of microorganisms.

However, final sequestration of metal ion depends on the biosorbent, available sorption sites, cell wall structure of microbial cell and various physicochemical parameters.

Bioremediation of Pesticides

Pesticides are the chemical substances use to kill or manage pests. These are widely used in agricultural fields, parks, forests, industrial sites, sport fields, *etc.*

Their mode of action is repulsion, mitigation, or destruction of pests/weeds. These can be classified into insecticides, herbicides, bactericides, fungicides, miticides, nematicides, and rodenticides.

Based on the chemical structure of pesticides, these can be categorized into organochlorines, organophosphorus, carbamates, chlorophenols, and synthetic pyrethroids.

When pesticides are applied to crops, they can reach the soil. Runoff from the soil and infiltration processes leads to contamination of waterbodies and groundwater. Also, pesticides are ubiquitous compounds, which are highly toxic and can cause abnormalities in human beings, and can also destroy flora and fauna.

Strategies for Pesticide Remediation

1. *Microbial Degradation of Pesticides*

Bacterial species which may biodegrade the pesticides belongs to *genera Flavobacterium, Arthobacter, Aztobacter, Burkholderia,* and *Pseudomonas*. The degradation of the pesticide is due to the oxidation of the parent compound which produces carbon dioxide and water, which provides energy to microorganisms. External factors like temperature, pH and availability of nutrients also affect the rate of degradation. Some pesticides are easily degraded; however, others are recalcitrant because of presence of anionic species in the compound.

Various fungi which have shown potential to degrade pesticides are *Flammulina velupites, Stereum hirsutum, Coriolus versicolor, Dichomitus squalens, Hypholoma fasciculare,* white rot fungi.

Enzymes play a major role in the degradation of pesticides through intrinsic detoxification and evolved metabolic resistance, via biodegradation by soil and water microorganisms. *P. putida* theoretical oxygen demand (TOD) enzyme is a representative of a much larger family of enzymes with application in the biocatalysis of environmentally relevant reactions. Fungal enzymes especially, oxidoreductases, laccase and peroxidases have prominent application in removal of polyaromatic hydrocarbons (PAHs) contaminants either in fresh, marine water or terrestrial.

In 1973, the first bacterium to degrade organophosphorus compounds was isolated from a soil sample from the Philippines and was identified as *Flavobacterium* sp. ATCC 27551. Since then, several bacteria, a few fungi and cyanobacteria, have been isolated that can use these compounds as a nutrient source.

Bioremediation is a promising approach for remediation of the soils that are affected by pesticides. This technology has proved again and again its potential to degrade not only pesticides but also the various recalcitrant compounds. So, time is to avail maximum benefit of this eco-friendly technology for better and safe future.

Bioremediation of Hydrocarbons

Hydrocarbons are compounds made up of carbon and hydrogen. Hydrocarbons are used in industries and daily life and these are the major energy providers as their usage has increased ten folds in the last decade. They pose a major threat to aquatic life as every year approximately 35 million barrels of oil is spilled across the oceans. Contamination of soil with oil spills is another major concern, as polluted soil is a serious hazard to the health of humans and also decreases overall productivity of agricultural land. In India, incident of oil spill occurred in Mumbai 2010, where oil spill from the ship contaminated the Arabian sea, another such incident occurred in 2014 in Sundarbans (Bangladesh) in 2014 where 350 tons of oil was spilled into the river Sela spread over more than 70 square km, thereby threatening the flora and fauna of that region. Oil spills due to leakages from joints of pipelines, accidents of tankers are common but are severely devastating.

Strategies for Removal of Hydrocarbon Contamination

Biodegradation of hydrocarbons involving the use of microorganisms is the transformation of organic contaminants to a less destructive and non – hazardous compounds which can be degraded further. There are two main methods of oil spill bioremediation using microorganisms:

1. **Bioaugmentation**: In this process, population of known oil-degrading bacteria are added to increase the number of existing microbial population. Indigenous or genetically modified microorganisms are added to the contaminated site to start the bioremediation. This method is very efficient when the indigenous microorganisms are unable to degrade the contaminants.
2. **Biostimulation**: Stimulating the growth of indigenous microorganisms by addition of growth factors like nutrients and optimizing the environmental parameters of contaminated site. The stimulants may be added to the subsurface through injection wells.

Other forms of treatment of the oil contaminated sites are:

1. **Land Farming**: Oil contaminated soil is spread over a bed, where it is stimulated by fertilizers to take full advantage of the activity of

microorganisms and enhance their chances of hydrocarbon degradation. The soil is rotated at a regular interval.

2. **Composting**: This is an Ex-situ method of bioremediation where the contaminated soil is added to organic substances like agricultural waste, manure. This in turn, stimulates the microbial population to degrade the hydrocarbon pollutants.
3. **Anaerobic degradation:** Addition of urea and ammonia, like fertilizers, are used in the bioremediation of oil spills which enhances their oxygen demand addition of oxygen is difficult, so in these sites, anaerobic microorganisms are used to perform bioremediation.

Hydrocarbon pollution removal is a real-world problem, to resolve it, a better understanding of the biodegradation mechanisms is needed and is of utmost importance. Microorganisms aided elimination of spilled oil from soil and water surfaces and sub-surfaces is a very cost effective and simple process that can be popularized for bioremediation.

Biomineralization

Microbial biomineralization refers to microorganisms mediated formation and deposition of minerals. It may be under direct or indirect microbial influence. It may be categorized as under:

1. Biologically Induced Mineralization (BIM)

Metabolic activity of the microorganisms triggers the extracellular processes which indirectly affects the nucleation and growth of biominerals. It may take place due to alterations in the chemical equilibrium of the surrounding environment or may be corelated to any particular metabolic products.

2. Biologically Controlled Mineralization (BCM)

In this the microorganisms directly BCM implies that the organism actively controls the nucleation site, growth, morphology and final location of the mineral. Mineral formation in BCM takes place in a closed, isolated environment.

Biofertilizers

To support the increasing human population and to fulfill their food requirements, it becomes necessary to increase the crop as well as land productivity. This concurrent production and supply of food can only be accomplished by the use of synthetic chemical fertilizers. However, increased dependence on chemical fertilizers, deteriorates the soil productivity, causing the environmental pollution. Also, these are very costly.

Biofertilizers are considered to be a safe substitute to chemical fertilizers as these are natural, nonpolluting, organic, renewable and cost effective. They improvise soil texture, pH, and other soil properties. They produce plant growth promoting substances *e.g.*, IAA amino acids, vitamins *etc.*

They have potential to fix atmospheric nitrogen in to nitrates. Biofertilizer is a mixture which contains living cells specially microorganisms or microbial preparations containing useful microorganisms in a viable state which assist the root system with good seed germination by providing essential nutrients. These living cells can also solubilize insoluble salts like phosphate and can also produce growth promoting substances for plants *e.g.*, vitamins and hormones.

Biofertilizers are also called as "Microbial inoculants", due to use of many nitrogen fixing bacteria and cyanobacteria.

Common biofertilizers such as *Azotobacter, Azospirillum, Rhizobium,* blue green algae *etc.* are good nitrogen fixer and *Bacillus megatherium var phosphaticum, Aspergillus awamori, Penicillium digitatum etc.* are good phosphate solubilizers.

Nitrogen Fixation

Leguminous plants have got root nodules, where atmospheric nitrogen fixation is being done by bacteria belonging to genera, *Rhizobium* (fast growing rhizobia), *Bradyshzodium* (slow growing rhizobia), *Sinorhizobium, Azorhizobium* and *Mesorhizobium* collectively called as rhizobia. Rhizobium is a gram negative, free living non sporulating, aerobic, motile and rod-shaped bacterium which is present in the soil. It occurs in the roots of leguminous plants and promotes nodule formation in the presence of leghemoglobin. Leghemoglobin promotes O_2 utilization and converts atmospheric nitrogen into ammonia in presence of phosphorus and molybdenum.

Nitrogen fixation is catalyzed by the enzyme 'nitrogenase'. The reduction of atmospheric nitrogen to ammonia by the nitrogenase enzymes is expressed as follows:

$$N_2 + 8H^+ + 6e- \rightarrow 2NH_4^{\ +}$$

Rhizobium resides in roots of beans, grams, groundnut and soyabean *etc.* It is a crop specific inoculant and can fix 15-20 kg N/ha and increase crop yield upto 20 per cent.

Cyanobacteria (Blue Green Algae)

Cyanobacteria, commonly called 'blue-green algae', are photopic in nature as they obtain their energy via photosynthesis. These are prokaryotic cells, as they lack membrane-enclosed chloroplasts. They play a significant role in enrichment of paddy field soil by fixing atmospheric nitrogen and supplying vitamin B complex and growth promoting substance which promotes plant growth.

Azolla-Anabaena Symbiosis

It is a free floating, aquatic fern present on the aquatic surface having a cyanobacterial symbiont *Anabaena azolla* in their leaves. Azolla fixes atmospheric nitrogen in association with nitrogen fixing cyanobacteria in paddy field. It is used as biofertilizer in India, USA, Sri Lanka, China, Indonesia, Bangladesh and many other countries. It can fix 40-60 Kg N/ha in a month and enhances 10-20 per cent yield of paddy crops. *Azolla* contributes nitrogen, phosphorus, potassium and organic carbon *etc.* to the crop. It can also survive in high temperature, water scarcity and can also be applied in heavy metal contaminated sites as these are metal tolerant.

Phosphate Solubilizing Bacteria

Pseudomonas fluorescens, Bacillus megatherium var. phosphaticum, Bacillus polymyxa are the bacteria have phosphate solubilising ability. USSR scientists invented the bacterial fertilizers named 'Phosphobacterin' containing cells of *Bacillus megatherium var. phosphaticum*. They can enhance approximately 10 to 20 per cent crop yield (Cooper, 1959). They can dissolve soil phosphate and make it available for crops.

Phosphate Solubilizing Fungi

Some fungal species also have phosphate dissolving ability *e.g., Aspergillus niger, Aspergillus awamori, Penicillium digitatum etc.*

Plant Growth Promoting Rhizobacteria (PGPR)

These are the rhizosphere bacteria which can increase plant growth by a wide variety of mechanisms like phosphate solubilization, biological nitrogen fixation, quorum sensing (QS) signal interference and inhibition of biofilm formation, phytohormone production, exhibiting antifungal activity, production of volatile organic compounds (VOCs), promoting beneficial plant-microbe symbioses, interference with pathogen toxin production *etc.* PGPR's offer an attractive way to replace the use of chemical fertilizers, pesticides and other supplements. Growth promoting substances are produced in large quantities by these microorganisms which influences the overall morphology of the plants.

They are also called as microbial pesticides *e.g. Bacillus* spp. and *Pseudomonas fluorescens*.

Mycorrhiza

Myco" – "rhiza" literally means "fungus" – "root" and defines the mutual symbiotic association between the plant and root fungus **mycorrhiza.**

These fungi grow on roots of the plants. Mycorrhizas are widely used as biofertilizers and biocides. They efficiently absorb nutrients like manganese, phosphorus, iron, zinc *etc.* from the soil and transfer it to the plants. They are also tolerant to high soil temperature and can increase the crop productivity by 30-40 per cent. Plant growth promoting substances are also produced by these fungi.

Mycorrhizas are of two types: Ectomycorrhiza and Endomycorrhiza.

1. **Ectomycorrhiza:** These occur in the roots of the higher plants *e.g.* gymnosperms and angiosperms. The hyphae of ectomycorrhizal fungi form a mantle around the root and also grow into the spaces between root cells - but do not penetrate the root cells. The hyphae form a net-like covering, called a Hartig net, around the cells.
2. **Endomycorrhiza (Vesicular-arbuscular mycorrhizas, or VAM):** They form symbiotic relationship with approximately 85 per cent of plant families. They occur commonly in the roots of crop plants. These fungi are able to penetrate the cortical cells and secrete extracellular enzymes. VAM fungal hyphae enhance the uptake of phosphorus and other nutrients that are responsible for plant growth stimulation including roots and shoot length.

Biopesticides

Agricultural productivity is severely affected by numerous pests like fungi, weeds and insects which reduces the crop yield. Chemical/synthetic pesticides resolve this crisis to a great extent. Dichloro-diphenyl-trichloroethane (DDT), followed by other organophosphate and carbamate pesticides were used in the earlier days which also brought green revolution and lead to increase in food production but the over dependence on chemical pesticides had detrimental effects on soil health, water quality, developed problems like insect resistance, genetic variation in plants and also raised many other environmental concerns. Therefore, ecofriendly alternative is the need of the hour.

Biopesticide is gaining interest because of its advantages associated with the environmental safety, target-specificity, efficacy, biodegradability and suitability in the integrated pest management (IPM) programs. Thus, biopesticides is one of the promising alternatives as it is target specific, more efficient, biodegradable and suitable in the integrated pest management (IPM) programs.

The most frequently used biopesticides are living organisms, which are pathogenic for the pest of interest. These include biofungicides (*Trichoderma*), bioherbicides (*Phytopthora*) and bioinsecticides (*Bacillus thuringiensis*).

Biopesticides fall under three major categories:

1. **Microbial pesticides**- These contain a microorganism (bacterium, fungus, virus, protozoan or alga) as the active ingredient. They can control many different kinds of pests, although each one is target specific. For example, some fungi can control some weeds while others can kill specific insects. The most extensively used microbial pesticides are variabilities of the bacterium *Bacillus thuringiensis*, or Bt, which can control certain insects in cabbage, potatoes, and other crops. Bt produces a protein that is harmful to specific insect pests. However, these microbial pesticides have to be constantly checked to ensure they do not acquire potential to harm non-target organisms, including human beings.
2. **Plant-pesticides**- These are pesticidal substances that plants produce as a result of transgenes which are inserted into the plants. For example, scientists can incorporate the gene of Bt pesticidal protein into the genetic material of plant. Then the plant, like the Bt bacterium synthesizes the substance that destroys the pest/insect.
3. **Biochemical pesticides** - Conventional pesticides usually kill or inactivate the whole pest. In contrast, biochemical pesticides control pests by non-toxic mechanisms. These include substances that interfere with growth or mating, such as plant growth regulators, or substances that repel or attract pests, such as pheromones.

Integrated Pest Management

Integrated pest management (IPM), also known as **integrated pest control (IPC)** is a broad-spectrum approach which **emphasizes on the** urgent need for sustainability of crop protection.

The UN's Food and Agriculture Organization defines IPM as "the careful consideration of all available pest control techniques and subsequent integration of appropriate measures that discourage the development of pest populations and keep pesticides and other interventions to levels that are economically justified and reduce or minimize risks to human health and the environment. IPM emphasizes the growth of a healthy crop with the least possible disruption to agro-ecosystems and encourages natural pest control mechanisms.".

IPM is an ecosystem-based strategy that focuses on long-term prevention of pests or their damage through a combination of techniques such as biological control, habitat manipulation, use of resistant varieties, intercropping, crop rotation' *etc.*

REFERENCES

1. Tahvonen O, Salo S. Economic growth and transitions between renewable and nonrenewable energy resources. European Economic Review. 2001 Aug 1;45(8): 1379-98.
2. Silva S, Soares I, Afonso O. Economic and environmental effects under resource scarcity and substitution between renewable and non-renewable resources. Energy Policy. 2013 Mar 1; 54: 113-24.
3. Chowdhury MN, Uddin S, Saleh S. Present scenario of renewable and non-renewable resources in Bangladesh: A compact analysis. International Journal of Sustainable and Green Energy. 2014;3(6): 164-78.
4. Güney T. Renewable energy, non-renewable energy and sustainable development. International Journal of Sustainable Development and World Ecology. 2019 Jul 4;26(5): 389-97.
5. Shalaby A. Biofuel: sources, extraction and determination. Liquid, gaseous and solid biofuels-conversion techniques. Croatia: InTech. 2013 Mar 20: 451-78.
6. Arshad M, Zia MA, Shah FA, Ahmad M. An overview of biofuel. Perspectives on water usage for biofuels production. 2018: 1-37.
7. Shishir TA, Mahbub N, Kamal NE. Review on bioremediation: a tool to resurrect the polluted rivers. Pollution. 2019 Jul 1;5(3): 555-68.
8. Zango Usman U, Mukesh Y, Vandana S, Sharma JK, Sanjay P, Sidhartha D, Sharma Anil K. Microbial bioremediation of heavy metals: Emerging trends and recent advances. Research Journal of Biotechnology Vol. 2020 Jan; 15: 1.
9. Yang Q, Li Z, Lu X, Duan Q, Huang L, Bi J. A review of soil heavy metal pollution from industrial and agricultural regions in China: Pollution and risk assessment. Science of the total environment. 2018 Nov 15;642: 690-700.
10. Adams GO, Fufeyin PT, Okoro SE, Ehinomen I. Bioremediation, biostimulation and bioaugmention: a review. International Journal of Environmental Bioremediation and Biodegradation. 2015;3(1): 28-39.
11. £awniczak £, WoŸniak-Karczewska M, Loibner AP, Heipieper HJ, Chrzanowski £. Microbial degradation of hydrocarbons–basic principles for bioremediation: a review. Molecules. 2020 Jan;25(4): 856.

12. Mazid M, Khan TA. Future of bio-fertilizers in Indian agriculture: an overview. International Journal of Agricultural and Food Research. 2015 May 1;3(3).
13. Brahmaprakash GP, Sahu PK. Biofertilizers for sustainability. Journal of the Indian Institute of Science. 2012 Dec 10; 92(1): 37-62.
14. Rai S, Shukla N. Biofertilizer: An alternative of synthetic fertilizers. Plant Archives. 2020; 20(2): 1374-9.
15. Gupta S, Dikshit AK. Biopesticides: An ecofriendly approach for pest control. Journal of Biopesticides. 2010; 3(Special Issue): 186.
16. Kumar S, Singh A. Biopesticides: present status and the future prospects. J Fertil Pestic. 2015;6(2): 100-29.
17. Chandler D, Bailey AS, Tatchell GM, Davidson G, Greaves J, Grant WP. The development, regulation and use of biopesticides for integrated pest management. Philosophical Transactions of the Royal Society B: Biological Sciences. 2011 Jul 12;366(1573): 1987-98.

Chapter 12

Genomics and Proteomics

Manish Shandilya[1]*, *Bhuvnesh Yadav*[1] *and Sonika Charak*[2]

[1] Department of Chemistry, Biochemistry and Forensic Science, Amity School of Applied Sciences, Amity University Haryana, Gurugram – 122 413, Haryana, India

[2] National Brain Research Centre, Manesar, Gurugram – 122 052, Haryana, India

*e-mail: shandilya.manish7@gmail.com

ABSTRACT

Biological molecules like DNA, RNA, and Proteins are responsible for major phenomena that happened in cells. To understand the fundamental concepts of these molecules provide us valuable mechanism those are being used or will be useful for numerous applications in the health industry, agriculture, and synthetic biology. These genomics, transcriptomics, and proteomics approaches are required multiple high throughput techniques like next-generation sequencing, microarray, chromatography, 2D electrophoresis, mass spectrometry, high end computational servers and software. Handling these sophisticated techniques required multiple inter-disciplinary expertise. Nowadays worldwide researchers are to connect these advanced techniques to decrease the time and money for analysis like LC-MS, Microarray MS, 2D PAGE MS. Therefore, in this chapter, we have tried to discuss the fundamental concepts, outlines of advanced techniques and analysis through the in-silico approach.

Keywords: *Genomics, Transcriptomics, Proteomics, Sequencing, Microarray, Mass spectrometer.*

1. Introduction and Structural Genomics

1.1 Introduction

Deoxyribonucleic acid (DNA) is the genetic material of cells. It carries information in a coded form from cell to cell and from parent to offspring. A gene is a linear array of nucleotides located in a particular position on a particular chromosome that encodes a specific functional product (a protein or RNA molecule). When a gene is active, its information is copied first into another nucleic acid, ribonucleic acid (RNA), which in turn directs the synthesis of the gene products, the specific proteins. This module introduces some basic concepts of DNA, proteins, genes and genomes.

1.2 Genes

Genes are the fundamental physical and functional units of heredity. Genes carry information for making all the proteins required by all organisms. These proteins determine other things, like how the organism looks, how well its body metabolizes food or fights infection, and sometimes even how it behaves. A gene is an ordered sequence of nucleotides located in a particular position on a particular chromosome that encodes a specific functional product (a protein or RNA molecule). Expressed genes include those that are transcribed into mRNA and then translated into protein and those that are transcribed into RNA but not translated into protein (tRNA and rRNA). The sequence of a strand of DNA corresponds to the amino acid sequence of a protein. This concept is explained by the central dogma of molecular biology. Information flows (except in reverse transcription) from DNA to RNA via the process of transcription, and then to protein via translation. Transcription is the making of an RNA molecule of a DNA template. Translation is the construction of an amino acid sequence (polypeptide) from an RNA molecule. An mRNA specifies amino acid sequence using the genetic code. It would be impossible for each amino acid to be specified by one nucleotide because there are only 4 nucleotides and 20 amino acids. Similarly, two nucleotide combinations could only specify 16 amino acids. The conclusion is that each amino acid is specified by a particular combination of three nucleotides, called a codon. To code for the 20 essential amino acids, a genetic code must consist of at least a 3-base set (triplet) of the 4 bases. If one considers the possibilities of arranging four things 3 at a time (4x4x4), we get 64 possible codons (a 3-base sequence on the mRNA that codes for either specific amino acid or a control word).

1.3 The Genomes

A genome is all the DNA in an organism, including its genes. In 1990, the Human Genome Project was launched by the U.S. Department of Energy and the National Institutes of Health. The project originally was planned to be completed in 15 years, but rapid technological advances have accelerated the draft completion date to 2001. The goals of the project are to identify all the genes in human DNA. To understand the fundamental concepts, worldwide researchers are also studying the genetic makeup of several nonhuman organisms. Because all organisms are related through similarities in DNA sequences, insights gained from nonhuman genomes often lead to new knowledge about human biology. These include the bacterium *Escherichia coli*, fruit fly (*Drosophila melanogaster*), brewer's yeast (*Saccharomyces cerevisiae*), *Caenorhabditis elegans*, *Arabidopsis thaliana*, *Chlamydomonas reinhardtii*, *Taeniopygia guttata*, the mouse (*Mus musculus*) and many more.

1.4 Genome Size and Sequence Complexity

The genome and the complexity of living beings. The genome of an organism is the whole DNA content of its cells, including genes and intergenic regions. In prokaryotes (Archaea and Bacteria) there is, in general, a linear relationship between genome size and the number of genes. The smallest genomes are found in symbionts and parasites, as they undergo a gene degradation process during adaptation to their new lifestyle. However, in eukaryotes there is no correlation between genome size and the complexity of the organism. This is known as the C-value paradox. The largest genome is found in an amoeba, a one-cell organism, with 686,000 Mb, 200-fold larger than the human genome and 20,000-fold larger than the one found in yeast. Now we know that most excess DNA is repetitive DNA, apparently lacking a function (selfish DNA) and whose possible role in genome evolution is still unknown. As we know, DNA is the basic material of genes; therefore, it is natural to think that more complex organisms will require more genes and will have more DNA. Accordingly, one might expect that: "more complex organisms have larger genomes and contain a larger number of genes". That is, throughout evolution an increase in genome sizes and the number of genes is expected.

1.5 Genome Ranges and Sizes

Figure 12.1 represents the range of sizes of the genome found in the three domains of life: bacteria, archaea and eukaryotes. It seems clear that prokaryotes are, in general, smaller than eukaryotes, except some large-sized bacteria and some very small-sized eukaryotes.

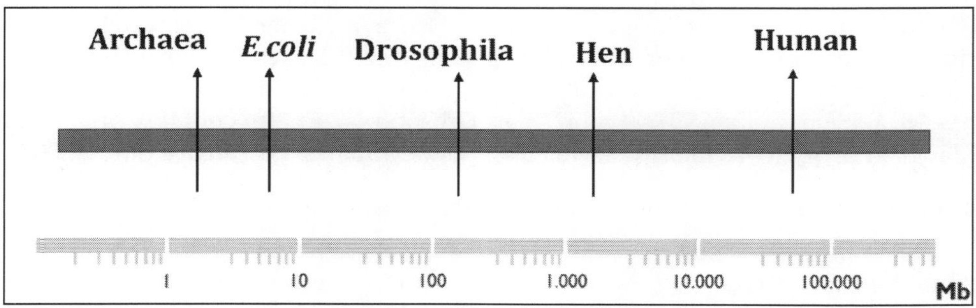

Figure 12.1: Range of Genome Size in Organisms of the Three Domains of Life.

1.6 Prokaryotes Genome: Bacteria and Archaea

According to published data, the size varies from 0.58 megabases (1 megabase (Mb) is one million base pairs (bp)) in the intracellular pathogen *Mycoplasma genitalium*, to more than 10 Mb in several species of cyanobacteria except *Bacillus megaterium*, which has a genome of 30 Mb. The second smallest genome published is that of *Buchnera sp.* APS, an endosymbiont of the cereal aphid *Acyrthosiphon pisum*, with a size of 641 kb.

1.7 Eukaryotes Genome: C-Value Paradox

You might expect more complex organisms to have progressively larger genomes, but eukaryotic genome size fails to correlate well with apparent complexity and instead varies wildly over more than a 100,000-fold range. Single-celled amoebae have some of the largest genomes, up to 100-fold larger than the human genome. This variation suggested that genomes can contain a substantial fraction of DNA other than genes and their regulatory sequences. C.A. Thomas Jr coined it as the 'C-value paradox' in 1971.

1.8 Gene DNA or Non-Gene DNA

We have known since the late 60s that the eukaryotic genome is composed of a large amount of repetitive DNA. Moreover, since the late 70s, we have known that genes are interrupted by non-coding sequences, introns, which must be removed before the ribosome synthesizes protein. We are talking in both cases about a seemingly superfluous DNA, which contributes to the wide variation in C-values and therefore explains the apparent paradox. The size and number of introns vary widely along the evolutionary scale, mammals being the ones with the highest number and larger size. Repetitive DNA also varies between organisms. Traditionally this DNA is classified as: highly repetitive, with sequences such as microsatellites and minisatellites; and moderately repetitive, where transposable elements, the sequences that constitute the clearest example of selfish DNA, are found.

1.9 Number of Genes and Complexity of the Organism

After completion of whole-genome sequencing, researchers will know with more or less accuracy the number of genes derived from these sequences, since what we had so far were indirect estimates. However, some data is proving to be surprising because, in some cases, there appears to be a clear correlation between the number of genes and the complexity of the organism. The nematode worm *C. elegans* has 18,000 genes, about 5,000 more than Drosophila, a more complex organism. Man has only twice as many genes as *C. elegans* (estimates indicated about 100,000).

1.10 Molecular Mechanisms that Alter Genome Size

Many mutational mechanisms can produce changes in genome size. Some of them occur on a large scale (whole genome duplication), while others occur on a very small scale (loss or gain of a few nucleotides). However, we must note that these mutations affect, in principle, a single cell, and if it is a gamete, the mutation may be transmitted to an offspring. The probability of one or the other occurring depends on evolutionary mechanisms such as natural selection or genetic drift (random). Chromosomal mechanisms often produce drastic changes with a single mutation. The mobile genetic elements or transposable elements are other causes of large variations in genome size. It has been estimated that the maize genome has been duplicated because of the transposable elements in the last three million years of its evolution. It is considered that the spontaneous insertions or deletions (indels) of a few nucleotides are one of the most important causes of the development of the size of the genome in the long term. The variation in the length of the DNA of the minisatellites and microsatellites is another mechanism that can alter the size of the genome. These sequences are formed by a unit of few nucleotides, repeated continuously from less than ten to several thousand times. The number of repeated units varies greatly, even in individuals of the same species. One of the most important processes in the increase of genome size in unicellular organisms, especially prokaryotes, is horizontal gene transfer. This process involves the introduction of a DNA fragment into the genome from another species, containing one or more genes. The DNA is introduced into the cell by different mechanisms and must then recombine with the genome. If the genes introduced confer some advantage to the organism, they remain like that, otherwise, they can mutate and become inactive. All these mutations arise periodically in many species, including humans. Many of them are disadvantageous and selective pressure progressively removes them from the population, others are individually neutral but maybe collectively beneficial or harmful, by increasing or decreasing the size of the genome.

1.11 Structural Features of the Genome

1.11.1 Typical Prokaryotic Gene Structural Elements

The coding region of structural genes don't split, but rRNA genes have spacers within them. The upstream elements from the start of the coding region include promoter elements. Nearly 50 to 100 nucleotides upstream of the start codon, is the first nucleotide at which transcription initiates, it means, it is at this site the first nucleotide is incorporated. This site is called transcriptional initiation site or START. Nearly 10 nucleotides upstream of the start, there is a sequence called TATAAT or Pribnow box. Any nucleotide present on the left of the start is denoted by the (-) symbol and the region is called the upstream element. The numbers are written as -10, -20, -35 *etc.* The start site is the first ends and symbolized by +1, any sequence to the right of the start is called downstream elements and numbered as +10, +35 and so on. At –35 there is another consensus sequence **TTGACA**. These two sequences are the most important promoter elements, if there is any change in their sequence and position, transcriptional initiation suffers.

1.11.2 Promoter

The meaning of a promoter essentially is a distinct sequence module recognized by RNA polymerase, which binds to the sequence tightly and initiates transcription by unwinding the helically coiled **DNA** into the transcriptional bubble. The said sequences not only facilitate the binding of the enzyme and also provide sequence information for the site at which the enzyme initiates transcription. If anyone of the consensus sequences is deleted or changed drastically, the enzyme won't bind, even if it binds, it initiates transcription at different positions.

-200 -65 -60 -35 -10 +1

I————I–//–I————I——I——I————I————A ->

Enhancers Activator TTGACA TATAT

RNA polymerase binding region

-35 –10 +1—>

TTGACA——TATAAT——C A T—

When prokaryotic RNA polymerase binds properly in a sequence context, it covers a length from –60 to +20 or a little more. It is this segment of the gene that is called Promoter. Whether it is a housekeeping gene or a special gene, either from prokaryote or eukaryote, the meaning and the function of the promoter are the same. So promoters act as defining a set of sequence structural elements, which positions the transcriptional apparatus to initiate the transcriptional process. For the RNA polymerase to recognize different genes, the promoter elements have recognition sequences, which are recognized by specific sigma factors that associate with the RNA-Polymerase.

In prokaryotes, there are other sequences upstream of the promoter, beyond –35 sequences. Such sequences may present at –65 to –60 or they may be present at –200 or they may be present at–1000 bp upstream or they may present in downstream regions. The –65 to –60 sequences have the binding position of certain factors, whose binding leads to the activation of the polymerase, which was hitherto remained inactive even though it is bound to correct promoter elements. This process is termed activation and the element as **activator elements**. The other sequence at -200 or -1000, is called an **enhancer**, as it enhances the rate of transcription by 100 to 200-fold. This is achieved through certain proteins bind to enhancer elements, and then contact RNA Holoenzyme by protein-protein interactions, by way of DNA bending or looping, and enhances the efficiency of the enzyme. The proteins that bind to DNA have specific **motifs** called DNA binding motifs, and also possess protein-protein interacting domains.

Domain: A part of the protein that is self-stabilizing and folds independently from the rest.

Motif: A small part of protein 3 D protein structure and their amino acid sequence shared among different proteins. Motifs are neither self-stabilizing nor folds independently. Although it has a characteristic functional feature in a protein.

1.12 Terminal Region of the Gene

At the end of the coding region that is the terminal region beyond the terminator codon (TER codon), there are certain sequences positioned from the TER codon which provide a sequence for the transcript to generate a secondary structure that facilitates the termination of transcription. One of the structural motifs that the sequence provides is the formation of the stem with GC-rich sequence and open-loop and terminates in 2 to 4 U sequences. In some of the transcriptional terminator sequences, there are specific sequences rich in Cs; they are a little longer and far away from the TER codon.

1.13 Eukaryotic Genome Structure

Genes which are expressed usually have **introns** that interrupt the coding sequences. A typical eukaryotic gene, therefore, consists of a set of sequences that appear in mature mRNA (called **exons**) interrupted by introns. The regions between genes are likewise not expressed, but may help with chromatin assembly, contain promoters. Intron sequences contain some common features. Most introns begin with the sequence GT (GU in RNA) and end with the sequence AG. Intron sequences may be large relative to coding sequences. The eukaryotic mRNA precursors must be **processed** to remove introns as well as to add the caps at the 52 end and polyadenylic acid (poly-A) sequences at the 32 end. Eukaryotic genes may be clustered but are independently controlled. Operons or polycistronic mRNAs do not exist in eukaryotes. This contrasts with prokaryotic genes, where a single control gene often acts on a whole cluster like, *lac*I controls the synthesis of β galactosidase, permease, and acetylase. Mammalian globin genes are the best example of clustered gene system. Two globin clusters exist in humans: the alpha cluster on chromosome 16 and the beta cluster on chromosome 11. These clusters, and the gene for the related protein myoglobin, probably arose by duplication of a primordial gene that encoded a single heme containing, oxygen binding protein. Within each cluster is a gene designated with the Greek letter Ψ is called **pseudogenes**. DNA sequences are related to a functional gene but containing one or more mutations so that it isn't expressed known as **pseudogenes**.

1.13.1 Organisation of Single Copy of Sequences

Single copy DNA has a unique sequence of DNA and codes for protein and are sites of transcription. The single-copy DNA sequences are mainly found in the **exons** as they are coding regions and are the sites for **transcription** to make mRNA. These are present in the **euchromatin** part as they are coding regions. These are similar in many individuals. The repetitive sequence of DNA has short repeated sequences of nucleotides, and these do not code for proteins. These are mainly found in the **introns** and other noncoding parts of the DNA. They do not code for protein synthesis. These are present in the **heterochromatin** part as they are noncoding regions. They are unique in different individuals.

Euchromatin: part of a chromosome that is involved in transcription

Heterochromatin: part of a chromosome that is not included in transcription and has suppressed genes

Introns: noncoding sections of an RNA transcript that are spliced out before the RNA molecule is translated into a protein.

Exons: the sections of DNA (or RNA) that code for proteins

1.14 Repetitive Sequences

In the human genome, various sized stretches of DNA sequences exist in variable copy numbers. These repetitive sequences may be in tandem orientation and/or dispersed throughout the genome. Repetitive sequences may be classified by function, dispersal patterns and sequence relatedness. Three different **repetitive sequences are** Macrosatellites, Minisatellites and Microsatellites. Macrosatellites are the largest of the tandem DNA repeats, located on one/multiple chromosomes. Macrosatellites are very long arrays, up to hundreds of kilobases, of tandemly repeated DNA. Minisatellites are tandemly repeated sequences of DNA, yielding a total length from less than 1 Kbp to 15 Kbp. One subset of minisatellites comprises the highly polymorphic arrays of short tandem repeats with no known function that serves as useful DNA markers referred to as **variable number tandem repeats (VNTRs)**. These sequences generally contain 1–5 Kbp of DNA of repeating units of 15– 100 nucleotides. Several minisatellites share enough sequence homology to be analyzed by a single probe yielding DNA fingerprints. Telomeric DNA sequences contain another subset of minisatellites. The telomeric sequences contain 10–15 kb of hexanucleotide repeats, most commonly TTAGGG in the human genome, at the termini of the chromosomes. These sequences are added by telomerase to ensure complete replication of the chromosome. **Microsatellites** are small arrays of short simple tandem repeats, primarily 4 bp or less. Different arrays are found dispersed throughout the genome, although dinucleotide CA/TG repeats are most common, yielding 0.5 per cent of the genome. Microsatellites have no known functions. However, CA/TG dinucleotide pairs can form the Z-DNA conformation *in vitro*, which is possibly indicative of function. Repeat unit **copy number variation** of microsatellites occurs by replication slippage yielding highly polymorphic DNA markers referred to as short tandem repeat polymorphisms (STRPs). STRPs are commonly used in commercial DNA fingerprinting kits. The expansion of trinucleotide repeats within genes has been associated with genetic disorders such as Huntington's disease, myotonic muscular dystrophy, Friedreich ataxia, and Fragile-X syndrome. **Transposable elements** are DNA sequences that are capable of changing their position within a genome. They can create or reverse mutations and hence modifying the cell's genetic identity and genome size.

2. Resources of Genome Study

2.1 DNA Markers

Segments of chromosomal DNA are known to be linked with heritable traits or diseases. Following are different types of DNA markers.

2.2.1 Restriction Fragment Length Polymorphisms (RFLPs)

RFLPs refer to variations found within a species in the length of DNA fragments generated by the specific endonuclease. RFLPs are the first type of DNA markers developed to distinguish individuals at the DNA level.

2.2.2 Amplified Fragment Leng0th Polymorphism (AFLP)

AFLPs are differences in restriction fragment lengths caused by SNPs (Single nucleotide polymorphism) or INDELs (Insertion–deletion mutations) that create or abolish restriction endonuclease recognition sites. AFLP assays are performed by selectively amplifying a pool of restriction fragments using PCR. RFLP technique was originally known as selective restriction fragment amplification.

2.2.3 Random Amplified Polymorphic DNA (RAPDs)

RAPD refers to polymorphism found within a species in the randomly amplified DNA generated by the restriction endonuclease enzyme. RAPDs are PCR-based DNA markers. RAPD marker assays are performed using a single DNA primer of arbitrary sequence.

2.2.4 Cleaved Amplified Polymorphic Sequences (CAPS)

CAPS polymorphisms are differences in restriction fragment lengths caused by SNPs or INDELs that create or abolish restriction endonuclease recognition sites in PCR amplicons produced by locus-specific oligonucleotide primers. CAPS assays are performed by digesting locus-specific PCR amplicons with one or more restriction enzymes and separating the digested DNA on agarose or polyacrylamide gels. The combination of CAPS with other markers increases the chance of finding a DNA polymorphism.

2.2.5 Simple Sequence Repeats (SSRs)

Simple sequence repeats (SSRs) or microsatellites are tandemly repeated mono-, di-, tri-, tetra-, penta-, and hexanucleotide. SSR length polymorphisms are caused by differences in the number of repeats. SSR loci are individually amplified by PCR using pairs of oligonucleotide primers specific to unique DNA sequences flanking the SSR sequence. Jeffreys (1985) showed that some restriction fragment length polymorphisms are caused by VNTRs. The name **"minisatellite"** was coined because of the similarity of VNTRs to larger satellite DNA repeats.

2.2.6 Single Strand Conformational Polymorphisms (SSCPs)

SSCPs refer to DNA polymorphisms produced by differential folding of single-stranded DNA mutations. The conformation of the folded DNA molecule is produced by intramolecular interactions and is thus a function of the DNA sequence. SSCP marker assays are performed using heat-denatured DNA on non-denaturing DNA sequencing gels.

2.2.7 Heteroduplex Analysis (HA)

It refers to DNA polymorphisms produced by separating homo-duplex from heteroduplex DNA using non-denaturing gel electrophoresis or partially denaturing high-performance liquid chromatography. Single-base mismatches between genotypes produce hetero-duplexes; thus, the presence of hetero-duplexes signals the presence of DNA polymorphisms. Heteroduplex analyses can be rapidly and efficiently performed on numerous genotypes before specific alleles are sequenced, thereby greatly reducing sequencing costs in SNP discovery and SNP marker development.

2.2.8 Single Nucleotide Polymorphism (SNP)

The variations which are found at a single nucleotide position are known as single nucleotide polymorphisms or SNP. Such variation results due to substitution, deletion or insertion. This type of polymorphism has two alleles and is also called biallelic loci. This is the most common class of DNA polymorphism.

The main features of SNP markers are given below.

1. SNP markers are highly polymorphic and mostly biallelic.
2. The genotyping throughput is very high.
3. SNP markers are locus-specific.

4. Such variation results due to substitution, deletion or insertion.
5. SNP markers are excellent long-term investments.
6. SNP markers can be used to pinpoint functional polymorphism.
7. This technique requires a small amount of DNA.

2.2.9 Expressed Sequence Tags (EST)

Expressed Sequence Tags (ESTs) are small pieces of DNA and their location and sequence on the chromosome are known. The term Expressed Sequence Tags (ESTs) was first used by Venter and his colleagues in 1991. Main features of EST markers are given below.

1. ESTs are short DNA sequences (200-500 nucleotide long).
2. They are a type of sequence tagged sites (STS).
3. ESTs consist of exons only.

2.2.10 Sequence Tagged Sites (STS)

In genomics, a sequence-tagged site (STS) is a short DNA sequence that has a single copy in a genome and whose location and base sequence are known. The main features of STS markers are given below.

1. STSs are short DNA sequences (200-500 nucleotide long).
2. STSs occur only once in the genome.
3. STSs are detected by PCR in the presence of all other genomic sequences.
4. STSs are derived from cDNAs.

2.3 Genetic and Physical Map

Using genetic and physical maps researchers can understand the gene arrangement and DNA markers on a chromosome. The relative distances between gene positions are calculated using recombination frequencies. However, a physical map is based on the number of nucleotide pairs between loci. These maps are useful to understand the vast genome organization of the various genomes.

2.4 Mapping Populations

A population that is apt for linkage mapping of genetic markers is known as mapping population and they are generally obtained from controlled crosses.

2.5 Genome Sequencing (Eukaryotic and prokaryotic) – Methods

In genome sequencing, the order of nucleotides in a genome or DNA has been identified by various methods. It is highly useful in plentiful applied fields like medical diagnosis, biotechnology, forensic biology, virology, *etc.* Following are famous methods used for genome sequencing:

A. Chemical Method

It is also called as Maxam–Gilbert sequencing method of DNA sequencing. In this method, chemical modification of specific nucleotides and cleavage of DNA adjacent to the modified nucleotides are generally performed for sequencing.

B. Chain Termination Method

It is also known as Sanger sequencing. In this method, single-stranded DNA template, a DNA primer, a DNA polymerase, normal deoxynucleotide triphosphates (dNTPs), and modified di-deoxynucleotide triphosphates (ddNTPs) are used for sequencing. Modified di-deoxynucleotide triphosphates lack a 3′-OH group and because that phosphodiester bond between two nucleotides will not occur wherever ddNTPs is incorporated. These modified ddNTPs are either radioactively or fluorescently labeled and useful in automated DNA Sequencing.

2.6 Strategies of Genome Sequencing

A. Whole-genome Sequencing

It is also called full genome sequencing, complete genome sequencing, or entire genome sequencing. In near future, it will be useful for predicting disease susceptibility and drug response. Full genome sequencing can provide the raw nucleotide sequences of an individual organism's DNA and will be useful for medicinal purpose.

B. De novo Sequencing

If there is no reference sequence available for alignment then it is called de novo Sequencing.

2.7 Human Genome Project

The Human Genome Project (HGP) was an international, collaborative research program whose goal was the complete mapping and understanding of all the genes of human beings.

2.7.1 Goals

The main goals of the Human Genome Project were first articulated in 1988 by a special committee of the U.S. National Academy of Sciences and later implemented through a detailed series of five-year plans jointly written by the National Institutes of Health and the Department of Energy. Congress funded both the NIH and the DOE to embark on further exploration of this concept, and the two government agencies formalized an agreement by signing a Memorandum of Understanding to "coordinate research and technical activities related to the human genome." James Watson was appointed to lead the NIH component. The following year, the office of Human Genome Research evolved into the National Centre for Human Genome Research. In 1990, the initial planning stage was completed with the publication of a joint research plan, "Understanding Our Genetic Inheritance: The Human Genome Project, The First Five Years, 1991-1995." This initial research plan set out specific goals for the first five years of what was then projected to be a 15-year research effort. HGP researchers deciphered the human genome in three major ways: determining the sequences of all the bases in our genome's DNA; making maps that show the locations of genes for major sections of all our chromosomes;

and producing what are called linkage maps, through which inherited traits can be tracked over generations.

2.7.2 Impact

The HGP has revealed that there are probably about 20,500 human genes. This crucial product of the HGP has given the world a resource of detailed information about the structure, organization and function of the complete set of human genes. The International Human Genome Sequencing Consortium published the first draft of the human genome in the journal *Nature* in February 2001 with the sequence of the entire genome's three billion base pairs approximately 90 percent complete. A startling finding of this first draft was that the number of human genes appeared to be significantly fewer than previous estimates, which ranged from 50,000 genes to as many as 140,000. The full sequence was completed and published in April 2003. The tools created through the HGP also continue to inform efforts to characterize the entire genomes of several other organisms used extensively in biological research, such as mice, fruit flies and flatworms and many more. These efforts support each other because most organisms have many similar, or "homologous," genes with similar functions. Therefore, the identification of the sequence or function of a gene in a model organism explains the various untouchable aspects of the various organism or human. Of course, information is only as good as the ability to use it. Therefore, advanced methods for widely spreading the information created by the HGP to various scientists are necessary to ensure the most rapid application of research results for the benefit of humanity.

2.8 Next Generation Sequencing

The procedure to determine the sequence of nucleotide in the fragment of DNA is termed DNA sequencing. The advanced version of the high throughput sequencing method with more accuracy, enhanced read length, increased speed, reduced time and the diminishing cost is called the Next Generation Sequencing. The progressive and improved version sequence of the whole genome with high speed and high throughput sequencing at a reduced cost are popularized as NEXT GENERATION SEQUENCING. It also known as Massively Parallel Sequencing. It is faster, cheaper and required much less time in template preparation. Three basic steps: library preparation, sequencing, and data analysis.

2.8.1 Pyrosequencing

Many sequenced genomes were determined using the dideoxy method. But now a great effort is being expended to find ways to sequence DNA more rapidly and more cheaply. Pyrosequencing is mainly based on detection of pyrophosphate release and the generation of light on nucleotide incorporation, rather than chain termination with dideoxynucleotides. This method is also called **sequencing by synthesis**.

2.8.2. Virtual Terminator (VT) Sequencing

In this sequencing virtual terminator nucleotides are nucleotide analogues that contain a fluorescent dye and chemically cleavable group 3′-O-azidomethyl group. Once it incorporates the VT analogues block further incorporation until the VT moiety is chemically removed. The VT was removed before the next cycle regenerating the 3′ OH group using reducing agent Tris 2 carboxyethyl phosphine.

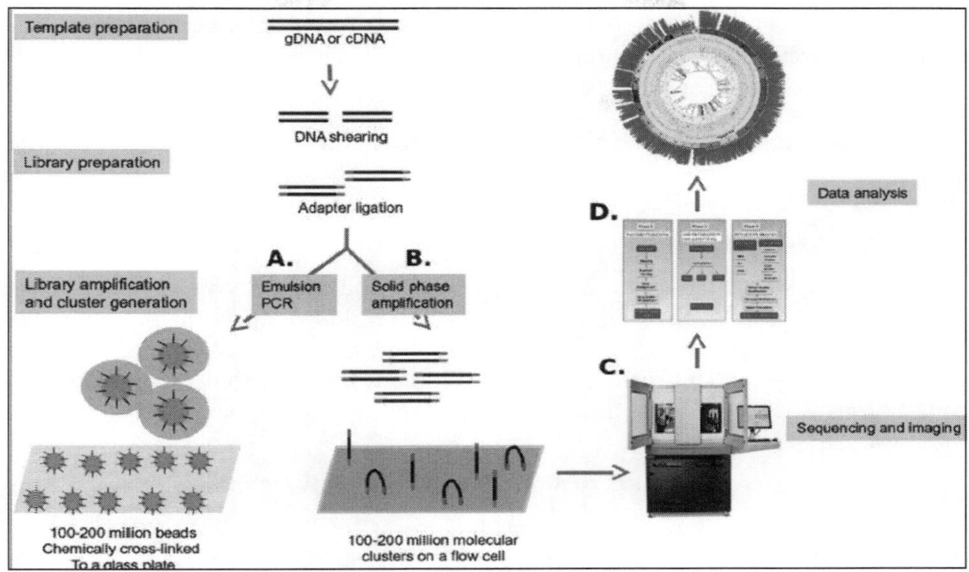

Figure 12.2. Overview of NGS.

2.8.3. Ion Torrent Sequencing

Ion Torrent uses ion semiconductor sequencing technology. The chip of Ion Torren is an ultrasensitive pH meter that senses hydrogen ions released when nucleotides are incorporated during DNA synthesis. Each ion chip comprises millions of ion-sensitive field-effect transistor (ISFET) sensors that allow parallel detection of multiple sequencing reactions.

2.8.4 Nanopore Sequencing

In nanopore sequencing, a single molecule of DNA or RNA can be sequenced without the requirement for PCR amplification or chemical labeling of the sample. Nanopore sequencing uses electrophoresis to transport an unknown sample through a slit of nm in diameter. A nanopore system always comprises an electrolytic solution when a constant electric field is applied, an electric current can be observed in the system. Sequencing is possible since, when close enough to nanopores, samples cause distinctive changes in electric current density across nanopore surfaces.

2.9 Genome Finishing

The acquisition of both cDNA and genomic DNA sequences sequencing fields has progressed so rapidly that multiple experimental data have errors, ambiguities, and incompleteness. Therefore, the next step for the large-scale sequencing data is required genome finishing. In this step, contiguous segments of sequence are ordered and linked to each other and any discrepancies among the reads are resolved.

2.9.1 GENOME ANNOTATION: Structural and Functional

'Structural' genome annotation is the process of identifying **genomic** elements like genes, promoters, and regulatory elements. 'Functional' genome annotation is the assigning of functions to structural elements.

3. Comparative and Functional Genomics

3.1 Overview of sequence analysis

3.1.1 Databases

Genomic sequence assemblies are updated periodically as new sequence becomes available. UCSC's Genome Browser ("Golden Path") (http://genome.ucsc.edu). UCSC is usually the first to display new assemblies, followed by NCBI and then Ensembl. UCSC also gives access to their older genome assemblies and annotations while NCBI and Ensembl do not. Following tools are used analysis of genomic sequences

NCBI's Map Viewer (http://www.ncbi.nlm.nih.gov/mapview/)

Ensembl (http://www.ensembl.org)

Genomes On Line Database (GOLD) (https://gold.jgi.doe.gov/) provide access to genomes and metagenomes projects.

MITOMAP (http://www.mitomap.org/) is a useful mitochondrial genome database.

3.1.2 Genome Browsers (NCBI, UCSC, ENSEMBL)

Genome browsers enable the user to visualize and browse whole genomes by annotated data including Genomic sequence, Genes, RefSeq mRNAs (non-redundant), GenBank mRNAs (redundant), ESTs (Expressed sequence tags), Gene predictions, SNPs (Single nucleotide polymorphisms), Homologous sequences from further organisms, STSs (Sequence tagged sites). Genome Workbench at NCBI can be used to analyze sequences of interest.

Tools for the comparison of genomic DNA in eukaryotes including:

MUMmer program lets two microbial genomes of interest for comparison on a dot plot. The output of MUMmer consists of a dot plot that exhibitions maximally unique matching subsequences (MUMs) among two genomes. One of the many variants of MUMmer is PROtein MUMmer (PROmer) is analogous to NUCmer (NUCleotide MUMmer), but utilizes six-frame translations of each nucleotide sequence, and thereby achieves a higher sensitivity in aligning distantly related sequences.

TaxPlot tool at NCBI permits the comparison of two genomes.

VISTA (Visualization Tools for Alignments)

PipMaker and MultiPipMaker ("Pip" stands for "percent identity plot.")

Integrative Genomics Viewer

3.2 Homologs, Paralogs, Orthologs, Synteny, Colinearity and Gene Displacement

3.2.1 Homologs

Homology is not measured in degrees, instead, homology indicates an evolutionary relationship. The term "homolog" may apply to the relationship between the followings:

- ☆ Genes that are separated by the event of speciation is called orthology.
- ☆ Genes that are separated by the event of genetic duplication are called paralogy.

3.2.2 Orthologs

Orthologs sequences are direct descendants of a sequence in a common ancestor. Their proteins may have similar biological function domain structure and three-dimensional structures.

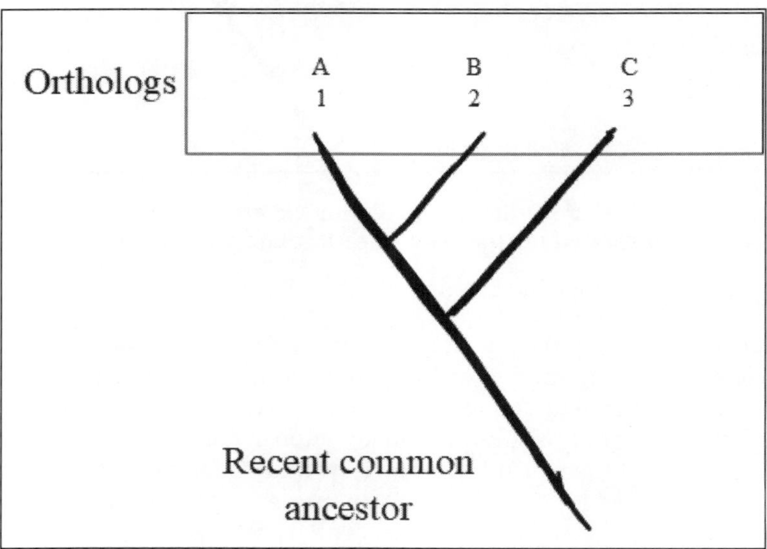

Figure 12.3: Descend A, B, C Genes 1, 2 and 3 are Orthologs Forms of one another.

3.2.3 Paralogs

Genes that are related by a gene duplication event in the last common ancestor. Descendants of these gene products result in different DNA sequences and biological functions by the accumulation of mutation in the duplicated genes.

3.2.4 Synteny

Synteny is the region of the genome that is similar to another organism's genome. Organisms that are recently diverged show more synteny, that is similar blocks of genes present in the same region in their genome. Synteny shows how genomic region is rearranged in the different organism during evolution. To analyze conserved synteny regions, or perhaps even larger regions of genomic DNA that do not necessarily contain protein-coding genes, pairwise and multiple sequence alignment of genomic DNA is necessary.

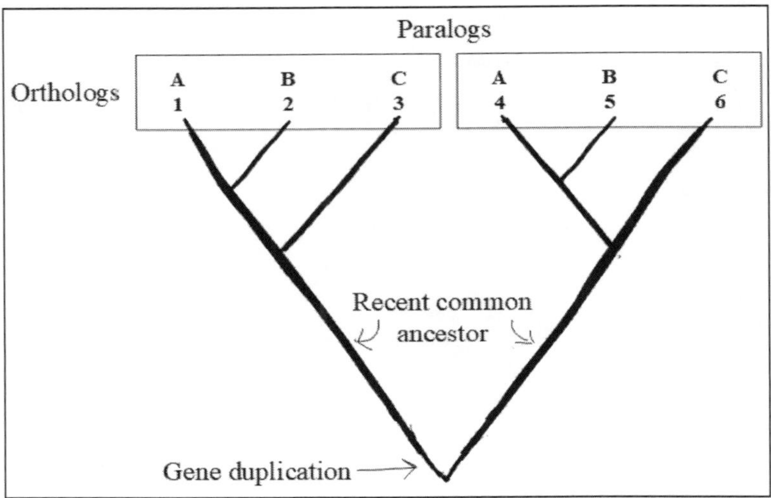

Figure 12.4: Genes 1-3 are Orthologous; Genes 4-6 are orthologous; Any pair of α and β genes are paralogous (genes related through a gene duplication event).

3.2.5 Colinearity

Colinearity is a very specific form of synteny, which requires a more common order of gene arrangement. Events like whole genome duplication or gene loss, reduces the amount of gene colinearity observed today, make it tougher to realize the nature and timing of previous polyploidization events. If an annotated genome shares extensive colinearity with a newly found organism genome, then this colinearity will be used for gene discovery in the newly found organism's genome.

3.3 Gene displacement

3.3.1 Implications of Comparative Genomics – Molecular Evolution and Multigene Family Evolution

Comparative genomics provides a tool to describe the relationship between two or more genomes, this can be achieved by alignment of genomes. The evolutionary relationship among organisms can also be depicted by phylogenetic tree construction.

3.3.2 Forward and Reverse Genetics (Tools and Methods – mutagenesis, knockouts/knock -ins, RNAi, morpholino), Genome-wide Expression Analysis

For the investigation of gene function, there are two contrasting approaches:

Forward genetics approach is used when a phenotype is known but the genetic basis is unknown. The genetic basis of a specific phenotype is deduced by introducing mutations in DNA by mutagenic chemicals or radiation. Mutation can also be introduced by insertional mutagenesis using a transposable element containing a marker. These transposons are made to transposes only once, randomly mobilized in the genome, these markers easily be identified and mapped. These mutations then are screened, usually, a complementation test to confirm that mutant phenotypes arise from the same genes and the mutations are recessive. Forward genetics is also termed as "top-down" approach because this starts with a phenotype (mutant organism) and encoding gene is deduced.

Reverse genetics is opposite to forward genetics. The reverse genetics approach is used to find out the phenotype of a gene. This approach employs techniques that deliberately change the genetic make-up of a gene, and thereby altering the phenotype.

Techniques involved in reverse genetics:

1. **Mutagenesis**: A technique by which mutation is introduced in either the promotor region or coding region of a gene to study the function of gene.
2. **Knock-outs**: Deletion of the target gene, causes permanent elimination of gene expression.
3. **Knock-ins**: Endogenous exon of a gene is replaced by an altered sequence of interest.
4. **RNA interference (RNAi)**: RNAi is used to silence target gene expression. RNAi bind to mRNA in a site-specific manner and with the help of enzymes such as RISC (RNA-induced silencing complex) and AGO_2 (Protein argonaute-2) causes cleavage of mRNA and thereby mRNA degradation. RNAi is a gene knock-down technique that means target gene expression is not eliminated.
5. **Morpholino**: It is a Phosphorodiamidate Morpholino Oligomer (PMO), an antisense oligomer, which is nucleic acid analogs use in gene knockdown techniques. Morpholino binds to mRNA or single-stranded DNA through complementary sequences. Unlike RNAi, Morpholino does not cause degradation of RNA rather then it forms Morpholine-RNA heteroduplex and causes blockage for protein synthesis.

Due to high throughput genome sequencing, most genes can be predicated computationally effortlessly by the presence of ORF, *etc.*, but gene's biological function in an organism can be revealed by reverse genetics approaches in wet-labs settings. **Reverse genetics** is also termed as the "bottom-down" approach because this starts with a genotype and its phenotype is deduced.

3.4 Genome-wide Expression Analysis

3.4.1 Concept of Epigenomics

Epigenomics use to define the epigenetic modifications made in a genome. Because of that epigenetics plays a vital role in the regulation of gene expression by histone modifications or by DNA methylation. The necessity of Epigenomics is as much as genomics and proteomics. Epigenomics modification can be detected through the use of various methods such as **Bisulfite** sequencing, Nanopore sequencing (a fast, real-time sequencing modern tool), *etc.*

Some of the available epigenomics database and browsers mentioned below:

WashU Epigenome Browser (http://epigenomegateway.wustl.edu/) – Also provide a VR (Virtual Reality) interaction on the website.

Roadmap Epigenomics Project (http://www.roadmapepigenomics.org/data/, https://egg2.wustl.edu/roadmap/web_portal/)

3.4.2 Concepts of Genome Evolution (Finding signatures of function, remodeling and applications)

Genome evolution is a process by which the genome changes its structure and it occurs due to continuous accumulation of mutations over time, duplications of the gene or whole genome (increase in ploidy, as seen in wheat), transposable elements, pseudogenes (segment of DNA which look similar to a gene but don't code of any gene product), exon shuffling (when two or more exons DNA of different genes combine or duplicates, results in new genes) and lateral gene transfer (also known as LGT). Lateral Gene Transfer (LGT) is the phenomenon in which an organism's genome acquires a gene from another organism directly, rather than by descent.

4. Transcriptomics and Gene Expression

4.1 Protein Expression Profiling

It is generally defined as the identification of expression of proteins in tissue in a given specific time and condition. It is an offshoot of DNA microarray and is very well inspired from it. Where DNA microarray utilizes multiple mRNAs, segments analyze the genome. But for the development of protein microarray cannot be done similar to DNA-based array which utilizes base pairing to showcase its result. For protein expression profiling protein microarrays are utilized which then work on the principle of antigen-antibody interaction to capture the proteins. The capturing antibodies are immobilized into an array (generally monoclonal antibodies). These antibodies are specific to a protein. The other method for this approach is to perform 2D gel electrophoresis. It is very useful for multiple types of analysis such as toxicology, drug design, cell function analysis *etc.*

4.2 Transcriptomics and Transcriptomes

It is the study of the transcriptome, which is the total RNA content of the cell at the given point of time is called the transcriptome of the cell. The transcriptome includes all forms of the RNA such as mRNA, tRNA, exons, introns, ribosomal RNA all of this is the transcriptome of the cell. It is dynamic as it varies from time to time. Even though all cells in the body have the genome and is the same in all but the reason for different functions and structure of the different cells of the same organisms is due to the difference in varying combination of the gene expression and this gene expression is related to the production of the mRNA. This can be used to compare and measure the transcriptome of various cells.

4.3 Gene Expression Profiling

Measuring the expression of multiple genes at once is considered gene expression profiling. mRNA expression is influenced by many environmental and regulatory factors that are responsible for the activation or the inactivation of the genes. Evidently in the same organism different cells will show different mRNA content at a given state time or may have different functions hence different mRNA build up. Gene expressed in a plasma cell will be different from genes expressed in nerve cells in the same organism though both of them have the same genetic material.

4.4 Tools for Gene Expression Profiling

4.4.1 Northern Blotting

It is a method to study the expression of RNA in a given tissue with the utilization of RNA hybridization. The total RNA is extracted from the sample tissue and is resolved in the agarose gel electrophoresis method based on their length. When the RNA is separated into bands, blotting is performed for further probing of the required RNA. This blotting is done on a membrane filter as the gel is fragile and is not helpful in the interaction of the probe and the RNA. When the RNA is transferred to the membrane with the help of capillary action, then the probes labeled with fluorescent or radiolabelled are used that has the complementary sequence to the target RNA was present in the membrane. Where ever the target RNA band is present, the probe will bind to it and with the presence of labeling on the probe, it will be detected. Different sequences can be detected and later be noted in a database. Similarly changing the conditions of the sample tissue grown will show the difference in the RNA content.

4.4.2 Subtractive Hybridization

It is a technique to identify the difference in the expression pattern in RNA in various cells and tissues of control and the test. Such as in the case of a disease we can try to find out what is the difference in the normal healthy person's RNA expression with the cells and tissue of the diseased state. It can also identify if any changes or rearrangements to the DNA have been caused. It is based on the tester-driver hybridization techniques where tester is the patient's nucleic material and the driver being the normal nucleic content such as in normal patients. The ratio of this hybridization is said to be 1 tester with 10 drivers (1:10) because to prevent any tester-tester hybridization. Also, to be noted only the complementary sequences in between the tester and the driver are to be used. When the tester driver hybridizes all the complementary parts of both sequences will combine leaving the single-stranded tester sequence that is unavailable in the driver sequence. Hence these uncombined sequences in the tester indicate some new sequence and can be the cause of the effect of disease in the patient.

It is to be noted that the driver is always RNA sample while DNA is utilized for the tester sample as it is more stable. For this procedure, mRNA is reverse transcribed for tester into single-stranded cDNA. After this hybridization is carried on and then the hybridized sequences are removed. The tester sequences that did not match (hybridized) are then put through sequence analysis.

4.4.3 Serial Analysis of Gene Expression (SAGE)

It is a method used in transcriptomics to generate an expression profile of a specific tissue. It can be employed in the analysis and identification of certain genes that are activated during different conditions provided to the same cells, which can be compared. SAGE uses cDNA which are achieved from the sample mRNA is tagged with 10-14bp long, short oligonucleotide linker tags that concatenate the cDNAs which is then sequenced. The more the number of tags that are present the more the expression of the particular gene. The benefit of such a technique is that thousands of the mRNA transcripts can be analyzed simultaneously with the frequency of each telling relative abundance of the mRNA during the presented condition.

4.4.4 Microarrays

It is the most common way to study the expression of a gene using mRNA. In Microarray, the mRNA is extracted from the cells and then this total RNA content is subjected to reverse transcriptase which uses the poly-A tail as its primer binding site. In a microarray multiple wells containing single-stranded DNA probes are

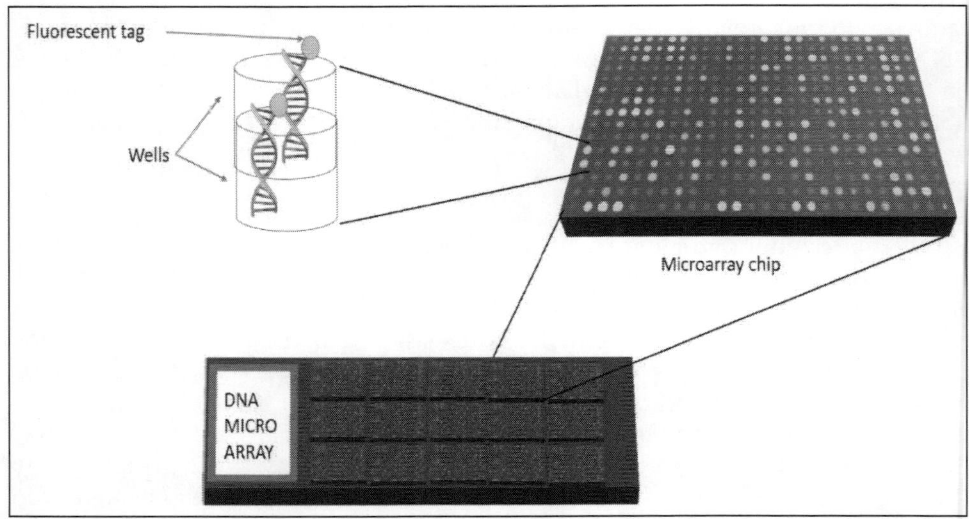

Figure 12.5: Schematic Diagram of Microarray.

present that are bound to the solid support. Each of the wells representing a particular gene as in the earlier step when the cDNA is formed, it is labeled with a fluorescent tag. When this cDNA finds a complementary probe in a well, they bind to the probe and the leftovers are then washed away. This causes only the bound DNA to be detected as fluorescent color in the well. This can be used as the positive confirmation for the gene that coded for this mRNA to be expressed. Microarray is a fast reliable method that can be utilized for seeing the expression of thousands of genes simultaneously.

5. Proteomics: Fundamentals and Interactomics

5.1 Proteome and Proteomics and its Applications

Proteome denotes all the proteins that are present at a specific point time in a cell/tissue in an organism. The proteome is the same for the same cell-type/tissue but different among different cell types/tissue and different organisms. Since cell has protein that is expressed by the constitutive gene which gives a similar result, however, different cell types have a range of diverse functions, therefore their proteomes are different. The identification and analyses of the proteome is known as **proteomics**. For example, comparing the proteome of kidney cells and liver cells of an organism. Proteomics is a vital tool for various studies that cannot be inferred using other omics techniques alone like genomics or transcriptomics. Other important research that can be carried out using proteomics is differential protein expression, Post-translational modifications and compartmentalization of the protein, *etc.*

5.2 Techniques Used for Proteomics Analysis

Proteomics techniques are able to analyze a large number of proteins at once (like 2D-GE, Mass spectrometry) and are sensitive to detect low abundant proteins (like protein microarray) and results can be later analyzed using various databases, for example, search for similar protein(s) in other organisms.

5.2.1 Separation of Proteins

For the separation of protein, one can use techniques like Isotachophoresis (based on ionic mobility), Gel electrophoresis, Iso-electric focusing (IEF), Zonal electrophoresis (based on electrophoretic mobility), Off-Gel electrophoresis (based on liquid-phase peptide isoelectric focusing), 2D liquid chromatography, reverse phase chromatography, *etc.* So in the following sections, we will discuss the routinely used protein separation techniques in proteomics.

5.2.1.1 Gel-based Methods

The gel-based method is based on electrophoresis

5.2.1.2 2D-GE (Two Dimensional Gel Electrophoresis)

5.2.1.2.1 2D-PAGE ((Two Dimensional Poly Acrylamide Gel Electrophoresis)

The SDS protein separation is based on the molecular weight and mass when the protein has a relatively large difference in molecular masses. It could not be used for proteins having similar molecular masses. 2D-PAGE is an electrophoretic technique that includes the first dimension for IEF (iso-electric focusing) in which separation of proteins is based on their Isoelectric point (pI), then in second dimension more resolution results in by SDS-PAGE so the separation is based on protein molecular weight. The cell extract is denatured by high urea concentration and then it is layered on a glass tube which is filled with polyacrylamide which is saturated with a solution of poly-ionic, polycationic and ampholytes. Based on the net charge the ampholytes will separate and forms a continuous gradient when placed in an electric field. The polyanionic and polycationic ampholytes will separate on the opposite ends. A pH. gradient is established by ampholytes. Until the protein reaches the isoelectric point that is net charge zero, charged proteins will migrate through the gradient. This resolution of proteins by one charge unit is called isoelectric focusing. It is carried in the acrylamide gel. To form the pH gradient, the gel contains ampholytes with a mixture of 8M urea and non-ionic detergent which will denature and maintains the protein solubility that is being analyzed. Thus, the denatured proteins in the gel are separated according to their isoelectric point. Proteins separated based on IEF can now be separated in the second dimension based on their size and mass. This step-wise resolution of proteins first by its charge and then by its mass can be used in the separation of cellular proteins.

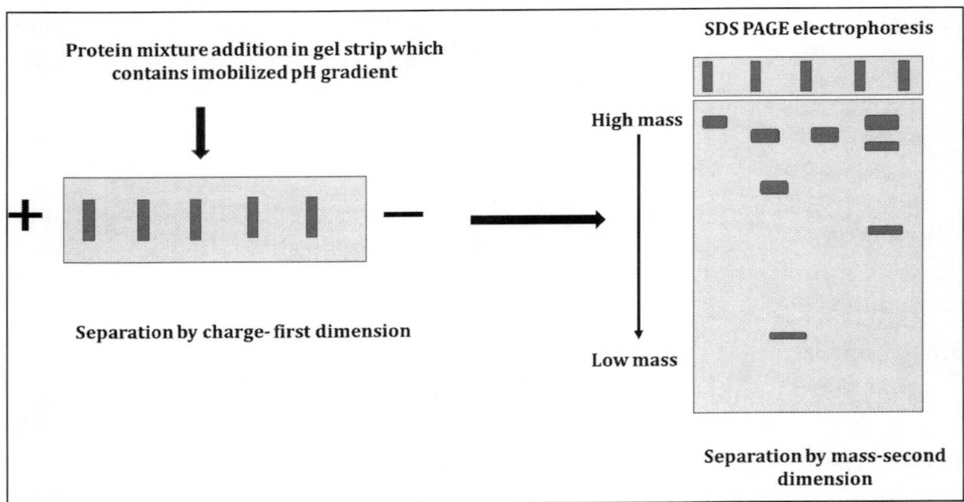

Figure 12.6: 2D Gel Electrophoresis.

5.2.1.2.2 2D-DIGE (Two Dimensional Differential Gel Electrophoresis)

There are numerous glitches in 2D-PAGE that causes gel to gel variation that may be due to technical variation, old TEMED use, impure Tris, streaking pattern on the gel (either due to presence of salts, *etc.*), abundant protein from the crude sample which can interfere and mask small proteins. These can give rise to bad gel results. To overcome these 2D-PAGE limitations Two-Dimensional Differential Gel Electrophoresis (2D-DIGE) was developed to reduce or eliminates gel to gel variation. 2D-DIGE is a modified technique of the conventional 2D-PAGE technique. In 2D-DIGE protein is labeled by fluorescent tags, these are N-hydroxy succinimidyl (NHS) ester derivatives of cyanine dyes Cy2, Cy3 and Cy5 are used. To avoid dye bias, labeling is done the other way around like in one experiment use of Cy3 for samples and Cy5 for control, while contrarily in another experiment. In 2 D-DIGE, before electrophoresis, dye labeled samples or control which excite and emit at different wavelengths, are then parted within the same 2D-PAGE gel based on charge and mass. An internal control (Cy2) in all sample sets is used for the normalization and elimination of gel variations.

5.2.1.2.3 2D-BN-PAGE

Two-Dimensional Blue Native Polyacrylamide Gel Electrophoresis (2D-BN-PAGE) is used for the separation of protein complexes from biological membranes under native conditions and determination of multi-protein complex composition, size and relative abundance. In this method, the first dimension is solubilization of protein complexes with a slight nonionic detergent such as digitonin or dodecyl maltoside or Coomassie brilliant blue G-250, then separation according to their size by non-denaturing (native) electrophoresis. The second dimension in this process is of denaturation condition utilizing SDS-PAGE to separate multi-protein complex of interest (two-dimensional (2D)-BN/SDS-PAGE).

5.2.1.2.4 Staining for Gel

Silver staining is more sensitive than Coomassie-blue stain but is not compatible when gel sample has to be used further in Mass spectrometry. SYPRO Ruby stain an endpoint stain can be able to detect post-translational modification of proteins like glycoproteins and is compatible with MS. Pro-Q Diamond- a fluorescent dye, able to detect phosphorylation (At Ser, The, Try) in proteins. It is sensitive down to the nanogram level.

5.2.2 Gel Free Method

Gel-free methods involve the use of chromatography.

5.2.2.1 HPLC

High-performance liquid chromatography also referred to as high-pressure liquid chromatography is a type of column chromatography. The mobile phase is liquid, so it is liquid chromatography. The stationary phase may be solid or liquid. When compared to traditional column chromatography it yields high performance and high speed because the mobile phase is pumped with high pressure. When the stationary phase is solid it is called adsorption chromatography. Depending upon the relative polarity of solvent and stationary phase the partition chromatography can be divided into 2 variants. When the mobile phase is nonpolar and the stationary phase is polar it is a normal phase but in the reversed-phase the mobile phase is polar, and the stationary phase is nonpolar. The most commonly used HPLC is the reversed-phase.

HPLC is an improved form of liquid chromatography because the solvent is forced under high pressure up to 400 atmospheres. The column packing material is made up of very small particles because it gives a greater surface area for interaction between the stationary phase and the molecules that are flowing past it. To provide a greater surface area many stationary phases are porous. Most of the HPLC performed used a stationary phase that was attached outside silica particles. Components of HPLC included gradient controller, pressure pump, column, detector, and recorder. The main aim of the pressure pump is to provide a constant pressure that moves to the solvent through the column. HPLC used in modern times has improved high-pressure systems for better separation. The columns of HPLC are prepared from stainless steel with dimensions of 5-100, 10-20 cm are most common. For analytic separation, the diameter of the column is 2.1, 3.2 or 4.5mm and for the preparative application, it is up to 30mm. The most common detectors used in HPLC are UV-Vis's absorbance detector, but other detectors can also be used.

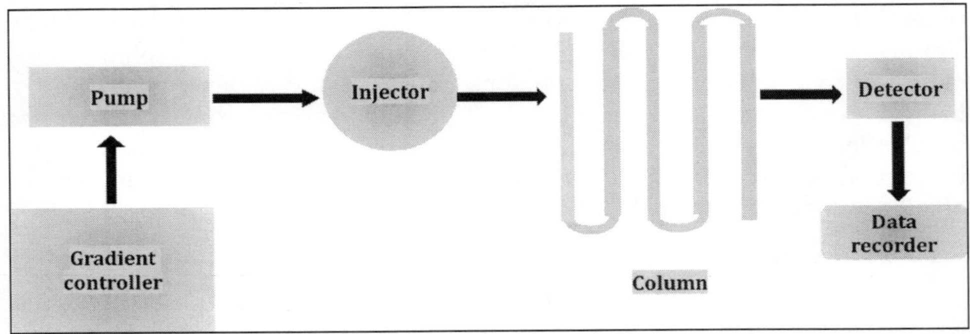

Figure 12.7: Schematic Representation of HPLC.

Benefits of using HPLC

1. It is powerful, adaptable and affordable.
2. It increases productivity from sample to instrument and from separation to reporting results.
3. Automates chromatography instruments.

Application

The main purpose of HPLC is to identify and purify a particular analyte which includes both qualitative and quantitative analysis.

1. It is used in water purification, detection of impurities in pharma industries.
2. Ion exchange chromatography of proteins, ligand exchange chromatography.
3. Anion exchange chromatography at high pH of oligosaccharides and carbohydrates.

5.2.2 Mass Spectrometry

It is the method of determining the molecular mass by the measurement of the mass to charge ratio of ions in the gas phase. In the ionization source, the ions are generated by either gain or loss of charge. It consists of three basic components: - Ionization Chamber, Detector, and Recorder. First, the sample is let inside through sample inlet, it then goes to ionization source followed by mass analyzer, detector, and recorder.

- **Ionization**- by bombardment with the stream of electrons there is knocking off one or more electrons to give off positive ions, most of which carry +1 charge.
- **Acceleration** – acceleration is done to maintain equal kinetic energy of the ions. There is voltage in decreasing order as the positive charge ions pass through the slit.
- **Deflection** – deflection of ions in the presence of a magnetic field because of their difference in masses. The lighter and more positive the ion is; it is deflected the most when compared to heavy mass ions.

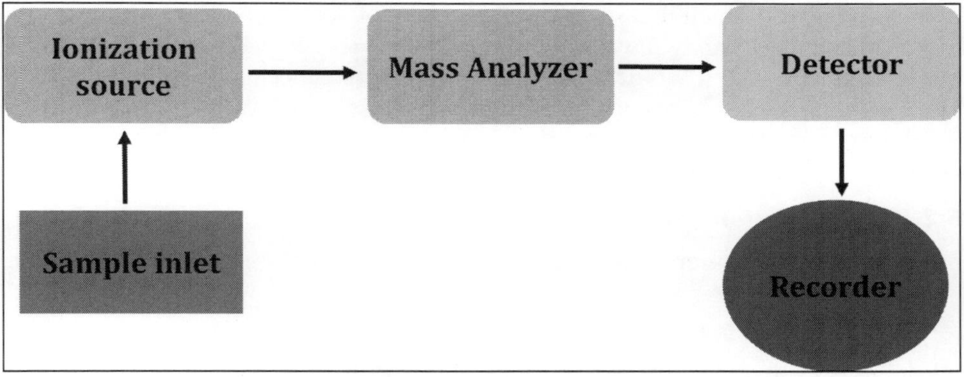

Figure 12.8: Schematic Diagram of Typical Mass Spectrometer.

5.2.2.1 Ionization Techniques

A. Electron Ionization

High energy electron beam strikes the molecule, it strips the electron from the molecule and forms a cation. It has a disadvantage that high molecular weight compounds cannot be determined.

B. Chemical Ionization

It is a process in which sample molecules are combined with ionized reagent gas, and when these sample molecules collide with ionized gas, the sample molecules become ionized by a method like an electron transfer, proton transfer adduct formation. The gas choice should be made closest to the proton affinity of reagent gas with that of the sample.

C. Desorption Ionization

High-intensity photons or high energy beam is bombarded on the sample which is dissolved in the matrix. When high-energy photons are used it is called

MALDI (matrix-assisted laser desorption). A non-volatile and inert matrix should be used in this case. The material that is commonly used are aromatic compounds with a carboxylic functional group. A solid matrix should be used because it absorbs laser radiation. It can be used for larger molecular weight molecules like proteins.

D. Electrospray Ionization

Polar volatile solvent is used for dissolution of the sample which is then pumped through narrow steel capacity. In the presence of an electric field, the sample is dispersed from the tip and forms highly charged droplets. The size becomes smaller because the solvent evaporates, and this leads to the release of ions free from solvent.

5.2.2.3 Mass Analysis

After the ionization of the sample, it is accelerated in the presence of an electric field and then reaches to mass analyzer where the separation of ions takes place by mass to charge ratio. TOF (Time –Of – Flight) is one of the most common types of mass analyzer which measures the flight time of ion. The velocity of ions with identical kinetic energy will vary according to their respective masses. That means the ion light in weight would reach the detector first since it has a high velocity. The ions that are large in size and high in weight would travel slowly and reach the detector late. Thus, the mass, charge and kinetic energy determine the arrival time of the ion to the detector.

5.2.2.4 Applications

1. It is used in environmental monitoring to check the quality of soil and water.
2. It is used in peptide sequencing by tandem mass spectroscopy.
3. All known and unknown amino acids can be sequenced according to their masses by tandem MS or MS/MS.
4. It can be used to detect residual gases in high vacuum systems.
5. It can be used in carbon dating of soil, rocks, and other radioactive processes.

5.2.3 Protein and Peptide Array

Protein microarray is one of the essential tools in proteomics. It is used for protein-protein interaction and to determine their functions. In this, a protein chip is used that has support surfaces like nitrocellulose/glass slide to which an array of captured protein is bound. A fluorescent dye labelled probe is added to the array. The fluorescent signal emitted by a reaction between probe and immobilized proteins is used for analysis. Analytical and protein microarray are two classes of protein microarray.

A. Analytical Microarray

Analytical microarray is also called antibody microarray. In this, the antibodies are arrayed in high density on a glass surface. For more specificity and increased affinity, it involves a signal amplification system and sandwich assay in which the primary antibody on the array captures antigen which is detected by a secondary antibody that recognizes different parts of antigens. For each antigen to be detected it requires highly specific antibodies.

B. *Functional Protein Microarray*

It is also called target protein assay. It is prepared through immobilizing an enormous number of proteins to assay enzymatic activity and detection of antibodies with their functions. The biochemical activity of the entire proteome can be studied in a single experiment. To maintain the functional interactions, the native structure of the protein should be preserved.

5.2.3.1 Applications

1. Diagnostics- used in antigen-antibody interaction in the blood sample.
2. Biomarker identification tool that can test a specific disease when proteins are treated as potential antigens.

   Example- coronavirus protein microarray which is produced by diagnosing SARS in which the array included the SARS coronavirus protein and five additional infectious coronaviruses.
3. Protein functional analysis- it identifies protein, protein phospholipid interactions and enzyme substrates and receptor ligands.
4. Proteomics- it is used in protein expression profiling that means identifying a particular protein in a cell, or which proteins are expressed in a particular cell.
5. Treatment Procedures- used in the treatment of autoimmune, cancer and allergies by the development of antigen-specific therapies and identifies molecules that could be used as a drug.

5.3 Qualitative and Quantitative Proteomics

5.3.1 Qualitative Proteomics

The main aspect of qualitative analysis is to identify the proteins, that are extracted from the cell (whole proteome). In this method after the extraction and isolation of whole proteins from the cells/tissue, we usually perform protease digestion and separation of peptides through various techniques like gel electrophoresis, 2D gel electrophoresis, liquid chromatography. The identification of the protein is done by Mass spectrometric analysis this analysis shows the abundance of certain amino acids in the peptide chain by plotting a graph of mass by charge hand-builds relative abundance. These are then combined to form the whole protein. With this information, we can compare the analyzed proteins that were found in the sample with protein databases that is available online. With the help of searching, we can also determine, whether this protein that was found has already been discovered and then compared with the existing one or maybe a discovery. The benefit is that we can create a database of such organisms and their proteome. Challenge existing database structures integrate new findings interpret and validate existing structures and proteomes that are present in a certain organism. Other approaches can be used by conducting protein immune assays such as utilizing microarray studies for these protein-protein interactions that can avail the possibility of system biological studies which help in the study of cellular functions and pathways. The major drawback of this approach to proteomics is that many organisms are complex and contain vast amounts of proteins and also single protein may have many variants in the same organisms. Defining their function becomes a tedious time-consuming laborious task.

5.3.2 Quantitative Proteomics

For the quantitative study of protein expression interactions or modifications, mass spectrometry has become a prominent technology. The most widely used MS-based proteomics is reversed phased liquid chromatography which is coupled to tandem mass spectrometry. Isotopic labeling of the proteins and peptides is also involved in quantitative proteomics, which can be differentiated by mass spectrometry. A considerable amount of data can be acquired from quantitative proteomics, it is, therefore, more often used in understanding protein kinetics and molecular mechanism of a given biological process. Modern quantitative proteomics methods such as liquid chromatography coupled to mass spectrometry (LC-MS) could measure their changes in the abundance of protein-specific post-translational modification (PTM), facilitating the location of the modified residue. Typically, quantitative proteomic analyses rely on MS for quantitating selected peptides, tandem mass spectrometry (MS/MS) is required for peptide identification. Ionized peptides are sampled to produce a precursor ion spectrum during the first round of MS (MS1) that represents all ionized peptides in the sample. Individually, ions are then selected to undergo collision-induced fragmentation (CID) and another round of MS (MS2), which produce a fragment ion spectrum for each precursor ion. These fragment spectra are compared to peptide databases and assessed specific peptide sequences, then computationally correlated into the anticipate protein sequence.

5.4 Proteome Mining

Proteome mining is an integral functional investigation utilized in proteomics. It is a method that is used for screening total protein content in an organism or proteome, drug discovery target identification. The method is based on the thought that every protein has natural ligands. The ligand binds to a protein in the active site of the organism is selected then immobilized on a bead which then is exposed to the whole proteome content. When they are presented with the proteome only the proteins that interact with the immobilized ligand bind to it the rest can be removed. Later on, these proteins can be further tested and sequenced using various methods such as protein electrophoresis, MS, *etc.* After sequencing and identification of the proteins, researchers correlate whether identified protein is relevant in the disease. These proteins will be further tested with different drugs that have a similar affinity as the immobilized ligand which is then selectively scanned with such iterations of the ligand these should be able to inhibit the protein that usually only functions when the natural ligand is bound to the new analogue. If that drug will compete and prevent the binding of the natural one to the protein, then this can be then utilized as a drug that will mitigate the effects of the protein on the host.

For determining whether the lead molecule is toxic or not the molecule can be interacted with the eluted proteins for checking whether they bind to it or not in different concentrations. They are tested to determine at which concentration the molecule may affect the other isolated proteins and their respective pathway in the organism. If the lead is only selective to one of the proteins, then it can be tested for potential drug

For *e.g.*, in a study for drug discovery for malaria which targeted purine binding proteins determining a molecule for protein kinase inhibition ATP was immobilized when the proteome of the organism was subjected to it many enzymes and proteins were attached such as dehydrogenases, heat shock proteins, protein kinases, *etc.* These were then structurally analyzed and differentiated into human purine interacting proteins which were disregarded the malarial ones were selected for further Drug Database Analysis.

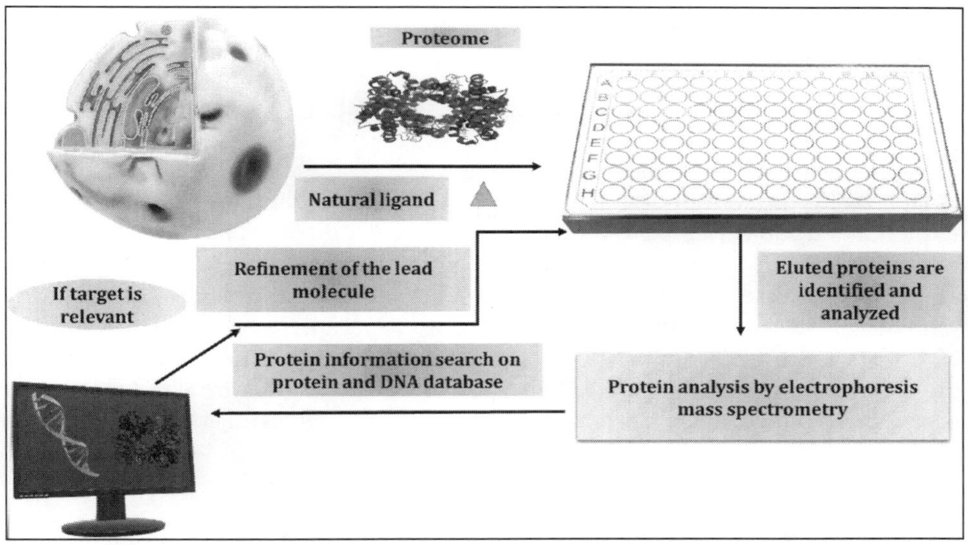

Figure 12.9: Process of Proteome Mining.

The benefit of such a study, first of all, is drug discovery against a pathogen during the refinement process. Multiple compounds can be found that attack multiple pathogenic proteins and pathways which then disables the pathogen to quickly develop immunity towards a single drug hence quite effective.

5.5 Computational Approach to Study Proteome

5.5.1 Data Banks

Most organisms have DNA as the basic genetic material some viruses are special cases where they have RNA as the genetic material. In the case of most organism's DNA is converted to RNA and then to the required protein, so basically all the information to form any protein possible by the organism is contained by the DNA which is then selectively transferred to RNA and then transcribed to protein. DNA functions as the storage unit, RNA as the transport and protein as the functional unit of an organism.

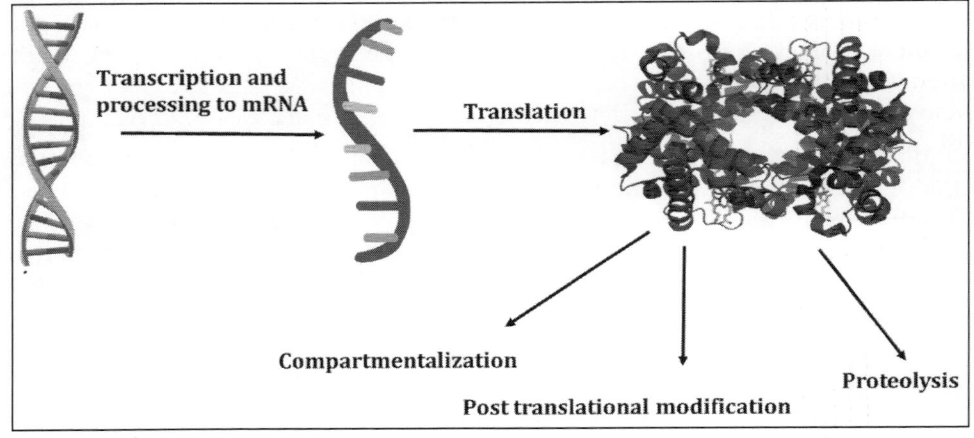

Figure 12.10: The Process of Biomolecules.

Nucleotide sequence data is available in various online data banks and different databases for all known organisms such as DNA data bank of Japan, nucleotide sequence databank at EMBL-EBI (European Molecular Biology Laboratory European Bioinformatics Institute), *etc.* They compile data received from data depositaries. These can be utilized for studying the DNA sequence and predicting possible peptide sequences. These are converted into a standard format that can be used by all. The National Centre for Biotechnology Information (NCBI) is another major database of the genome for many organisms. It also hosts DNA, RNA and protein sequences of organisms from various taxonomic classification such as plants, bacteria plasmids viruses, *etc.*

5.5.2 Nucleotide to Peptide Sequence Converting Tools

A codon (trinucleotide sequence) in DNA codes for a specific amino acid but also one amino acid is coded by different codons with this information from DNA peptide sequences can be predicted.

There are multiple software's that can convert DNA sequence to peptide sequence like Expasy translate tool. But with a catch that is RNA in higher eukaryotic organisms have introns to tackle this, some databanks have the sequence with only the part that will be transcribed or simply have databases with expressed protein sequences.

5.5.3 Structure Functional Studies: Structural Database

In an organism, the protein 3D structure is the functional form and is very small to study visually even by the best microscopes available to compensate and to study the structural features of the protein. A Protein Data Bank (PDB) is maintained by Brookhaven national laboratory in New York. They include collaborative studies done by various scientists utilizing X-ray crystallographic,

NMR, Cryo-Electron Microscopic structures. These databases are useful for studying structural orientation, conformation, overall size and shape components present in the structure. It is also an essential tool in studying protein-ligand interactions and changes caused due to this interaction in the protein. Modeling software such as Chimera, Pymol, *etc.* can be used to visualize and analyze the structure and predict interactions with other molecules for drug discovery and various other purposes. Many protein relations can be found out using the basic local alignment tool (BLAST) where positions in amino acid sequences that are conserved are aligned and highlighted showing relationships between different organism's proteins.

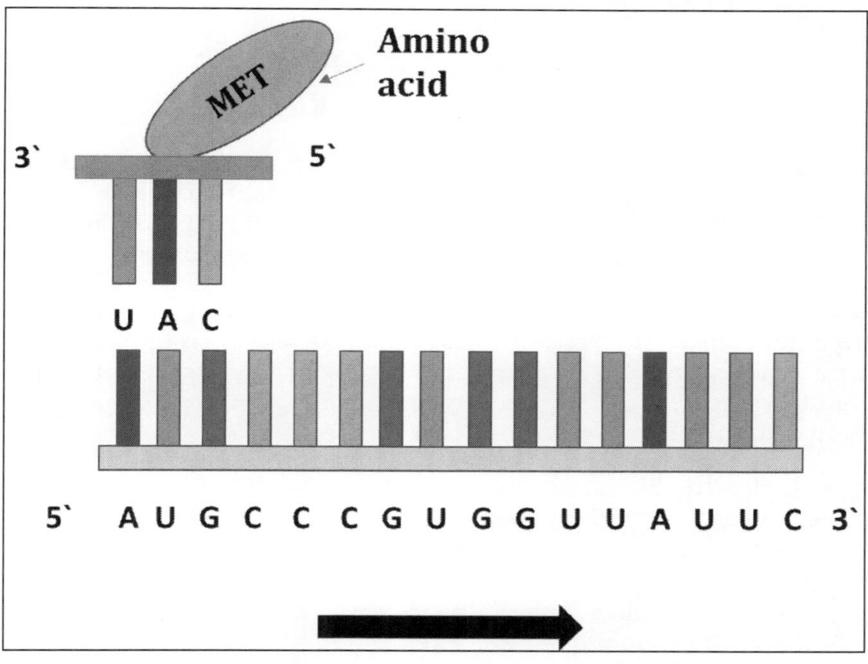

Figure 12.11: Transcription of mRNA begins with AUG, in Eukaryotes, it Codes for Methionine.

5.5.4 Archives for Proteins

Uniport is one of the most famous protein database archives. It provides free access to all publicly available and verified proteins which are manually checked and updated regularly. It was developed in conjugation with the Swiss Institute of Bioinformatics (SIB), Department of Bioinformatics, Structural Biology of the Geneva University, European Bioinformatics Institute (EBI) and the Georgetown University Medical Centre's Protein Information Resource (PIR). They have done collaborative work to make this online database. Since 2003, the data contained in them not only gives the protein sequence but also the functional domains information on binding sites, post-translational modifications, 3D structures and similarities to other proteins.

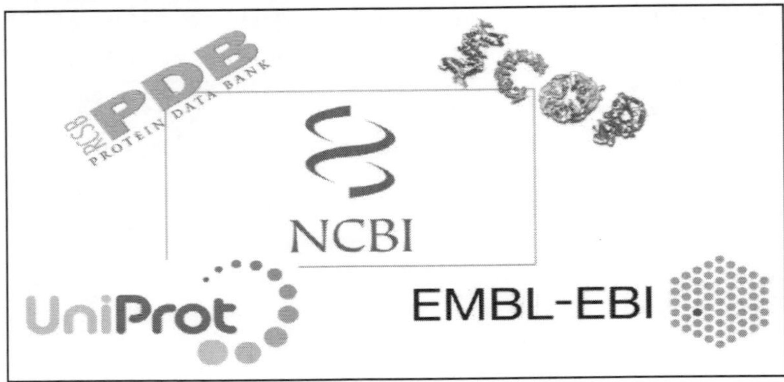

Figure 12.12: Protein Databases.

For visualization and storage of macromolecular protein in the online format, Protein Data Bank (PDB) is considered the most important and major tool though its main function is to provide the user with a set of atomic coordinates which when viewed with certain software such as VMD can be visualized with known atomic resolution, also it has information on the protein, its related literature and publications structural information on the protein and presence of any molecules other than the protein. It is a free access website created by joint efforts of Molecular Structure Database at the European Bioinformatics Institute (EBI) and the Protein Data Bank, Japan hosted at the Osaka University and distributed by Research Collaboratory for Structural Bioinformatics (RCSB).

SCOP (Structural Classification of Proteins) is another database that deals with the classification of the protein's structurally and provides a hierarchical classification of the proteins structural similarity such as by domain, families super families and at lasts by folds (alpha helixes and beta sheets containing structures). Other classification includes in the bases protein function which can be viewed on Gene Ontology Consortium

5.6 Protein Mapping

Protein mapping can be divided based on protein expression or protein interaction mapping.

5.6.1 Protein Expression Mapping

Protein expression mapping is a quantitative method to study the whole cell or tissue protein expression patterns by utilizing 2D gel electrophoresis, mass spectrometry, LC-tandem mass spectrometry or gel electrophoresis with Isotope labeling. By utilizing the 2D gel electrophoresis technique, proteins can be separated and the protein of interest spotted on the gel is cut, and for further analysis mass spectrometry is performed. Mass spectrometry gives further details about protein/peptide's sequence and also post-translational modification on protein/peptides. However, quantitative analysis of proteins by gel electrophoresis is a challenge due to poor gel to gel reducibility and that low amount of protein that is expressed hide by the larger amount of protein that expresses in the cell. So, to compensate for this, the labeling method is used.

5.6.1.1 Isotope Labelling

In isotope labeling, we can utilize metabolic labeling of proteins with radioactive amino acids or stable isotopes. For example, identifying disease biomarkers, stable isotope labeling by amino acids in cell culture (SILAC) can be used, which provides isotopicaly labeled forms of amino acids used to estimate protein levels. While SILAC labelling is for culture system, another method Isotope-coded affinity tag (ICAT) labeling is for all proteins, specifically cystine residue of proteins. ICAT labeling method that uses chemical labeling reagents for quantitative proteomics by mass spectrometry. These chemical probes are consisting of 3 different compounds. ICAT allows us to detect, quantify, and identify the proteins from complex mixtures by labeling specific moieties of protein and thus reducing complexity. We can compare our protein expression mapping to a variety of protein expression profiles that happen in cells or tissues under various environmental or disease conditions. This can also be achieved by uploading this experimental data to the protein expression profile database. As nearly all cellular functions of cells determined by their protein, this comparison allows us to understand how each protein expression change alters during different states of cell or environment, whether it is upregulated or downregulated, and whether it has post-translational modifications or not. Diagnosis of the disease can also be carried out by diagnostic markers like specific proteins that define the specific disease.

5.6.2 Protein Interaction Mapping

Protein-protein interaction (PPI) mapping involves the study of interactions that happens between proteins that are encoded by cells on a proteome scale. Interactions of protein also give an idea about the function of a protein like signaling, multi-protein complexes. As a result, creating a PPI map of the cell would be very beneficial to understanding its biological processes. Protein interaction mapping can be studied experimentally by techniques such as Two-hybrid systems or Three-hybrid systems, Phage display, Co-IP. Protein interaction data, and Protein-protein interaction (PPI) or Protein-ligand interaction (PLI) networks can be predicted or generated using bioinformatics tools.

5.7 Two-Hybrid Methods and Variations

The two-hybrid screening method, also known as the yeast two-hybrid system or protein trap capture system, is an *in-vivo* technique for studying large-scale protein-protein or protein–DNA interactions by studying physical interactions (or binding) between two proteins or a single protein and a DNA molecule, respectively. The development of the yeast two-hybrid system is based on the eukaryotic transcription regulation process, which involves the involvement of transcriptional activators.

Eukaryotic transcription activation factors contain two different domains the DNA binding domain (BD) and DNA transcription activation domain (AD). The DNA binding domain (BD) and the DNA transcription activation domain (AD) are two distinct domains contains in eukaryotic transcription activation factors.

These two domains can be separated independently; the functions have no bearing on one another. Only when the two are sufficiently close can the complete transcriptional activator activity be achieved, allowing the downstream genes to be transcribed; based on this principle, a yeast two-hybrid system can be designed.

Protein X and protein Y are constructed into fusion plasmids with BD and AD domains, and the plasmids are transferred to homozygous yeast cells for expression. Then, if there is no interaction between the two proteins the downstream genes or the reporter genes will not be transcribed for expression. If the two proteins interact, BD and AD become spatially closed, and a downstream reporter gene is transcribed.

By determining whether or not the reporter is expressed, the interaction between the two proteins can be determined. And these reporter genes, such as ADE2, HIS3, or lac Z, are commonly used. As a result, when interacting proteins are present, reporter gene expression is activated to confirm the presence of interactions.

5.8 Phage Display

Phage display is a technique for studying PPIs (protein protein interactions). The most common application of this technique is the fusion of peptides or proteins to a minor or major coat protein of a filamentous bacteriophage (M 13 bacteriophage). In filamentous phage display, random peptides are fused to the N-terminus of gene III or gene VIII of phage protein. Minor coat of phase is gene III protein present in 3-5 copies per phase, located at the phage's tip. Where else, the major coat protein is gene VIII protein, which exist in 2700 copies per phage particle. Because the fusion protein's gene is packaged within the same phage, there is a direct link between the phenotype like the ligand binding characteristics of a displayed protein. The targeting ligand can be immobilized on the solid phase. Phage displaying a protein that interacts with the target is enriched by affinity purification in a process called panning. After multiple rounds of panning, the phage is used to infect *E. coli* and the identity of the selected inserts is determined by DNA sequencing. This allows for the rapid screening of large libraries of peptides with random amino acid sequences for desired ligand binding properties. Furthermore, a large number of mutants of a displayed protein can be screened for variants with different ligand-binding properties.

5.9 Co-IP

Co-immunoprecipitation is a common classical method based on antigen-antibody interaction specificity. The interaction of two known proteins is used in co-immunoprecipitation to detect the interaction of unknown proteins. When cells are lysed many of the protein-protein interactions that exist in intact cells are preserved. If there is an XY protein complex in the cell and acts or the bait protein is immunoprecipitated with an anti X antibody, then the protein Y or the target protein bound to X is also precipitated therefore anti-X antibody is added to the cell lysate to precipitate protein acts and then western blot is used to detect the presence of protein Y in the precipitate. Hence, the presence of a Y protein in western blot indicates the presence of protein-XY interactions.

5.10 Bioinformatics Tools for PPIs

Based on genome sequence data, computational approaches have been developed to predict functional interactions between proteins. These approaches have the advantage of being able to quickly generate interaction maps for a variety of organisms. Tools for Structure-Based PPI Prediction are PrISE (PRediction of Protein-Protein Interface Residues Using Structural Elements), InterPreTS (Interaction Prediction Through Tertiary Structure), iLoops, Struct2Net, PRISM 2.0 (Protein Interactions by Structural Matching 2.0), ImproViser- for automated peptide mapping of quantitative proteomics data in the protXML data. IntAct - Analysis tools for molecular interaction data, STRING or String db - Uses a spring model to generate the network images.

5.11 Protein – (Protein/ligand) Interaction Networks

Protein interaction networks show that interactions occur not only between proteins involved in different cellular processes but also between proteins involved in the same process. These links may be crucial for sharing information and thereby coordinating global responses to environmental stimuli. Protein-protein interaction networks (PPIN) are depictions of the physical interaction between protein-protein or protein-ligand in the cell. These studies provide a global view of how cells perform their processes in a coordinated way. The total PPI that happens in a cell is called Interactome.

6. Structure-Omics and Cellular Proteomic: Gel Electrophoresis and MS

6.1 2D Proteomics

The 2D gel electrophoresis is used to analyze thousands of proteins with higher resolution. It has two steps in which the proteins are separated which is first by isoelectric focusing that is separated according to their pI value then they are separated according to their molecular weight. For the rapid identification of protein separated through 2D gel electrophoresis, mass spectrometry is used. Methods of ionization like MALDI (matrix-assisted laser desorption ionization), TOF MS, ESI (electron spray ionization) are widely used and highly sensitive techniques.

6.2 Microarray and MS

DNA microarray does not provide any direct information about changes in protein functions. In most biological functions proteins are effector molecules therefore it is critical to evaluate the protein function. Especially protein-protein interactions analysis in system biology has the limitation of traditional methods. To analyze broad ranges of interactions in systems biology, nowadays a new approach using protein microarray combined with mass spectrometry is being used by various researchers.

6.3 SAGE and Microarray

SAGE stands for serial analysis of gene expression it creates cDNA from mRNA then is used for amplification and sequencing. The expression of gene patterns in cells, animal tissues can be determined by using both SAGE and microarray. The data of microarray of cDNA is very closely related to data produced by SAGE for higher gene expression levels, the combination of both is used widely in determining gene levels of expression.

6.4 3D Structure Determination

6.4.1 X-RAY

X-ray radiation determines the 3D structure by electron distribution in a crystallized molecule. The crystal diffracts the X-rays of different intensities. X-ray crystallography is one of the most sensitive methods for protein structure visualization because it provides one of the best resolutions as the X-ray wavelength is of the same length as of covalent bond. It requires highly purified protein crystals. Therefore, before X-ray diffraction, protein crystallization is a very important step. The components of protein crystallography include the crystal, the X-rays and the detector. The diffracted X-rays are detected by the detector. The basic principle is the scattering of X-rays by the electrons and the number of the electron is proportional to the wave scattered by the electron. The scattered beam is formed by the contribution of each atom. The scattered waves are then detected by the detector or the X-ray film. In protein X-ray diffraction analysis, researchers uses a static crystal therefore we cannot identify the dynamics of proteins through X-ray crystallography.

6.4.2 NMR

NMR stands for nuclear magnetic resonance; it is a technique that reveals the structure of molecules in highly concentrated solutions. The principle behind this is the nuclei of the atom are intrinsically magnetic. It is mainly used in analytic chemistry to determine the purity of the sample. The basic principle behind NMR is that all nuclei are electrically charged and many have spin, in the presence of an external magnetic field energy transfer takes place from base to upper energy level. The transfer of energy takes place at the definite wavelength which corresponds to the radio frequency, the energy emitted is of the same frequency as spin returns to base. NMR of protein samples is performed in a highly purified state only. Approximate 1000 µl of a few mM concentration of purified samples is required. The source of proteins can be natural or recombinant. Although NMR of recombinant proteins is easier as researcher can purify sufficient concentration of protein and isotopic labeling is also possible. Generally, in protein, multidimensional NMR experiments are performed to identify the structural parameters. In addition to this NMR gives dynamic information of protein.

6.4.3 PDB

It means protein data bank, it describes the 3-D structure of a protein, nucleic acids in a text file. The text file of PDB provides information about the coordinates of atoms, secondary structure, amino acid locations, atoms connectivity with distances. It includes all the structures that are obtained by NMR or X-ray crystallography. There is a worldwide collaboration of protein data bank Europe, a protein data bank of Japan, RCSB PDB. The PDB structures for a better and clear understanding can be visualized in many software, the structures could be ball and stick, ribbon, *etc.* Each solved protein structure either by X-ray crystallography or NMR or cryogenic electron microscopy has a designated unique PDB ID, which could never be the same for two proteins. NCBI and uniport which are freely available give high-quality information about protein sequences and their IDs.

6.4.4 Pfam

Pfam is a database that provides complete information about the domains and family of the proteins. For the determination of the domain, one has to upload the respective protein sequence in the software. One can also find multiple alignments, domain architecture, species distribution in Pfam. The family of Pfam has seed alignment which means it contains a set of sequences one can enter. Hidden Markov Model (HMM) is built by a seed sequence. Pfam generates a high level of a grouping called clans, thus a clan is defining as the collection of data in Pfam which are structurally and sequentially related or similar.

6.4.5 SMART

A simple modular architecture research tool, it is a database that identify and analyze the domains of the protein and its sequences. SMART is the collection of 1204 domain models. For the detection of protein domain in a protein sequence, SMART uses HMM (hidden Markova model) which is built from multiple sequence alignment. For the specific domain architecture identification, architecture SMART is used by AND/NOT logic. Proteins with the identical domain as a query SMART is used. SMART has relatively high specificity that detects domains from the sequences.

6.4.6 Modeller

It is a bioinformatic tool used in homology modeling for determining tertiary protein structure or quaternary which is very rare. The method used in Modeller is inspired by NMR (nuclear magnetic resonance), which then creates the density function for each atom location in the protein. Based on the alignment with the template, it predicts the 3D structure of the target given protein. The steps are as involves finding some similarity between the template and the target, alignment and building a model.

6.5 High Throughput Cloning

It is performed to obtain a high yield of recombinant protein. Restriction-free cloning is a PCR-based method in which a fragment of DNA is inserted into vector at a random position independent of restriction sites. The polymerases used today have less error rates but have high fidelity. This method does not require any pre-treatment of vectors; thus, this method has high potential in the field of biotechnology, or structural biology. Ligation independent cloning (LIC) is very important and efficient method in high throughput cloning, single-stranded complementary overhangs are generated by treating linear plasmid with DNA insert. Any vector can be made compatible with the LIC system, proteins with different affinity tags proteins are produced by using the same PCR product insert.

There is minimal addition of amino acids added to proteins by LIC sequences, and it can later be modified if necessary, which is an important step in N to C terminal extension.

6.6 Structure to Functional Analysis

6.6.1 Homology modeling

Homology modeling is done with similar sequences of known structures that is identifies homologous protein structures. It is performed by alignment of the query sequence with template sequence the templates are searched using databases such as by BLAST/FASTA. It is the most accurate for all but requires a similar template for the accomplishment of the modeling process.

6.6.2 *ab initio* Modeling

Models that do not have any similar homologous sequences are prepared using the method of *ab initio* modeling which involves the construction of a protein model from the scratch. Because of this its productivity is low and the success rate is only restricted to lesser than 1000 residues. *ab initio* modeling does it by scanning multiple energy functions that give altered conformations. The lowest energy-containing and the most thermodynamically stable conformation is selected for modeling.

6.6.3 Protein Threading

It is also known as fold recognition. It is a method that uses similar folds of a known protein as a template for building models. Its efficacy is average compared to homology modeling but is better than *ab initio* modeling and needs less computational power. Individual amino acids are threaded on the protein and estimated how well the target sequence fits the template. The best fit is selected and used for model formation.

6.6.4 Post Translational Modification (PTM)

Post-translational modification fundamentally is an enzymatic alteration of proteins which is followed by protein biosynthesis. The synthesizing of the proteins by translating mRNA into polypeptide chains, which could undergo PTM to the nature of mature proteins product. PTMs are vital components in cell signaling. Also, PTM is increasing the functional diversity of the proteome with the help of the covalent addition of functional groups. Generally, these modifications including such as glycosylation, nitrosylation, methylation, acetylation, phosphorylation, ubiquitination, lipidation and proteolysis, *etc.* Understanding and identifying PTMs are important in the study of cell biology and disease treatment and prevention. The increasing complexity from the level of the genome to the proteome is additionally facilitated by protein post-translational modifications (PTMs). PTMs are the chemical modifications that play a key role in functional proteomics because they are regulating the activity, interaction and localization with the help of the other cellular molecules such as proteins, lipids, nucleic acids (DNA and RNA) and cofactors.

6.6.5 Protein Engineering

It is a method by which researchers can modify/change the sequence by utilizing insertion substitution or deletion of nucleotides at the transcriptional level. This enables to creation of new proteins that are better suitable for the task that is to be performed. For example, CRISPR/CAS9 recently has been proven as a powerful tool for editing plant genomes for inducing targeted mutagenesis in crops. This is done to get more yield per crop or could be used to make crops resistant to certain diseases and pests. Directed protein evolution also falls under protein engineering. In this multiple sequence, diversification is studied by amino acid substitution. These are then screened for potential sequences whose structure and functions are suitable for further experiments and their goals. These steps of diversification and screening are repeated multiple times to narrow down the sequence to the experimental goal.

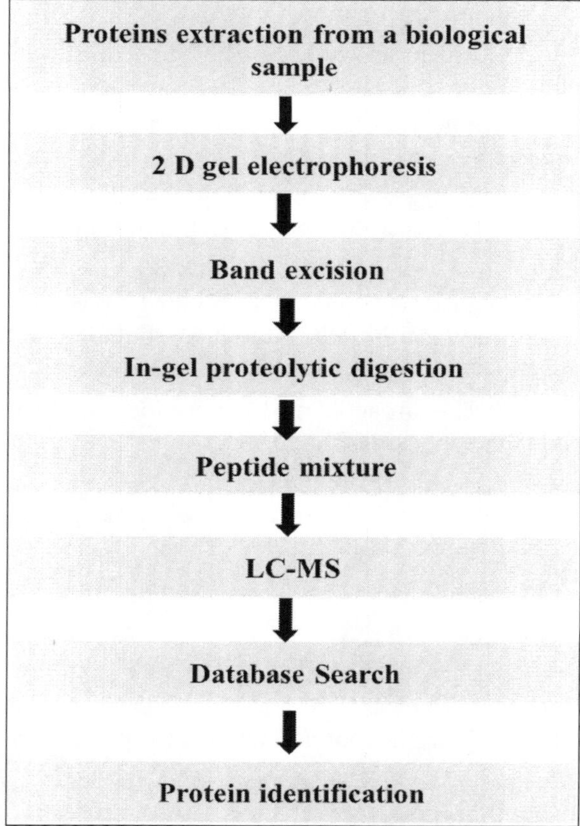

Figure 12.13: Flowchart Showing Proteomics Workflows.

6.7 Proteomics Workflows

The workflow of the proteomics experiment involves protein extraction and isolation from a biological sample followed by enzymatic digestion (usually trypsin),

MS analysis, and peptide identification. Generally, isolated peptide mixture is further fractionated by HPLC (high-performance liquid chromatography) with the different columns (usually reverse-phase chromatography), followed by ESI-MS (electrospray ionization-mass spectroscopy) analysis. Although, the mixture of ESI-MS and LC are usually named as LC-MS/MS. Analysis of a protein by using this approach not only provides protein identity but also able to get peptide sequencing information. Other benefits of mass spectrometric analysis are characterization and identification of post-translation modification in proteins. It could be a great challenge to completely identify the PTM patterns at any given time in cells, tissues, and organisms. Therefore, MS-based proteomics becomes the method of choice for characterization and detection of PTM.

REFERENCES

1. Batzer, M. A. Genome Organization: Human.
2. Amparo, L., and Silva Francisco, J. (2013). The size of the genome and the complexity of living beings. Metode, 32.
3. Shafee, T., and Lowe, R. (2017). Eukaryotic and prokaryotic gene structure. WikiJournal of Medicine, 4(1), 2.
4. Alberts, B., Johnson, A., Lewis, J., Raff, M., Roberts, K., and Walter, P. (2002). How genetic switches work. In Molecular Biology of the Cell. 4th edition. Garland Science.
5. Donis-Keller, H., Green, P., Helms, C., Cartinhour, S., Weiffenbach, B., Stephens, Keith TP, Bowden DW, Smith DR, Lander ES, Botstein D. (1987). A genetic linkage map of the human genome. Cell, 51(2), 319-337.
6. Mardis, E. R. (2008). The impact of next-generation sequencing technology on genetics. Trends in genetics, 24(3), 133-141.
7. Barchi, L., Lanteri, S., Portis, E., Acquadro, A., Valè, G., Toppino, L., and Rotino, G. L. (2011). Identification of SNP and SSR markers in eggplant using RAD tag sequencing. BMC genomics, 12(1), 1-9.
8. Pevsner, J. (2015). Bioinformatics and functional genomics. John Wiley and Sons.
9. Baxevanis, A. (2005). Current Topics in Genome Analysis Spring 2005 Week 4 Biological Sequence Analysis I. Current Topics in Genome Analysis.
10. Thomas, A. (2013). Thrive in genetics. Oxford University Press.
11. Amaya, M., Baer, A., Voss, K., Campbell, C., Mueller, C., Bailey, C., Kehn Hall, K., Petricoin III, E. and Narayanan, A. (2014). Proteomic strategies for the discovery of novel diagnostic and therapeutic targets for infectious diseases. Pathogens and disease, 71(2), 177-189.
12. Beretov, J., Wasinger, V. C., Graham, P. H., Millar, E. K., Kearsley, J. H., and Li, Y. (2014). Proteomics for breast cancer urine biomarkers. Advances in clinical chemistry, 63, 123-167.

13. Beretov, J., Wasinger, V. C., Graham, P. H., Millar, E. K., Kearsley, J. H., and Li, Y. (2014). Proteomics for breast cancer urine biomarkers. Advances in clinical chemistry, 63, 123-167.

14. Kikuchi, S., Bédard, J., and Nakai, M. (2011). One-and two-dimensional blue native-PAGE and immunodetection of low-abundance chloroplast membrane protein complexes. In Chloroplast Research in Arabidopsis (pp. 3-17). Humana Press, Totowa, NJ.

15. Liu, Y., Liao, J., and Lu, Q. (2015). Laboratory Methods in Epigenetics. In Epigenetics and Dermatology (pp. 7-35). Academic Press.

16. Fakruddin, M., Chowdhury, A. B. H. I. J. I. T., Hossain, M. N., Mannan, K. S., and Mazumda, R. M. (2012). Pyrosequencing-principles and applications. Int J Life Sci Pharma Res, 2(1), L-65.

17. Mardis, E., McPherson, J., Martienssen, R., Wilson, R. K., and McCombie, W. R. (2002). What is finished, and why does it matter. Genome research, 12(5), 669-671.

18. Bharagava, R. N., Purchase, D., Saxena, G., and Mulla, S. I. (2019). Applications of metagenomics in microbial bioremediation of pollutants: from genomics to environmental cleanup. In Microbial diversity in the genomic era (pp. 459-477). Academic Press.

Chapter 13

Biostatisics

Amresh Prakash

Amity Institute of Integrative Sciences and Health,
Amity University Haryana, Gurugram (Manesar) – 122 413, Haryana, India
e-mail: aprakash@ggn.amity.edu

ABSTRACT

Statistics is a branch of applied mathematics which deals with the collection, classification, analysis, and interpretation of data. The course aims to develop competency and expertise in the application of statistical methods applied to biological data obtained in experimental techniques. This includes designing of the biological experiments, data collection and analysis followed by results interpretation.

Keywords: *Mean, Median, Mode, Probability, Correlation, Regression, Normal distribution, Poisson distribution, ANOVA.*

Preliminary Concepts and Measures of Central Tendency

Introduction to Statistics and Application in Biology (Biostatistics)

Statistics

A branch of applied mathematics which deals with the collection, classification, analysis, and interpretation of data.

Application

(i) to understand the nature of variability

(ii) helps in deriving general laws from small samples.

(iii) designing the experiments and,
(iv) validation of experiments

Statistics broadly can be classified into two categories.

1. Pure Statistics
2. Applied Statistics

Pure Statistics

(a) Descriptive statistics
(b) Analytical statistics
(c) Inductive statistics
(d) Inferential statistics

(a) Descriptive Statistics

It describe and summarize the main feature of the data *e.g.*, measure of central tendency (Mean, Median, mode); measure of dispersion, range, standard deviation, mean deviation. It explains the characteristics of the data and reduce the complexities of the data into simple and logical summaries.

- ☆ Displaying data.
- ☆ Frequency distribution tables.
- ☆ Graphs or pictorial presentation of data.
- ☆ Tables.

(b) Analytical Statistics

To compare the different variables (Boys, Girls). It helps to establish the functional relationship between variables (data). *e.g.*, Correlation (relationship), Regression (dependencies).

(c) Inductive Statistics

Inductive statistics (or inductive reasoning) is a branch of statistics that deals with taking samples from a larger population and using that data to: draw conclusions, make decisions, forecast and, predict future behavior. To generate conclusions on the basis of random observations. Involves logic or reasoning: Computational-Intelligence.

(d) Inferential Statistics

Inferential statistical techniques are used to test the hypotheses and on that basis, it is decided whether the hypotheses are accepted or rejected. Description of data through mere descriptive analysis does not provide conclusive results. It only helps to describe the properties of a specific sample under study. Thus, in order to obtain conclusive results, hypotheses formulated is tested in the research. These hypotheses are tested statistically with the help of statistical techniques. It is used for the **Complex analysis and Quality Control**.

The nature and purpose of statistical inference:

(i) The process of testing hypothesis
- ☆ False-positive and false-negative errors.
- ☆ The null hypothesis and alternative hypothesis
- ☆ The alpha level and p value
- ☆ Variation in individual observations and in multiple samples.

(ii) Tests of statistical significance

(iii) Choosing an appropriate statistical test.

(iv) Making inferences from continuous (parametric) data.

(v) Making inferences from ordinal data.

(vi) Making inferences from dichotomous and nominal (nonparametric) data.

Basic Concepts

Variables

Data is a set of values of qualitative or quantitative variables. A variable is a characteristic or condition that can change or take on different values. Most research begins with a general question about the relationship between two variables for a specific group of individuals. Examples: body weight, age, test, height, education level, income...

Let's assume x and y are two variables, so given "x" calculate the value of "y" which we have learnt from the school times. You have learnt variables a, b, c, ...etc. Thus, the Quantity or Characteristic which can vary from one individual to another.

*Data are the basic building blocks of statistics and refers to the individual values presented, measured, or observed.

Population vs Sample

Data can be derived from a total population or a sample.

A population is the universe of units or values being studied. It can consist of individuals, objects, events, observations, or any other grouping.

A sample is a selected part of a population.

The following are some of the common types of samples:

a) Simple random sample
b) Systematic selected sample
c) Stratified selected sample
d) Cluster selected sample
e) Nonrandomly selected, or convenience sample.

Ungrouped vs Grouped Data

1. Ungrouped data are presented or observed individually. An example of ungrouped data is the following list of weights (in pounds) for six men: 140, 150, 150, 150, 160, and 160.
2. Grouped data are presented in groups consisting of identical data by frequency. An example of grouped data is the following list of weights for the six men noted above: 140 lb (one man), 150 lb (three men), and 160 lb (two men).

Measures of Central Tendency

Whenever one wishes to evaluate the outcome of study, it is crucial that the attributes of the sample that could have influenced it be described.

Three statistics, the mode, median, and mean, provide a means of describing the "typical" individual within a sample. These statistics are frequently referred to as "measures of central tendency".

- ✰ Measures of central tendency are characteristics that describe the middle or most commonly occurring values in a series.
- ✰ They tell us the point about which items have a tendency to cluster. Such a measure is considered as the most representative figure for the entire mass of data.
- ✰ They are used as summary measures for the series. The series can consist of a sample of observations or a total population, and the vales can be grouped or ungrouped.
- ✰ Measure of central tendency is also known as statistical average.

1. Mode

The mode of a data set is that value that occurs with the greatest frequency. A series may have no mode (*i.e.,* no value occurs more than once) or it may have several modes (*i.e.,* several values equally occur at a higher frequency than the other values in the series).

Whenever there are two nonadjacent scores with the same frequency and they are the highest in the distribution, each score may be referred to as the **'mode'** and the distribution is **'bimodal'**. In **truly bimodal distribution**, the population contains two sub-groups, each of which has a different distribution that peaks at a different point.

More than one mode can also be produced artificially by what is known as digit preference, when observers tend to favor certain numbers over others. For example, persons who measure blood pressure values tend to favor even numbers, particularly those ending in 0 (*e.g.,* 120 mm Hg).

Calculation

The mode is calculated by determining which value or values occur most in a series.

Example

Consider the following data. Patients who had received routine periodontal scaling were given a common pain-relieving drug and were asked to record the minutes to 100 per cent pain relief. Note that "minutes to pain relief" is a continuous variable that is measured on the ratio scale. The patients recorded the following data:

Minutes to 100 per cent pain relief:

15, 14, 10, 18, 8, 10, 12, 16, 10, 8, 13

First, make an array, that is, arrange the values in ascending order:

8 8 10 10 10 12 13 14 15 16 18

By inspection, we already know two descriptive measures belonging to this data: N=11 and mode=10.

Application and Characteristics

1. The primary value of the mode lies in its ease of computation and in its convenience as a quick indicator of a central value in a distribution.
2. The mode is useful in practical epidemiological work, such as determining the peak of disease occurrence in the investigation of a disease.
3. The mode is the most difficult measure of central tendency to manipulate mathematically, that is, it is not amenable to algebraic treatment; no analytic concepts are based on the mode.
4. It is also the least reliable because with successive samplings from the same population the magnitude of the mode fluctuates significantly more than the median or mean.

It is possible, for example, that a change in just one score can substantially change the value of the modal score.

2. Median

The median is the middle of the quartiles (the values that divide the series into quarters) and the middle of the percentiles (the values that divide the series into defined percentages).

Calculation

a) In a series with an odd number of values, the values in the series are arranged from lowest to highest, and the value that divides the series in half is the median.

b) In a series with even number of values, the two values that divide the series in half are determined, and the arithmetic mean of these values is the median.

c) An alternative method for calculating the median is to determine the 50 per cent value on a cumulative frequency curve.

Example

In the above example of data series of minutes to 100 per cent pain relief,

8 8 10 10 10 12 13 14 15 16 18

determine which value cuts the array into equal portions. In this array, there are five data points below 12 and there are five data points above 12. Thus, the median is 12.

8 8 10 10 10 **12** 13 14 15 16 18

If the number of observations is even, unlike the preceding example, simply take the midpoint of the two values that would straddle the center of the data set.

Consider the following data set with N=10:

8 8 10 10 10 13 14 15 16 18

$$Median = \frac{10 + 13}{2} = 11.5$$

Applications and Characteristics

1. The median is not sensitive to one or more extreme values in a series; therefore, in a series with an extreme value, the median is a more representative measure of central tendency than the arithmetic mean.
2. It is not frequently used in sampling statistics. In terms of sampling fluctuation, the median is superior to the mode but less stable than the mean. For this reason, and because the median does not possess convenient algebraic properties, it is not used as often as the mean.
3. Median is a positional average and is used only in the context of qualitative phenomena, for example, in estimating intelligence, *etc.*, which are often encountered in sociological fields.
4. Median is not useful where items need to be assigned relative importance and weights.
5. The median is used in cumulative frequency graphs and in survival analysis.

3. Arithmetic Mean

The arithmetic mean, or simply, the mean, is the sum of all values in a series divided by the actual number of values in a series.

The symbol for the mean is a capital letter X with a bar above it: $\bar{X}$ or "X-bar".

Calculation

The arithmetic mean is determined as,

$$\bar{X} = \frac{\Sigma X}{N}$$

Using the minutes to pain relief, N = 11 and ΣX = 134.

Therefore, $\bar{X}$ = 134/11 = 12.2 min.

Properties of the Mean

1. The mean of a sample is an unbiased estimator of the mean of the population from which it came.
2. The mean is the mathematical expectation. As such, it is different from the mode, which is the value observed most often.
3. The sum of the squared deviations of the observations from the mean is **smaller** than the sum of the squared deviations from any other number.
4. The sum of the squared deviations from the mean is **fixed** for a given set of observations. This property is not unique to the mean, but it is a necessary property of any good measure of central tendency.

Applications and Characteristics

1. The arithmetic mean is useful when performing **analytic manipulation**. With the exception of a situation where extreme scores occur in the distribution, the mean is generally the best measure of central tendency.
   - ☆ The values of mean tend to fluctuate least from sample to sample.
   - ☆ It is amenable to algebraic treatment and it possesses known mathematical relationships with other statistics.
   - ☆ Hence, it is used in further statistical calculations. Thus, in most situations the mean is more likely to be used than either the mode or the median.
2. The mean can be conceptualized as a **fulcrum** such that the distribution of scores around it is in perfect balance. Since the scores above and below the mean are in perfect balance, it follows that the algebraic sum of the observations of these scores from the mean is 0.
3. Whereas the median counts each score, no matter what its magnitude, as only one score, the mean takes into account the absolute magnitude of the score. The median, therefore, does not balance the halves of the distribution except when the distribution is exactly symmetrical; in which case the mean and the median have identical values.

Grouped Data: Mean, Median and Meode

(i) Data is Grouped on the Basis of Occurring Frequency

Calculate Mean, Median and Mode from the following grouped data

X	Frequency
0	1
1	5
2	10
3	6
4	3

x (1)	Frequency (f) (2)	$f \cdot x$ (3) = (2) × (1)	cf (5)
0	1	0	1
1	5	5	6
2	10	20	16
3	6	18	22
4	3	12	25
---	---	---	---
	$n = 25$	$\sum f \cdot x = 55$	--

Mean $\bar{x} = \dfrac{\sum fx}{n}$

$= \dfrac{55}{25}$

$= 2.2$

Median :

M = value of $\left(\dfrac{n}{2}\right)^{th}$ observation

= value of $\left(\dfrac{25}{2}\right)^{th}$ observation

= value of 12th observation

x (1)	Frequency (f) (2)	$f \cdot x$ (3) = (2) × (1)	cf (5)
0	1	0	1
1	5	5	6
2	10	20	16
3	6	18	22
4	3	12	25
---	---	---	---
	$n = 25$	$\sum f \cdot x = 55$	--

From the column of cumulative frequency cf, we find that the 12th observation is 2.

Hence, the median of the data is 2.

Mode

In the given table we can see that the frequency of observation 2 is maximum *i.e.*, 10

Thus, define as the mode for the given data.

Therefore, Mode (Z)= 2

(ii) Grouped Data on the Basis of Class Frequency

Examples

Class	*Frequency*
2-4	3
4-6	4
6-8	2
8-10	1

Solution

Class(1)	Frequency (f) (2)	Mid value(x) (3)	f.x(4)=(2)x(3)	Cf(6)
2-4	3	3	9	3
4=6	4	5	20	7
6-8	2	7	14	9
8-10	1	9	9	10
———	———	———	———	———
———	n=10	———	$\sum fX = 52$	———

We have $\sum f * x = 52$; and value of n= 10

$$Mean = \frac{\sum fx}{n}$$

$$= \frac{52}{10} = 5.2$$

To find Median Class

= value of $\left(\frac{n}{2}\right)$ *th obdervation*

= value of $\left(\frac{n}{2}\right)$ *th observation*

= value of 5th observation

From the column of cumulative frequency cf, we find that the 5th observation lies in the class 4 - 6.

∴ The median class is 4 - 6.

Now,

∴ L = lower boundary point of median class = 4

∴ n = Total frequency = 10

∴ cf = Cumulative frequency of the class preceding the median class = 3

∴ f = Frequency of the median class = 4

∴ c = class length of median class = 2

Median $M = L + \frac{\frac{n}{2} - cf}{f} \cdot c$

$= 4 + \frac{5 - 3}{4} \cdot 2$

$= 4 + \frac{2}{4} \cdot 2$

$= 4 + 1$

$= 5$

Solution:

Class (1)	Frequency (f) (2)	Mid value (x) (3)	$f \cdot x$ (4) = (2) × (3)	cf (6)
2-4	3	3	9	3
4-6	4	5	20	7
6-8	2	7	14	9
8-10	1	9	9	10
---	---	---	---	---
--	$n = 10$	--	$\sum f \cdot x = 52$	--

To find the Mode Class

Here, maximum frequency is 4.

Therefore, the mode class is 4-6. And,

L = lower boundary point of mode class = 4

f_1 = frequency of the mode class= 4

f_0 = frequency of the preceding class= 4

f_2 = frequency of the succeeding class= 4

c – class length of mode class = 2

$$Z = L + \left(\frac{f_1 - f_0}{2 \cdot f_1 - f_0 - f_2}\right) \cdot c$$

$$= 4 + \left(\frac{4 - 3}{2 \cdot 4 - 3 - 2}\right) \cdot 2$$

$$= 4 + \left(\frac{1}{3}\right) \cdot 2$$

$$= 4 + 0.6667$$

$$= 4.6667$$

Solution:

Class (1)	Frequency (f) (2)	Mid value (x) (3)	$f \cdot x$ (4) = (2) × (3)	cf (6)
2-4	3	3	9	3
4-6	4	5	20	7
6-8	2	7	14	9
8-10	1	9	9	10
---	---	---	---	---
--	$n = 10$	--	$\sum f \cdot x = 52$	--

Quartiles are values that divide your data into quarters.

Find the interquartile range of data set : 4, 4, 10, 11, 15, 7, 14, 12, 6

Arrange the data : 4, 4, 6, 7, 10, 11, 12, 14, 15

Arrange the data : 4, 4, 6, 7, **10**, 11, 12, 14, 15

Arrange the data : 4, 4, 6, 7, **10**, 11, 12, 14, 15

Arrange the data : 4, 4, 6, 7, **10**, 11, 12, 14, 15

Mean for 1st half: (4 + 6)/2 = 5
Mean for 2nd half: (12 +14)/2 =13

So, IQR = Mean for 2 nd Half – Mean for 1st half

IQR = 13 -5 = 8

Example: Based on the grouped data below, find the median:

Time to travel to work	Frequency
1 – 10	8
11 – 20	14
21 – 30	12
31 – 40	9
41 – 50	7

Solution:

Class (1)	Frequency (f) (2)	Mid value (x) (3)	$f \cdot x$ (4) = (2) × (3)	cf (6)
2-4	3	3	9	3
4-6	4	5	20	7
6-8	2	7	14	9
8-10	1	9	9	10
---	---	---	---	---
--	$n = 10$	--	$\sum f \cdot x = 52$	--

Median $M = L + \dfrac{\frac{n}{2} - cf}{f} \cdot c$

$= 4 + \dfrac{5 - 3}{4} \cdot 2$

$= 4 + \dfrac{2}{4} \cdot 2$

$= 4 + 1$

$= 5$

1st Step: Construct the cumulative frequency distribution

Time to travel to work	Frequency	Cumulative Frequency
1 – 10	8	8
11 – 20	14	22
21 – 30	12	34
31 – 40	9	43
41 – 50	7	50

$$\frac{n}{2} = \frac{50}{2} = 25 \longrightarrow \text{ class median is the 3}^{\text{rd}} \text{ class}$$

$$\text{So,} \quad F = 22, \quad f_m = 12, \quad L_m = 20.5 \text{ and } i = 10$$

Therefore,

$$\text{Median} = L_m + \left(\frac{\frac{n}{2} - F}{f_m} \right) i$$

$$= 21.5 + \left(\frac{25 - 22}{12} \right) 10$$

$$= 24$$

Thus, 25 persons take less than 24 minutes to travel to work and another 25 persons take more than 24 minutes to travel to work.

Percentiles can also be used to split your dataset into portions to measure dispersion and identify the average of the values (known as the central tendency). Certain meaningful percentiles are referred to by their own terms. Here are some:

- **Median:** The 50th percentile, in which half the values of a data set are above the 50th percentile, and half are below.
- **Quartile:** Values that split the data set into quarters based on percentiles. The first quartile is referred to as Q1, or the lower quartile. This value is the 25th percentile, in which the lower quarter of the values fall below the 25th percentile while three quarters are above it.
- The second quartile, or Q2, is the value at the 50th percentile. This is the median of the data set.

- Q3, the third quartile, is referred to as the 'upper quartile' and is the value of the 75th percentile, meaning only 25 per cent of values in the set are above this value.
- **Interquartile range:** Used to measure the dispersion of values, this is meant to show the middle half of the data. One quarter of the data values sit above this number, and one quarter falls below. The IQR is calculated by finding the difference between the first quartile and the third quartile (Q3 – Q1). The larger the IQR, the more spread out the values.

Quartiles	Deciles
$Q_1 = P_{25}$	$D_1 = P_{10}$
$Q_2 = P_{50}$	$D_2 = P_{20}$
$Q_3 = P_{75}$	$D_3 = P_{30}$
	•
	•
	•
	$D_9 = P_{90}$

Interquartile Range: $Q_3 - Q_1$

Semi-interquartile Range: $\frac{Q_3 - Q_1}{2}$

Midquartile: $\frac{Q_1 + Q_3}{2}$

10–90 Percentile Range: $P_{90} - P_{10}$

Example:

find the quartiles Q1, Q2, and Q3 of the following data 20, 30, 25, 23, 22, 32, 36

Solution:

Arrange data in ascending form, and n = 7 odd number

Ascending arrangement
20
22
23
25
30
32
36

q1 = (1/4) x n
= (1/4) x 7 = 1.75

q1 = 2
Q1 = 22

q2 = (2/4) x n
= (2/4) x 7 = 3.5

q2 = 4
Q2 = 25

q3 = (3/4) x n
= (3/4) x 7 = 5.25

q3 = 6
Q3 = 32

Example:

find the quartiles Q1, Q2, and Q3 of the following data 20, 30, 25, 23, 22, 32, 36, 18

Solution:

Arrange data in ascending form, and n = 8 even number

Ascending arrangement
18
20
22
23
25
30
32
36

q1 = (1/4) x n
= (1/4) x 8 = 2

q1 = mean of (2), and (3)

Q1 = (20+22)x(1/2) = 21

q2 = (2/4) x n
= (2/4) x 8 = 4

q2 = mean of (4), and (5)

Q2 = (23+25)x(1/2) = 24

q3 = (3/4) x n
= (3/4) x 8 = 6

q3 = mean of (6), and (7)

Q3 = (30+32)x(1/2) = 31

Example:

find the desiles D1, D5, and D8 of the following data 20, 30, 25, 23, 22, 32, 36

Solution:

Arrange data in ascending form, and n = 7 odd number

Ascending arrangement
20
22
23
25
30
32
36

d1 = (1/10) x n
= (1/10) x 7 = 0.7

d1 = 1

D1 = 20

d5 = (5/10) x n
= (5/10) x 7 = 3.5

d5 = 4

D5 = 25

d8 = (8/10) x n
= (8/10) x 7 = 5.6

d8 = 6

D8 = 32

Example:

find the desiles D1, D5, and D8 of the following data 20, 30, 25, 23, 22, 32, 36, 18

Solution:

Arrange data in ascending form, and n = 8 even number

Ascending arrangement

18
20
22
23
25
30
32
36

d1 = (1/10) x n
= (1/10) x 8 = 0.8

d1 = 1

D1 = 18

d5 = (5/10) x n
= (5/10) x 8 = 4

d5 = mean of (4), and (5)

D5 = (23+25)x(1/2) = 24

d8 = (8/10) x n
= (8/10) x 8 = 6.4

d8 = 7

D8 = 32

Example:

find the percentiles P8, P50, and P85 of the following data 20, 30, 25, 23, 22, 32, 36

Solution:

Arrange data in ascending form, and n = 7 odd number

Ascending arrangement

20
22
23
25
30
32
36

p8 = (8/100) x n
= (8/100) x 7 = 0.56

p8 = 1

P8 = 20

p50 = (50/100) x n
= (50/100) x 7 = 3.5

p50 = 4

P50 = 25

p85 = (85/100) x n
= (85/100) x 7 = 5.95

p85 = 6

P85 = 32

Example:

find the percentiles P8, P50, and P85 of the following data 20, 30, 25, 23, 22, 32, 36, 18

Solution:

Arrange data in ascending form, and n = 8 even number

Ascending arrangement
18
20
22
23
25
30
32
36

p8 = (8/100) x n
= (8/100) x 8 = 0.64

p8 = 1
P8 = 18

p50 = (50/100) x n
= (50/100) x 8 = 4

p50 = mean of (4), and (5)
P50 = (23+25)x(1/2) = 24

p85 = (85/100) x n
= (85/100) x 8 = 6.8

p85 = 7
P85 = 32

Using the same method of calculation as in the Median, we can get Q_1 and Q_3 equation as follows:

$$Q_1 = L_{Q_1} + \left(\frac{\frac{n}{4} - F}{f_{Q_1}} \right) i \qquad Q_3 = L_{Q_3} + \left(\frac{\frac{3n}{4} - F}{f_{Q_3}} \right) i$$

Quartiles

Using the same method of calculation as in the Median, we can get Q_1 and Q_3 equation as follows:

$$Q_1 = L_{Q_1} + \left(\frac{\frac{n}{4} - F}{f_{Q_1}} \right) i \qquad Q_3 = L_{Q_3} + \left(\frac{\frac{3n}{4} - F}{f_{Q_3}} \right) i$$

Example: Based on the grouped data below, find the Interquartile Range

Time to travel to work	Frequency
1 – 10	8
11 – 20	14
21 – 30	12
31 – 40	9
41 – 50	7

***1st Step:** Construct the cumulative frequency distribution*

Time to travel to work	*Frequency*	*Cumulative Frequency*
1 – 10	*8*	*8*
11 – 20	*14*	*22*
21 – 30	*12*	*34*
31 – 40	*9*	*43*
41 – 50	*7*	*50*

2nd Step: Determine the Q_1 and Q_3

$$\text{Class } Q_1 = \frac{n}{4} = \frac{50}{4} = 12.5$$

Class Q_1 is the 2nd class

Therefore,

$$Q_1 = L_{Q_1} + \left(\frac{\frac{n}{4} - F}{f_{Q_1}}\right) i$$

$$= 10.5 + \left(\frac{12.5 - 8}{14}\right) 10$$

$$= 13.7143$$

$$\text{Class } Q_3 = \frac{3n}{4} = \frac{3(50)}{4} = 37.5$$

$$Q_3 = L_{Q_3} + \left(\frac{\frac{n}{4} - F}{f_{Q_3}}\right) i$$

Class Q_3 is the 4th class

Therefore,

$$= 30.5 + \left(\frac{37.5 - 34}{9}\right) 10$$

$$= 34.3889$$

Interquartile Range

$$IQR = Q_3 - Q_1$$

$IQR = Q_3 - Q_1$

calculate the IQ

$IQR = Q_3 - Q_1 = 34.3889 - 13.7143 = 20.6746$

Summary

Measure of **central tendency** is a value that represents a typical, or central, entry of a data set. The most common measures of central tendency are:

- **Mean (Average):** The sum of all the data entries divided by the number of entries.

  Population Mean: $\mu = \frac{\Sigma x}{N}$ Sample Mean: $\bar{x} = \frac{\Sigma x}{n}$

- **Median:** The value that lies in the **middle** of the data when the data set is **ordered.** If the data set has an odd number of entries, then the median is the middle data entry. If the data has an even number of entries, then the median is obtained by adding the two numbers in the middle and dividing result by two.
- **Mode**: The data entry that occurs with the **greatest frequency**. A data set may have one mode, more than one mode, or no mode. If no entry is repeated the data set has no mode.
- **Outliers** are not just greatest and least values, but values that are very different from the pattern established by the rest of the data. Outliers affect the mean. When outliers are present it is best to use the median as the measure of central tendency.

Measures of Dispersion

Measures of central tendency provide useful information about the typical performance for a group of data. To understand the data more completely, it is necessary to know how the members of the data set arrange themselves about the central or typical value.

The following questions must be answered:

1. How spread out are the data points?
2. How stable are the values in the group?

The descriptive tools known as measures of dispersion answer these questions by quantifying the variability of the values within a group. Hence, they are the characteristics that are used to describe the spread, variation, and scatter of a series of values. The series can consist of observations or a total population, and the values can be grouped or ungrouped.

Range

The range is the difference between the highest and lowest values in a series.

Range = Maximum – Minimum.

More usual, however, is the interpretation of the range as simply the statement of the minimum and maximum values:

Range = (Minimum, Maximum)

For the sample of minutes to 100 per cent pain relief,

8 8 10 10 10 12 13 14 15 16 58

Range = (8, 18) or Range = 18-8 = 10 min

Application and Characteristics

1. The range is used to measure data spread.
2. The range presents the exact lower and upper boundaries of a set of data points and thus quickly lends perspective regarding the variable's distribution.
3. The range is usually reported along with the sample median (not the mean).
4. The range provides no information concerning the scatter within the series.

5. The range can be deemed unstable because it is affected by one extremely high score or one extremely low value. Also, only two values are considered, and these happen to be the extreme scores of the distribution. The measure of spread known as standard deviation addresses this disadvantage of the range.

**Mean deviation, variance, and standard deviation are three measures of dispersion based on the mean.

Although mean deviation is seldom used, a discussion of it provides a better understanding of the concept of dispersion.

Mean Deviation about their median M is given by

$$\text{M.D (M)} = \frac{|x_i - \text{M}|}{n}$$

$$\overline{x} = \frac{\Sigma x}{n} = \frac{5+10+15+20}{4} = \frac{50}{4} = 12.5$$

Data	$x - \overline{x}$	$(x - \overline{x})^2$
5	**5 – (12.5) = –7.5**	$(-7.5)^2 = 56.25$
10	**10 – (12.5) = –2.5**	$(-2.5)^2 = 6.25$
15	**15 – (12.5) = 2.5**	$(2.5)^2 = 6.25$
20	**20 – (12.5) = 7.5**	$(7.5)^2 = 56.25$
		$\Sigma(x - \overline{x})^2 = 125.01$

(ii) Mean deviation for discrete frequency distribution

Let the given data consist of discrete observations $x_1, x_2, \ldots, x_n$ occurring with frequencies $f_1, f_2, \ldots, f_n$, respectively. In this case

$$\text{M.D } (\overline{x}) = \frac{f_i\,|x_i - \overline{x}|}{f_i} = \frac{f_i\,|x_i - \overline{x}|}{\text{N}}$$

$$\text{M.D (M)} = \frac{f_i\,|x_i - \text{M}|}{\text{N}}$$

And, we know here "N" is $f_{i.}$

Variance: Let x1, x2, ……, xn be n observations with $\overline{X}$ as the mean. The variance, denoted by σ^2, is given by

$$\sigma^2 = \frac{1}{n} (x_i - \bar{x})^2$$

Standard Deviation: If σ^2 is the variance, then σ, is called the standard deviation is given by

$$\sigma = \sqrt{\frac{1}{n} (x_i - \bar{x})^2}$$

Standard deviation for a discrete frequency distribution is given by,

$$\sigma = \sqrt{\frac{1}{n} f_i (x_i - \bar{x})^2}$$

Standard deviation of a continuous frequency distribution (grouped data) is given by,

$$\sigma = \sqrt{\frac{1}{N} \quad f_i (x_i - \bar{x})^2}$$

Coefficient of Variation

Coefficient of variation (relative standard deviation: RSD): It is sometimes useful to **describe variability** by expressing the **standard deviation** as a proportion of **mean**, usually expressed in a percentage term. It is defined as,

$$Coefficient\ of\ variation\ (CV) = \frac{Standard\ deviation}{Mean} \times 100$$

Significance: Useful for comparing distribution in respect of their variability, homogeneity, uniformity or consistency.

Standard Deviation

$$\text{Standard Deviation} = \sigma = \sqrt{\frac{\Sigma(x-\mu)^2}{N}}$$

$$SD = \sigma = \sqrt{\frac{\Sigma X^2}{N} - \left(\frac{\Sigma X}{N}\right)^2}$$

$$SD = \sigma = \sqrt{\frac{\Sigma fd^2}{N} - \left(\frac{\Sigma fd}{N}\right)^2}$$

Comparison

$$\text{Variance } (\sigma^2) = \frac{(x_i - \overline{x})^2}{n}$$

$$CV\ of\ X = \frac{Standard\ deviation\ (\sigma_X)}{Mean\ of\ X\ (\overline{X})} \times 100$$

$$CV\ of\ Y = \frac{Standard\ deviation\ (\sigma_Y)}{Mean\ of\ Y\ (\overline{Y})} \times 100$$

$\overline{X} = 45; \overline{Y} = 60$

$\sigma_X = 9.0\ \sigma_Y = 18$

Question: Life of bulbs produced by two factories A and B are given below:

Length of life (in hours)	Factory A (Number of bulbs)	Factory B (Number of bulbs)
550 - 650	10	8
650 - 750	22	60
750 - 850	52	24
850 - 950	20	16
950 - 1050	16	12
	120	120

Calculate that the bulbs of which factory are more consistent from the point of view of length of life?

Length of Life (hrs)	*Mid Value (xi)*
550-650	600
650-750	700
750-850	800
850-950	900
950-1050	1000

Length of Life (hrs)	*Mid Value (xi)*	
550-650	600	-2
650-750	700	-1
750-850	800	0
850-950	900	1
950-1050	1000	2

Length of Life (hrs)	*Mid Value (xi)*		*Factory A*	*Factory B*
550-650	600	-2	10 -20 40	
650-750	700	-1	22 -22 22	
750-850	800	0	52 0 0	
850-950	900	1	20 20 20	
950-1050	1000	2	16 32 64	

For Factory A

$$\text{Mean } (\bar{x}) = 800 + \frac{10}{120} \times 100 = 816.67 \text{ hours}$$

$$= A + \frac{f_i y_i}{f_i} \times 100$$

$$\text{S.D.} = \frac{100}{120}\sqrt{120\,(146) - 100} = 109.98$$

Therefore, Coefficient of variation (C.V.) = $\frac{\text{S.D.}}{\bar{x}} \times 100 = \frac{109.98}{816.67} \times 100 = 13.47$

Question: Following are the marks obtained, out of 100, by two students Ravi and Babita in 10 tests.

Ravi	25	50	45	30	70	42	36	48	35	60
Babita	10	70	50	20	95	55	42	60	48	80

Who is more intelligent and who is more consistent

Combined Mean and Standard Deviation

$$\textit{Combined Mean}, \bar{X}_{AB} = \frac{N_A\bar{X}_A + N_B\bar{X}_B}{N_A + N_B}$$

Here, $\bar{X}_{AB}$ is the new mean which is the combined mean of A and B. Now to calculate the variance *i.e.*, how random variable ($\bar{X}_A$ and $\bar{X}_B$) from the mean value ($\bar{X}_{AB}$). Therefore,

$d_A = \bar{X}_A - \bar{X}_{AB}$

$d_B = \bar{X}_B - \bar{X}_{AB}$

$$Standard\ deviation\ (\sigma_{AB}) = \sqrt{\frac{N_A\left((\sigma_A^2) + (d_A^2)\right) + N_B\left((\sigma_B^2) + (d_B^2)\right)}{N_A + N_B}}$$

1. The average wages of 100 workers in a company A is Rs. 460 per day and, the average wages of 80 workers in a company B is Rs. 489 per day. Calculate which factory shows greater variability in the distribution of wages. Calculate the combined mead and deviation. S.D., 50 and 40, respectively.
2. A sample of 150 vales has mean 40 and standard deviation (S.D.) is 26. A second sample of 100 values from the same population has mean 55 and S.D. is 35. Find the mean and standard deviation of the combined sample.

Correlation is a statistical method that determines the degree of relationship between two different variables. It is also known as a "bivariate" statistic, with bi- meaning two and variate indicating variable or variance. The two variables are usually a pair of scores for a person or object. The relationship between any two variables are can vary from strong to weak or none. When a relationship is strong, this means that knowing a person's or object's score on one variable helps to predict their score on the second variable. In other words, if a person has a high score of variable A (compared to all the other peoples' scores on A, then they are likely to have a high score on variable B (compared to the other peoples' scores on B). The latter would be considered a strong positive correlation. If the correlation or relationship between variable A and B is a weak one, then knowing a person's score on variable A does not help to predict their score on variable B. One very nice feature of the correlation coefficient is that it can only range from –1.00 to +1.00.

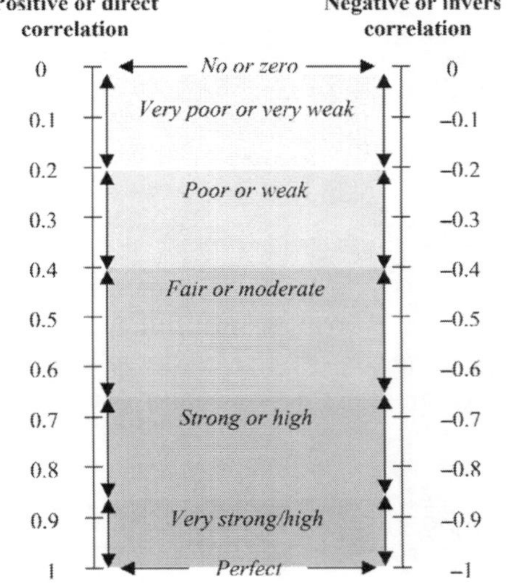

Correlation coefficient / Pearson's correlation coefficient: To express the strength of the relationship

This coefficient is generally used when variables are of quantitative nature, that is, ratio or interval scale variables.

Pearson's correlation coefficient is denoted by r and is defined by,

$$r = \frac{n\sum XY - \sum X \sum Y}{\sqrt{[n(\sum X^2) - (\sum X)^2\,][n(\sum Y^2) - (\sum Y)^2\,]}}$$

The value of r always lies between –1 and 1 inclusive, that is, $-1 \leq -r \leq +1$.

Example:

X	Y	X^2	Y^2	XY
15	10	225	100	150
12	25	144	625	300
8	17	64	289	136
8	11	64	121	88
7	13	49	169	91
7	17	49	289	119
7	20	49	400	140
6	13	36	169	78
5	9	25	81	45
3	15	9	225	45
78	150	714	2468	1192

For the bivariate/bivariable data X and Y, the correlation coefficient/Karl Pearson's Coefficient(r), we formula as given below (here, n is the number of variables which is 10)

$$r = \frac{n\sum XY - \sum X \sum Y}{\sqrt{[n(\sum X^2) - (\sum X)^2\,][n(\sum Y^2) - (\sum Y)^2\,]}}$$

$$= \frac{10 \times 1192 - 78 \times 150}{\sqrt{[10 \times 714 - (78)^2][10 \times 2468 - (150)^2]}} = \frac{220}{1517} = 0.145$$

To solve such questions, first make table as given above, this will also help you to remember formula.

Correlation and Regression

Correlation defines the relation (co-relation) between two variables, whereas, regression defines the dependency. Using regression, we can estimate the value of X for given Y (given value of Y other than the values given in above table), similarly, we can estimate Y for any given value of X. Simple regression/linear regression can represented using straight line equation ($y=a+bx$), where, a is intercept and b is slope. Since, Y and X is given in question. Thus, we have to calculate the value of **a** and **b**.

$$b = \frac{n\,(\sum XY) - (\sum X)(\sum Y)}{n(\sum X^2) - (\sum X)^2} = \frac{10 \times 1192 - 78 \times 150}{10 \times 714 - (78)^2} = \frac{220}{1056} = 0.20$$

$$\text{and, } a = \frac{\sum Y - b\,(\sum X)}{n} = \frac{150 - (0.20 \times 78)}{10} = \frac{134.4}{10} = 13.4$$

Thus, c, now we have values of $a = 13.4$ and $b = 0.20$

Therefore, regression equation Y = 13.4 + 0.20 X using this you can estimate the value of Y for the given value of X.

Question: The yield of a particular crop on a farm is thought to depend principally on the amount of rainfall in the growing season. The values of the yield Y, in tonnes per acre, and the rainfall X, in centimetres, for seven successive years are given in the table below.

Rainfall (cm)	12.3	13.7	14.5	11.2	13.2	14.1	12.0
Yield (tonnes per acre)	6.25	8.02	8.42	5.27	7.21	8.71	5.68

Calculate the linear correlation coefficient and interpret your result.

Introduction to Probability

People use the term probability many times each day. For example, physician says that a patient has a 50-50 chance of surviving a certain operation. Another physician may say that she is 95 per cent certain that a patient has a particular disease.

By Definition

If an event can occur in N mutually exclusive and equally likely ways, and if m of these possesses a trait, E, the probability of the occurrence of E is read as

$$P(E) = m/N$$

Experiment ==> any planned process of data collection. It consists of a number of trials (replications) under the same condition.

Sample space: collection of unique, non-overlapping possible outcomes of a random circumstance.

Simple event: one outcome in the sample space; a possible outcome of a random circumstance.

Event: a collection of one or more simple events in the sample space; often written as A, B, C, and so on....

Representation

= {*male, female; head, tail; success, failure*}

Complement ==> sometimes, we want to know the probability that an event will not happen; an event opposite to the event of interest is called a complementary event.

If A is an event, its complement is the probability of the complement is AC or A.

Example: The complement of male event is the female; head is for tail *etc.*

$$P(A) + P(\bar{A}) = 1$$

Experiments, Outcomes, Events and Sample Spaces

Events and Venn Diagrams

Example

No. of Times the Coin is Tossed	*No. of Times Head Comes Up*	*No. of Times Tail Comes Up*
10		

Fraction of outcomes as "head"

Fraction of outcomes as "tail"

Total no. of trails

$$\frac{\text{No. of outcomes as head (H)}}{\text{No. of outcomes as tail (T)}}$$

$$\frac{No.\ of\ times\ a\ head\ (H) comes\ up}{Total\ no.\ of\ times\ the\ coin\ is\ tossed\ (no.\ of\ trails)}$$

Heads on both coins = (H,H) = HH
Head on first coin and Tail on the other = (H,T) = HT
Tail on first coin and Head on the other = (T,H) = TH
Tail on both coins = (T,T) = TT
Thus, the sample space is S = {HH, HT, TH, TT}

Similarly, the no. of times a die is thrown.

No. of Times a Die is Thrown	No. of Times these Scores Turn Up					
	1	2	3	4	5	6
10/20/30						

$$\frac{No.\ of\ times\ 1\ turned\ up}{Total\ no.\ of\ times\ the\ die\ is\ thrown\ (no.\ of\ trails)}$$

$$\frac{No.\ of\ times\ 1\ (any\ no.\ 1-6) turned\ up}{Total\ no.\ of\ times\ the\ die\ is\ thrown\ (no.\ of\ trails)}$$

Let n be the total number of trials. The *empirical probability/experimental probability* P(E) of an event E happening, is given by,

$$P\ (E) = \frac{No.\ of\ trials\ in\ which\ the\ event\ event\ happened}{The\ total\ no.\ of\ trials}$$

So, in the previous class we have seen the probability (P) of outcomes as Head (H) and Tail (T), as ½ and ½.

$$P\ (H) + P\ (T) = \frac{1}{2} + \frac{1}{2} = 1$$

Therefore, in this case we can say that probability of H= ½, and prob. of T =½.

If the prob. of success is denoted by p and then the prob. of failure by q, then we can write that $p + q = 1$.

Therefore, $q = 1 - p$.

$$\sum_{i=0}^{n} p + (1 - p) = 1$$

And, the value p will be range between 0 and 1 ($0 \leq p \leq 1$).

Types of Events

1. Impossible and Sure Events

The empty set ϕ and the sample space S describe the event. Since, ϕ describe the impossible events, thus S = whole sample space, and is called the sure event.

Ex. Consider the experiment of rolling a die. The associated sample space (S) will be:

S = {1, 2, 3, 4, 5, 6}

So, any number > 6 will be define as, empty set corresponding to the event E. Thus, the event E= ϕ is an impossible event.

2. Simple Event

If an event E has only one sample point of a sample space, it is called a simple (or elementary) event. In a sample space containing n distinct elements, there are exactly n simple events. *Ex.* tossing two coins. The associated sample space (S) will be:

S={HH, HT, TH, TT}

So, There are four simple events corresponding to this sample space. These are E1= {HH}, E2={HT}, E3= { TH} and E4={TT}.

3. Compound Event

If an event has more than one sample point, it is called a Compound event. Ex., in the experiment of "tossing a coin thrice" the events

Compound events

E1: 'Exactly one head appeared' ={HTT,THT,TTH} E2: 'Atleast one head appeared' ={HTT,THT, TTH, HHT, HTH, THH, HHH} E3: 'Atmost one head appeared' = {TTT, THT, HTT, TTH}

Since, each of the above subsets contain more than one sample point, hence they are all compound events.

Complementary Event

For every event A, there corresponds another event A2 called the complementary event to A. It is also called the *event 'not* A' ($\bar{A}$). For example, take the experiment of tossing three coins. An associated sample space is

S = {HHH, HHT, HTH, THH, HTT, THT, TTH, TTT}

Ex.

If event A={HTH, HHT, THH} be the event 'only one tail appears'

Then in event A what is not occurred.......................wrt— S.

A' ($\bar{A}$) = {HHH, HTT, THT, TTH, TTT}

Then we can write $\bar{A} = S - A$

That means subsets of $\bar{A}$ belongs (∈) to = S, but not belongs (∉) to *A*.

Another event is union of two sets A and B denoted by A ∪ B: It contains all those elements which are either in A or in B or in both:

For example,

A = {(6,1), (6,2}, (6,3), (6,4), (6,5), (6,6)}, and B = {(5,6), (6,5), (6,6)}

A ∪ B:

But in case of the event 'A and B' *i.e.*, the intersection of two sets A ∩ B is the set of those elements which are common to both A and B. *i.e.*, which belong to both 'A and B'.

Here, A and B are two events, so the set A ∩ B denotes the event 'A and B'

Ex. A = {(6,1), (6,2}, (6,3), (6,4), (6,5), (6,6)}, and B = {(5,6), (6,5), (6,6)}

so A ∩ B = {(6,5), (6,6)}

We can see one another event that is 'A but not B' : We know that A–B is the set of all those elements which are in A but not in B. Therefore, the set A–B may denote the event 'A but not B'. And, it is denoted as A – B = A ∩ B´.

Ex. Consider the experiment of rolling a die. Let A be the event 'getting a prime number', B be the event 'getting an odd number'. Write the sets representing the events,

(i) A or B
(ii) A and B
(iii) A but not B
(iv) 'not A'.

Here we have S = {1, 2, 3, 4, 5, 6}, A = {2, 3, 5} and B = {1, 3, 5}

Therefore,

(i) A or B' = A ∪ B = {1, 2, 3, 5}
(ii) 'A and B' = A ∩ B = {3,5}
(iii) 'A but not B' = A – B = {2}
(iv) 'not A' = A2 = {1,4,6}

The sample space of the experiment is S = {HHH, HHT, HTH, THH, HTT, THT, TTH, TTT} and A = {TTT}, B = {HTT, THT, TTH}, C = {HHT, HTH, THH, HHH}

Question

Find out A ∪ B ∪ C

Answer

A ∪ B ∪ C = {TTT, HTT, THT, TTH, HHT, HTH, THH, HHH} = S

Another question

Find out A ∩ B = ?, A ∩ C = ? and B ∩ C = ?

Given, A = {TTT},

B = {HTT, THT, TTH},

C = {HHT, HTH, THH, HHH}

Probability and Venn Diagram

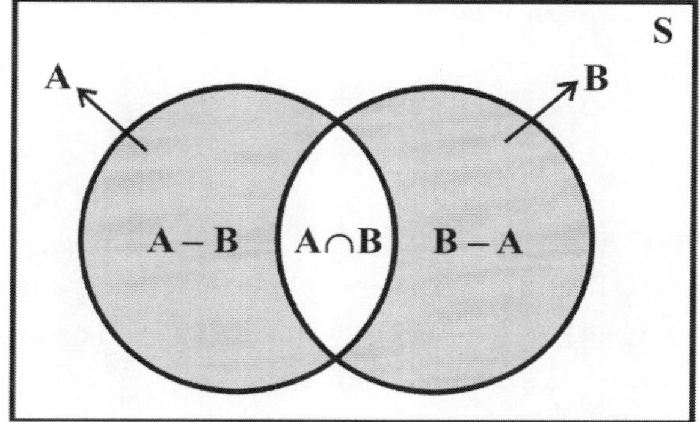

$$P(A \cup B) = P(A) + P(B) - P(A \cap B)$$

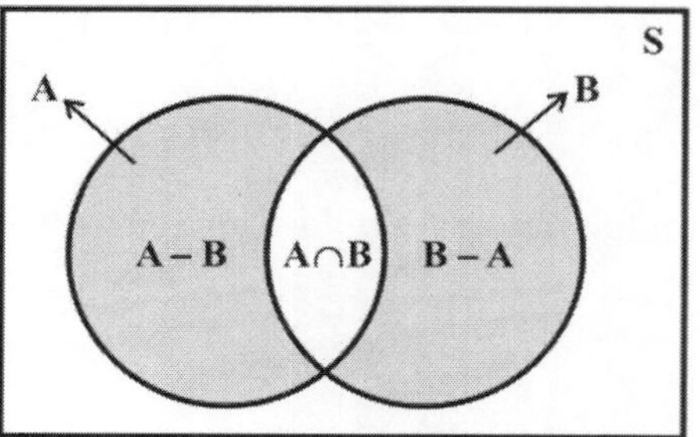

If A and B are disjoint sets, i.e., they are mutually exclusive events, then $A \cap B = \phi$

Therefore $P(A \cap B) = P(\phi) = 0$

Thus, for mutually exclusive events A and B, we have

$$P(A \cup B) = P(A) + P(B),$$

Probabilityof event 'not A' Consider the event A = {2, 4, 6, 8} associated with the experiment of drawing a card from a deck of ten cards numbered from 1 to 10. Clearly the sample space is S = {1, 2, 3, ...,10}

If all the outcomes 1, 2, ...,10 are considered to be equally likely, then the probability of each outcome is $\frac{1}{10}$.
Now if we are looking for P (A)

Then, $P(A) = P(2) + P(4) + P(6) + P(8) \quad = \frac{1}{10} + \frac{1}{10} + \frac{1}{10} + \frac{1}{10} = \frac{4}{10} = \frac{2}{5}$

And, if we are looking for event "not $\bar{A}$" or P(A')
= P(1) + P(3) + P(5) + P(7) + P(9) + P (10)

That is $\frac{6}{10} = \frac{3}{5}$ *which can be obtained as* $1 - \frac{2}{5} = 1 - P(A)$.

So, what we can conclude,
We can conclude that A' and A are mutually exclusive and exhaustive events *i.e.*,

$$A \cap A' = \phi \text{ and } A \cup A' = S$$

$$P(A \cup A') = P(S)$$
$$P(A) + P(A') = 1,$$

Permutation: An arrangement of objects in a specific sequence.
For Ex. A horse (H), cow (C), and sheep (S) could be arranged linearly in Six different ways: H, C, S; H, S, C; C, H, S; C,S,H; S,H,C; S,C,H.

$k_1 = 3, k_2 = 2, k_3 = 1$

which is, $(k_1)(k_2)(k_3)$= (3)(2)(1)= 6 ways to align

$${}_nP_n = n(n-1)(n-2)\ldots.(3)(2)(1)$$

$${}_nP_n = n!$$

Question

In how many sequences can six photographs be arranged on a page?

$${}_nP_n = n!$$

$= 6! = 720$

For circular arrangements...

$${}_nP'_n = \frac{n!}{n} = (n-1)!$$

Fewer than *n* Position:

The number of permutations of *n* objects taken X at a time: In how many different ways can a sequence of four slides be chosen from a collection of six slides?

$$_nP_X = \frac{n!}{(n-X)!} = \frac{6!}{(6-4)!} = 360$$

Combinations

$$_nC_X \text{ or } {}^nC_r = \frac{_nP_X}{X!} = \frac{n!}{X!(n-X)!}$$

Ex.: Of a total of ten animals (mice), eight are to be used in a lab. expt. How many different combinations of eight animals may be formed from ten?Of a total of ten animals (mice), eight are to be used in a lab. expt. How many different combinations of eight animals may be formed from ten?

$$_{10}C_8 = \frac{_nP_X}{X!} = \frac{10!}{8!(10-8)!} = 45$$

Ex: One card is drawn from a well shuffled deck of 52 cards. If each outcome is equally likely, calculate the probability that the card will be

(i) a diamond

(ii) not an ace

(iii)a black card (i.e., a club or, a spade)

(iv)not a diamond

(v) not a black card.

When a card is drawn from a well shuffled deck of 52 cards, the number of possible outcomes is 52.

(i) Let A be the event 'the card drawn is a diamond'

Clearly the number of elements in set A is 13.

$$Therefore, P(A) = \frac{13}{52} = \frac{1}{4}$$

(ii) We assume that the event 'Card drawn is an ace' is B

Therefore 'Card drawn is not an ace' should be B'.

$$We\ know\ that\ P\ (B') = 1 - P(B)$$

$$= 1 - \frac{4}{52} = 1 - \frac{1}{13} = \frac{12}{13}$$

(iii) Let C denote the event 'card drawn is black card', Therefore, number of elements in the set C = 26

$$1.e., P(C) = \frac{26}{52} = \frac{1}{2}$$

$$Thus, Prob. of\ a\ black\ card = \frac{1}{2}$$

(iv) We assumed in (i) above that A is the event 'card drawn is a diamond', so the event 'card drawn is not a diamond' may be denoted as A' or 'not A'

Now $P(\text{not } A) = 1 - P(A) = 1 - \frac{1}{4} = \frac{3}{4}$

(v) The event 'card drawn is not a black card' may be denoted as C′ or 'not C'

We know that $P(\text{not } C) = 1 - P(C) = 1 - \frac{1}{2} = \frac{1}{2}$

Therefore, Probability of not a black card $= \frac{1}{2}$

Two students Anil and Ashima appeared in an examination. The probability that Anil will qualify the examination is 0.05 and that Ashima will qualify the examination is 0.10. The probability that both will qualify the examination is 0.02. Find the probability that

(a) Both Anil and Ashima will not qualify the examination.
(b) Atleast one of them will not qualify the examination and
(c) Only one of them will qualify the examination.

Let E and F denote the events that Anil and Ashima will qualify the examination, respectively. Given that

$$P(E) = 0.05,\ P(F) = 0.10 \text{ and } P(E \cap F) = 0.02$$

$$P(E) = 0.05,\ P(F) = 0.10 \text{ and } P(E \cap F) = 0.02$$

(a) The event 'both Anil and Ashima will not qualify the examination' may be expressed as $E' \cap F'$.

Since, E' is 'not E', i.e., Anil will not qualify the examination and F' is 'not F', i.e., Ashima will not qualify the examination.

Also $\quad E' \cap F' = (E \cup F)'$ (by Demorgan's Law)

Now $\quad P(E \cup F) = P(E) + P(F) - P(E \cap F)$

or $\quad P(E \cup F) = 0.05 + 0.10 - 0.02 = 0.13$

Therefore $P(E' \cap F') = P(E \cup F)' = 1 - P(E \cup F) = 1 - 0.13 = 0.87$

(b) P (atleast one of them will not qualify)

= 1 – P(both of them will qualify)

= 1 – 0.02 = 0.98

(c) The event only one of them will qualify the examination is same as the event either (Anil will qualify, and Ashima will not qualify) or (Anil will not qualify and Ashima will qualify) i.e., $E \cap F'$ or $E' \cap F$, where $E \cap F'$ and $E' \cap F$ are mutually exclusive.

Therefore, P(only one of them will qualify) $= P(E \cap F' \text{ or } E' \cap F)$

$= P(E \cap F') + P(E' \cap F) = P(E) - P(E \cap F) + P(F) - P(E \cap F)$

$= 0.05 - 0.02 + 0.10 - 0.02 = 0.11$

Ex: A deck of playing cards is composed of 52 cards, with thirteen cards in each of four suits called club, diamonds, hearts, and spades. In each suit there is one Card each of following denominations: ace (A), 2, 3, 4, 5, 6, 7, 8, 9, 10, jack (J), Queen (q) and king (K).

(i) What is the probability of selecting at random a Diamonds from the deck of 52 cards?

(ii) What is the prob. Of selecting at random a king from the deck?

(iii) What is the prob. Of selecting at random a diamond or a king?

Conditional Probability

$$P(event A,\ given\ event\ B) = \frac{P\ (A\ and\ B\ jointly)}{P\ (B)}$$

$$P(event A,\ given\ event\ B) = \frac{frequency\ of\ events\ A\ and\ B\ jointly}{frequency\ of\ event\ B}$$

So, the prob. Of randomly selecting a queen, with the specification that the card is a diamond, is

P (queen, given it is diamond) = P (queen of diamond)/P (diamond)

$$P\ (\text{queen, given it is diamond}) = \frac{1/52}{13/52} = \frac{0.02}{0.25} = 0.08$$

$$P(event A,\ given\ event\ B) = \frac{frequency\ of\ events\ A\ and\ B\ jointly}{frequency\ of\ event\ B} = \frac{1}{13}$$

Question

Either allele A or a may occur at a particular genetic locus. An offspring receives one of its alleles from each of its parents. If one parent possesses alleles 'A' and 'a' and the other parent possesses 'a' and 'a':

(a) What is the probability of an offspring receiving an A and a?

(b) What is the probability of an offspring receiving two a alleles?

(c) What is the probability of an offspring receiving two A alleles?

Bayes Theorem

Let A and B be two events from a (countable) sample space Ω, and $P : \Omega \to [0, 1]$ a probability distribution on Ω, such that $0 < P(A) < 1$, and $P(B) > 0$. Then

$$P(A \mid B) = \frac{P(B \mid A)P(A)}{P(B \mid A)P(A) + P(B \mid \overline{A})P(\overline{A})}$$

Let A and B be events such that $0 < P(A) < 1$ and $P(B) > 0$.

By definition, $P(A \mid B) = \frac{P(A \cap B)}{P(B)}$. So: $P(A \cap B) = P(A \mid B)P(B)$

Likewise, $P(B \cap A) = P(B \mid A)P(A)$.

Likewise, $P(B \cap \overline{A}) = P(B \mid \overline{A})P(\overline{A})$. (Note that $P(\overline{A}) > 0$.)

Note that $P(A \mid B)P(B) = P(A \cap B) = P(B \mid A)P(A)$. So,

$$P(A \mid B) = \frac{P(B \mid A)P(A)}{P(B)}$$

Furthermore,

$$\begin{aligned} P(B) &= P((B \cap A) \cup (B \cap \overline{A})) = P(B \cap A) + P(B \cap \overline{A}) \\ &= P(B \mid A)P(A) + P(B \mid \overline{A})P(\overline{A}) \end{aligned}$$

So, $$P(A \mid B) = \frac{P(B \mid A)P(A)}{P(B \mid A)P(A) + P(B \mid \overline{A})P(\overline{A})}$$

Problem

Suppose it has been observed empirically that the word "Congratulations" occurs in 1 out of 10 spam emails, but that "Congratulations" only occurs in 1 out of 1000 non-spam emails. Suppose it has also been observed empirically that about 4 out of 10 emails are spam.

In Bayesian Spam Filtering, these empirical probabilities are interpreted as genuine probabilities in order to help estimate the probability that a incoming email is spam.

Suppose we get a new email that contains "Congratulations". Let **C** be the event that a new email contains "Congratulations". Let **S** be the event that a new email is spam

Bayesian solution: By Bayes' Theorem:

$$P(S \mid C) = \frac{P(C \mid S)P(S)}{P(C \mid S)P(S) + P(C \mid \overline{S})P(\overline{S})}$$

From the "empirical probabilities", we get the estimates:

$P(C \mid S) \approx 1/10; \quad P(C \mid \overline{S}) \approx 1/1000;$

$P(S) \approx 4/10; \quad P(\overline{S}) \approx 6/10.$

So, we estimate that:

$$P(S \mid C) \approx \frac{(1/10)(4/10)}{(1/10)(4/10) + (1/1000) * (6/10)}$$

$$\approx \frac{.04}{.0406} \approx 0.985$$

So, with "high probability", such an email is spam.

Normal Distribution

Properties of Normal Distributions

A **continuous random variable** has an infinite number of possible values that can be represented by an interval on the number line.

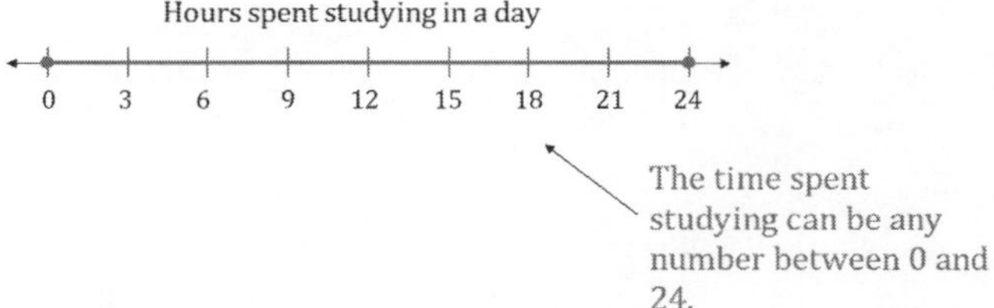

The probability distribution of a continuous random variable is called a **continuous probability distribution.**

Measure of Position z-score

Z Score (or standard score) the number of standard deviations a score is above or below the mean

$$z = \frac{X - \bar{X}}{\sigma} \qquad z = \frac{x - \mu}{\sigma}$$

Interpreting Z Scores

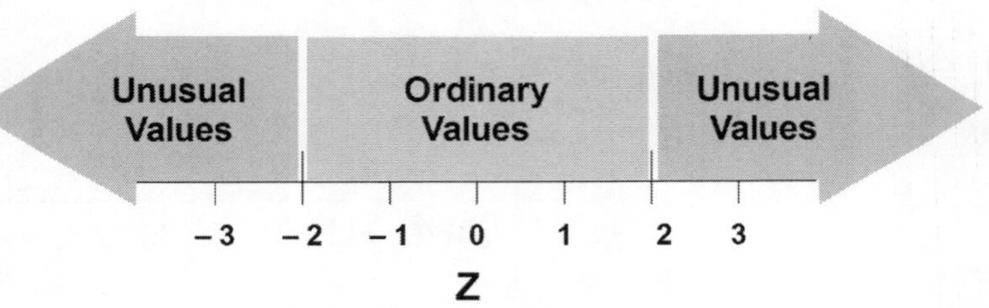

The most important probability distribution in statistics is the **normal distribution.**

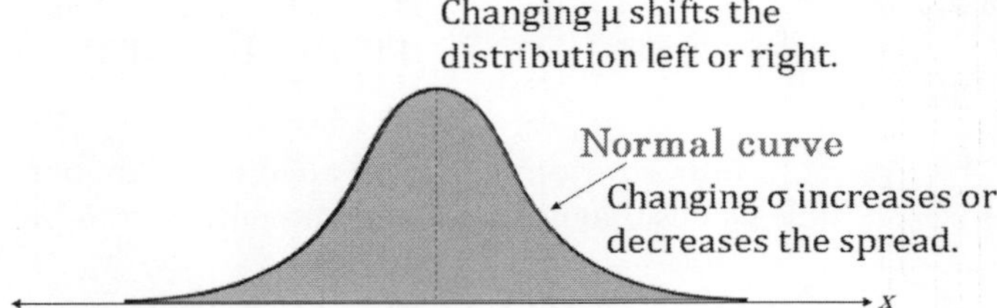

A normal distribution is a continuous probability distribution for a random variable, x. The graph of a normal distribution is called the **normalcurve.**

The Normal Distribution: as mathematical function (pdf)

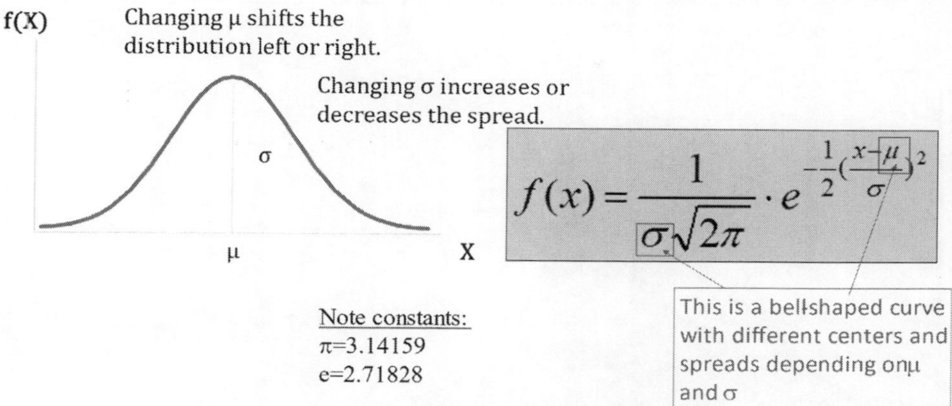

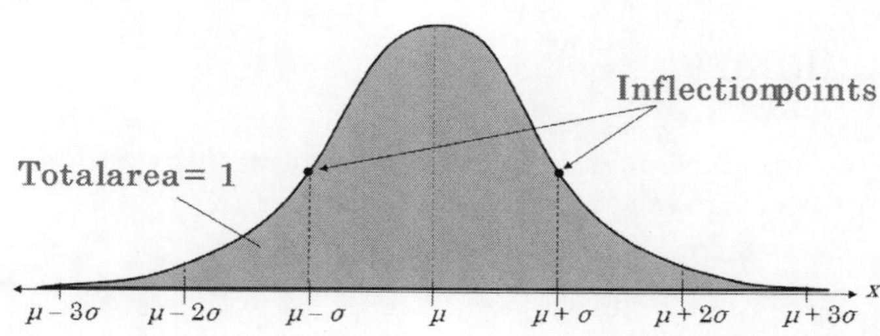

If x is a continuous random variable having a normal distribution with mean μ and standard deviation σ, you can graph a normal curve with the equation

It's a probability function, so no matter what the values of μ and σ, must integrate to 1!

$$\int_{-\infty}^{+\infty}\frac{1}{\sigma\sqrt{2\pi}}\cdot e^{-\frac{1}{2}(\frac{x-\mu}{\sigma})^2}\,dx=1$$

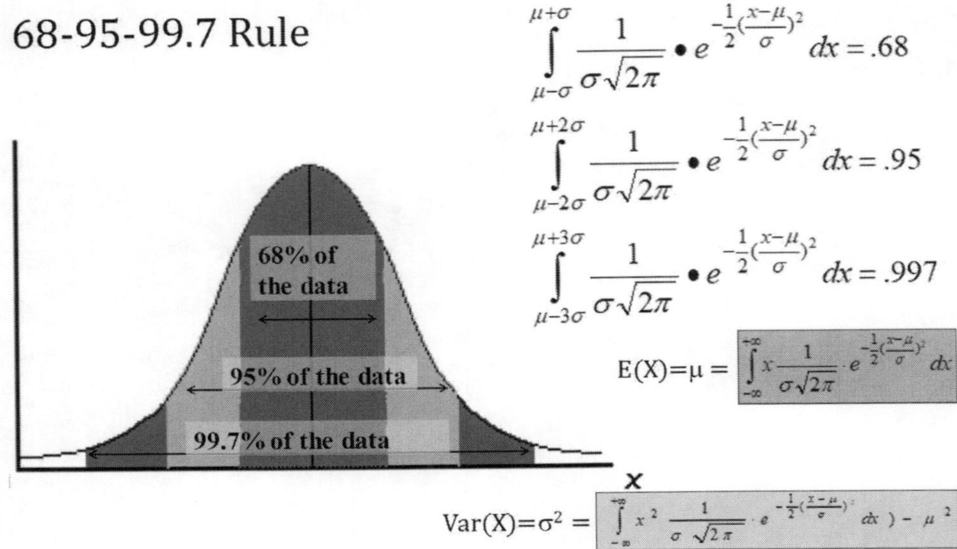

Summary:

The **standard normal distribution** is a normal distribution with a mean of 0 and a standard deviation of 1.

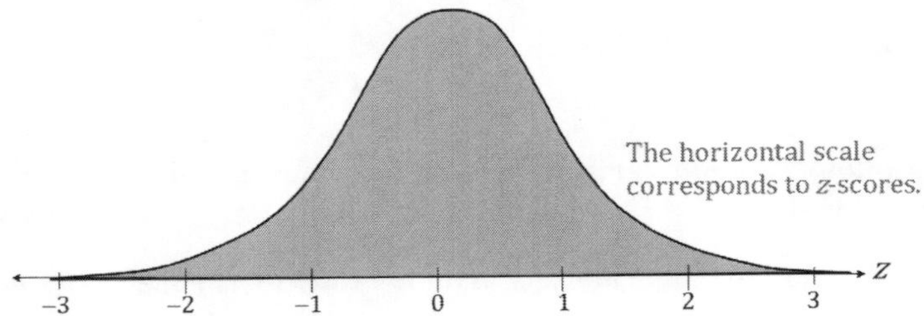

Any value can be transformed into a z-score by using the formula

$$z = \frac{\text{Value - Mean}}{\text{Standard deviation}} = \frac{x - \mu}{\sigma}.$$

Example

Calculating the proportions of a Normal Dist. of Bone Lengths, where, $\mu = 60$ mm and σ=10 mm.

Q 1.

What proportion of the population of bone length is larger than 66 mm?

We know for the normal dist.

$$Z = \frac{X_i - \mu}{\sigma}$$

From the given question, we have to calculate, P (X_i >66 mm).

Therefore, putting the values of mean (μ)= 60 mm and SD (σ) = 10 mm,

We have, $Z = \frac{X_i - \mu}{\sigma} = \frac{66\ mm - 60\ mm}{10 mm}$ = 0.60 #Z is the distribution

So, P (X_i >66 mm) = P (Z >0.60) = 0.2743 or 27 per cent #value will be provided in ques.

**This question can be asked as, what is the probability of picking, at random from this population, a bone larger than 66 mm?

Q2. If there are 2000 bone lengths in this population, how many of them are greater than 66 mm?

Sol. Population of bone lengths greater than 66 mm = (0.2743) (2000)= 549

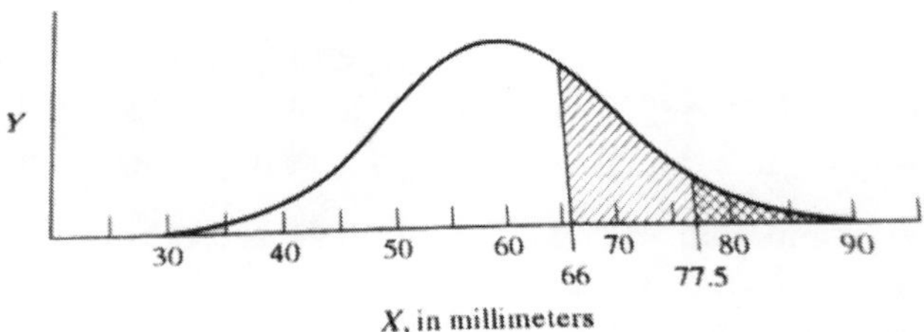

Q3. What is the population is smaller than 66 mm?

Sol.: P (X_i < 66 mm) = 1.000 −P (Xi >66 mm) = 1.000 −0.2743=0.7257

Q2. What proportion of this population lies between 60 and 66 mm?

We are looking for, P (60 mm< X_i < 66 mm)

Total prob. of population, ... right hand to mean (μ = 60 mm) is 0.5000. And the prob. Of population greater than 66 mm is 0.2743

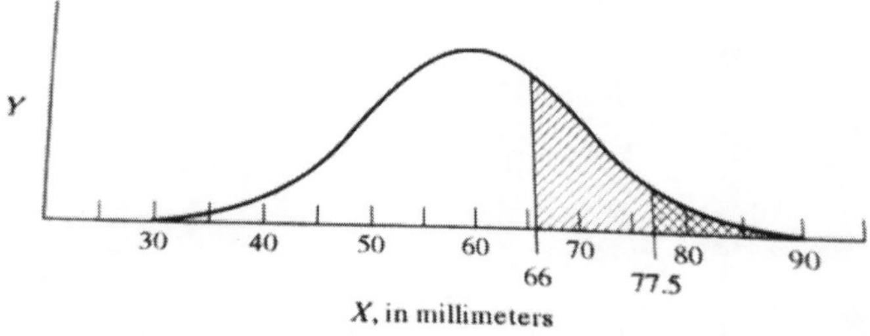

Therefore, P (60 mm< X_i < 66 mm) = 0.5000 – 0.2743 = 0.2257

Q 2.

What proportion of the area under the normal curve lies to the right of 77.5 mm?

We are looking for, P (X_i > 77.5 mm) **for that we need the value of P (Z)**

So, $Z = \frac{X_i - \mu}{\sigma} = \frac{77.5\,mm - 60\,mm}{10mm} = 1.75$

P (X_i > 77.5 mm) = P (Z > 1.75) = 0.0401 or 4.01 per cent

Binomial Distribution

Suppose the random variable (R.V.) X= number of getting head (H) from flipping 5 coins. times. Since, it is a coin, therefore, for each flip you have two possibilities, either 'H' or 'T'. There is equally likely probability (ELP) that you will get 'H' or 'T' for each coin.

Outcomes: THHTT, HHTTT, ... *that is equal to* $2^5 = 32$.

If we are looking for the probability of not getting a single head 'H' *i.e.*, P (X=0). Given that from the 32 equally probability as outcomes, looking for not getting a single 'H'. This is going to be equal to $\frac{1}{32}$ ELP. So, for this, to think in term of Binomial Coefficient, and combination and all that it is much easier to just reason through it. Just think in terms of R.V., this will build up for the binomial distribution. So, we can get a **sense** of where the name come from.

Writing in those term, P (X=0) $= \frac{5C_0}{32}$ *i.e.*, $\frac{nC_X}{32}$; from the 5 flips, choosing zero '0' of them to be head 'H'.

P (X=0) $= \frac{nC_X}{32} = \frac{5C_0}{32} = \frac{1}{32}$ $[5C_0 = \frac{5!}{0!(5-0)!} = \frac{5!}{5!} = \frac{5\times4\times3\times2\times1}{5\times4\times3\times2\times1} = 1]$ # by definition 0!=1

So, the probability of not getting a single head 'H' is equal to $\frac{1}{32}$.

The probability of not getting a single Tail 'T' **or** the probability of getting all heads (H,H,H,H,H).

P (X=5) $= \frac{nC_X}{32} = \frac{5C_5}{32} = \frac{1}{32}$ $[5C_5 = \frac{5!}{5!(5-5)!} = \frac{5!}{5!} = \frac{5\times4\times3\times2\times1}{5\times4\times3\times2\times1} = 1]$

P (X=0) $= \frac{5C_0}{32} = \frac{1}{32}$ P(X=1) $= \frac{5C_1}{32} = \frac{5}{32}$ P (X=2) $= \frac{5C_2}{32} = \frac{10}{32}$

P(X=3) $= \frac{5C_3}{32} = \frac{10}{32}$ P (X=4) $= \frac{5C_4}{32} = \frac{5}{32}$ P (X=5) $= \frac{5C_5}{32} = \frac{1}{32}$

Thus, you can get the binomial coefficient using combination.

The notion of Binomial distribution defines as, X ~ B (n, p); x=0, 1, 2, ..., n n = number of trials

p = probability of success

$P\ (X = x) = \binom{n}{x} p^x (1-p)^{n-x}$

or $P\ (X = k) = \binom{n}{k} p^k (1-p)^{n-k}$

It can be also written as,

$P\ (X = k) = \binom{n}{k} p^k (q)^{n-k}$

$*\ p\ is\ the\ prob.of\ success\ and\ q\ is\ prob.of\ failure$

For X~ B (n,p)

The expected value (mean), E(X) = np

Variance, V (X) = npq

Standard deviation (σ^2) = $\sqrt{npq}$

Poisson Distribution

Poisson Process

Suppose X= no. of car passes in an hour.

Let 100 cars passes in one hour or any given time period, or no car passed in an hour (any given time period). Here, every hour is complementary just like any other hour, that is really no differentiation from one second to the other in terms of probability, that a car arrives or passed.

Another case: Assume that a bunch of cars passed in one hour, that in no way does the number of cars that pass in one period affect or correlate or some how influence the number of cars, they are really **independent**. Given that it provides an idea to model of some type of a **distribution**.

Measure this variable, average them in bunch of hours, and it is to be a pretty good estimator for the actual mean of population or since it is a random variable (R.V.), The expected value of this R.V. is define as λ (average change in the given tome period), *i.e.*, E (X) = λ (letter lamda).

We have seen in previous chapter that in the case of binomial distribution (B.D.), the expected value of R.V. is equal to the number of trials *i.e.*, E (X) = np.

Here, in case of Poisson process, E (X) = λ = np.

That is true, λ defines the cars passes in per hour, λ cars/hour or λ/60 cars/ minutes.

Further, E (X) = λ = np

where, n is the number of trials and p is probability of success. Therefore,

$$p = \frac{\lambda}{n}$$

Considering the binomial distribution, we can write,

$$P\ (X = k) = \binom{n}{k}\ p^k (q)^{n-k}$$

Now put the value of p, that is $p = \frac{\lambda}{n}$.

Therefore,

$$P\ (X = k) = \binom{n}{k}\ (\lambda/\text{n})^k (1 - \lambda/\text{n})^{n-k}$$

Applying calculus,

$$\lim_{k \to \infty} \left(1 + \frac{a}{x}\right)^x = e^a$$

For the Poisson distribution,

$$\boldsymbol{P\ (X = k) = \frac{\lambda^k\ e^{-\lambda}}{k!}}$$

So, let $\lambda = 9$ cars/hour

Find, P (X=2)

$$P\ (X = 2) = \frac{9^2\ e^{-9}}{2!}$$

Pearson's Chi Square Test (Goodness of fit)

It is used to really test how well theoretical distribution explain observed one.

The **chi-square (χ^2) test for goodness-of-fit** uses frequency data from a sample to test hypotheses about the shape or proportions of a population. Each individual in the sample is classified into one category on the scale of measurement. The data, called **observed frequencies**, simply count how many individuals from the sample are in each category.

- ☆ The null hypothesis specifies the proportion of the population that should be in each category.
- ☆ The proportions from the null hypothesis are used to compute **expected frequencies** that describe how the sample would appear if it were in perfect agreement with the null hypothesis.

$$\chi^2 = \sum \frac{(O_i - E_i)^2}{E_i}$$

O_i = *observed value*

E_i = *expected value*

Example

Let, Salima is thinking of buying a restaurant and asks about the distribution of lunch customers. The owner provides row 1 below. Sal records the data in row 2 himself one week.

	M	T	W	T	F	S	
Owner's distribution	.1	.1	.15	.2	.3	.15	1.00 (100 per cent)
Observed # of customers (cust.)	30	14	34	45	57	20	Total # of cust. 200
Expected	**20**	**20**	**30**	**40**	**60**	**30**	

The chi-square goodness-of-fit test on the null hypotheses:

H_0: the owner's distribution is correct.

H_A: the owner's distribution is not correct.

Here,

$$\chi^2 = \frac{(30-20)^2}{20} + \frac{(14-20)^2}{20} + \frac{(34-30)^2}{30} + \frac{(45-40)^2}{40} + \frac{(57-60)^2}{60} + \frac{(20-30)^2}{30}$$

$$\chi^2 = \frac{(10)^2}{20} + \frac{(-6)^2}{20} + \frac{(4)^2}{30} + \frac{(5)^2}{40} + \frac{(-3)^2}{60} + \frac{(-10)^2}{30}$$

$$\chi^2 = \frac{100}{20} + \frac{36}{20} + \frac{16}{30} + \frac{25}{40} + \frac{9}{60} + \frac{100}{30} = 11.44$$

However, the value of $\chi^2_{\alpha,\, df=n-1}$ from χ^2 distribution table as given below

$\chi^2_{0.05,5} = 11.07$ that mean that $\chi^2_{c(\text{critical value})} = 11.07$

Therefore, $\chi^2 > \chi^2_c = 11.07$ thus, null hypothesis is rejected.

The degree of freedom (d.f.) here are going to be n-1 *i.e.*, 6-1 = 5 and given at the significant level of 5 per cent ($\alpha = 0.05$). Look at the chi-squared distribution table at $\alpha = 0.05$ and d.f. = 5, the chi-squared value is 11.07. It means that the probability of getting at least as extreme as 11.07 is 5 per cent. This probability is less likely than the probability at significant level, thus, the null hypothesis is rejected.

Percentage Points of the Chi-Square Distribution

Degrees of Freedom	Probability of a larger value of x^2								
	0.99	0.95	0.90	0.75	0.50	0.25	0.10	0.05	0.01
1	0.000	0.004	0.016	0.102	0.455	1.32	2.71	3.84	6.63
2	0.020	0.103	0.211	0.575	1.386	2.77	4.61	5.99	9.21
3	0.115	0.352	0.584	1.212	2.366	4.11	6.25	7.81	11.34
4	0.297	0.711	1.064	1.923	3.357	5.39	7.78	9.49	13.28
5	0.554	1.145	1.610	2.675	4.351	6.63	9.24	11.07	15.09
6	0.872	1.635	2.204	3.455	5.348	7.84	10.64	12.59	16.81
7	1.239	2.167	2.833	4.255	6.346	9.04	12.02	14.07	18.48
8	1.647	2.733	3.490	5.071	7.344	10.22	13.36	15.51	20.09
9	2.088	3.325	4.168	5.899	8.343	11.39	14.68	16.92	21.67

REFERENCES

1. Biostatistics: A manual of Statistical Methodology for use in Health, Nutrition and Anthropology, K. Visweswara Rao. Publisher: Jaypee Brothers Biostatistics: A foundation for analysis in the Health Sciences, W.W. Daniel, Publisher: John Wiley and Sons
2. Fundamentals of Mathematical Statistics, S.C. Gupta and V.K. Kapoor, Publisher: S.Chand and Co.
3. Statistical Analysis, Kaushal, T.L. Publisher: Kalyani Publishers
4. Statistical Methods, Potri, D. Kalyani Publishers.
5. Mathematical Statistics, H.C. Saxena, and V.K. Kapoor: S. Chand and Company
6. Biostatistics, P.N. Arora and P.K. Malhan, Publisher: Himalaya Publishing House.
7. Introduction to Biostatistics, Ronald N. Forthfer and Eun Sun Lee, Publisher: Elsevier.
8. Statistical Methodology, S.P. Gupta, Publisher: S. Chand and Co.
9. Fundamentals of Statistics, S.C. Gupta. Publisher: S.Chand and Co.
10. H. A. STURGES, "The Choice of a Class Interval," Journal of the American Statistical Association, 21 (1926),65–66.
11. HELEN M. WALKER, "Degrees of Freedom," Journal of Educational Psychology, 31 (1940), 253–269.
12. ROB J. HYNDMAN and YANAN FAN, "Sample Quantiles in Statistical Packages," The American Statistician, 50 (1996), 361–365.
13. JOHN W. TUKEY, Exploratory Data Analysis, Addison-Wesley, Reading, MA, 1977.

Chapter 14

Bioinformatics and Computational Biology

Jinny Tomar

Amity Institute of Biotechnology, Amity University Haryana, Gurugram (Manesar) – 122 413, Haryana, India
e-mail: jinny.tomar@gmail.com

ABSTRACT

Bioinformatics has emerged as a field with wide applicability in life sciences. This module allows one to understand the basics of bioinformatics, its application. The base of bioinformatics is biological data, which can be in the form of nucleotide sequence, protein sequence, protein structure etc. Extraction of the correct data holds the key, as the entire analysis will be based on whether the exact data has been obtained using the different biological databases. Thus, information about the prominent biological databases helps a lot. The next important step in the field of Bioinformatics is sequence analysis, which is basically understanding the query data in hand. Sequence analysis is preceded by sequence alignment, which allows the user to understand the biological relevance of aligning sequences. It is usually the comparative study which facilitate the prediction about the different parameters under study. This indicates predictions can be made based on the similarity in the sequence data, which can be prediction about the secondary structure information of proteins, their tertiary structure prediction and even the prediction of the possible functions. The study of evolution also has been facilitated with the various phylogenetic tools provided by Bioinformatics.

Keywords: *Bioinformatics, Biological databases, Sequence alignment, Phylogenetic analysis, Structure prediction, Molecular modeling.*

1. Basics of Bioinformatics

Bioinformatics as the name indicates is referred as an interdisciplinary field, which not only allows the storage of biological data, rather it also involves the assembly, analysis and dissemination of the acquired data using tools to interpret biologically relevant information.

The term Bioinformatics was introduced by Paulien Hogeweg and Ben Hisper in 1970s as the study of informatics processes in Biotic systems.

1.1 Scope of Bioinformatics

1.1.1. Medicine/Drug Designing and Development

The time, cost factor involved in the process of drug designing and development had been reduced dramatically with the help of bioinformatics. Computer aided drug designing (CADD) allows the user to design ligand molecule according to the structure of the target molecule/receptor molecule. In case of the new infections which have arisen, one can choose molecules available in the chemical libraries. Using combinatorial chemistry approach, the process of identifying and validating lead molecule has eased.

The concept of personalized medicine could also be practiced based on comparative studies which were possible due to the sequencing of the human genome data. The identification of the normal state of gene expression in a healthy individual and comparison with the diseased state, has allowed us to choose better therapeutic practices based on individuals.

1.1.2. Agriculture Sciences

Use of databases providing details of the genetic makeup of the plant resources. Application of bioinformatics in agriculture is also known as Agri-informatics, which facilitate us to understand the plants, studying the various factors like biotic and abiotic stress and their response and even how one can improve the quality of soil using the nutrients or microbes enhancing the soil quality.

1.1.3. Animal Based Studies

Sequencing the various animal genomes has enabled us to have a better understanding of the genetic diseases. The genomic data of farm animals have allowed us to improve the production of livestock, improvement in terms of their health and efficiency.

1.1.4. Plant Based Studies

With the advent of bioinformatics based studies, plant genomes have been studied, which allowed identification and study of specific gene expression contributing to drought resistance or antibiotic resistance or even improvement of specific characteristics in the plant yield. In certain cases, researchers were able to increase the nutritional content of plant-based product by either enhancing the micronutrients, vitamin content or other minerals.

1.1.5. Environment

Bioremediation guides us in reducing the soil pollutants using the natural processes, where different microbes break down the different contaminants.

Different Biological databases provide information related to the genomes of microbes which can convert the specific pollutant contributing to the degradation of soil, water into less complex and easily degradable compounds. The study of their pathways, gene- gene interaction, data related to the proteins getting expressed using comparative genomics can provide new direction to the field of bioremediation.

To work in Bioinformatics, one requires specific type of dataset for example, either nucleotide sequences or amino acid sequences or protein structural dataset. Such data is available in Biological Databases, those repositories which deals with biological information.

Although several life science related fields, involve analysis using bioinformatic based databases and tools. Few of them are listed below:

1.2 Biological Databases

Biological databases play a very crucial role in bioinformatic based analysis, as choosing the right data forms the basis of any study. Biological databases can be defined as a storehouse of biological data with a user-friendly interface. Biological databases allow indexing of data, proper organization of the data and further optimizing it.

Biological databases can be broadly divided as sequence databases or structure databases based on type of data

1.2.1 Sequence Databases

These biological databases facilitate the user to access nucleotide and protein (amino acid) sequence data. In case of nucleotide sequence data, three organization which are working in close coordination under International Nucleotide Sequence Database Collaboration (INSD) are: National Centre for Biotechnology Information (NCBI) (GenBank), European Molecular Biology Laboratory (EMBL) -European Bioinformatics Institute (EBI) and DNA Databank of Japan (DDBJ)

1.2.1.1. National Centre for Biotechnology Information (NCBI) (www.ncbi.nlm.nih.gov)

NCBI is one such organization which provides numerous genomic and biomedical information to the user, and the data has been categorically divided into different databases and to analyze the data, different tools are also available. The different types of data divided into six major division: Literature data, Genes related Data, Protein data, Genomic data, Clinical data as well as information about the chemical nature of Compounds under PubChem.

GenBank is an NIH initiative which consists of all the publicly available nucleotide sequences. Each entry is given a unique Accession number, which can be used for further analysis. Users can even submit new sequences in the databank using submission tools like BankIt and even via submission portal.

1.2.1.2. European Molecular Biology Laboratory (EMBL)-European Bioinformatics Institute (EBI) (www.embl.org)

EMBL- EBI provides a series of scientific and technical services to scientific community. EMBL services are in the field of genomics, proteomics, structural biology, metabolomics chemical biology and even in vivo gene editing, imaging.

The EMBL-EBI tools deal with DNA/RNA dataset, study of structures, Gene Expressions, Chemical Biology, Literature, Protein sequence dataset and so on. The structural biology and imaging unit provides Electron microscopy, Light microscopy services to the researchers. In the Multi-Omics facilities, different groups dealing with Genomics core, Proteomics Core, Metabolomics Core and Flow cytometry work together. Likewise, the Chemical Biology services, In vivo gene editing services and Sample preparation for High throughput Crystallization, Histology and Protein Expression and purification groups work to facilitate the researchers according to their requirement by timely processing these tasks.

1.2.1.3. DNA Databank of Japan (DDBJ) (www.ddbj.nig.ac.jp)

DDBJ Centre and Bioinformation enables the user to access the sequence data and provide tools for analysis purpose. DDBJ has NIG supercomputer and user can access the server by following the guidelines set by DDBJ using an authorised account.

The services offered by DDBJ has been categorized into database- total nine in number, analysis-seven main tools, search- fifteen different tools for the same, submission- ten tools, Annotation, and the data of the two Centres of DDBJ- Database Centre for Life Science (DBCLS) and National Bioscience Database Centre.

To analyze the dataset, one may opt for either of these tools: BLAST, ClustalW, DFAST, MAFFT, Maser, VecScreen and WABI, likewise the database includes data under AGD, BioProject, BioSample, DDBJ, DRA, GEA, JGA, JVar and NHA.

1.2.1.4. Protein Information Resource (PIR) (www.proteininformationresource.org)

PIR is a Uniprot consortium member, which is an integrated resource for providing genomic, proteomic and system biology data. The three main databases under this head are: PRO (Protein Ontology), iPTMnet (Integrated Protein PTM Resource) and iProLINK (Literature Information and Knowledge). PRO provides information about proteins which are evolutionary related, their location and their interaction with other proteins. iPTMnet, as the name indicates talks about the post translational modification of proteins. iProLINK on the other hand integrates the Protein Literature, associated information by providing knowledge based on different databases, literature, association-based studies using PubMed, iSimp, pGenN *etc.*

1.2.2 Structure Database

This category highlights the database which provide the three-dimensional structural information about the biological macromolecule. These databases also include tools for visualizing the structure, allows downloading the structure in different formats and even facilitate the users to analyze the data for example: Protein Data Bank (PDB)

1.2.2.1 Protein Data Bank (PDB) (www.rcsb.org)

This is a well-known database, which allows the user to perform number of activities like depositing the structure in PDB, preparing the protein data, validation of the protein data and finally depositing in the databank. The search segment in PDB, facilitate the user from basic to advanced search, even browsing by annotation, by ligands and even identifying the Drugs and Drug targets. In the Visualization section, the protein 3D structure can be visualized, the protein feature view and genome view. To analyze the data, the numerous options available with PDB are pairwise structure alignment, protein symmetry-based studies, mapping of genomic position to proteins under study, get detailed information about the quality of macromolecule structure and so on. One can even download the structural information like coordinates and experimental data, sequences in varied formats and so on.

1.2.3. Other Databases

This category is quite vivid as databases which provide information about protein family, domains, interaction can be placed under this. This may also include organism specific databases which have detailed information about specific organism like SGD (Saccharomyces Genome database) *etc.*

1.2.3.1 Universal Protein Resource (Uniprot) (www.uniprot.org)

UniProt allows the researchers to retrieve literature data, provides information about the diseases and the related proteins, and even the subcellular locations of the proteins under study. One can analyze the data using sequence alignment tools or can-do peptide search and can even retrieve specific proteins using the identification number.

Uniprot is a composite database, which basically is a collaboration of European Bioinformatics Institute (EMBL- EBI), Swiss Institute of Bioinformatics (SIB) and the Protein Information Resource (PIR). The UniProt database has UniPort knowledgebase database (UniProtKB), the UniProt Reference Cluster (UniRef) and UniProt Archive (UniParc).

1.2.3.2 Prosite (www.prosite.expasy.org)

It is a database providing information about protein families and protein domains. The proteins are placed together based on similarities between the sequences and highlighting the conserved sequences responsible for a specific function or a specific structure. Since a protein signature is defined, thus that can be used further to identify an unknown protein sequence.

1.2.3.3. STRING (www.string-db.org)

STRING database predicts protein-protein interactions based on functional as well as physical interactions of the proteins under study. The interactions defined by STRING can be based on either of the sources: high throughput lab experimentation, conserved sequence expressions, genomic context predictions, automated text mining and existing knowledge in other databases.

1.2.3.4. Kyoto Encyclopedia of Genes and Genomes (KEGG) (www.genome.jp)

This database is a resource to provide information about the high-level functions of a biological system, like information about the pathways involved, genes and proteins, biochemical reactions, disease related network, human diseases, information about specific drugs, small molecules, functional orthologs *etc.*

Analysis of the different datasets can be done using KEGG Mapper, BLAST, annotation tools: BlastKOALA, GhostKOALA, KofamKOALA.

2. Sequence Analysis

Sequence analysis involves analysis of sequences which starts with sequence alignment. Sequence alignment can be defined as the arrangement of the sequences to find similarities and dissimilarities in the dataset under study.

2.1. Types of Sequence Alignment

Depending upon the number of sequences under study one can study them as:

2.1.1 Pairwise Sequence Alignment

When two sequences are aligned to locate the similar regions, which could be due to structural, functional, and evolutionary relatedness.

2.1.2 Multiple Sequence Alignment

When more than two sequences either protein or nucleic acid of similar length are studied together, so that evolutionary relationship can be inferred. There are three main ways to perform Multiple sequence alignment.: Dynamic Programming approach, Progressive method, and Iterative method.

Depending upon the region of the sequence considered, the two main categories are:

2.1.3. Local Alignment

In this alignment, part of the sequence shows matches, that is regions showing more similarities.

2.1.4. Global Alignment

When the alignment includes the matching of residues of two sequences across their entire length.

2.2. Method of Sequence Alignment

2.2.1. Dot Matrix

It represents a pairwise system in which two sequences are arranged across x and y axis, wherever there is a match, a dot is assigned.

In this graph, the dots represent the point where the two sequences show match of a nucleotide base pair or amino acid residue.

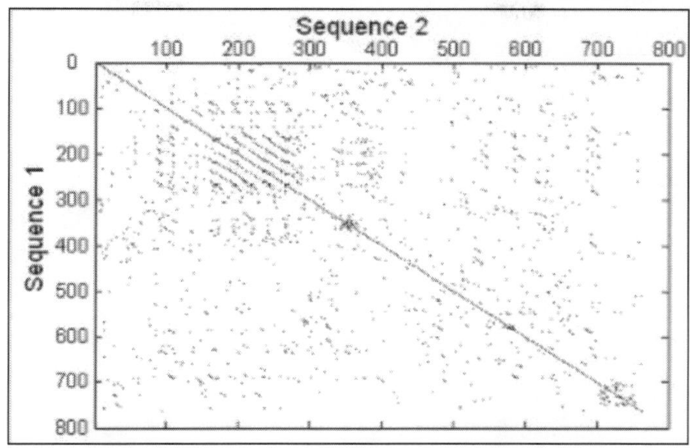

Figure 14.1L DOTPLOT Showing Sequences at x- axis and y-axis.

The dots are joined to form one diagonal, the diagonal covering the maximum number of dots is the best match across the sequences under study. Since the dot plots were having multiple diagonals and it was difficult to analyze the data, thus another concept was introduced, the concept of scoring matrices

2.2.2. Dynamic Programming

It is found useful in alignment of the sequences as it involves the breaking of the task of sequence alignment into sub tasks, and then solving each task using recursive methods and finally constructing an optimal solution by combining the sub parts. It was introduced by Richard Bellman in 1940. This is done by following three main steps of Initialization, filling up of the matrix using scoring matrices and trace back

2.2.3. Scoring matrices

In the process of alignment, the score are given to each position and it is the match or mismatch at specific position which is counted, this implies each position in the alignment matrix has a specific value, which depends on the factors whether:

i) The sequences are showing match at that position- same base pair or amino acid residue in both the sequences at that position.
ii) The score if there is a mismatch
iii) The value at the specific position if there is a gap. Gaps were introduced to extend the matches between the sequences under study.

The criteria define the best match as the highest scoring segment between the sequences while deducting the gap penalty.

The two most widely used matrices are: Point/Percent Accepted Mutation Matrix (PAM) and Block Substitution Matrices (BLOSUM). PAM was introduced by Dayhoff *et al.*,1978 and BLOSUM matrices was given Henikoff and Henikoff, 1992.

These matrices provide relative substitutability of amino acid residues/nucleotide base pair in the context of evolution.

PAM1 matrix specifies one point mutation accepted per 100 amino acid residues, while BLOSUM62 denotes minimum of 62 per cent similarity in the dataset

2.3. Tools for Sequence Alignment

The tools for sequence alignment- Pairwise as well as Multiple sequence alignment has been highlighted in this table, along with the name of the algorithm on which these are based

Table 14.1: Highlighting the Tools and Algorithm for Pairwise and Multiple Sequence Alignment

Multiple Sequence Alignment	*Pairwise Sequence Alignment*
Compares more than two sequences	Compare two sequences
Tools are based on: Dynamic Programming, Progressive alignment, Iterative alignment	Tools work on the following algorithm: Needleman Wunsch for Global Alignment and Smith Waterman for Local Alignment
CLUSTAL, MUSCLE, MAFFT, T-COFFEE *etc.*	BLAST, EMBOSS- Needle, EMBOSS- Water

2.3.1. Basic Local Alignment Search Tool (BLAST) (BLAST Basic Local Alignment Search Tool (nih.gov))

BLAST find regions of similarity in the sequences under study, the query sequence is aligned with the sequence database, to find statistically significant matches. BLAST works on the concept of local alignment.

Table 14.2: The Variants of BLAST

Variants of BLAST	
Blastn	Align nucleotide sequence with Nucleotide database
Blastp	Aligns protein sequence with protein database
Blastx	Aligns translated nucleotide with protein database
tblastn	Align protein sequence with translated nucleotide

2.3.2. Clustal W/Clustal Omega (www.clustal.org))

Clustal W is a multiple sequence alignment program for DNA or protein data. It allows the user to enter sequence data in multiple formats: Clustal, GCG-MSF, Fasta, EMBL-SWISSPROT and so on. Likewise, the output is also available in multiple formats. In this program, all sequences are aligned and compared to each other, based on that a dendrogram is generated and the final alignment shows the association among the sequences.

3. Phylogenetic Analysis

Phylogenetic analysis is the study of evolution, it is defined as the branch which enables to establish ancestral relationship based on phenetic or genetic characters or the distance of evolution.

Phylogenetic analysis which depicts ancestral relationship is shown in the form of trees. These trees like representation are known as **Phylogram/Dendrogram/ Cladogram** and so on. The trees generated may or may not represents origin, thus the ones highlighting the origin are known as rooted trees and the one with out an origin is known as unrooted tree.

Table 14.3: Common Terminologies in Phylogenetic Analysis (*Courtesy*: Prof. David Gilbert, University of Glasgow, Bioinformatics Research Centre)

Phylum	A primary division of a kingdom, as of the animal kingdom, ranking next above a class in size
Taxon	Any named group of organisms
Clade	a group of biological taxa or species that share features inherited from a common ancestor; A monophyletic taxon; a group of organisms which includes the most recent common ancestor of all its members and all of the descendants of that most recent common ancestor. From the Greek word "klados", meaning branch or twig.
Tree	A data structure consisting of nodes which may contain other nodes via its branches. Unlike a tree in nature, the root node is usually represented at the top of the structure and does not have a parent node. All other nodes have a single parent. Nodes having no child nodes are called leaf nodes
Dendrogram	Any branching diagram (or tree) (cf. cladogram, phylogram, phenogram); A dendrogram is a 'tree-like' diagram that summaries the process of clustering. Similar cases are joined by links whose position in the diagram is determined by the level of similarity between the cases. A treelike figure used to represent graphically a hierarchy. (dendron - greek 'tree
Orthologues	homologues produced by speciation. Tend to have similar function
Paralogues	homologues produced by gene duplication. Tend to have different functions
Xenologues	homologues resulting from horizontal gene transfer between 2 organisms
Horizontal (Lateral) gene transfer	When the bacteria have obtained naked DNA, genes from surrounding by getting infected from virus and even in case of cross-species mating
Ultrametric tree	A linearized tree, where the amount of change is reflected in terms of time, all the tree tips are equidistant from the root
Cladogram	These represents the cladistics, with respect to the recent most relative, no time scale is followed in this case
Phylogram	In these trees the branch length represents the amount of change
Outgroup	The outgroup should be a sequence (or set of sequences) known to be less closely related to the rest of the sequences than they are to each other.

3.1. Methods to Perform Phylogenetic Analysis

There are two main approaches to perform Phylogenetic tree reconstruction: Character Based Method and Distance Based Method.

3.1.1. Character Based Method

These methods determine the ancestral relationship based on the kind of changes accumulated in the sequences/taxon/cade under study. This represents the nonsynonymous substitution over synonymous substitution acquired over a period. Use the aligned characters, such as DNA or protein sequences, directly during tree inference – based on substitutions.

3.1.1.1. Maximum Parsimony (MP)

Parsimony is the most popular method for reconstructing ancestral relationships. Parsimony involves evaluating all possible trees and giving each a score based on the number of evolutionary changes that are needed to explain the observed data. The best tree is the one that requires the fewest base changes for all sequences to derive from a common ancestor.

Parsimony allows the use of all known evolutionary information in building a tree. In contrast, distance methods compress all the differences between pairs of sequences into a single number.

3.1.1.2. Maximum Likelihood Estimation (ML)

Felsenstein proposed a method for finding the maximum likelihood phylogeny relating observed DNA or protein sequences. Phylogenies are usually formulated in a probalistic framework and are statistically testable.

The maximum likelihood tree is the one that gives the observed genomes the highest probability of occurring under our specified model.

3.1.2. Distance Based Methods

When the phylogenetic study is based on the number of changes acquired by the taxon/specie/terminal/Node under study over a period of time leading to an entire new taxon, one can use distance based methods. In these methods, data is transformed into pairwise distances (dissimilarities), and then we use that matrix for tree building.

3.1.2.1. Neighbor Joining Method (NJ Method)

The Neighbor Joining method is the most popular way to build trees from distance measurements and it was given by Saitou and Nei in 1987. Neighbor Joining has given the best results in simulation studies, and it is the most computationally efficient of the distance algorithms. The distance matrix is adjusted for differences in the rate of evolution of each taxon (branch). Neighbor Joining corrects the UPGMA method for its (frequently invalid) assumption that the same rate of evolution applies to each branch of a tree.

3.1.2.2. Minimum Evolution (ME)

In this method the tree with the shortest sum of the branch length is considered, as it is assumed that nature permits minimum number of changes to be incorporated for healthy survival of a specie. This method is faster than the character-based methods and is preferred in the analysis of rate of change-based analysis and can also be used for immunological dataset as well. Although, it has a limitation, it is slower in comparison to methods based on clustering approach.

3.1.2.3. *Unweighted Pair Group Method using Arithmetic Average*

The distance between two taxa is calculated as the average distance between two sequences. This can also be applied on indirectly measured distances and is able to yield results faster. There are no specific optimization criteria, thus identifying whether the system worked properly or not is a difficult task.

Many multiple alignment programs such as PILEUP use a variant of UPGMA to create a dendrogram of DNA sequences which is then used to guide the multiple alignment algorithm. PHYLIP programs DNADIST and PROTDIST calculate absolute pairwise distances between a group of sequences. Then the GCG program GROWTREE uses UPGMA to build a tree.

3.2. Probabilistic Model of Evolution/Evolutionary Models

There are different evolutionary models which describe the evolution of a single site within a set of sequences. They are often based on the simplifying assumption that different sites evolve independently and are identically distributed. This assumption may be justifiable if the sites can be assumed to be evolving neutrally.

If the primary effect of natural selection on the evolution of the sequences is to constrain some sites, then models of among-site rate-heterogeneity can be used.

3.3. Tree Building and Tree Evaluation

This is a crucial step in predicting the right evolutionary tree. Among the many, the two prominent statistical methods, which can evaluate the phylogenetic tree are: Boot strapping and Jack knife method.

Among this bootstrapping is the widely known method. It is a re-sampling tree evaluation method that works with distance, parsimony and maximum likelihood. It was given by Felsenstein in 1985.

Table 14.4: List of Tools which can be Used to Perform Phylogenetic Analysis

Name of the Software	*Description*
PHYLIP	It is a free package that includes 30 programs that compute various phylogenetic algorithms on different kinds of data.
MEGA	Software for statistical analysis of molecular evolution. It includes different tree visualization features
PAUP	Inferring phylogenies based on parsimony and distance based method
iTOL - interactive Tree Of Life	annotate trees with various types of data and export to various graphical formats; scriptable through a batch interface
GCG package	The GCG package (available at most research institutions) contains a full set of programs for phylogenetic analysis including simple distance-based clustering
POWER	Phylogenetic web Repeator is an online tool for reconstructing phylogenetic trees
Phylogeny.Fr	Allows user to choose the mode of working of the tool, from one click mode to A la Carte mode

The result obtained by boot strapping gives the proportion of bootstrap replicates, that is the number of times a particular branch appears in the tree.

4. Structure Prediction

Protein structure prediction means predicting the 3dimensional structure of the biomolecule. Usually, the 3D structure of biomolecule is determined by high resolution structure determination methods like: X-ray crystallography, Nuclear Magnetic Resonance or by Lower resolution structure determination- Cryo-Electron microscopy. Additionally, bioinformatics-based approaches are also used to predict the 3D structure of biomolecules, these are referred as hypothetical structures.

4.1. Secondary and Tertiary Structure Prediction Methods of Protein

Computer Simulation Based on Energy Calculation/Ab Initio Nethod

- ✰ Based on physio-chemical principles
- ✰ Thermodynamic equilibrium with a minimum free energy
- ✰ Global minimum free energy of protein surface

Knowledge Based Approaches

- ✰ **Homology Based Approach -/Comparative (homology) modeling:** Determine if there is a sequence homology between the target and one or more known structures. Obtain the most accurate structural model for the target, consistent with the known set.
- ✰ **Fold recognition/Threading:** It enables to recognize a known fold in a domain within the target protein. Using a threading algorithm to detect common structures even in the absence of high sequence similarity. The target protein sequence is threaded through templates from the structure database. Alternative sequence structure alignments are scored using conformational energy calculation, based on statistics of known structures. Highest scores are used to determine the locations of the folds.
- ✰ **Hierarchical Methods-Free Modeling**

4.2 Structure Representation and Coordinate System

In molecular modeling, the concept of molecular mechanics plays an important role, as it enables to understand the atom –atom coordinates. It provides a description of each atom in a molecule in terms of its atomic number, bond length, bond angle, and dihedral angle, the so-called internal coordinates.

A Cartesian coordinate system is a coordinate system that specifies each point uniquely in a plane in terms of numerical coordinates, with respect to two lines or reference line which may be known as *coordinate axis* and the point where the axis meet is known as *origin*

4.3 Molecular Modeling

It may be defined as a process which helps to mimic the structure and behavior of biomolecules using certain methods and techniques. Primarily, molecular modeling in bioinformatics refers to the designing of the proteins whose structure have not been made available.

There are different approaches which help to design models for protein structure prediction. As the function of a biomolecule is determined by its 3d structure and its physico-chemical properties.

The visualization, modeling, simulation of molecular structures and their properties are crucial for structural bioinformatics.

4.3.1. Steps Involved in Homology Modeling

1. Identify related structures (using PDB sequence as database)
2. Select templates (alignment via BLAST)
3. Align target sequence with templates and correction (when sequence similarity is low, other sequences can be referred)
4. Backbone generation (coordinate of the template are copied to the target)
5. Loop Modeling (regions created by insertions/deletions that lead to gaps need to be modeled, by either finding loops or ab initio methods
6. Side chain Modeling (all possible conformations can be searched for every torsion angle, to check the lowest energy state)
7. Model Optimization (Energy minimization procedure on the entire model is done

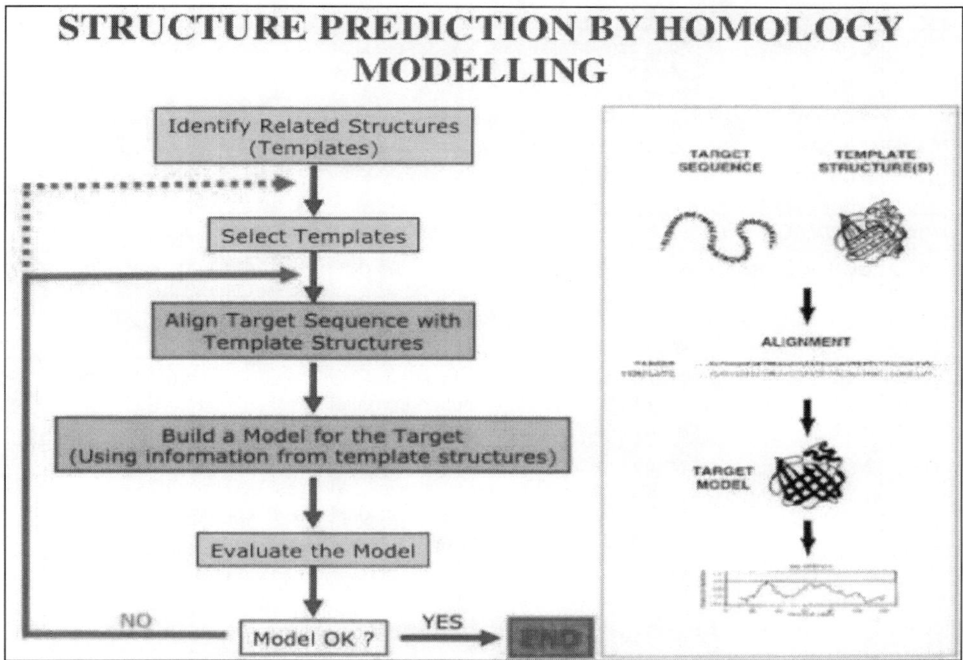

Figure 14.2: Molecular Modeling (Image courtesy: slideshare.net/75836997).

8. Model Validation (To remove the chances of errors in calculating the bong angles, bong lengths, chemical properties and so on)

4.3.2. Important Databases for Molecular Modeling

- ☆ MMDB [(Molecular Modeling DataBase) (Macromolecular Structures Resource Group (nih.gov)]
- ☆ PDB (Protein DataBank) (www.rcsb.org)
- ☆ SWISS-MODEL (SWISS-MODEL - SIB Swiss Institute of Bioinformatics | Expasy)
- ☆ ChemDB [ChemDB Web Interface Index (uci.edu)]
- ☆ BindingDB [Binding Database (bindingdb.org)]
- ☆ MODBASE [ModBase Help (ucsf.edu)]

4.3.3. Tools for Molecular Modeling

Table 14.5: Online Tools for Bioinformatics-Based Structure Prediction

Sl.No.	*Software Name*	*Task Done*	*Website*	*Free*
1	ChemSketch	Fast 2-D graphical molecule builder and 3-D viewer. Contains simplified CHARMM for fast stable inaccurate optimization of single molecules up to 1000 atom	http://www.acdlabs.com/resources/freeware/chemsketch/	Free
2	CHARMM	Chemistry at HARvard Macromolecular Mechanics studiesumerous conformational and path sampling methods, free energy estimates, molecular minimization, dynamics, and analysis techniques, and model-building capabilities	http://www.charmm.org/	
3	GROMACS	High performance molecular grpahics	www.gromacs.org	Free
4	UCSF Chimera	Visually appealing viewer, amino acid rotamers and other building, includes Antechamber and Ambertools sub-programs	http://www.cgl.ucsf.edu/chimera/index.html	
5	ArgusLab	3D molecule builder that allows the user to build and manipulate complex structures	http://www.arguslab.com/	
6	MODBASE	database of annotated comparative protein structure models for all available protein sequences matched to at least one known protein structure.	http://modbase.compbio.ucsf.edu/modbase-cgi/index.cgi	

4.3.4. Evaluation of Internal Energy of Biomolecule

Steric energy calculation in molecular mechanics corresponds to an internal energy calculation. The steric energy of a molecule is the sum of the bonded and nonbonded terms (Van der Waals energy, and the electrostatic energy). The steric energy of a molecule can be used to calculate the enthalpy of formation, (the bond energy), or enthalpy (which is the energy needed to make all the chemical bonds in the molecule starting from the elements in their standards states) as well as the energy of translation and rotation of the molecule.

The energy of translation (x, y, z motion of the center of mass of the molecule) is 3/2RT. The rotational energy of a non-linear molecule is also 3/2RT (1/2RT for each rotational axis).

The lowest energy conformation is the set of bond lengths and angles that gives the smallest steric energy.

4.3.5. Energy Minimization of Small Molecules

Energy Minimization based methods in their pure form, make no priori assumptions and attempt to locate global minima. This includes the collective mathematical expression which is known as a potential function and is related to the system internal energy (U), a thermodynamic quantity equal to the sum of potential and kinetic energies.

Molecular potential energy is a sum of energy terms that describe the deviation of bond lengths, bond angles and torsion angles away from equilibrium values, including the non-bonded pairs of atoms describing van der Waals and electrostatic interactions.

Methods which minimize the potential energy are known as energy minimization techniques (*e.g.*, steepest descent and conjugate gradient), while methods that model the behaviour of the system with respect to time are known as molecular dynamics.

Broadly classified in two divisions:

Static Minimization Methods

- ☆ Classical many potential-potential can be constructed
- ☆ Assume that atoms in protein are in static form
- ☆ Problems (large number of variables and minima and validity of potentials)

Dynamical Minimization Methods

- ☆ Motions of atoms also considered
- ☆ Monte Carlo simulation (stochastics in nature, time is not considered)
- ☆ Molecular Dynamics (time, quantum mechanical, classical equation.)

Limitations

- ☆ Large number of degree of freedom
- ☆ Interaction potential is not good enough to model

4.3.6. Local and Global Minima

The object of energy minimization is to find the lowest energy conformation of a molecule.

The goal of energy minimization is simply to find the local energy minimum, *i.e.*, the bottom of the energy well occupied by the initial conformation. The energy at this local minimum may be much higher than the energy of the global minimum.

There is only one global minimum of the energy surface, but many local minima.

A minimization is considered converged if the root mean squared deviation of the gradient (GRMS) is very close to zero (the necessary condition for a function to have a local minimum is that all its first derivatives are zero.

4.3.7. Molecular Docking

In the field of molecular modeling, docking is a method which predicts the preferred orientation of one molecule with respect to second molecule when they come in close association with each other to form a stable complex.

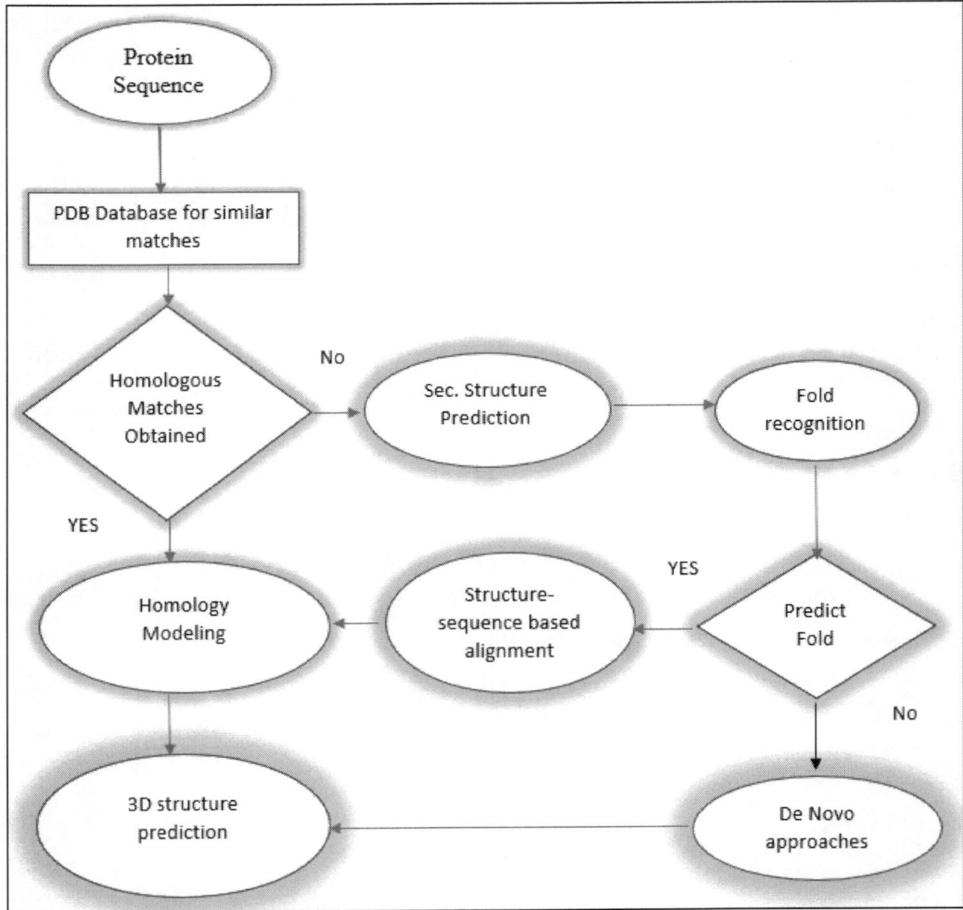

Figure 14.3: Overall Process of Structure Prediction of Biomolecule, Involving the Decision Taking Steps.

This orientation enables to predict the strength of association or binding affinity between two molecules using certain features such as scoring functions.

Docking is frequently used to predict the binding orientation of small molecule drug candidates to their protein targets to predict the affinity and activity of the small molecule.

There are mainly two types of Docking

1. **Protein-Protein Docking**: Both molecules usually considered rigid, 6 degrees of freedom, the energetics of possible binding conformations need to be checked
2. **Protein-Ligand Docking**: Flexible ligand, rigid-receptor, either reduce flexible ligand to rigid fragments connected, then studying the conformational space using monte-carlo methods or molecular dynamics

REFERENCES

1. Altschul, S.F., Gish, W., Miller, W., Myers, E.W. and Lipman, D.J. (1990) "Basic local alignment search tool." J. Mol. Biol. 215: 403-410.
2. Benman H.M., Westbrook J., Feng Z., Gilliland G., Bhat T.N., Weissig H., Shindyalov I.N., Bourne P. E., 2000, The Protein Data Bank, Nucleic Acid Research, 28, 235-242.
3. Bateman Alex. The UniProt Consortium, UniProt: a worldwide hub of protein knowledge, Nucleic Acids Research, Volume 47, Issue D1, 08 January 2019, Pages D506–D515, https: //doi.org/10.1093/nar/gky1049.
4. Chen J, Swamidass SJ, Dou Y, Bruand J, Baldi P. ChemDB: a public database of small molecules and related chemoinformatics resources. Bioinformatics. 2005 Nov 15;21(22): 4133-9. doi: 10.1093/bioinformatics/bti683. Epub 2005 Sep 20. PMID: 16174682.
5. Chung-Yen Lin, Fan-Kai Lin, Chieh Hua Lin, Li-Wei Lai, Hsiu-Jun Hsu, Shu-Hwa Chen, Chao A. Hsiung, POWER: PhylOgenetic WEb Repeater–an integrated and user-optimized framework for biomolecular phylogenetic analysis, Nucleic Acids Research, Volume 33, Issue suppl_2, 1 July 2005, Pages W553–W556, https: //doi.org/10.1093/nar/gki494
6. Gary O. Spessard. ACD Labs/LogP dB 3.5 and ChemSketch 3.5. Journal of Chemical Information and Computer Sciences 1998 38 (6), 1250-1253.DOI: 10.1021/ci980264t
7. Hingamp P, van den Broek AE, Stoesser G, Baker W. The EMBL Nucleotide Sequence Database. Contributing and accessing data. Mol Biotechnol. 1999 Oct;12(3): 255-67. doi: 10.1385/MB: 12: 3: 255. PMID: 10631682.
8. J. Felsenstein. 1989. PHYLIP - Phylogeny Inference Package (Version 3.2). Cladistics. 5: 164-166.
9. Larkin MA, Blackshields G, Brown NP, Chenna R, McGettigan PA, McWilliam H, Valentin F, Wallace IM, Wilm A, Lopez R, Thompson JD, Gibson TJ, Higgins

DG. Clustal W and Clustal X version 2.0. Bioinformatics. 2007 Nov 1;23(21): 2947-8. doi: 10.1093/bioinformatics/btm404. Epub 2007 Sep 10. PMID: 17846036.

10. Lin, Chung-Yen and Lin, Fan-Kai and Lin, Chieh and Lai, Li-Wei and Hsu, Hsiu-Jun and Chen, Shu-Hwa and Hsiung, Chao. (2005). POWER: PhylOgenetic WEb Repeater - An integrated and user-optimized framework for biomolecular phylogenetic analysis. Nucleic acids research. 33. W553-6. 10.1093/nar/gki494

11. S. Jo, T. Kim, V.G. Iyer, and W. Im (2008) CHARMM-GUI: A Web-based Graphical User Interface for CHARMM. J. Comput. Chem. 29: 1859-1865

12. The NCBI Handbook [Internet]. 2nd edition. Bethesda (MD): National Center for Biotechnology Information (US); 2013-. Available from: https: //www.ncbi.nlm.nih.gov/books/NBK143764/

13. Tingjian Zhang, Yuxuan Li, Ping Gao, Qi Shao, Mingshan Shao, Meng Zhang, Jinxiao Zhang, Xiaohui Duan, Zhao Liu, Lin Gan, Haohuan Fu, Wei Xue, Weiguo Liu, and Guangwen Yang. 2019. SW_GROMACS: accelerate GROMACS on Sunway TaihuLight. In Proceedings of the International Conference for High Performance Computing, Networking, Storage and Analysis (SC '19). Association for Computing Machinery, New York, NY, USA, Article 66, 1–14. DOI: https: //doi.org/10.1145/3295500.3356190

14. Ursula Pieper, Narayanan Eswar, Fred P. Davis, Hannes Braberg, M. S. Madhusudhan, Andrea Rossi, Marc Marti-Renom, Rachel Karchin, Ben M. Webb, David Eramian, Min-Yi Shen, Libusha Kelly, Francisco Melo, Andrej Sali, MODBASE: a database of annotated comparative protein structure models and associated resources, Nucleic Acids Research, Volume 34, Issue suppl_1, 1 January 2006, Pages D291–D295, https: //doi.org/10.1093/nar/gkj059.

15. Waterhouse, A., Bertoni, M., Bienert, S., Studer, G., Tauriello, G., Gumienny, R., Heer, F.T., de Beer, T.A.P., Rempfer, C., Bordoli, L., Lepore, R., Schwede, T. SWISS-MODEL: homology modelling of protein structures and complexes. Nucleic Acids Res. 46, W296-W303 (2018).

16. Winona C. Barker, John S. Garavelli, Peter B. McGarvey, Christopher R. Marzec, Bruce C. Orcutt, Geetha Y. Srinivasarao, Lai-Su L. Yeh, Robert S. Ledley, Hans-Werner Mewes, Friedhelm Pfeiffer, Akira Tsugita, Cathy Wu, The PIR-International Protein Sequence Database, Nucleic Acids Research, Volume 27, Issue 1, 1 January 1999, Pages 39–43, https: //doi.org/10.1093/nar/27.1.39

17. Yang Z, Lasker K, Schneidman-Duhovny D, Webb B, Huang CC, Pettersen EF, Goddard TD, Meng EC, Sali A, Ferrin TE. UCSF Chimera, MODELLER, and IMP: An integrated modeling system. J Struct Biol. 2012 Sep;179(3): 269-78.

Chapter 15

Biophysics and Structural Biology

*Ramendra Pati Pandey, Ghousepeer and Anjali Priyadarshini**

SRM University, Delhi-NCR, Rajiv Gandhi Education City, Sonepat – 131 029, Haryana, India

**e-mail: anjalipriyadarshini1@gmail.com*

ABSTRACT

The macromolecules present in a biological system have varied functions. The function is closely related to their structure. The structure is a function of the surrounding environment too. So it becomes very important to know about the structure and information about the surrounding environment of the macromolecules. Moreover there are medications which impact the exceptionally fundamental elements of living beings, like protein biosynthesis, nucleic acid replication and quality articulation, broadly referred to as antibiotics. So the information about interaction of these drugs at molecular level requires fundamental knowledge of structure and function of molecules involved. All of such studies is facilitated by techniques such as spectroscopy, NMR, CD XRD etc. This chapter gives a comprehensive knowledge about the various aspects of the macromolecules and the techniques used to study them.

Keywords: *Protein, DNA, RNA, NMR, XRD, CD, Alpha helix, Beta turn, DNA-drug interaction, DNA-protein interaction.*

Introduction

A biomolecule or organic atom is an approximately utilized term for molecules present in creatures that are crucial for at least one regularly organic cycles, like cell division, morphogenesis, or development. Biomolecules incorporate enormous macromolecules (or polyanions) like proteins, starches, lipids, and nucleic acids, just as little molecules like essential metabolites, auxiliary metabolites and characteristic items. A more broad name for this class of material is natural materials. Biochemical reactions in living cells depend on molecular collaborations between proteins, nucleic acids, sugars, lipids, and low sub-atomic weight ligands. Understanding these communications is an essential to understanding the advancement of living beings, the movement of disease, and the powerlessness of host life forms to infection causing microorganisms. Likewise, it is significant for planning new treatments. Biomolecules are a significant component of living life forms, those biomolecules are frequently endogenous, delivered inside the organic entity Biomolecular interactions, including contacts between organic macromolecules (protein/protein or protein/nucleic acids) and protein-ligand cooperations are fundamental to natural chemistry. A significant test in cell and molecular biology research is to comprehend the connection between the primary highlights of natural macromolecules and their capacity. A comprehension of the instruments that control cellular cycles requires information on how protein exercises, cooperations and complex development are controlled at explicit destinations and times in the cell. Data on how macromolecules collect into buildings and separate over the long haul is needed to characterize biomolecular restricting. These can be very not normal for those of mass material of a similar creation in light of the fact that the nanoparticle's successful surface charge, soundness, dissolvability, and hydration are incredibly influenced by the neighborhood milieu's pH, ionic strength, temperature, and natural/sub-molecular organization (*e.g.*, proteins, lipids, sugars, surfactants). These interactions includes DNA-Protein interaction, DNA-drug interactions, protein-protein interactions.

Proteins and nucleic acids are two most important biomolecules from the perspective of biophysics and structural biology. The following sections summarize the essential information regarding their structure, function and the techniques used to study them.

1. Proteins

A significant proportion of the genes in our genome code for proteins, which comprise of amino acids held together by peptide bonds. α-carboxyl group of one amino acid reacts with α-amino group of another amino acid to form a peptide bond.

1.1 Levels of Structural Organization in Proteins

1. **Primary structure** describes the order of amino acids in the polypeptide chain and the location of disulfide bonds (if any).
2. **Secondary structure** refers to particularly stable arrangements of amino acid residues giving rise to recurring structural patterns.
3. **Tertiary structure** describes the three-dimensional folding of a polypeptide.
4. **Quaternary structure** results when the proteins comprise of two or more polypeptide chains, their arrangement in space is defined by this structural level.

1.2 Fundamentals of the Peptide Bond

Linus Pauling and Robert Corey were the first to provide essential insights into the nature of peptide bond. Their careful analysis of X-ray diffraction data from simple dipeptides and tripeptides revealed that the peptide C–N bond is somewhat shorter than the amine C–N bond, and secondly, atoms associated with the peptide bond are coplanar. This results in partial sharing of two pairs of electrons between the carbonyl oxygen and the amide nitrogen. Thus, the oxygen has a partial negative charge, and the nitrogen possesses a partial positive charge leading to a dipole situation. Furthermore, the oxygen atom of the carbonyl group and the hydrogen atomof the amide nitrogen are in trans positions with respect to each other. C–N bonds are thus, unable to rotate freely due to the partial double-bond character. However, rotation can happen around the N–Cα and the Cα–C bonds. The bond angles resulting from rotations at Cα are labeled ϕ for the N–Cα bond, and Ψ for the Cα–C bond. These angles are also referred as torsion angles and dihedral angles in the context of a peptide bond. Even though ϕ and Ψ can theoretically take up values between-180°and +180°,many such values are prohibited due to possible steric interference taking place between atoms in the polypeptide backbone and side chains of the amino acids.

1.3 Different Types of Secondary Structures in Proteins

1.3.1 α-helix

The α-helix is the most common and stable conformation for a polypeptide chain. It is the most abundant helical conformation in the case of globular proteins accounting for about 32-38 per cent of all residues. The overall structure is stabilized by a hydrogen bond between the hydrogen atom attached to the electronegative nitrogen atom of a peptide bond and the electronegative carbonyl oxygen atom of the fourth amino acid on the amino-terminal side of that peptide bond. Except the peptide bonds near the ends of the helix, every peptide bond participates in such a pattern of hydrogen bonding. Each turn is formed by 3.6 residues and each successive turn of the helix is held to adjacent turns by about3-4 hydrogen bonds. The hydrogen bonds that extend throughout provides considerable stability to the helical structure. The alpha helices are usually of the right-handed type and left-handed alpha helices are a rarity, mainly due to the fact that amino acids in the proteins are of L-type.

Five different kinds of factors/constraints influence the formation and stability of an alpha helix:

1. *The electrostatic repulsion (or attraction) between successive amino acid residues with charged R groups.* Continuous block of similarly charged amino acids in a polypeptide is usually unfavorable for the formation of an alpha helix.
2. *The bulkiness of adjacent R groups.* The bulk and shape of certain amino acids like cysteine, asparagine, serine, and threonine can also destabilize an helix if they are close together in the chain.
3. *The interactions between R groups spaced three (or four) residues apart.* The twist of an α-helix ensures critical interactions between side chains of

amino acids that are 3-4 residues away. For instance, a positively charged amino acid is frequently seen three residues away from a negatively charged amino acid, allowing an ion pair to form. In a similar manner, hydrophobic interaction often results between two aromatic amino acid residues are similarly spaced.

4. *The occurrence of proline and glycine.* This is probably the most important feature to consider. The nitrogen atom in the case of proline is part of a rigid ring, which hinders any rotation about the N–Cα bond. This results in a kink or a break in the helix. Furthermore, proline being an imino acid instead of amino acid, its nitrogen atom which participates in the peptide bond has no hydrogen to take part in hydrogen bonds with other residues. Due to these reasons, occurrence of proline within an alpha-helix is extremely rare. Glycine on the other hand, due to its very small side chain often assumes coiled structures different from an alpha-helix, when present in blocks.
5. *The interaction between amino acid residues at the ends of the helical segment and the electric dipole inherent to the helix.* As mentioned before, there exists a small electric dipole in each peptide bond. With the help of hydrogen bonds in the helix, these dipoles are connected, and a resultant net dipole extends along the helix. Since the amino acids near the ends do not completely participate in the helix hydrogen bonds, a partial positive and a partial negative charge reside on the peptide amino and carbonyl groups near the amino-terminal and carboxyl-terminal ends of the helix, respectively. As a result of this, to ensure stability, negatively charged amino acids are often located near the amino terminus of the helix, and positively charged amino acids are situated at the carboxyl-terminal end of the helix.

1.3.2 Other Helical Structures

Besides α-helix, some other helical structures are also seen in the proteins. Even though they are rare and only occur at specific regions, they have structural and functional consequence. The following table summarizes and contrasts the features of the various helical structures in proteins.

Table 15.1: The Different Types of Helical Structures found in Proteins. 3.10 helices are typically observed as extensions of α-helices found at either their N- or C- termini. Like the 3.10 helix, one turn of pi helix is sometimes found at the ends of regular alpha helices.

Helix Type	*Frequency*	*phi*	*psi*	*Length of Helical Turn (Å)*	*Residue/ Turn*	*CO.HN Hydrogen Bond (i= residue position)*
Alpha	Abundant	-57.8°	-47°	5.4-5.5	3.6	i, i+4
3.10	Infrequent	-74°	-4°	6.0	3.0	i, i+3
pi	Rare	-57.1°	-69.7°	5.0	4.4	i, i+5

1.3.3 β-conformation

In the case of β-conformation, the peptide backbone is extended into a zigzag like structure rather than helix. The zigzag polypeptide chains are often arranged side by side to form a pleated structure, referred to as a β-sheet. Unlike an α-helix, in this case, hydrogen bonds are formed between adjacent segments of polypeptide chain. The individual segments forming a β-sheet can be from the same polypeptide chain and can be segments from different polypeptide chains too. When from the same polypeptide chain, the segments could be in proximity and far apart in certain cases. The R groups of adjacent amino acids protrude from the zigzag structure in opposite directions, creating the alternating pattern which is signature of the β-pleats. When two or more β-sheets are layered close together within a protein, the R groups of the amino acid residues on the touching surfaces should not be bulky, as this can lead to steric clashes. The adjacent polypeptide chains in a β-sheet can be either parallel (having the same amino-to-carboxyl orientation) or antiparallel (opposite amino-to-carboxyl orientation).The repeat period is shorter for the parallel conformation (6.5 Å), compared to the antiparallel conformation having a value of 7 Å. Furthermore, the hydrogen bonding patterns also appear distinct in appearance.

1.3.4 β-turns

β-turns connect the ends of two adjacent segments of an antiparallel β-sheet. The structure is typically made of four amino acid residues, with the carbonyl oxygen of the first residue forming a hydrogen bond with the amino-group hydrogen of the fourth. The peptide groups of the central two residues do not participate in any inter-residue hydrogen bonding. Two amino acids, glycine and proline residues frequently feature in β-turns. Glycine has a very small side chain, hence due to its flexibility it can fit in turns easily. In proline, the peptide bond involving the imino nitrogen can take up a cis configuration that favors formation of a tight turn. There are broadly two categories of β-turns-Type I and type II. Type I β-turns are more frequent compared to the type IIβ-turns. Secondly, the type II β-turns always have Gly as the third residue. Notably, the geometry of hydrogen bond also is distinct in both types.

1.4 Tertiary Structure

Tertiary structure describes the overall three-dimensional arrangement of all atoms present in a protein. Proteins are broadly classified into two major groups based on this perspective: (1) fibrous proteins; polypeptide chains are arranged in the form of long strands or sheets, and globular proteins; herein the polypeptide is folded into a spherical or globular form. While the fibrous proteins are largely made up of a single type of secondary structure; globular proteins usually are comprised of several types of secondary structures. In terms of the their function, the fibrous proteins are typically meant to provide and maintain structure and shape. Enzymes on the other hand are typical examples of globular proteins.

1.5 Ramachandran Plot

Ramachandran plot is a fundamental tool involved in the analysis of protein structures. It is a plot to visualize the energetically allowed regions for backbone

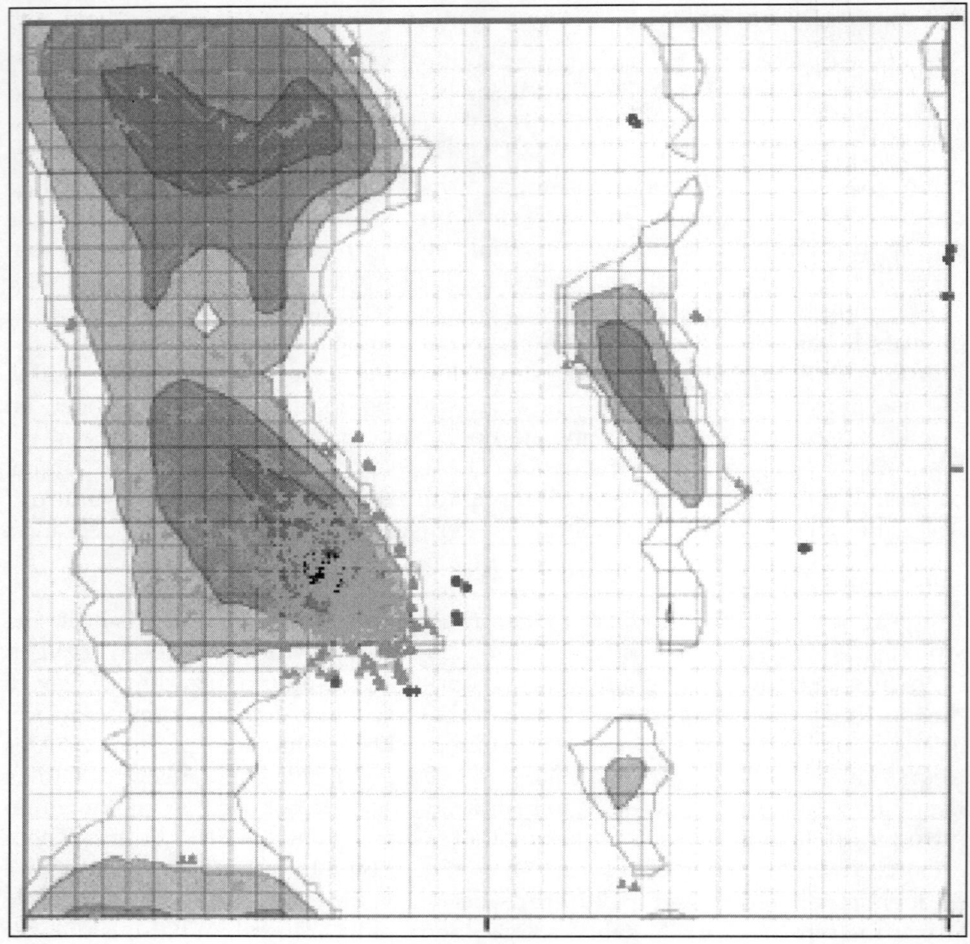

Figure 15.1: A Typical Ramachandran Plot for a Protein Structure (PDB ID: 1pv6) prepared using. online tool available at https://zlab.umassmed.edu/bu/rama/index.pl. Dots represent the amino acids of the protein. Black, dark grey, grey and light grey represent the highly preferred conformations. White with black grid represents preferred conformations. White with grey grid represents questionable conformations. Highly preferred observations shown as green crosses. Preferred observations are shown in brown triangles and questionable observations are shown as red circles.

dihedral angles ϕ against Ψ of amino acid residues in a protein structure. As mentioned before, certain rotations around the peptide chain can bring atoms too close to each other resulting in steric repulsion. In such cases, Ramachandran plot serves as an important tool to judge the quality of 3D-structures. A high-resolution structure should have the torsion angles within the allowed regions of the plot. However, theoretical calculations and observations in protein structures might vary in certain cases. For instance, the average ϕ and Ψ values for α-helices and β-sheets should ideally be around -57°,-47° and -80°, +150°, respectively. However, the experimental structures deduced show significant fluctuation in the values. Another interesting case is often seen with glycine. Glycine side chain which is of a negligible size allows for higher conformational flexibility in the polypeptide chain, thus, making otherwise forbidden rotation angles accessible.

1.6 Structural Motifs

Before understanding the various structural motifs, the basic understanding of difference between a motif and a domain is important.

Table 15.2: Difference Between a Motif and a Domain

Sl.No.	Motif	Domain
1.	A supersecondary structure of a protein	Tertiary structure of the protein
2.	Not stable independently	Stable independently
3.	Made of secondary structural elements and their connection in between	Independently folding unit of the 3D structure
4.	Mainly have structural function	Mainly have functional importance

Some basic types of structural motifs commonly seen in the proteins include:

a) β-α-β motif: These motifs are common in parallel beta sheets; wherein parallel beta strands are often connected by small alpha helical segments.

b) β-hairpin motif: These are one of the simplest structural motifs and are often present in globular proteins. They are present as short loop regions between antiparallel hydrogen bonded beta-strands.

c) α-α motif: It is made of two alpha helices connected by a short loop.

d) Greek key motif: It is made up of four adjacent antiparallel beta strands folded upon itself to give appearance of a Greek key, hence the name.

Besides some of the basic structural motif types, certain structural motifs are essentially seen in the DNA binding or regulatory proteins. All these motifs have distinct signatures which are relevant for specific interactions with the DNA molecule. These motifs recognize specific DNA sequence because their surface is extensively complementary to the special surface features of the double helix in that region. A significant number of number of contacts with the DNA, involving hydrogen bonds, ionic bonds, and hydrophobic interactions are usually established. With several such contacts at the protein-DNA interface, both specific and very strong interactions are conferred. Some common examples are highlighted below:

a) Helix-turn-helix Motif

This motif is one of the most common motifs seen in gene regulatory proteins. The basic structure comprises of two helices connected by a turn. The C-terminal α-helix is called the recognition helix and it participates in sequence-specific interaction with the DNA. The recognition helix recognizes and fits into the major groove of DNA, wherein it interacts with the edges of the base pairs. The interaction involves a series of hydrogen bonds and also Van der Waals interactions. The N-terminal α-helix essentially acts as a structural component that helps position the recognition helix for its interaction with the major groove. In most of the cases, these motifs function as dimers. For instance, the λ repressor of lambda-phage utilizes two helix-turn-helix motifs to interact with DNA.

b) Zinc-finger Motif

One common form of zinc-finger is present in the Cys-Cys-His-His family of zinc finger proteins. The three-dimensional structure of this type of zinc finger is comprised of an antiparallel β-sheet followed by an α-helix. Four amino acids, namely two cysteine and two histidine residues coordinate with a zinc atom and hold one end of the α-helix firmly to one end of the β-sheet. Like the helix-turn-helix motif, zinc-fingers also participate as multimers while interacting with DNA, thus increasing the strength and specificity of the interactions. Another form of zinc finger is present in the family of certain intracellular receptor proteins, wherein instead of one β-sheet and oneα-helix, two alpha helices coordinate with the zinc atom. Although structurally distinct, both use zinc as a structural element, and both use an α-helix to recognize the major groove of the DNA.

c) Leucine-zipper Motif

The motif is comprised of two α helices, one from each monomer, which are joined together to form a short coiled-coil (hence, the name). These helices are held close together with the help of hydrophobic interactions between the side chains of non-polar amino acid residues, (mostly leucines) that extend from one side of each helix. At some distance from the dimerization interface, the two α helices separate from each other to form a Y-shaped structure, allowing the side chains of the amino acid residues to establish specific contacts with the major groove of DNA. Each arm of the Y can be from same proteins (homodimer) or different proteins (heterodimer).

d) Helix-loop-helix Motif

This type of DNA-binding motif has an overall structural resemblance to the leucine zipper. The motif consists of 2 alpha helices, a short one connected by a loop to a second, longer one. The flexibility of this loop allows one helix to fold back and pack against the other. This two-helix structure binds both to DNA as well as to another helix-loop-helix motif from a second protein. This second helix-loop-helix containing protein can be the same (a homodimer) or different (a heterodimer). The two longer alpha- helices extending from the dimerization interface make specific contacts with the major groove of the DNA.

2. Nucleic Acids

Nucleic acids are built from nucleotides which essentially contain three components: a nitrogenous base, a pentose sugar, and a phosphate. The molecule without the phosphate group is called a nucleoside. The nitrogenous bases are of further two types, the pyrimidine and purine. Nucleic acids contain two types of pentose sugars. While the DNA contains nucleotide units with 2′-deoxy-D-ribose, the nucleotide units of RNA contain D-ribose. The pentose sugars are also in their β-furanose form. Both DNA and RNA contain two major purines, adenine and guanine. and two major pyrimidines. Out of the two pyrimidines, one is cytosine, but the second one is different in both types of nucleic acids. Thymine present in DNA is replaced by a uracil in RNA.

The phosphate groups play an important role in connecting the successive nucleotides of DNA and RNA. The 5′-phosphate group of one nucleotide unit is linked to the 3′-OH group of the next nucleotide creating via a phosphodiester linkage.

2.1 Structure of DNA

It was Rosalind Franklin and Maurice Wilkins who laid the foundation for solving the structure of DNA. They utilized X-ray diffraction studies to reveal the typical diffraction pattern of a DNA molecule. It was clear from the pattern that that DNA molecules are helical in shape and possess two periodicities along their long axis, a primary one of 3.4 Å and a secondary one of 34 Å. Watson and Crick utilized this knowledge as a template and exploited other already available information like the Chargaff's rule (no. of A=T and G=C in a DNA molecule)to propose the 3D-model of DNA. As per the model, two helical strands are wound around the same axis to form a right-handed double helical structure of DNA. The sugar-phosphate backbone faces the exterior of the double helix and contacts the surrounding water. Nitrogenous bases from both strands are stacked inside the double helix. The offset pairing of the two strands creates a major groove and minor groove on the surface of the duplex. Nitrogenous base of one nucleotide from one strand pairs with a base of the other strand within the same plane. To take Chargaff's rule into account, Watson and Crick proposed that a G always should pair with C and A should always pair with T, better known as the complimentary pairing. Notably, three hydrogen bonds form between G and C, and two can form between A and T. They also arrived at a conclusion after extensive analysis that the proposed model appears conclusive when the strands of DNA run antiparallel to each other. In other words, 5,3-phosphodiester bonds of the two strands run in the opposite directions.

2.2 Other Forms of DNA

The Watson-Crick structure described above is referred to as the B form of DNA, or B-DNA. The B form is the most stable form for a DNA molecule under physiological conditions and is used as the standard point of reference for studying the structural features. However, two other structural variants are also known for DNA and have been well studies with the help of crystal structures. These forms are denoted as the A and Z forms. Table 15.3 summarizes its features and contrasts them with features of the B form.

Table 15.3: Table Summarizing the Features of different Structural Forms of DNA

	A Form	B Form	Z Form
Helical sense	Right-handed	Right-handed	Left-handed
Diameter	~26 Å	~20 Å	~18 Å
Base pairs per helical turn	11	10.5	12
Helix rise per base pair	2.6 Å	3.4 Å	3.7 Å
Sugar pucker conformation	C-3' endo	C-2' endo	C-2' endo for pyrimidines; C-3' endo for purines
Glycosyl bond conformation	Anti	Anti	Anti for pyrimidines, syn for purines
Occurrence	favored in solutions devoid of water	physiological conditions	Alternating pyrimidines and purines, namely G and C

2.3 Unusual Structures of DNA

Under many conditions, some unusual structures of DNA that involve three to four strands can develop. Besides the usual base pairing seen in DNA structures, better known as Watson-Crick base pair, a few additional hydrogen bonds can be formed by the nucleotides. For example, a cytidine residue (if protonated) can pair with the guanosine residue of a Ga"C nucleotide pair, and a thymidine can pair with the adenosine of an A=T pair. Three atoms of the purines, namely, N-7, *O*6, and *N*6 of purines, participate in the hydrogen bonding and result in the formation of triplex DNA. These atoms are referred to as Hoogsteen positions, and the resultant non-Watson-Crick type pairing is regarded as Hoogsteen pairing. One example, Ca"G^{a}%C^{+} typically forms under low pH conditions, because there is requirement of a protonated cytosine.

Four DNA strands can also pair to form a special type of tetraplex/quadruplex structure, when the DNA sequences are richly populated with guanosine residues. This G quadruplex is relatively much more stable than other unusual structures that are known. The G-quadruplex can also be intramolecular as well as intermolecular.

Another kind of unusual structure is called as the i-motif. i-motifs are four-stranded DNA structures held together by hemi-protonated and intercalated cytosine base pairs (C:C+).Initially it was thought that i-motif structures can only develop at acidic pH values due to the requirement of hemi-protonated base pairs. However, recent studies have shown that phenomenon such as molecular crowding favors G quadruplex and i- motif formation. i-motif structures are usually located in the regulatory regions of the genome and both G4 and i-motif structures play complementary roles in the regulation of gene expression.

2.4 Structure of RNA

The single-stranded RNA which is product of transcription assumes a right-handed helical conformation which primarily is stabilized by base stacking interactions, which are stronger between two purines than between a purine and pyrimidine or between two pyrimidines. Any self-complementary sequences in the molecule produce more complex structures.

3. Denaturation of Proteins and Nucleic acids: Effects of Temperature, pH *etc.*

Denaturation of proteins involves the disruption of the secondary and tertiary structures. Since the effect of denaturants are not strong enough to break peptide bonds, the primary structure remains intact after the denaturation process. However, denaturation can disrupt the secondary structure elements like the alpha-helices and beta sheets and result in a more random shape. Some of the common denaturants and their effects are summarized below:

Table 14.4: Table Summarizing the Effect of different Denaturing Conditions on the Protein Structure. Information partly compiled from: https://chem.libretexts.org/

	Effect on Protein Structure
Temperatures above 50°C or ultraviolet (UV) radiation	Heat or UV radiation supplies kinetic energy which cause the atoms to vibrate more rapidly and disrupting the relatively weak hydrogen bonding and dispersion forces.
Use of organic compounds, such as ethyl alcohol	These compounds can engage inhydrogen bonding with protein molecules, disrupting intramolecular hydrogen bonding within the protein.
Salts of heavy metal ions, such as mercury, silver, and lead	These ions can form strong bonds with the carboxyl groups and SH groups of the negatively charged amino acids and cysteine, respectively, disrupting the native linkages.
Urea	Urea causes protein denaturation in multiple ways. One primary mechanism involves hydrogen bonding of urea to polarized areas of charge, like the peptide groups. This results in weakening of the intermolecular bonds and interactions, thus altering the overall secondary and tertiary structure.

Native DNA solutions are highly viscous at room temperature and neutral pH conditions. When such a solution is subjected to extremes of pH or to temperatures above 80 to 90°C, the DNA undergone a physical change and the viscosity of the solution changes drastically. Much similar to proteins, heat and extremes of pH also result in denaturation or melting of double helical DNA. This phenomenon includes loss of the hydrogen bonds between the base pairs as well as the hydrophobic interactions between the stacked bases. As a result, the double helical structure unwinds to form two single strands, which can be completely or partially separated from each other. Like the protein denaturation process, covalent bonds in the DNA remain intact.

Thermal denaturation studies provide crucial insights into the secondary structure of DNA molecules. Since G and C base pairs are held together by three hydrogen bonds compared to A and T, which are only held together by two hydrogen bonds, a DNA sample with a high GC content will require much more energy to separate the strands, leading to a higher DNA melting temperature. UV-vis Spectrophotometry is generally used to monitor the thermal denaturation of

DNA, wherein the sample is heated to allow the determination of the DNA melting temperature.

4. Biomolecular Interactions

DNA-Protein Interaction

Among proteins and nucleic acids interaction control the controlled and coordinated articulation of the genome in cell metabolism, replication, and improvement functional classes of DNA-associating proteins can be partitioned further into those which communicate with explicit nucleotide successions or locales and those which connect with the DNA non-arrangement explicitly. we should be worried about both the chemical types sorts of functional groups accessible on every macromolecule and the overall demeanor of these groups in space. From this viewpoint similar sorts of configurational and compound thinking should be applied to the DNA-protein interaction issue as have generally been utilized in thinking about the particularity of the communication among proteins and their substrates and inhibitors. The prospects inborn in the tertiary structure and subunit communications of globular proteins are basically boundless, and along these lines we will move toward the issue by considering the varieties conceivable in the more mentally manageable accomplice: the DNA. We should briefly understand the structure of DNA that characterize the conformational, chemical, and thermodynamic features in solution. There are few structural aspects in DNA-PROTEIN interaction process by inspecting the DNA molecule as it might appear to a protein (*e.g.* repressor) in search of a specific sequence of bases (*e.g.* an operator site) with which to interact.

Pathway is used by proteins in searching for the interaction site Most biologically critical connections among protein and DNA happen under conditions in which the local, twofold helical structure addresses the **thermodynamically** preferred DNA structure. However proteins exist that tight spot explicitly to one or the other local or random coil (single-stranded) DNA districts under these conditions. The last sort, which we call liquefying 'proteins, promptly approach a degree of grouping explicitness controlled by contrasts in the neighborhood solidness of the local DNA twofold helix. Accordingly the free energy of restricting of a protein to a single strand of DNA in an area ordinarily twofold abandoned under the predominant natural conditions should at any rate balance the free energy preferring the local over the arbitrary curl conformity at that locus. Inorganic ions, dyes, *etc.* illustrate interaction modes available with DNA for ligands these might serve as models for certain types of functional groups found in proteins, these also defines other interactive specificities of which DNA is capable.

4.1 Different Level of Specificity for DNA-Protein Interaction

In Binding site specification We first consider the framework in quite a while of supreme particularity; *i.e.*, we expect a protein that can totally (and as it were) segregate between the four data components of DNA. There are four authoritative nucleotide deposits (A, T, G, and C) in single-abandoned DNA and four kinds of base sets (APT, T-A, G-C, and C(G) in twofold abandoned DNA. The last will be our essential concentration here. A particular restricting site is perceived as far as explicit arrangements of base sets. A contingent likelihood approach[10] can be utilized to decide the negligible length (n) of a arrangement of acknowledgment components (base sets) needed to determine a site, with the goal that the normal recurrence with which that site returns indiscriminately inside the genome is not as much as solidarity. For E. coli DNA this negligible length is - 12 base sets, expecting a twofold abandoned succession inside a genome of generally speaking creation A = T = G = C. This methodology accepts that the general grouping of the genome can be treated as synthetically (however clearly not hereditarily) arbitrary and that each base pair is completely indicated (as far as base-pair type). Unknown loci can, obviously, intrude on the general succession in characterized positions, however these loci won't check toward n. Essentially, determination just at the degree of R-Y (purine-pyrimidine) (versus Y-R) base sets can happen; such loci are weighted less in setting up.

After the binding site specification now the sequence should be recognized there are two mechanism **primary** and **secondary sequence recognition mechanism.** In **primary sequence recognition mechanism** The molecular mechanism that can unambiguously perceive and segregate singular base sets in twofold abandoned DNA is complementary hydrogen-holding through the major or minor scores of the twofold helix. These acknowledgment examples of hydrogen-bond donors and acceptors on DNA have been unequivocally recorded by Seeman *et al.*, and have been introduced in an especially basic and valuable "stick-figure" portrayal. Such acknowledgment relies upon the cooperation of the pertinent hydrogen-bond donor and acceptor gatherings of the DNA base pair with a complementary matrix of hydrogen bond acceptor and donor bunches gave by suitably situated amino corrosive and peptide utilitarian gatherings in the restricting site of the administrative protein. This hydrogen-reinforced acknowledgment matrix approach has all the more as of late been utilized by crystallographers in finding cooperation in explicit protein nucleic corrosive association buildings. Contrary in **Secondary sequence recognition mechanism** When the issue isn't the total ID of a specific sequence of base pairs by an administrative protein, other recognition components, at a "lower level" of detail, can likewise become an integral factor. Subsequently DNA "districts" can be segregated at the level of strandedness (*e.g.*, single-versus twofold stranded), groove math and optional construction (*e.g.*, B-versus Z-structure DNA, *etc.*, in light of contrasts in protein restricting fondness. The starting points of these fondness contrasts can be steric, conformational, or electrostatic and may reflect underlying results of provincial contrasts in base-pair arrangement. Models incorporate the favored restricting of tetraalkylammonium particles to dA*dT groupings in the (major) furrow of B-DNA, the favored restricting of the anti-toxins netropsin and distamycin in the minor notches of poly(dAdT) what's more, dA-dT-rich groupings of B-structure DNA, the nonspecific restricting of E. coli lac repressor to twofold abandoned DNA, the particular restricting of phage T4 quality 32-encoded protein to single-abandoned DNA and RNA, and the differential sensitivities of quality explicit eukaryotic DNA districts to endonucleases[21]. Such communications clearly give a proportion of local restricting particularity. Be that as it may, they don't convey sufficient primary data to give an instrument to the essential acknowledgment of explicit base-pair groupings by proteins. Such acknowledgment should begin in hydrogen-holding bonds

For affinity Tolerating the idea that particular objective site acknowledgment does surely include the "reading," by an administrative protein, of a explicit cluster of hydrogen-holding benefactors and acceptors in the major and minor sections of the DNA twofold helix, we next think about the topic of quantitative explicitness or segregation, which can likewise be named "the issue of the different locales." This issue exists since segregation between, for model, "right" and "wrong" base sets can't be absolute. Maybe there is some limited level of liking of the protein for the "right" site and some lower (yet nonzero) and dynamically diminishing partiality for different locales with decreasing levels of homology with the right one. To the degree that the incredible prevalence of wrong destinations can contend with the administrative objective for protein and in this manner diminish the free protein focus, the successful liking of protein for the right destinations will likewise be decreased.

4.2 Analysis of DNA-Protein Interaction

Electromobility shift measure is a basic, proficient, and quick strategy for the investigation of explicit DNA–protein associations. It depends on the decrease in the electrophoretic versatility gave to a DNA part by a cooperating protein. The procedure is reasonable to subjective, quantitative, and dynamic examinations. It can additionally be utilized to dissect conformational changes. This is based on the basic reasoning that particles of varying size, sub-atomic weight, and charge will have diverse electrophoretic mobilities in a non denaturing gel lattice. On account of a DNA– protein complex, the presence of a DNA-binding protein will cause the complex to relocate in an unexpected way (generally more gradually) comparative with the free DNA, and will subsequently cause a shift apparent upon identification.

4.3 DNA-drug Interactions

The DNA- Drug interaction has been to designed specifically for rare diseases and to target their action at the DNA level. Uncommon strategies have now been created to give exact record of the exact area of ligand-DNA adducts on DNA that is target. The acknowledgment of one sort of molecule by another is key also, a typical component of every single living life form. The replication of DNA and its record to RNA, which gives the format to protein amalgamation, is maybe extraordinary compared to other known illustration of molecular recognition. These nonprotein molecules that are known to tie DNA atoms incorporates common items like anti-microbials, antitumor *etc.* what's more, other optional metabolites from microbes and growths and plants, manufactured mixtures, *viz.*; CC 1065, copper phenanthroline complex, Alkylnitroso-urea and homopyrimidine oligonucleotides· The cooperation of generally little particles of this kind with DNA may prompt a "valuable" results like antibacterial and anticancer action, yet may likewise include unfortunate natural reactions, for example, carcinogenesis or mutagenesis.

4.3.1 Methods of Drug Interaction

these interactions can hinder the cycles identified with DNA through replication and transcription in the accompanying ways which includes, Inhibition of Template Functions, Inhibition of polymerase function, Inhibitor complexing with template and inhibits polymerase function, Triple-helix formers. In Inhibition of Template Functions there are different **Intercalators,**

Noncovalent Binding Formers and Covalent Binding Formers

Intercalators which are planar molecules with 3-4 fused aromatic rings this has ability to intercalating between stacked nucleic acid base pairs. The intercalating drugs are Actinomycin D Anthracylins *e.g.*, Duanomycins Nogalomycins Cinnerubins Pyrromycins Rhodomycins Profavine, Acridine, and Ethidium.

In **Noncovalent complex formers** There are a group of compounds like distamycin, netropsin, A3, chromomycin A3, SN18071, mithramycin, hedamycin, olivomycin, pluramycin and rubiflavin. distamycin A3, Netrospin are generally long, adaptable, molecules with at least one emphatically charged end gatherings and a number of proton giver and acceptor bunches along their length. Minor groove covers are normally isohelical with B-DNA and fit cozily inside the minor section stood firm on in footing by a mix of hydrogen bonds, van der Waals powers, and electrostatic connections.

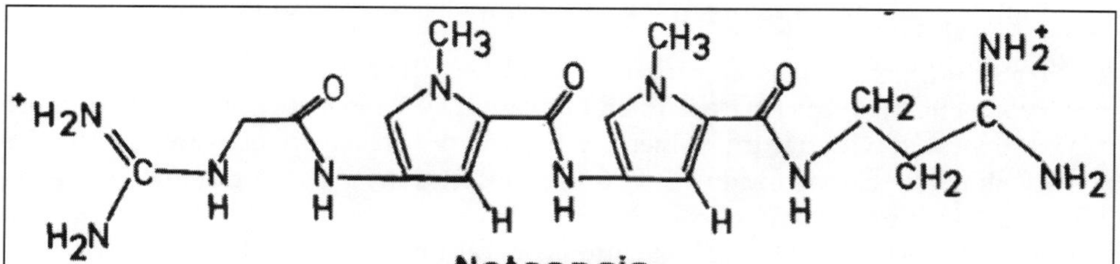

Figure 15.2: The Structure of the DNA Interactive Ligands Netropsin.

The succession selectivity of netropsin-like folios for A-T rich locale of DNA is a typical element, and one clarification is that steric obstacle may result from projection of guanine C2-NH2 bunch into the minor groove at GC destinations. On the other hand, A-T rich arrangements may compare to destinations of most extreme sub-atomic electrostatic potential (MEP) in the minor score, which may draw in ligands, particularly those with cationic utilitarian gatherings. The bisquaternary heterocycle SN18071 can't structure hydrogen bonds yet at the same time ties in the minor section with a comparable AT selectivity, obviously affirming the part of electrostatic fascination. Be that as it may, a netropsin subsidiary without cationic end gatherings can still tie to poly(dA)- poly(dt) oligomers, exhibiting that electrostatic fascination or communications are not fundamental for restricting. As of late, it has been recommended that the inclination for restricting is for a more equivalent dispersion of GC and AT base sets.

Chromomycin A3, mithramycin and olivomycin are additionally intercalated into DNA and are firmly related anti-toxins having indistinguishable components of activity and are considered collectively. The sugar sidechains contrast in three anti-toxins and the chromophore of olivomycin is somewhat extraordinary.

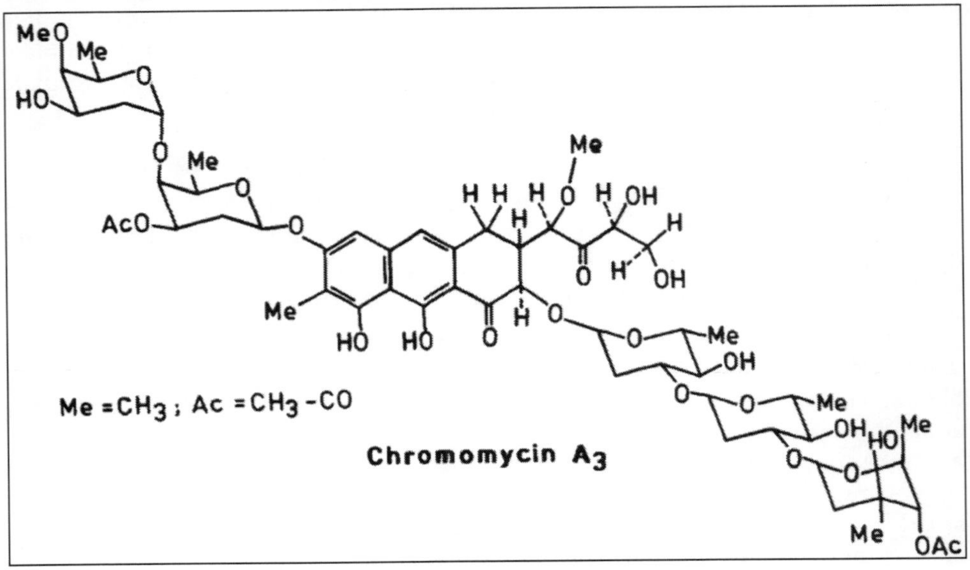

Figure 15.3: The Structure of the DNA Interactive Ligand Chromomycin A_3.

These antigens are intense inhibitors of record in the two prokaryotes and eukaryotes. Stable edifices are framed between DNA also, anti-infection yet these can be separated with natural solvents which demonstrates that covalent securities are not shaped. Like actinomycin D these medications are additionally requiring 2-NH2 gatherings of G in helical DNA for complex development however vary in requiring the presence of divalent cation for communication like Mg^{2+} particles.

In **Covalent binding formers** natural products along with carbinolamines, epoxide, imines, aziridines with Electrophilic utilitarian gatherings are equipped for covalent collaboration with DNA. Nitrogen mustards, for example, mechlorethamine address one of the easiest classes of covalent folios, and numerous mixtures of this family are clinically helpful anticancer medications. They act by crosslinking DNA through covalent bonds to G N-7 iotas in the significant depression and display selectivity for a guanine flanked by two different guanines.

The alkylating species is by and large viewed as the cyclic aziridinium particle and the selectivity can be seen by estimation showing that the most noteworthy MEP at a G N-7 of a focal G in a GGG grouping is more prominent than other agent trios like AGA or TGT.

Mitomycin C is illustrative of anti-microbials which tie to a DNA format by covalent linkage. Upon enactment by synthetic or enzymatic decrease mitomycin turns into a bisfunctional alkylating specialist that can frame covalent bonds with numerous kinds of natural particles, including nucleic acids.

As a bisfunctional alkylating specialist, mitomycin incites crosslinks between the correlative strands of the DNA, subsequently guaranteeing unconstrained renaturation of the DNA when the strands are in part isolated. It ties to N-2 or N-7 of G in minor score or significant furrow through carbocation species.

Table 15.5: Covalent Binding Drug Compounds along with their Binding Action

Covalent Binding Drug Compounds	*Binding Action*
Mitomycin C	To N2 of N-7 of G in minor or major groove via carbocation species
Alkylinitrosourea	To N-7 of G in major groove via carbocation species
Aflatoxin B1 oxide	To N-7 of G in minor groove via an epoxide (formed through metabolism) (24)
Anthramycin	To N2 of G in minor groove via a carbinolamine moiety (25-27)
Mitozolamides	To N-7 of G in major groove

For **Inhibition of Polymerase Function** Two firmly related anti-infection agents, Rifamycin B and Rifampicin are intense inhibitors of prokaryotic RNA polymerase: Rifamycin B is delivered by *Streptomyces mediterrani* and rifampicin is its semisynthetic subsidiary. It is unmistakable for prokaryotic RNA polymerase however doesn't by any means influence eukaryotic RNA. It is utilized against gram-positive microorganisms and furthermore in tuberculosis. The RNA polymerase comprises of two α, β and one σ subunit: The σ subunit has a limiting site for this medication. This medication doesn't restrain the extension interaction, however the consolidation of the initial purine nucleotide into RNA is obstructed. This inactivates RNA polymerase and this inactivated catalyst consistently stays bound to the DNA, along these lines impeding the limiting of uninhibited catalyst

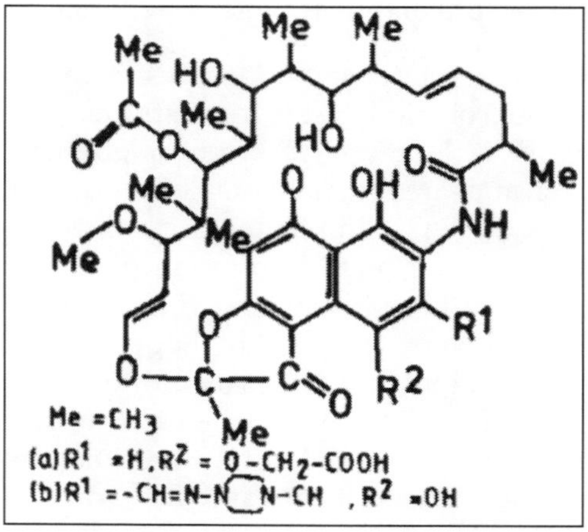

Figure 15.4: The Structure of the DNA Interactive Ligand (a) Ri famycin B (b) Rifampicin.

For **Inhibitor Complexing with Template and Inhibiting Polymerase Function** an intense LUTEOSKYRIN which is hepatotoxic discharged from the growth mat Penicillium islandicum, related with yellow rice, contains an indistinguishable pair of 4-membered ring frameworks. This communicates with DNA yet just within the sight of stoichiometric mounts of Mg^{2+}. As with the chromomycin-like anti-toxins, Luteoskyrin Mg^{2+} complex is framed first and this accordingly ties to DNA. It can frame two unmistakable sorts of buildings with DNA. Complex I is shaped quickly with single-abandoned nucleic acids containing purine bases. To shape complex I in any event 5-6 nucleotide long oligonucleotides ought to be available, which proposes that a particular compliance is needed for this limiting. Complex II is shaped with twofold abandoned nucleic acids. For complex I development any purine buildup in a polynucleotide is a possible site however, neither the idea of the purine nor the idea of the sugar is significant. It is a strong inhibitor of *E. coli* RNA polymerase.

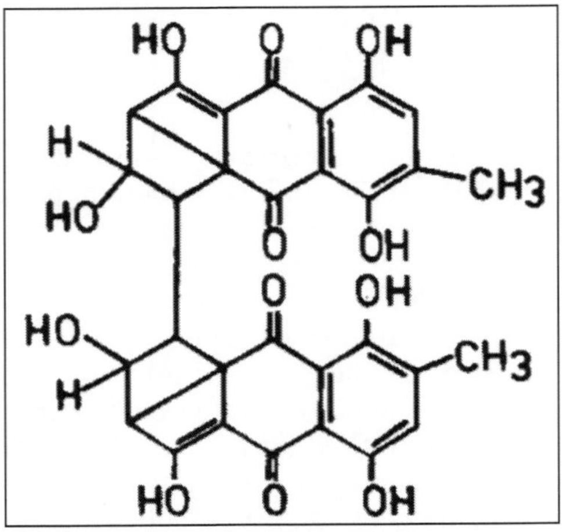

HO O OH H HO CH3 O OH O OH HO H CH3 HO O OH

Figure 15.5: The Structure of the DNA Interactive Ligand LUTEOSKYRIN.

In Triple-Helix Formation interaction includes the development of a "Triple Helix." Triple helix formers or trio DNA, a triple strand type of DNA was created by Alexander Rich in 1957. Homopyrimidrine oligonucleotides of 10-20 base combines long have been appeared to shape stable edifices in the significant section at homopurine with GC and AT complementarity. Specialists in a few labs are investigating the utilization of trio DNA to produce another kind of "molecular scissors" for cutting DNA. It has been exhibited as of late that trio DNA can be produced at explicit destinations on normally happening qualities, and this can upset quality record. The first test confirmation of the chance of the utilization of trio DNA in treatment came 5 years prior when Hogan and Hay Balor partners appeared that, at any rate in a test-tube test, trio development could specifically repress an objective quality. This was corresponded with constraint of the action of the human myc quality. One of the objectives of this kind of exploration work is to foster explicit tests that can perceive a specific grouping of base sets with a view to change quality articulation. There is specific interest in creating ligands with GC particularity since the greater part of the realized mixtures are AT particular. This interest begun from the finding that locales of high GC content are normal in genomes of vertebrates, including people, and 5′ flanks of certain oncogenes.

4.4 Protein- Protein Interactions

To control various biological phenomena which includes cell to cell interactions and metabolic process proteins undergo Protein to protein interactions (PPI). In humans, disturbances of the normal patterns of PPIs and protein complexes can be causative or demonstrative of a disease state. PPIs incorporate heterogeneous strategies generally and the chance of their guideline is colossal. Different communications and the result of these connections are expected to recognize the better comprehension of PPIs inside the cell. Test judgments of connections between proteins are done at either an enormous or limited scope with two primary innovations that produce various kinds of PPI information. The procedures that action direct actual collaborations between protein sets are "binary" strategies, while the strategies that action actual communications among gatherings of proteins, without pairwise assurance of protein accomplices, are "co-complex" techniques. The frequently utilized parallel and co-complex systems are, separately, yeast two-mixture (Y2H) and pair partiality refinement coupled to mass spectrometry (TAP-MS). Both are broadly applied in huge scope examinations. Co-complex techniques measure both immediate and roundabout connections between proteins. The most well-known methodology depends on the pre-choice of one protein labeled with a sub-atomic marker (the trap protein), which is utilized to catch or "fish out" a gathering of proteins (prey proteins) trailed by a biochemical strategy to "pull-down" and separate them from a blend. Along these lines, what happens is a co-purging of protein gatherings. Another regular co-complex methodology, in light of protein counter acting agent acknowledgment, is co-inmunoprecipitation (CoIP). The trial results got with co-complex techniques are unique in relation to those got with parallel strategies. Information got from co-complex examinations can't be straightforwardly allocated a twofold translation. A calculation or model is expected to make an interpretation of gathering based perceptions into pairwise collaborations. The spoke model is most regularly utilized, as it delivers the insignificant number of bogus positives. An illustration of organizations got from Y2H versus TAP-MS outlines the distinctions that must be surely known by any analyst delivering or breaking down PPI information.

4.4.1 Interactions of Hemoglobin and Myoglobin

Hemoglobin (Hb) fills in as oxygen transporter in red blood cells. In the physiologically dynamic protein, every one of the four subunits contains a ferrous heme iron (FeII) that is composed by a proximal histidine. Oxygen restricting happens at the inverse face of the heme, where O_2 can involve the leftover coordination site while additionally framing a H-bond with a distal histidine. The oxygen-soaked protein (with four O_2 bound) is alluded to as HbO_2. Myoglobin (Mb) is a monomeric oxygen stockpiling protein that displays a tertiary design basically the same as that of the Hb subunits. Ligand collaborations in Mb are similar to those talked about above for Hb. Oxygen restricting to FeII heme creates MbO_2, while carbon monoxide openness yields MbCO. Mb auto-oxidation produces water-bound FeIII Mb that promptly converts to MbCN within the sight of CN–. A key contrast among Hb and Mb is the noncooperative restricting component of the last mentioned, leading to O_2 restricting profiles that are exaggerated instead of sigmoidal. The oxygen conveyed by hemeproteins, for example, hemoglobin and myoglobin is bound straightforwardly to the ferrous iron (Fe^{2+}) iota of the heme prosthetic gathering. Oxidation of the iron to the ferric (Fe^{3+}) state delivers the atom unequipped for ordinary oxygen restricting.

4.4.2 G-protein Coupled Receptors

Most metabotropic receptors are G protein-coupled receptors (GPCRs). The GPCR family includes around 800 human receptors that are coordinated into five subfamilies, to be specific classes A (the biggest gathering), B, C, frizzled, and bond. Thinking about the construction, GPCRs have a comparable compliance showing an exceptional seven TM (7TM) α-helical locale, an extracellular amino-terminal section and an intracellular carboxy-terminal tail. While the area that is confined in the extracellular segment permits the ligand(s) – receptor connection, the TM district is liable to a conformational change when the limiting with a ligand happens; this change is then sent to the intracellular locale of the GPCR answerable for actuating the flagging course. GPCR monomers can perceive/translate signals specifically, an inborn versatility portrays GPCR monomers motioning, indeed GPCR enactment can decide the beginning of various sign transduction designs, similar to the G proteins or potentially arrestin pathways. Moreover, it is set up that GPCRs can practically associate by sharing flagging pathways or by components of transactivation

By these biomolecular interactions with the scientific strategies we have had comprehend the method of acknowledgment of DNA sequencing by these different medications and identifying different ligands binding site. This agreement can be used to plan explicit medications for a particular infection. These medications will be extraordinary for a specific quality and of conceivable use in treatment. Specificity of protein-nucleic acid interactions involved in the regulation (at the DNA level) of biological function.

5. UV-VIS Spectroscopy

Electromagnetic radiation spans a wide range of energy levels in a continuum called the electromagnetic spectrum. Each part of this spectrum may be characterized by a specific range of wavelengths. Living organisms are constantly exposed to a wide range of electromagnetic radiation from the Sun or other stars. Man-made sources of radiation include heated filaments of the type found in ordinary light bulbs. We can select for different parts of the electromagnetic spectrum using a prism or similar device. Depending on its energy content, radiation from different parts of the electromagnetic spectrum may interact with biomolecules in a wide variety of ways. Electromagnetic radiation therefore provides a useful means to probe the chemical structure of biomolecules. In this chapter we will look at the electromagnetic spectrum and describe some of the experimental information it is possible to derive from studying interactions between electromagnetic radiation and biomolecules.

We have seen that light from the Sun is white but, when it impacts on a coloured object, some of this light is absorbed and it is the reflected or nonabsorbed light which gives us the sensation of colour. If light in the ultraviolet/visible part of the electromagnetic spectrum is passed through a sample in solution, some light energy may also be absorb molecules (or parts of molecules) capable of absorbing light are called chromophores. This is known as an absorption spectroscopy experiment and it is of use because the particular frequencies at which light is absorbed are affected by both the structure and the environment of the chromophore. Light energy is used to promote electrons from the ground state to various excited states. Each chemical structure absorbs slightly different frequencies of light since each has a characteristic electronic structure (*i.e.* pattern of electron distribution). The ground and excited electronic energy levels each contain many vibrational energy levels differing from each other by smaller energy increments than those between the electronic energy levels. Excited electrons can return to the ground state by vibrational transitions through these smaller energy increments.

The light energy absorbed therefore appears ultimately as heat in the solution. The absorption phenomenon may be quantified by the Beer–Lambert law:

$$\log I_0/I = \varepsilon \cdot c \cdot l$$

where I_0 is the intensity of incident light, I is the intensity of transmitted light, c is the molar concentration and l is the length of the light path (usually 1 cm). ε is the molar extinction coefficient. The term [$\log I_0/I$] is the absorbance (Aλ) at a particular wavelength or frequency.

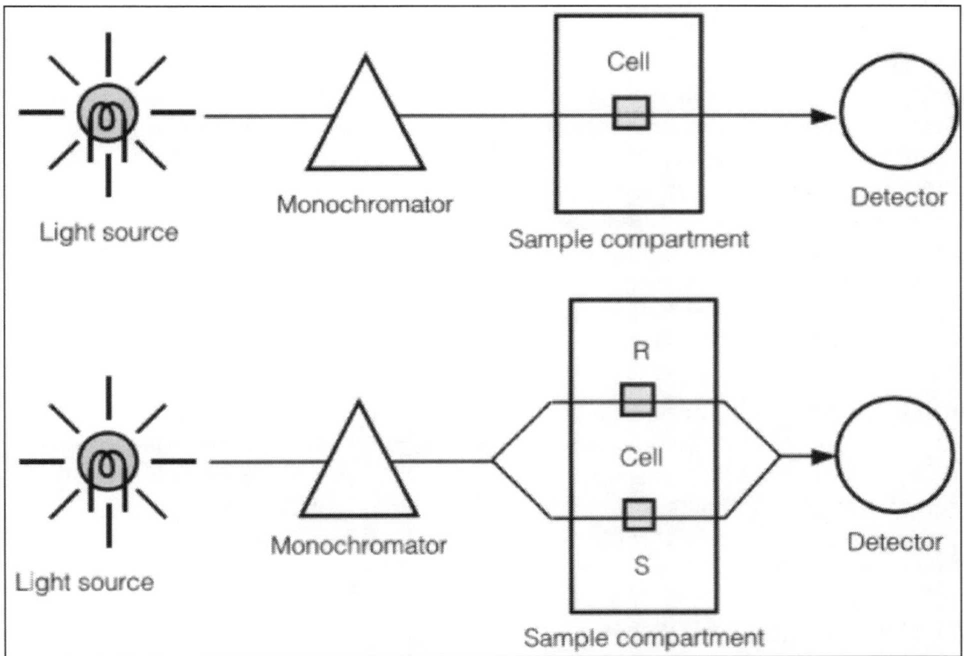

Figure 15.6: Working of UV-VIS Spectrophotometer.

A plot of Aλ or ε versus wavelength or frequency is known as an absorption spectrum. Wavelengths corresponding to maxima in such spectra are denoted by λmax. Under standard conditions, this spectrum is a fixed property of a pure chromophore and may therefore be used in identification of previously-characterized molecules. Moreover, since absorbance is directly dependent on molar concentration, it may be used as a measure of concentration provided a standard curve for that chromophore is also available. Absorbance is an especially appropriate scale for measuring interactions between light and molecules in solution in that, when no light is absorbed, this term has a value of 0. When light is absorbed, the absorbance value increases. In theory, the parameter is linear and can reach a maximum of infinity.

Applications of Absorption Spectroscopy Since many biomolecules possess distinct absorption spectra, absorption spectroscopy has a wide range of applications in biochemistry. Advantage is frequently taken of the Beer–Lambert law to carry out quantitative measurements. If the value of ε is known, it is possible to calculate concentrations directly from absorbance readings at specific wavelengths. In enzyme assays the concentration of either substrate or product may be measured to allow calculation of rates of enzyme-catalyzed reactions. These measurements may be continuous (*i.e.* the reaction is monitored continuously in the light-beam of a spectrophotometer) or stopped (*i.e.* the reaction is halted at various time-points and spectroscopic measurements are performed separately from the reaction producing product or consuming substrate). For example, reduction of NAD to NADH + H+ by oxidoreductase enzymes is conveniently followed by continuous measurement of A340. NADH has a strong λmax at this wavelength while NAD does not. Other quantitative applications of absorbance measurements include measurement of concentrations of biomolecules with the aid of a standard curve. A second type of application involves structural studies of biopolymers such as proteins and DNA. These are complex biomacromolecules and their assembly and unfolding are of considerable research interest. Chromophores, which are part of these molecules, are very sensitive to their immediate environment. We can often follow assembly/denaturation processes in such molecules, therefore, simply by monitoring absorbance changes at particular wavelengths, since these processes will alter the precise environment of the chromophore.

6. Circular Dichorism

In the early nineteenth century the French physicist Jean Baptiste Biot observed that solutions of some organic molecules appeared to rotate the plane of polarization of plane polarized light, a phenomenon referred to as optical rotatory dispersion. We now know that this is a consequence of the fact that each enantiomer of an optically active molecule interacts differently with left and right circularly polarized light. By convention, laevorotation is designated as (–) while dextrorotation is denoted by (+). A 50 : 50 mixture of equal amounts of d and l-enantiomers does not rotate the plane of polarization nor does a solution of an achiral molecule such as glycine. Light passing through a chromophore solution may interact with the sample in two main ways. The light may be refracted or delayed on passage through the solution or it may be absorbed. Refraction is quantified by the refractive index, n, of the solution while absorption is quantified by the molar extinction coefficient, ε. If the light is plane polarized and the sample is optically active, each enantiomer may interact differently with the left and right circularly polarized components of the light beam. ORD arises from the fact that there is a specific refractive index for left (nL) and right (nR) circularly polarized light:

$$nL = nR$$

The difference in refractive index at any wavelength may be expressed as an eqation. Similarly, optically active samples have distinct molar extinction coefficients for left (εL) and right (εR) circularly polarized light. This is called circular dichroism (CD):

$$\varepsilon L = \varepsilon R$$

The difference between εL and εR may be expressed as ε. Combining equations with the Beer–Lambert law) means that there is a difference in the absorbance of left and right circularly polarized light

$$A = \varepsilon \cdot c \cdot l$$

If ε or A or ellipticity is plotted against wavelength (λ), a CD spectrum is obtained. The CD spectrum of one enantiomer is a mirror image of that of the other and is related to the corresponding ORD spectrum (and vice versa) by a mathematical transformation called the general Kronig–Kramers transformation. Both ORD and CD spectra are evidence for optical activity in the sample and both reflect structure of molecules in the sample, especially of chiral biopolymers such as proteins and nucleic acids. In practice, ORD has now largely been superseded by CD spectroscopy.

7. Fluorescence Spectroscopy

Because vibrational energy levels of the ground and excited states of most chromophores overlap, they can return to the ground state by a series of nonradiative transitions. Some chromophores are quite rigid and inflexible molecules however, and may have a limited range of vibrational energy levels. In such molecules, the vibrational energy levels of the excited state often do not overlap with those of the ground state. When chromophores of this type absorb light, it is not possible for them to return to the ground state by simply losing their excess energy as heat. Instead, they undergo a radiative transition in which a portion of the absorbed energy is re-emitted as light. This phenomenon is called fluorescence and such chromophores are called fluors or fluorophores. Since at least some of the light energy initially absorbed is lost in transitions between vibrational energy levels, the light energy emitted is always of longer wavelength (*i.e.* lower energy) than that absorbed. This means that fluors have a characteristic fluorescence or emission spectrum as well as a characteristic absorbance spectrum. The excited state lifetime of a fluor (*i.e.* the period of time spent in the excited state) is usually very short (ranging from 0.5 to 8 ns). However, in certain cases the period of time spent in the excited state may be significantly longer ranging up to 2 s. The latter situation can arise as a consequence of a phenomenon associated with electrons called magnetic spin. Some heavy atoms possessing even numbers of electrons in their singlet ground state can have two unpaired electrons stably occupying different orbitals in a triplet state of slightly higher energy than the ground state (*e.g.* molecular oxygen). In such atoms, it is possible for a transition to occur between the singlet ground state (where the electrons are antiparallel and paired) to an excited state (where the electrons are parallel and unpaired). When this molecule returns to the ground state a radiative triplet-singlet transition occurs which is a much slower process than fluorescence called phosphorescence. Radiation emitted as a result of this transition is at an even longer wavelength than radiation emitted during fluorescence because the lowest-energy triplet state typically has only slightly higher energy than the lowest-energy singlet state. A third phenomenon resulting in radiative transitions called chemiluminescence occurs in molecules which can be promoted to an excited state as a result of a chemical reaction and which then return to the ground state with the emission of light. Molecules such as luciferin and luminol show this property and, when used as substrates by the enzymes firefly luciferase and peroxidase, respectively, emit light which may be measured or detected.

8. NMR and X-ray Crystallography

X-ray crystallography and nuclear magnetic resonance (NMR) spectroscopy are the most powerful and predominant techniques used to experimentally determine the three-dimensional structures of biological macromolecules at near atomic resolution. X-ray diffraction (XRD) studies require a crystalisable protein, whereas NMR is suitable for macromolecules in solution. XRD has no size limitations and provides the most precise atomic detail, whereas information about the dynamics of the molecule may be limited. NMR excels in cases where no protein crystals can be obtained and it provides solution state dynamics, but in turn delivers lower resolution structures and is in general limited to molecular weights below approximately 50 kDa. The two techniques can deliver complementary information. Approximately 90 per cent of the experimentally determined macromolecular structures deposited in Protein Data Bank are crystal structures, with NMR dominating the <10 kDa molecular weight range. XRD and NMR are complimentary structure determination methods. XRD has no size limitations and provides the most precise atomic detail, whereas information about the dynamics of the molecule may be limited. NMR excels in cases where no protein crystals can be obtained and it provides solution state dynamics, but in turn delivers less detail and in general practice is limited to molecular weights below approximately 50 kDa.

Atoms and molecules have a variety of quantized energy levels (*e.g.* electronic, vibrational and rotational). Many spectroscopic techniques take advantage of transitions between these energy levels with different E values being related to particular frequency-ranges of the electromagnetic spectrum by. A further property of atoms which is quantized is magnetic spin and nuclear magnetic resonance (NMR) spectroscopy is a spectroscopic technique which takes advantage of this fact. To explain the physical basis of NMR we can use the hydrogen nucleus, 1H, as a good example (this type of NMR is called proton NMR). However, as will become clear, magnetic spin is a property of many different types of atoms. The 1H nucleus may be regarded as a spinning positive charge. This generates a magnetic field which will have a magnetic spin moment, μ. If an external magnetic field (field-strength, B0) is applied to such a nucleus, it can orientate itself either with (parallel) or against (antiparallel) this field in much the same way as a bar-magnet does in the Earth's magnetic field on the macroscopic scale. These two orientations are referred to as spin states and are distinguishable by their different spin quantum numbers, mI, which are, respectively, –1/2 and +1/2. The magnetic spin moment 'wobbles' or precesses around the axis of the external magnetic field by an angle, θ, and rotates around this axis with a particular frequency, ω, which is called the Larmor frequency.

The second widespread technique for determination of three-dimensional structure of biomacromolecules is based on the study of X-ray diffraction patterns by crystals of protein/DNA called X-ray crystallography. The technique is equally applicable to structure determination of small molecules such as those encountered in organic/inorganic chemistry and is based on the fact that atoms diffract X-rays in a pattern which is dependent on their location in three dimensional space. The reason X-rays are used is that their wavelength range is of the same order of magnitude as chemical bonds thus allowing us to 'see' at a resolution equivalent to interatomic distances (*i.e.* 0.8–2.5 A). To detect diffracted ° X-rays with high enough sensitivity, it is essential that many atoms contribute to the diffraction pattern obtained. In practice, this means that the molecule under investigation must be present in the ordered three-dimensional array of a crystal so that many equivalent atoms in different molecules contribute to the diffraction pattern. In the case of biomacromolecules, it is often difficult to obtain crystals of adequate quality and this is a major limitation of this approach to structure determination. In particular, it means that biomolecules which do not form crystals (*e.g.* intrinsic membrane-bound proteins) are not immediately amenable to study by this technique. Notwithstanding this limitation, X-ray crystallography has resulted in determination of three-dimensional structures for thousands of proteins and is still far more widely used than multi-dimensional NMR for high-resolution structure determination. It has made a number of major contributions to biochemistry such as the demonstration that enzymes are protein in nature, the Watson–Crick model of DNA (although diffraction in this case was by DNA fibres) and understanding the molecular basis of phenomena such as allosterism and protein/DNA interactions. Moreover, structures derived from X-ray crystallography provide the major experimental link between structure and function underlying most modern biochemistry and molecular biology.

In order to determine molecular structure it is necessary to use X-rays because the wavelength of this radiation is of a similar order of magnitude as atoms and covalent bond-lengths. The diffraction pattern obtained contains the information we use to calculate this molecular structure. However, the diffraction pattern is a two-dimensional array of 'spots' of particular position and intensity. In order to convert this into a three-dimensional structure it is necessary to collect a data set of many such diffraction patterns from a single crystal (the precise number required depends on the symmetry and other characteristics of the crystal). Repeated exposure to the high-energy X-ray beam can sometimes lead to deterioration of the crystal during the experiment which can preclude the collection of a complete data set. In such cases it is often necessary to rescreen in an attempt to obtain more robust crystals, perhaps in a different crystal form. The electrons of atoms are responsible for diffraction of X-rays. This is due to an interaction between the X-ray electromagnetic wave and the electron. The electric vector of the electromagnetic wave induces an oscillation in the electron of a frequency identical to that of the wave. This results in emission of secondary radiation of a wavelength and frequency identical to that of the incident X-ray but 180° out of phase with it which is known as coherent scattering. A related process called anomalous scattering can occur if the frequency of the incident beam happens to be near that of a naturally occurring oscillation in the electron. This latter phenomenon can be useful in determining the phase of scattered beams. Since electrons are responsible for diffraction, there is a close relationship between the intensity with which incident X-rays are diffracted and the atomic number (Z) of the atom which diffracts them. This may be quantified by the scattering factor, f, which is related to the angle of incidence. The scattering factor is a ratio between the intensity of scattering of X-rays by an atom and that of a single electron in the same experimental circumstances. Relative values for some atoms of biological interest are; 1H (1), 12C (6), 16O (8) and 54Fe. This means that heavy metals diffract with much greater intensity than other atoms and that hydrogen diffracts so weakly that it is usually not detectable. For this reason the actual structure we calculate from X-ray diffraction patterns is an electron density map representing the location of C, N, S, O and other nonhydrogen atoms. Because of the similar scattering factors for N, O and C it can be difficult to distinguish side-chains of aspartate, glutamine and threonine from each other in electron density maps of proteins. The detection system for scattered X-rays should record both the position of the diffraction spot and its intensity as well as the overall diffraction pattern. X-ray diffraction patterns may be detected on photographic film since X-rays, like visible light, interact with film causing deposition of metallic silver. The intensity of each spot can be estimated relative to standard spots or by using a densitometer. The film is mounted in a camera which is orientated in a known angle relative to the incident beam and crystal. Alternatively, diffracted beams may be detected using electronic detectors such as the area detector. These convert spot intensities and position to an electrical charge which is recorded. Electronic detectors have a number of advantages over film; they are more sensitive which shortens the time necessary to collect a diffraction pattern (and hence shortens the exposure time of the crystal to the X-ray beam). Moreover, the data can be stored electronically in a computer-readable form which eliminates any requirement for a densitometer and again saves time. Once the crystal has been exposed to the X-ray beam, the diffraction pattern is collected and stored electronically. The detector is then erased, the crystal rotated slightly and a second diffraction pattern collected. In this way, a data-set of diffraction patterns is built up for the crystal. Because most of the incident beam passes straight through the crystal without being scattered, this would saturate the detector limiting its sensitivity. Accordingly, the detector is shielded from the direct incident beam by a circular piece of lead called a beam stop. More recently, detectors with an X-ray-sensitive phosphor screen coupled to a charge coupled device have become available

Bragg's Law

As with all electromagnetic radiation waves, diffraction can result in interference between diffracted waves which results in the waves either reinforcing or weakening each other depending on their relative phases. These phenomena are characteristic of wave functions and are known as constructive and destructive interference, respectively. In an X-ray diffraction experiment, a complicated pattern of scattering of X-ray beams is observed in which both of these processes occur simultaneously. The pattern of interference depends on the distribution of atoms in the sample through which X-rays pass. Since crystals are highly ordered arrays of atoms, systematic interference patterns occur which may be thought of as 'encoding' information on relative three-dimensional atomic locations. In 1913 Bragg proposed that a crystal may be regarded as a series of planes which behave as 'mirrors' reflecting X-rays. In a real crystal, these lattice planes cut through the crystal lattice in three dimensions. In practice this means that the diffracted beams detected in an X-ray diffraction pattern (sometimes called Bragg reflections) are those originating from successive lattice planes which obey Bragg's law and reinforce each other by constructive interference with a single reflection arising from each equivalent lattice plane in the crystal.

Acknowledgement

We acknowledge the assistance of Dr. Atanu Banerjee from Amity University Haryana in drafting the protein structure and function modules.

REFERENCES

1. Bunge, M. (1979). *Treatise on Basic Philosophy*, vol. 4. Ontology II: A World of Systems, p. 61-2.
2. Voon, C. H.; Sam, S. T. (2019). "2.1 Biosensors". *Nanobiosensors for Biomolecular Targeting*. Elsevier. ISBN 978-0-12-813900-4.
3. Piehler J. New methodologies for measuring protein interactions in vivo and in vitro. Curr Opin Struct Biol 2005;15(1): 4-14.
4. von Hippel PH, McGhee JD. DNA-protein interactions. Annual review of biochemistry. 1972 Jul;41(1): 231-300.
5. Prabhakar P, Kayastha AM. Mechanism of DNA-drug interactions. Applied biochemistry and biotechnology. 1994 Apr;47(1): 39-55.
6. Kuzmanov, U., Emili, A. Protein-protein interaction networks: probing disease mechanisms using model systems. *Genome Med* 5, 37 (2013). https: //doi.org/10.1186/gm441
7. Garner, M.M.and Revzin, A. (1981). A gel electrophoresis method for quantifying the binding of proteins to specific DNA regions: application to components of the Escherichia coli lactose operon regulatory system. Nucleic Acids Res. 9, 3047 – 3060.
8. Gaudreault M, Gingras ME, Lessard M, Leclerc S, Guérin SL. Electrophoretic mobility shift assays for the analysis of DNA-protein interactions. InDNA-Protein Interactions 2009 (pp. 15-35). Humana Press.
9. von Hippel, P. H. 1969. 1. Cell. Physiol. 74: Suppl. 1, 235
10. von Hippel, P. H. (1979) in Biological Regulation and Development, ed. Goldberger, R. F. (Plenum, New York), Vol. 1, pp. 279-347.
11. Von Hippel PH, Berg OG. On the specificity of DNA-protein interactions. Proceedings of the National Academy of Sciences. 1986 Mar 1;83(6): 1608-12.
12. Yarun, M. (1969) Annu. Rev. Biochem. 38, 841-880.

13. von Hippel, P. H. and McGhee, J. D. (1972) Annu. Rev. Biochem. 41, 231-300.
14. Seeman, N. C., Rosenberg, J. M. and Rich, A. (1976) Proc. Natd. Acad. Sci. USA 73, 804-808.
15. Woodbury, C. P., Jr., and von Hippel, P. H. (1981) in The Restriction Enzymes, ed. Chirikjian, J. (Elsevier, Amsterdam), Vol. 1, pp. 181-207.
16. Melchior, W. B., Jr., and von Hippel, P. H. (1973) Proc. Natl. Acad. Sci. USA 70, 298-302.
17. 10. Kopka, M. L., Yoon, C., Goodsell, D., Pjura, P. and Dickerson, R. E. (1985) Proc. Natd. Acad. Sci. USA 82, 1376-1380.
18. 11. deHaseth, P. L., Lohman, T. M. and Record, M. T., Jr. (1977) Biochemistry 16, 4783-4790.
19. 12. Revzin, A. and von Hippel, P. H. (1977) Biochemistry 16, 4769-4776.
20. 13. Kowalczykowski, S. C., Lonberg, N., Newport, J. W. and von Hippel, P. H. (1981) J. Mol. Biol. 145, 75-104.
21. 14. Weintraub, H. and Groudine, M. (1976) Science 193, 848-856.
22. Thurston, D. E. and Thompson, A. S. (1990), Chem. Britain 8, 767.
23. Rawn, D. (1989), Text-Book of Biochemistry, Neff Patterson, Burlington, p. 829.
24. Zubay, G. (1989), Text-Book of Biochemistry, Macmillen, New York, pp. 792 and 924.
25. Fok, J. and Waring, M. J. (1972), Mol. Pharmacol. 8, 65.
26. Goldberg, I. H. and Friedman, P. A. (1971), Ann. Rev. Biochem. 40, 772.
27. Warpehoski, M. A. and Hurley, L. H. (1988), Chem. Res. Toxicol. 1, 315.
28. Barton, J. K. (1986), Science 233, 727.
29. Taylor, J. S., Schultz, P. G., and Dervan, P. B. (1984), Tetrahedron 40, 457.
30. Denny, W. A., Baguley, B. C., and Cain, B. F. (1983), in Molecular Aspects of Anticancer Drug Action, Neidle, S. and Waring, M. J., eds., Macmillian, London, p. 1.
31. Pullman, B. (1989), in Advances in Drug Research, vol. 18, Academic, New York, p. 1.
32. Ward, D. C., Reich, E., and Goldberg, I. G. (1965), Science 149, 1259.
33. Behr, W., Honikel, K., and Hertmann, G. (1969), Eur. J. Biochem. 9, 82.
34. Kamiyama, M. (1968),]. Biochem. 63, 563.
35. Umezawa, H. (1978), in Bleomycin: Current Status and New Developments, Carter, S. K., Crooke, S. T., and Umezawa, H., eds., Academic Press, New York, p. 15.
36. Goldberg, I. H. and Friedman, P. A. (1971), Ann. Rev. Biochem. 40, 772.
37. Moffat, A. S. (1991), Science 252, 1374.

38. Hurley, L. H. (1989), J. Med. Chem. 32, 2027.

39. Dervan, P. B. (1986), Science 232, 464.

40. Braun P, Gingras AC. History of protein-protein interactions: From egg-white to complex networks. Proteomics. 2012;12(10): 1478-1498. DOI: 10.1002/pmic.201100563

41. Zhang A. Protein Interaction Networks: Computational Analysis. New York, NY: Cambridge University Press; 2009

42. Yu H, Braun P, Yildirim MA, Lemmens I, Venkatesan K, *et al.*, High-quality binary protein interaction map of the yeast interactome network. *Science.* 2008;322: 104–110

43. Suter B, Kittanakom S, Stagljar I. Two-hybrid technologies in proteomics research. *Curr Opin Biotechnol.* 2008;19: 316–323.

44. Berggard T, Linse S, James P. Methods for the detection and analysis of protein-protein interactions. *Proteomics.* 2007;7: 2833–2842.

45. Mackay JP, Sunde M, Lowry JA, Crossley M, Matthews JM. Protein interactions: is seeing believing? *Trends Biochem Sci.* 2007;32: 530–531.

46. Hakes L, Robertson DL, Oliver SG, Lovell SC. Protein interactions from complexes: a structural perspective. *Comp Funct Genomics.* 2007: 49356.

47. Dickerson, R. E.; Geis, I. Hemoglobin: Structure, Function, Evolution, and Pathology; The Benjamin/Cummings Publishing Company, Inc.: Menlo Park, CA, 1983.

48. Antonini, E.; Brunori, M. Hemoglobin and Myoglobin in Their Reactions With Ligands; North-Holland Publishing Company: Amsterdam, The Netherlands, 1971.

49. Degtyarenko, I.; Biarnes, X.; Nieminen, R. M.; Rovira, C. Coord. Chem. Rev. 2008, 252, 1497–1513.

50. Sigfridsson, E.; Ryde, U. JBIC, J. Biol. Inorg. Chem. 1999, 4, 99– 110.

51. Olson, J. S.; Phillips, G. N., Jr. JBIC, J. Biol. Inorg. Chem. 1997, 2, 544–552.

52. Ackers, G. K.; Doyle, M. L.; Myers, D.; Daugherty, M. A. Science 1992, 255, 54–63.

53. Arcovito, A.; Benfatto, M.; Cianci, M.; Hasnain, S. S.; Nienhaus, K.; Nienhaus, G. U.; Savino, C.; Strange, R. W.; Vallone, B.; Della Longa, S. Proc. Natl. Acad. Sci. U. S. A. 2007, 104, 6211–6216.

54. Maurus, R.; Overall, C. M.; Bogumil, R.; Luo, Y.; Mauk, A. G.; Smith, M.; Brayer, G. D. Biochim. Biophys. Acta, Protein Struct. Mol. Enzymol. 1997, 1341, 1–13.

55. McLendon, G.; Sandberg, K. J. Biol. Chem. 1978, 253, 3913– 3917.

56. Fersht, A. R. Structure and Mechanism in Protein Science; W. H. Freeman and Co.: New York, 1999.

57. Foord, S. M. (2002). Receptor classification: post genome. *Curr. Opin. Pharmacol.* 2, 561–566. doi: 10.1016/S1471-4892(02)00214-X

58. Tuteja, N. (2009). Signaling through G protein coupled receptors. *Plant Signal. Behav.* 4, 942–947. doi: 10.4161/psb.4.10.9530

59. Schonenbach, N. S., Hussain, S., and O'Malley, M. A. (2015). Structure and function of G protein-coupled receptor oligomers: implications for drug discovery. *Wiley Interdiscip. Rev. Nanomed. Nanobiotechnol.* 7, 408–427. doi: 10.1002/wnan.1319

60. Stockert, J. A., and Devi, L. A. (2015). Advancements in therapeutically targeting orphan GPCRs. *Front. Pharmacol.* 6: 100. doi: 10.3389/fphar.2015.00100

61. Bayburt, T. H., Leitz, A. J., Xie, G., Oprian, D. D., and Sligar, S. G. (2007). Transducin activation by nanoscale lipid bilayers containing one and two rhodopsins. *J. Biol. Chem.* 282, 14875–14881. doi: 10.1074/jbc.M701433200.

62. Pauling L, Corey RB. A proposed structure for the nucleic acids. Proceedings of the National Academy of Sciences of the United States of America. 1953 Feb;39(2): 84.

63. Rook MS, Treiber DK, Williamson JR. An optimal Mg2+ concentration for kinetic folding of the Tetrahymena ribozyme. Proceedings of the National Academy of Sciences. 1999 Oct 26;96(22): 12471-6.

64. Varani G. Exceptionally stable nucleic acid hairpins. Annual review of biophysics and biomolecular structure. 1995 Jun;24(1): 379-404.

65. Driessen RP, Sitters G, Laurens N, Moolenaar GF, Wuite GJ, Goosen N, Dame RT. Effect of temperature on the intrinsic flexibility of DNA and its interaction with architectural proteins. Biochemistry. 2014 Oct 21;53(41): 6430-8.

66. S. E. Wolkenberg, D. L. Boger, Chem. Rev. 2002, 102, 2477.

67. Wu P, Nakano SI, Sugimoto N. Temperature dependence of thermodynamic properties for DNA/DNA and RNA/DNA duplex formation. European journal of biochemistry. 2002 Jun;269(12): 2821-30.

Chapter 16

Fermentation Technology and Downstream Processing

*Kumar Gaurav**

Amity Institute of Biotechnology, Amity University Haryana, Gurugram (Manesar) – 122 413, Haryana, India
**e-mail: kgaurav1@ggn.amity.edu*

ABSTRACT

A phenomenal growth has been observed in last decades in the field of biochemical engineering where development of variety of biologically important products from different micro organisms took place. Downstream processing is a collective technique that involves the isolation and purification of a biological product from an organism and further developing it into useful products like antibiotics etc. This chapter will give an insight into the various steps involved in full scale process design of such product development process including separation and purification, various operating techniques and equipments required. The first step for large scale production of microbial products is cell disruption to release these biological products. Various methods are available to carry out the cell disruptions which are discussed in the following sections. This step is followed by separation of insoluble particles from culture broth. For achieving this objective, different methods such as filtration, centrifugation, coagulation and flocculation are applied depending on the nature of microorganism taken. These will be discussed in detail along with the details of equipments used for each technique. Finally product recovery is discussed where different techniques such as precipitation, adsorption, chromatography and dialysis are applied. The mathematical equations related to above techniques are also discussed in detail.

Keywords: *Cell disruption, Flocculation, Centrifugation, Affinity chromatography, Adsorption.*

1. Introduction

Downstream processing, the act of getting the purified final product from a soup of cultured cells, accounts for forty to fifty percent of biopharmaceutical manufacturing cost. The recovery and purification of a fermentation product is essential to any commercial process. Products may the biomass itself, an extracellular component, or an intracellular. Down stream processing has been given an orphan treatment due to low investment and a lack of interest by scientist resulting in it being a long-standing market barrier. Lack of specialized apparatus/instruments and automation systems has ultimately resulted into the main hindrance of this technology. Last decade or so has been a considerable improvement in the purification methods that has led to the growth of biopharmaceutical market, in addition to other advantages that the biologicals represent.

2. Cell Disruption

For the release of intracellular products, cell disruption is an essential part of the downstream processes. It results into the extraction and retrieval of the desired biological products. These biological products need to be released maximally and without affecting its property or activity. Several types of cell disruption methods exist which are basically categorized into mechanical methods and non- mechanical methods.

I. Mechanical Methods

1. Cavitation
2. Shearing (liquid/solid)
3. Impingement
4. Freeze-thaw
5. Ultrasonication

II. Non-mechanical Methods

A. *Physical*

1. Thermolysis
2. Decompression
3. Osmotic shock

B. *Chemical*

1. Detergents
2. Solvents
3. Alkali treatment

C. *Enzymatic Methods*

2.1 Mechanical Methods

1. Cavitation refers to creation of cavities inside homogenous liquid media. The bursting of these cavities can result into localized high pressure and temperature which could be sufficient to cause the disintegration of cell wall resulting into the extraction of desired biological product. This technique is advantageous as compared to others as it does not require high level of energy consumption.

2. **Shearing:** In this process, cell suspension is agitated at a very high speed, thus creating shearing force which leads to cell disruption. It includes high pressure homogenizers (HPH). High shear force is generated by forcing the liquid media through a small valve/orifice at high pressure which is then used to disrupt the cell.
3. **Impingement:** This is a technique where the suspended cells in liquid media are forced to strike a stationary surface at high velocity and pressure resulting into the disruption of cells. This technique is useful even when cells are at a low concentration.
4. **Freeze-thawing:** Freezing and thawing of a microbial cell slurry results into disruption of cells due to formation of ice crystals. This method is slow and in some cases, also results into loss of activity of the product extracted.
5. **Ultrasonication:** This method makes use of ultrasonic waves to cause cell disruption but results into issues related to temperature control. It is also not cost effective so cannot be used for large-scale operations.

2.2 Non-Mechanical Methods

A. Physical

1. **Thermolysis**: In this treatment, high temperature is used to disrupt the cell wall thereby release intracellular products and inactivates the cell. But this process is extremely unreliable as the solubility of protein varies with the temperature
2. **Decompression:** This is a process where a subcritical gas is mixed with the cell suspension and after entering the cell, it expands resulting into the cell disruption.
3. **Osmotic shock:** A cell properly functions at a particular pH and salt concentrations. If any significant deviation in these optimal conditions takes place, cell disruption will occur. In this treatment, cells are exposed to extreme deviations (first to high salt concentration and then to low salt concentration) from their optimal condition which leads to cell lysis.

B. Chemical

1. **Detergents:** etergents directly damage the cell wall resulting into release of intracellular content. They can be cationic, anionic or non ionic. The most commonly used detergents for cell lysis are sodium dodecyl sulphate (SDS) and Triton X100. The limitation of this process is that these detergents affect purification step.
2. **Solvents:** Certain chemical solvents like dimethyl sulphoxide, certain alcohols, toluene *etc.* can also cause cell distruption by extracting cell wall's lipid component. But the drawback associated is that it causes denaturation of certain proteins.

3. **Alkali treatment:** Cell wall can also be hydrolysed using alkali compounds. But the limitation of this process is that the cost of neutralization is very high and moreover, certain products may not of stable in alkaline conditions.

C. Enzyme Treatment

Certain enzymes such as lysozyme can be used to lyse cell walls of bacteria. The cells may be treated with Ethylene diamine tetra acetic acid (EDTA) or by freezing and thawing before treatment with lysozyme. EDTA is a chelating agent and its high levels will extract divalent ions that are part of the cell envelope. Enzymatic hydrolysis is an expensive methods and is not very widely used in industry.

3. Solid-Liquid Separation

The first step in any product recovery is usually the separation of insoluble particles from the culture broth. The methods employed for this purpose are (1) filtration, (2) centrifugation, (3) coagulation and flocculation.

3.1 Filtration

It is a process that separate solid from a liquid by forcing the liquid through a filter medium. It is probably the simplest and cheapest method for separation of solids and cells from culture broth. This broth is passed through a filter medium, and a filter cake is formed as a result of deposition of solids on the filter surface.

Two Types of Filtration

1. **Conventional filtration:** With addition of filter cake
2. **Microfiltration:** Without addition of filter cake

General Theory for Filtration

General theory for filtration involves the three steps:

1. **Darcy's law :** The equation for fluid mechanics.
2. The equation for incompressible cakes.
3. The equation for compressible cakes

1. Darcy's Law

The equation for fluid mechanics

Darcy's law explains the relation between pressure drop and flow rate

$$v \alpha \frac{\Delta p}{\mu l}$$

$$v = k \frac{\Delta p}{\mu l} \quad (1)$$

where,

v = velocity of fluid

k = Proportional constant called as Darcy's law permeability of the bed

Δp = Change in pressure through the bed of the thickness l.

μ = liquid's viscosity

l = Thickness of the bed

For a batch filtration,

Velocity can be written as,

$$v = \frac{1}{A}\frac{dV}{dt} \qquad (2)$$

where,

v = Total volume of the filtrate

t = time

The resistance (l/k) to include the contribution of cake and filter medium

$$\frac{1}{k} = R_M + R_C \qquad (3)$$

where,

R_M = Resistance of the filter medium

R_C = Resistance of the accumulated biomass

From equation 1 and 2

$$v = k = \frac{\Delta p}{\mu l} = \frac{1}{A}\frac{dV}{dt} \qquad (4)$$

Substituting the value of (l/k) in equation 4

$$\frac{1}{A}\frac{dV}{dt} = \frac{\Delta p}{\mu (R_M + R_C)}$$

$$\frac{1}{A}\frac{dV}{dt} = \frac{\Delta p}{\mu (R_M + R_C)}$$

where,

R_M (medium resistance) is a constant and its is independent of cake.

R_C (cake resistance) varies with amount filtered V.

The exact nature of this variation depends on whether the cake in incompressible or not.

2. The Equation for Incompressible Cakes

In case of incompressible cakes, the thickness of cake is directly proportional to the volume of filtrate and inversely proportional to the filter area. As a result, the cake's resistance R_C is described by the equation

$$R_C = \alpha \rho_0 \left(\frac{V}{A}\right) \quad (1)$$

where,

α = Specific cake resistance (dimension is length/mass)

ρ_0 = Mass of cake solids per volume of filtrate

$$\frac{1}{A}\frac{dV}{dt} = \frac{\Delta p}{\mu (R_M + R_C)}$$

Substituting the value of R_C from equation 1 in the above equation

$$\frac{1}{A}\frac{dV}{dt} = \frac{\Delta p}{\mu \left(R_M + \alpha \rho 0 \left(\frac{V}{A}\right)\right.} \quad (2)$$

This equation is subject to the initial condition

t = 0, V = 0

This condition says that at the start of the experiment, no solution has been filtered.

The equation 2 is easily integrated and rearranged to give

$$\left(\frac{At}{V}\right) = K \left(\frac{V}{A}\right) + B \quad (3)$$

where,

$$K = \frac{\mu \alpha \rho 0}{2 \Delta \rho}$$

and

$$B = \frac{\mu R_M}{\Delta \rho}$$

Thus a plot of (At/V) versus (V/A) should be linear. The slope K is a function of the pressure drop $\Delta \rho$ and the properties of the cake, represented by α and ρ_0. The intercept B should be independent of the properties of the cake, but it is proportional to the medium's resistance R_M. Often, this medium resistance is insignificant, so the equation 3 becomes simpler still :

$$t = \left(\frac{\mu \alpha \rho 0}{2 \Delta \rho}\right) \left(\frac{V}{A}\right)^2$$

These equations, valid for incompressible cakes.

3. The Equation for Compressible Cakes

All cakes formed of biological materials are compressible. As these cakes compress, filtration rate drop.

To estimate the effect of compressibility, we assume the cake resistance α is a function of pressure drop.

$$\alpha = \alpha' (\Delta \rho)^s$$

where,

α' = Constant related largely to the size and shape of the particles forming cake

s = Cake compressibility

Varies from, 0 for a rigid, incompressible cake; 1 for highly compressible cake (In practice s ranges form 0.1 to 0.8).

Values of s and α' are most easily determined by plotting the logarithm of α versus logarithm of $\Delta \rho$

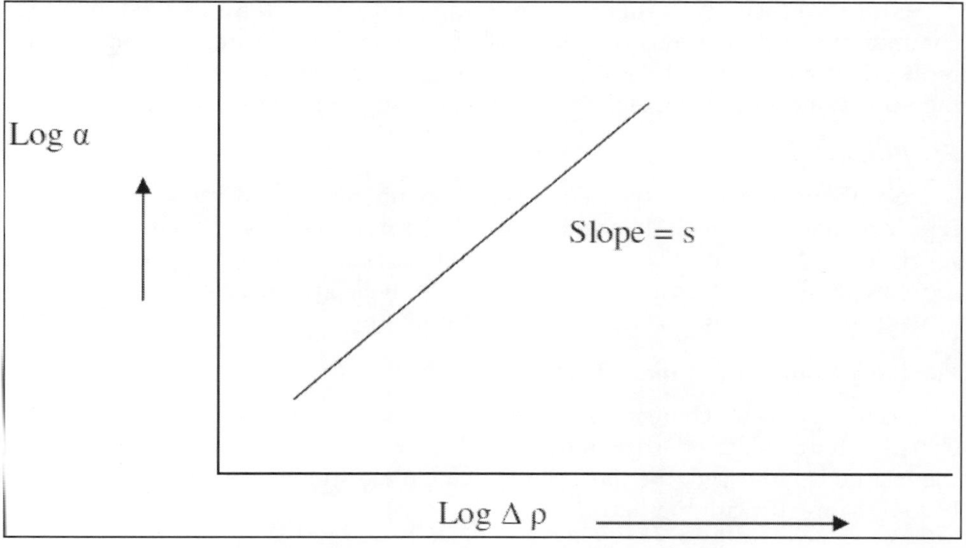

Pre-treatment of Fermentation Broth before Filtration

Improving the filtration characteristic of fermentation broth.

Fermentation broth and other biological solution are notoriously hard to filter. The reason for this is high viscosity (non-Newtonian) of fermentation broth or highly compressible filter cakes. These cakes can deform into an impermeable mat. This is especially true of mycelial microorganisms, but may apply to any bacterial broth.

As a result these biological feeds often require pretreatments like heating, coagulation and flocculation and adsorption on filter aids. These pretreatment are also useful for centrifugation and sedimentation.

1. Heating
2. Coagulation and Flocculation
3. Adsorption on filter aids

1. Heating

Simplest and least expensive method, is to heat the feed. Such heating can not only improve the handling characteristic but also may pasteurize it. *e.g.* ovalalbumin solution. Heating of the solution causes the denaturation of protein and it becomes easier to filter.

2. Coagulation and Flocculation

Addition of **electrolytes** (**simple** and **synthetic polyelectrolytes**), **acid** and **bases** to promote coagulation and flocculation and becomes easier to filter.

For Coagulation

Simple electrolytes act by screening the electrostatic repulsion which commonly exists between colloidal particles. When the electrostatic repulsion is reduced, attractive London- Vander waals forces predominate. The colloids can then coagulate as larger, denser particle which are more easily filtered.

For Flocculation

Synthetic polyelectrolytes added as pretreatment can both reduce electrostatic repulsion and adsorb on adjacent particles, forming bridges between them. As a result, the colloidal particles flocculate as large, less dense aggregates which are more easily filtered. Commercially available polyelectrolytes are polyacrylamide, ployethylenimines and polyamine derivatives.

For both Coagulation and Flocculation

Acid and **bases** change the pH and hence the charge on the particles. If the charge is reduced, the particle may coagulate and hence become easier to filter. If the charge is increased, the particle may coagulate still less, and the solution can become more difficult to filter.

3. Adsorption on Filter Aids

For improving the filtration characteristic of fermentation broth is the addition of solid filter aids to the broth prior to filtration.

Colloids

Colloids in the broth adsorb on particles filter aid and hence reduce **two of the chief problem** in filtration prior to filtration

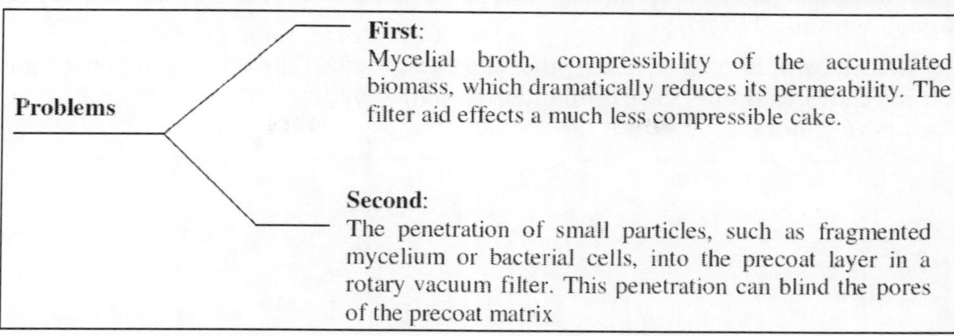

Two types of filter aids which have been found most effective for pretreatment are

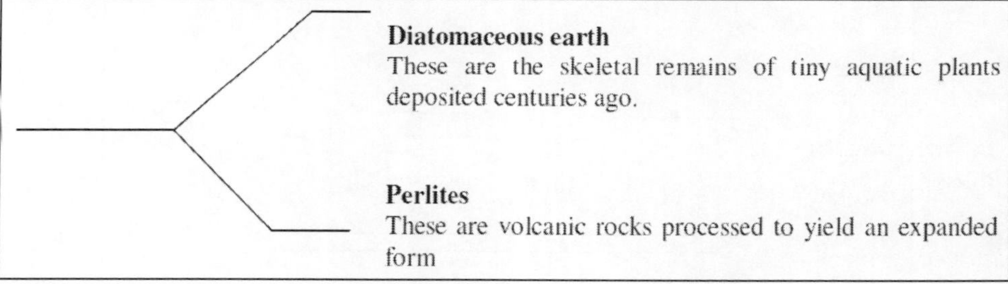

Disadvantages of filter aids

There can be disadvantages to using filter aids to enhance filtration.

e.g. **1** Particle size increases flow increases but filtrate clarity decreases.

e.g. **2** The aminoglycoside antibiotics may irreversibly binds to diatomaceous earth.

Equipment for Conventional Filtration

There are filter commonly used filter

1. Conventional filters
2. Rotary vacuum filter

Conventional Filters

There are different types of conventional filter are

1. Plate and frame filter (commonly used)
2. Horizontal filter
3. Vertical filter
4. Candle filter

Rotary Vacuum Filter

This type of filter is used for large scale commercial operations whenever the solid is difficult to filter. They are often automated, they have a lower labor cost. The filter includes;

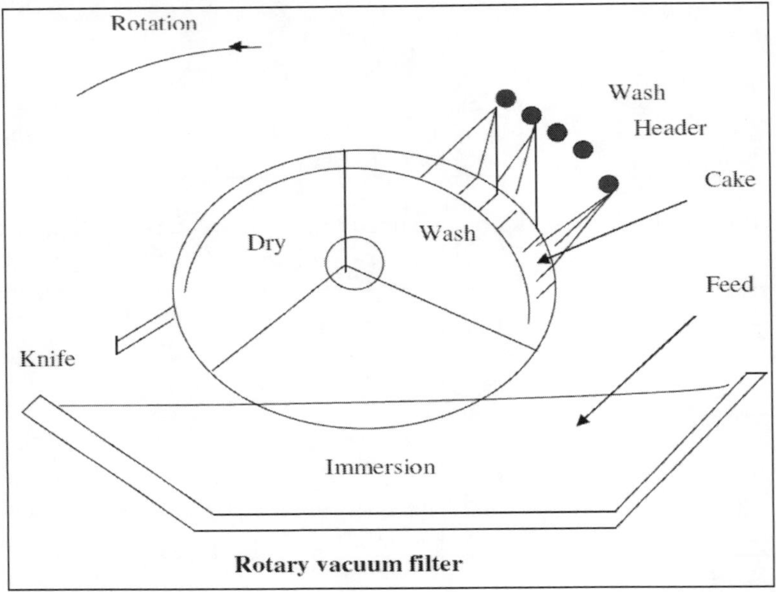

Rotary vacuum filter

1. *Rotating Drum*

Rotating drum, shown from the end. Pressure outside the drum is atmosphere, but inside the drum, it is partial vacuum. The drum is partially submerged in the beer and rotates at a low speed during the operation. During operation, solids are retained on the surface of the drum forming the cake whereas liquid passes through the filter cloth. When the cake rotates out of the beer, it is washed, dried, and removed.

2. *Knife*

A simple knife or doctor blade supplemented by an air blowback through the filter medium.

3. *Precoating of Filter*

Precoating of the filter is application of a layer of diatomaceous earth or some other inert microporous material to the filter itself. This coated filter is used with a beer to which still more inert material has been added.

Mechanism of Action

As the drum rotates, a thin layer of biomass and filter aid accumulates on the surface of the precoat and continues to build during the cake formation segment of the cycle.

The cake is then washed and again water is added followed by shaving off of thin layer of accumulated biomass and ultimately a fresh surface of precoat becomes available for next cycle. The depth of cut of by doctor blade depends on the penetration of the filtered particles. Vacuum is maintained throughout the entire filtration cycle. When the bed of precoat is depleted, a new layer is applied and further filtration proceeds.

Microfiltration (Filtration without filter cake)

Filtration without a cake is a part of the process called microfiltration. It is used to concentrate insolubles.

3.2 Centrifugation

The difference in the density of solid to be separated and the surrounding medium is the basis of this technique. This technique requires more expensive equipment than filtration.

Sedimentation is a technique where particles in a suspension are allowed to settle under the influence of gravity. This is usually a very slow process. When this settling of particles is accelerated with a centrifugal field, the process is called centrifugation.

Sedimentation = Under the influence of gravity.

Centrifugation = Under the influence of centrifugal field.

Settling of Solids

When solids particle moves through an infinite continuum, two forces mainly affect their velocity.

Two Forces

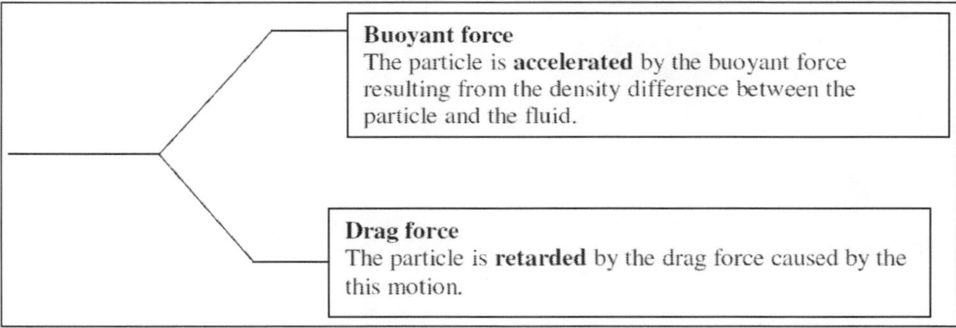

When buoyant force is equal to drag force the particle moves at a constant velocity.

Buoyant Force

The buoyancy force acting on the spherical biological particle is given by

$$F_B = \left[\frac{4}{3}\pi R^3 \rho_S - \rho\right] a$$

$$F_B = \left[\frac{4}{3}\pi R^3 \rho_S - \rho\right] a \quad (1)$$

diameter (d) = 2 radius (R), then equation 1 can be written as

$$F_B = \left[\frac{\pi d^3 \rho_S - \rho}{6}\right] a$$

F_B (force) = mass (m) x acceleration (a) (2)

$$\text{Density} = \frac{\text{Mass}}{\text{Volume}}$$

Mass = Volume x density

$$m = \frac{4}{3}\pi R^3 \times \rho_s - \rho \text{ (For the spherical particle)}$$

Substituting the value of mass (m) in equation 2

$$F_B = \frac{4}{3}\pi R^3 (\rho_s - \rho)\, a$$

$$F_B = [\frac{4}{3}\pi R^3 (\rho_s - \rho)]\, a$$

where,

R = Radius of the sphere

ρ_s = Density of the sphere

ρ = Density of the fluid

a = Acceleration due to some applied force

Drag Force

The drag force F_D acting on the a single sphere in dilute solution is given by Stokes law:

$$F_D = 6\pi r \eta v \quad (3)$$

$$F_D = 6\pi r \mu v$$

$$F_D = 3\pi d \mu v \quad \text{(Diameter = 2 Radius)}$$

$$F_D = 3\pi d \mu v$$

where,

μ = Viscosity of fluid

v = Velocity of fluid

The relation is accurate only if the sphere is small. Quantitatively, this means that

$$\frac{d\,v\,\rho}{\mu} < 1$$

The dimensionless quantity (d v ρ/μ) called Reynolds number characterizes the flow around the sphere.

When the spherical particle begins to move in solution, the drag force is small because the particle's velocity is small. As a result, the particle accelerates until the drag and buoyancy forces are equal. Under these condition equation 1 and equation 2

$$\frac{4}{3}\pi R^3 (\rho_s - \rho)\, a = 6\,\pi\, r\, \mu\, v$$

$$v = v_g$$

$$6\,\pi\, r\, \mu\, v_g = \frac{4}{3}\pi R^3 (\rho_s - \rho)\, a$$

$$v_g = \frac{4}{18\mu} R^2 (\rho_s - \rho)\, a$$

$$v_g = \frac{4}{18\mu} R^2 (\rho_s - \rho)\, g$$

$$v_g \frac{4}{18\mu} = R^2 (\rho_s - \rho)\, g \qquad (4)$$

$$v_g = \frac{1}{18\mu} d^2 (\rho_s - \rho)\, g$$

This relation gives the steady state or terminal velocity of the sphere.

There is two limit of equation 4

First,

For **Settling,** the acceleration is due to gravity (g)

$$v_g = \frac{4}{18\mu} R^2 (\rho_s - \rho)\, g$$

For **Centrifugation**, the acceleration is different

$$v_\omega = \frac{4}{18\mu} R^2 (\rho_s - \rho)\, r\omega^2$$

where,

ω = Angular rotation (rad/sec)

r = The radial distance from the center of the centrifuge to the sphere

$$v_{\omega} = \frac{1}{18\mu} d^2 (\rho_s - \rho) r\omega^2$$

Centrifuges

There are three basics types of centrifuges,

1. Tubular bowl centrifuge
2. Disc centrifuge
3. Basket centrifuge

1. Tubular Bowl Centrifuge

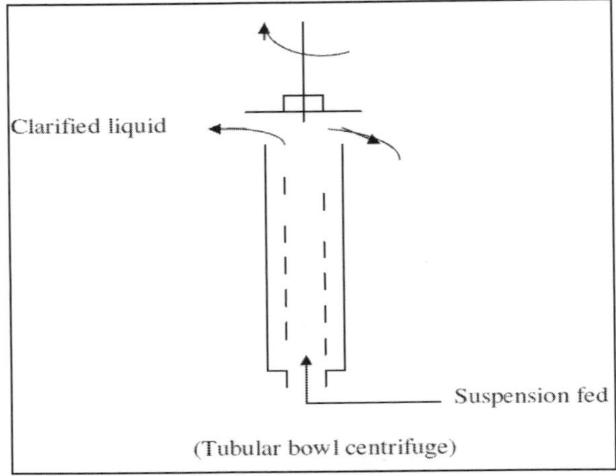

(Tubular bowl centrifuge)

This is a simple centrifuge that provides high centrifugal force. It is used for the protein work. In this case, clear liquid is removed from the top and solids deposits are removed manually.

Analysis of Tubular Bowl Centrifuge

The analysis depends on finding the position of a typical particle as a function of time.

Let us assume that the distance between particle and bottom of the centrifuge is z and the axis of rotation is r. This position is between the liquid surface R_1 and the bowl radius R_0.

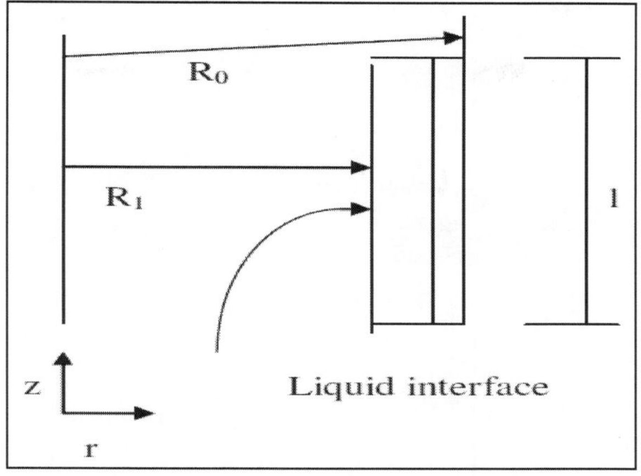

The particle is moving in both the z and r directions.

Its **movement in the z direction** comes from convection of the feed pumped in the bottom of the centrifuge

$$v_z = \frac{dz}{dt} = \frac{Q}{\pi\left(R_0^2 - R_1^2\right)} \tag{1}$$

The particle movement in the r direction is related to its radial position r by

$$v_r = \frac{dr}{dt} = \frac{1}{18\,\mu} d^2\left(\rho_S - \rho\right) r\omega^2$$

Rewrite the equation in terms of velocity of particle settling under the influence of gravity

$$v_r = \frac{dr}{dt} = v_g\left(\frac{r\,\omega^2}{g}\right) \tag{2}$$

Combining the equation 1 and equation 2

$$v_{rz} = \frac{dr}{dz} = \frac{dr/dt}{dz/dt} = v_g\left(\frac{r\,\omega^2}{g}\right)\pi\frac{\left(R_0^2 - R_1^2\right)}{Q} \tag{3}$$

If v_g is large, the particle will quickly reach the wall; if Q is increased, the particle will be swept farther up the tube.

These particle enter the centrifuge at $r = R_1$ and do not reach $r = R_0$ until the end of the unit, at z = l. Integrate the equation 3 and rearrangement of the equation.

$$Q = \frac{\pi\, l\left(R_0^2 - R_1^2\right) v_g\; r\,\omega^2}{g \ln(R_0 - R_1)}$$

Where R is an average radius about equal to R_0 and R_1 then

$$Q = \frac{v_g\,[2\,\pi\,lR^2\omega^2]}{g}$$

2. Disc Centrifuge

In this type of centrifuge, several discs are there which separate the whole centrifuge into different settling zones. The central tube is used to feed the slurry and clear liquid moves upwards while solids settle down.

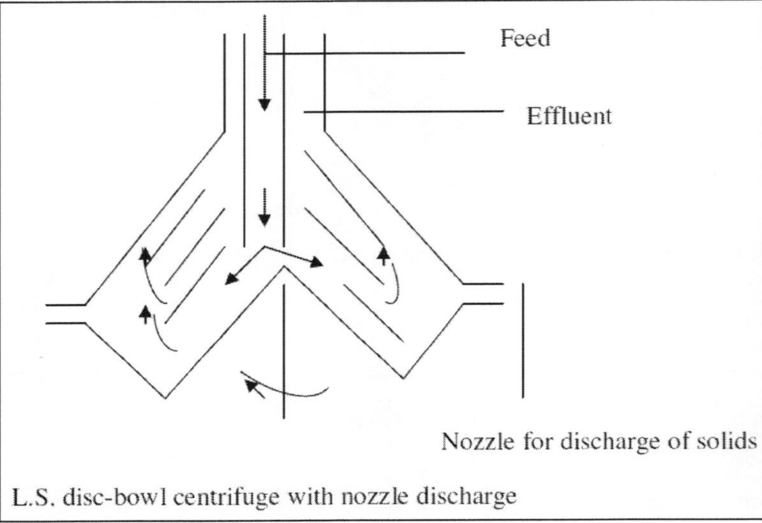

L.S. disc-bowl centrifuge with nozzle discharge

3. Basket Centrifuge

In this type of centrifuges, a filter media (usually made of nylon, cotton *etc.*) supported over a mesh is kept inside a rotating basket. The centrifugal force pushes the liquid, from the slurry, out through this filter media and solids are retained inside the basket which can then manually be separated.

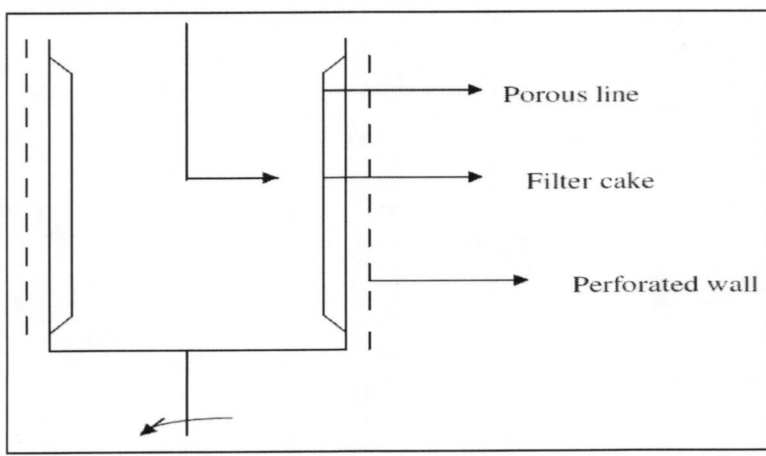

3.3 Coagulation and Flocculation

These are usually used to form cell aggregates before centrifugation, gravity settling, or filtration to improve the performance of these separation process.

Coagulation is basically destabilization of colloidal system by action of certain coagulants which are generally some electrolytes. Whereas, flocculation is aggregation of micro-flocs into larger flocs and their settling on the base.

4. Separation of Soluble Products/Product Recovery

Recovery of extracellular proteins or microbial products such as antibiotics and amino acids is carried out from the clarified medium. After centrifugation, the soluble proteins are separated from cell debris. Various methods available for extracting these protein from supernatant are precipitation, liquid-liquid extraction, adsorption, ultrafiltration, and chromatography.

4.1 Precipitation

Precipitation is the first step of purification of intracellular material after cell disruption. Proteins in fermentation broth can be separated from other components by precipitation.

The two major methods used for protein precipitation are as follows:

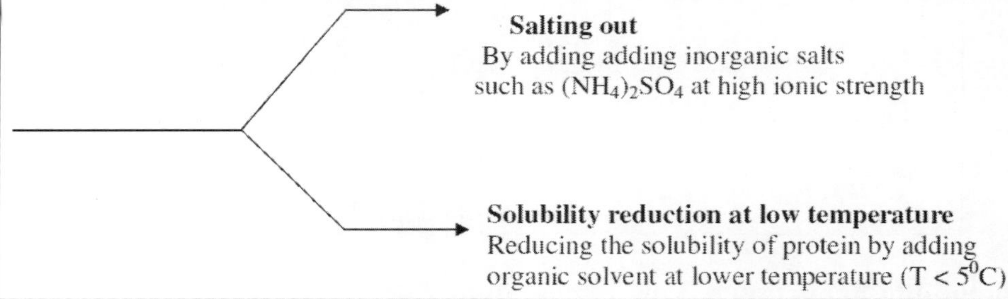

Salting Out

In this process, the ionic strength of protein is increased by adding salts such as ammonium sulfate. It is preferred because it is cheap, highly soluble and less toxic. The added ion interacts with water molecules resulting into the precipitation of protein molecule.

Solubility of protein is a function of ionic strength of solution

$$S = f(I)$$

$$\log \frac{S}{S_0} = -K_S' (I)$$

where,

S = Solubility of protein in solution (g/L)

S_0 = Solubility of protein when I = 0, I is the ionic strength of solution.

K'_S = Salting-out constant, which is a function of temperature and pH

The ionic strength of solution (I) is given as

$$I = \frac{1}{2} \Sigma C_i Z_i^2$$

where,

C_i = Molar concentration of the ionic species (mol/L)

Z_i = Charges (valences) on ions.

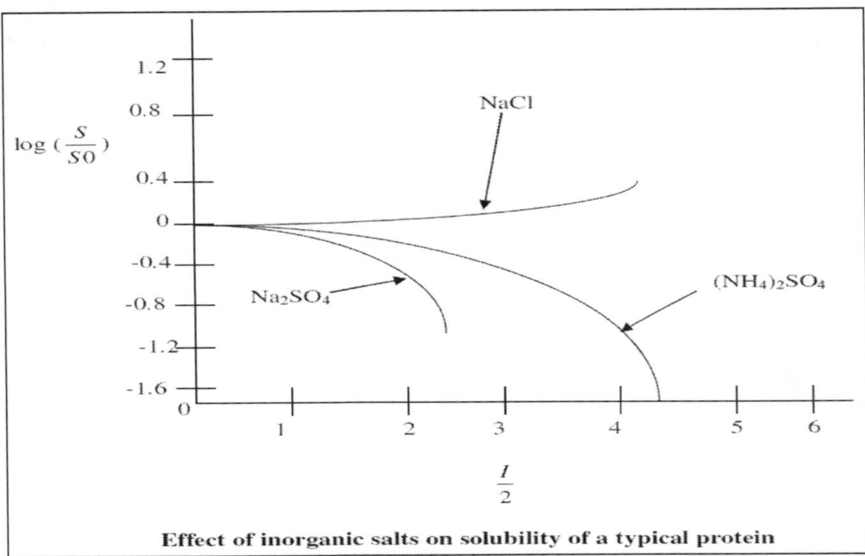

Effect of inorganic salts on solubility of a typical protein

Solubility Reduction at Low Temperature

Addition of certain organic solvents such as acetone and ethanol at low temperature (T<5°C), causes the precipitation of protein by reducing its solubility and dielectric constant of the solution. Solubility of protein is a function of dielectric constant of solution is given by

$$\log \frac{S}{S_0} = -K'/D^2_S$$

Solvent may cause denaturation of protein. Solvent precipitation can be used with salt addition, pH adjustment and low temperature to improve precipitation.

Isoelectric Precipitation

Isoelectric precipitation is the precipitation of protein at their Isoelectric point, which is the pH at which protein have no net charge. It is defined as

$$pI = \frac{1}{2}(p_{k1} + p_{k2})$$

when pH = pI, protein becomes free of charge and precipitates.

This method is effective for proteins with high surface hydrophobicity(*i.e.* a nonpolar surface). This method is inexpensive, but low pH values may result in the denaturation of protein.

4.2 Aqueous Two-Phase Extraction (ATPE)

This liquid- liquid fractionation technique is one of the key separation methods used for isolating many pharmaceutical compounds from plant and animal sources. It has gained attention due to ease in its operation and high recovery yield. Separation of proteins between two phases depends on their molecular weight and charge. Two major types of ATPE are combination of polymer-polymer or polymer-salt (as shown in table below).

Component 1	*Component 2*
Polypropylene glycol	Polyvinyl alcohol Dextran
Polyethylene glycol	Magnesium sulphate Sodium sulphate Ammonium sulphate Ficoll

Water is the main component in ATPE. Insoluble solids remain in one phase and proteins in other phase, each containing 85-99 per cent water.

Other techniques such as precipitation or crystallisation are further helpful in product removal from the partitioned phases.

Partition coefficient (K) may defined as

$$K = \frac{C_{Au}}{C_{Al}}$$

where,

C_{Au} and C_{Al} are equlibrium concentrations of component A in the upper and lower phases, respectively

If K> 1, component A favours the upper phase and *vice versa*.

4.3 Adsorption

It can be used to separate the target molecule from a complex mixture or to concentrate the biological products. This process can be carried out by making a bed of adsorbent column and passing the culture broth through it. The desired product, held by the adsorbent, can be eluted.

Common Adsorbents

There are two major groups of adsorbents that are used for biological molecules: carbons and synthetic resins.

Carbons or Activated Charcoal

The activated charcoal is a commercial products and are not manufactured specifically for bioseperations. But they are widely used as they have large surface area per unit weight.

Synthetic Resins

For low molecular weight compounds (such as vitamins, antibiotics *etc.*), synthetic polymer based resins are used as adsorbents. The polymer usually contain fixed charge and effectively adsorb both ionic and inionic as well as nonpolar solutes.

Resin based on acrylic ester often adsorb hydrophillic solutes. Clay are rarely used. Silica gel and alumina can be used to remove water, but these are good choice for the dilute solution.

Adsorption Isotherm

There are three isotherm:

1. Linear isotherm
2. Freundlich isotherm
3. Langmuir isotherm

1. *Linear Isotherm*

If we plot the graph between the adsorbed concentration (q) and solution concentration (y), there is linear relationship between them

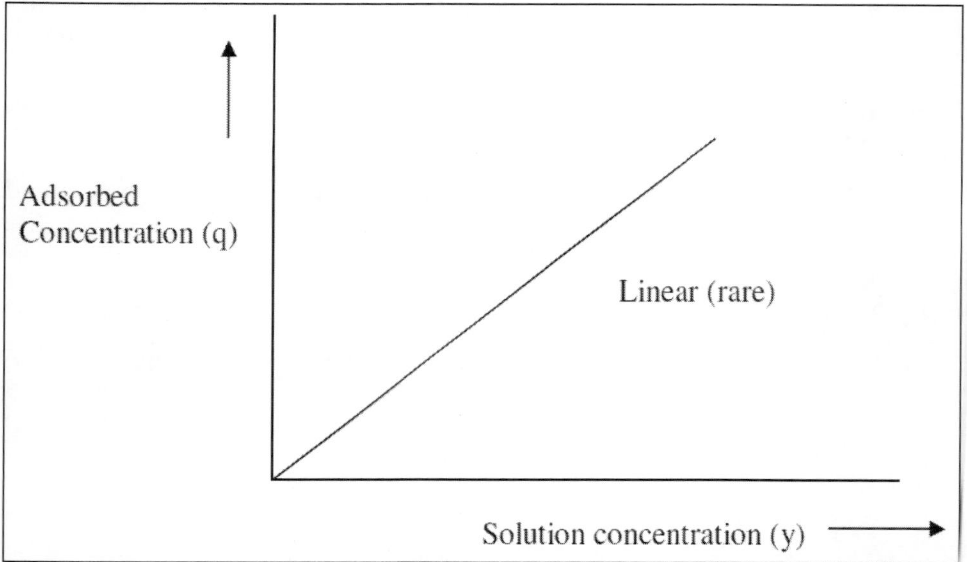

Linear isotherm is given by;

$q = K\,y$

where,

q = Amount of solute adsorbed per amount of adsorbent.

y = Solute concentration in solution.

K = Equilibrium constant.

Linear isotherm is not common; it may be approximate the other isotherm over a limited range of concentration.

2. Freundlich Isotherm

Freundlich isotherm describes the adsorption of a wide variety of antibiotics, steroids and hormones. It is given by;

$q = K\,y^n$

where,

q = Amount of solute adsorbed per amount of adsorbent.

y = Solute concentration in solution.

The constants n and K must be determined experimentally.

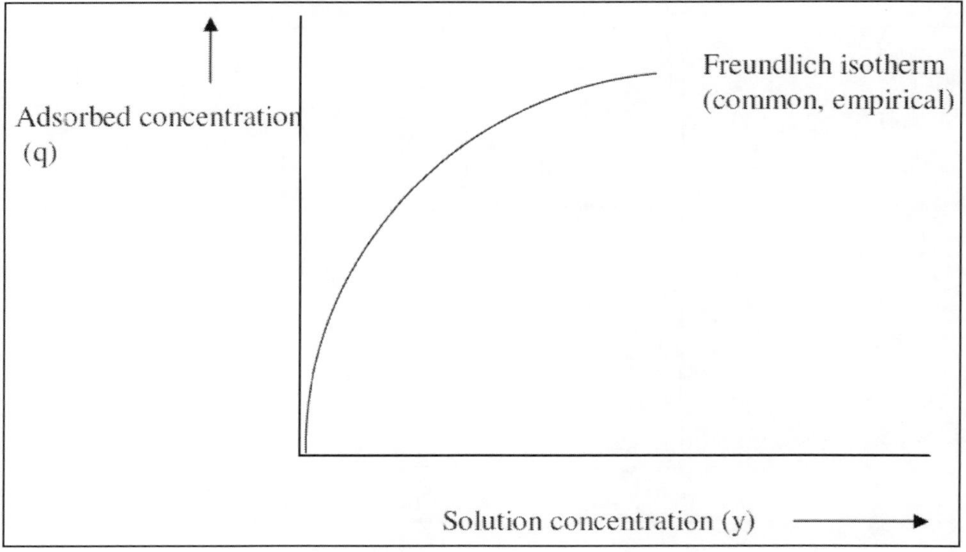

$q = K\,y^n$

Taking the log of above equation

$\text{Log}\ q = \log k + n \log y$

These constants are best determined by means of a log-log plot of q versus y. The slope of such a plot is the dimensionless exponent n.

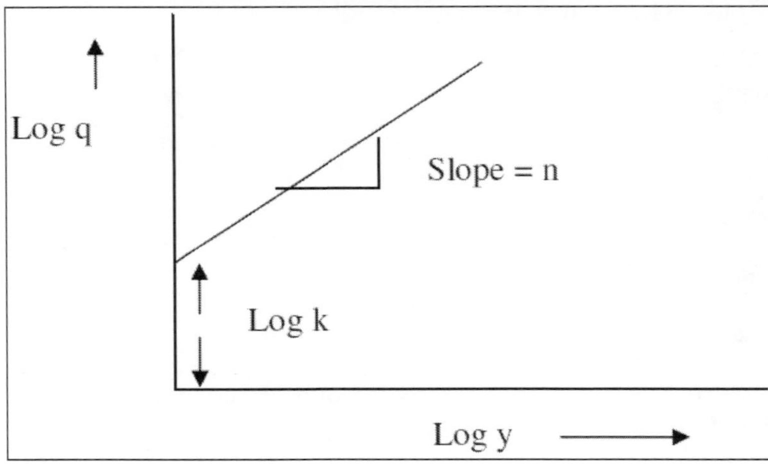

If the adsorption is favourable, then n< 1.

If the adsorption is unfavourable, then n> 1.

3. *Langmuir Isotherm*

Langmuir isotherm is often used to correlate adsorption data for proteins. It is given by;

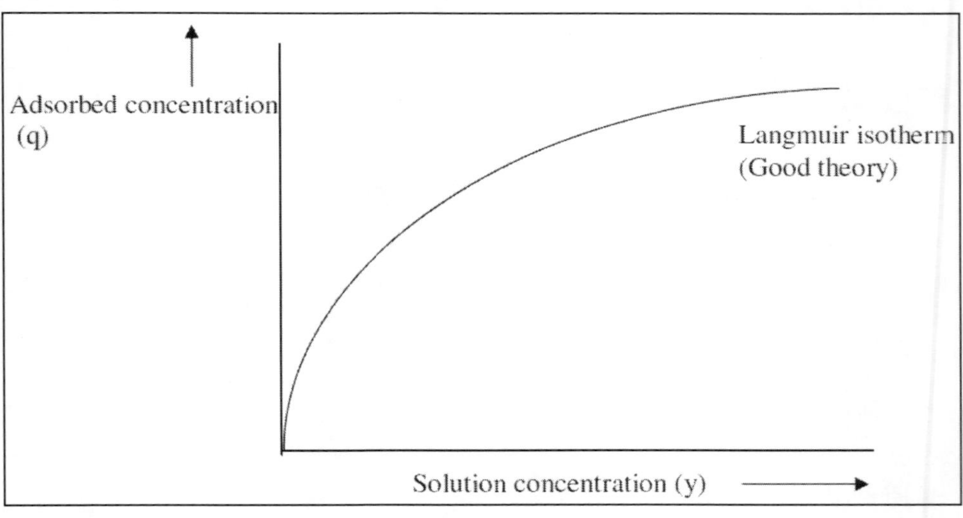

$$q = \frac{q_o\, y}{K + y}$$

where,

q = Amount of solute adsorbed per amount of adsorbent.

y = Solute concentration in solution.

The constants q_0 and K must be determined experimentally.

$$q = \frac{q_0\, y}{K + y}$$

Inversing the above equation

$$\frac{1}{q} = \frac{K}{q_0\, y} + \frac{y}{q_0\, y}$$

$$\frac{1}{q} = \frac{K}{q_0\, y} + \frac{1}{q_0}$$

$Y = m\,x + c$

The plot of (1/q) and (1/y).

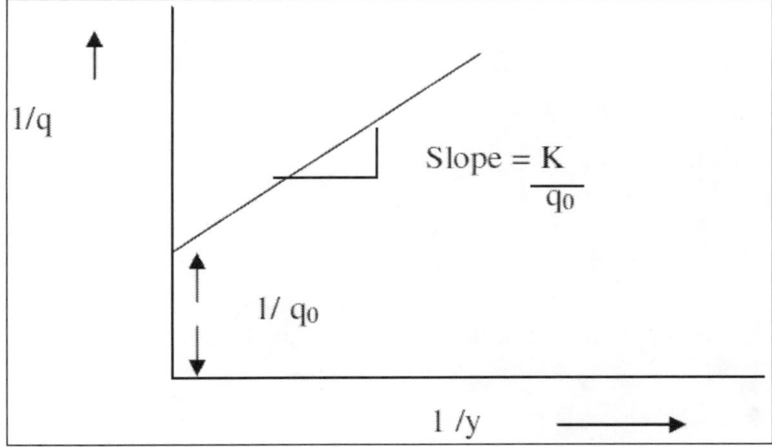

The intercept of such a plot is $(1/q_0)$ and the slope is K/q_0.

The dimension of q_0 = q and K = Y dimension.

The theoretical basis of Langmuir isotherm depends on the chemical reaction between solute and vacant sites on the adsorbent surface.

Solute + Vacant site = Filled site

If this reaction is at equilibrium, then it is described by an equilibrium constant K

$$K = \frac{[\text{Solute}]\,[\text{Vacant site}]}{[\text{Filled site}]}$$

Moreover, the total number of active sites must be fixed

[Total site] = [Vacant site] + [Filled site]

Combing the last two equation

$$[\text{Filled site}] = \frac{[\text{Total site}]\,[\text{Solute}]}{K + [\text{Solute}]}$$

Ion Exchange Isotherm

Ion exchange reaction on a resin for which

$Na^+ + HR \longleftrightarrow NaR + H^+$

where,

HR = Ion exchange sites fitted with a proton.

NaR = Ion exchange sites fitted with a sodium ion.

This implies that all sites are filled, with either a proton or a sodium ion.

At the equilibrium,

$$K = \frac{[NaR][H^+]}{[Na^+][HR]}$$

The total concentration of ionic groups R^- on the resin is fixed.

$[R^-] = [NaR] + [HR]$

Thus

$$[NaR] = \frac{K\,[R^-]\,[Na^+]}{[H^+] + K\,[Na^+]}$$

Sodium adsorption will imitate the Langmuir isotherm in a buffer solution (pH constant).

Affinity Adsorption

It depends on interactions between solute and resin, rather than the London-van der walls forces responsible for conventional adsorption or the electrostatic interactions of ion exchange. Affinity adsorption is much more selective.

The adsorbent consists of two parts;

1. Support
2. Ligand

The support bound to ligand by covalent or ionic bond, but it does not interact with the solute. In contrast the bound ligands do react with the solute. When the solute is macromolecular, the interaction often involves several adjacent sites on the adsorbent. Such interaction involves "Lock and Key" mechanism.

Affinity adsorption processes often show Langmuir isotherms, but this anticipated behaviour should be checked experimentally.

4.4 Chromatography

Principle of Chromatography

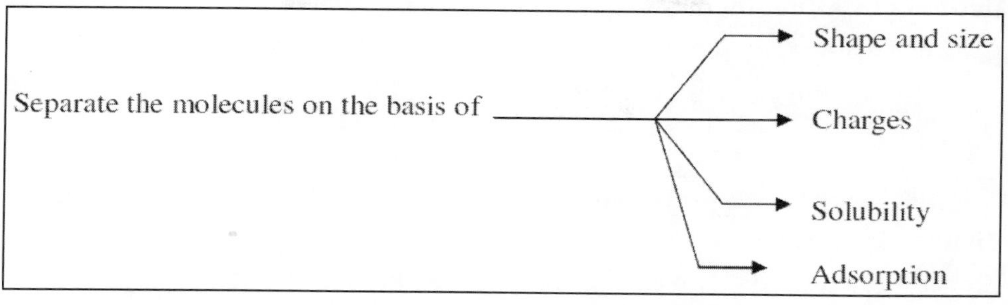

Shape and size → Gel filtration chromatography

Charge → Ion-exchange chromatography

Solubility → Partition chromatography

Adsorption → Adsorption chromatography

Chromatography, there is the interaction between three factors.

1. Stationary phase (column, paper or thin layer)
2. Mobile phase (Liquid or gas) flow over or through the stationary phase.
3. Molecules to be separated (Protein or Biomolecule).

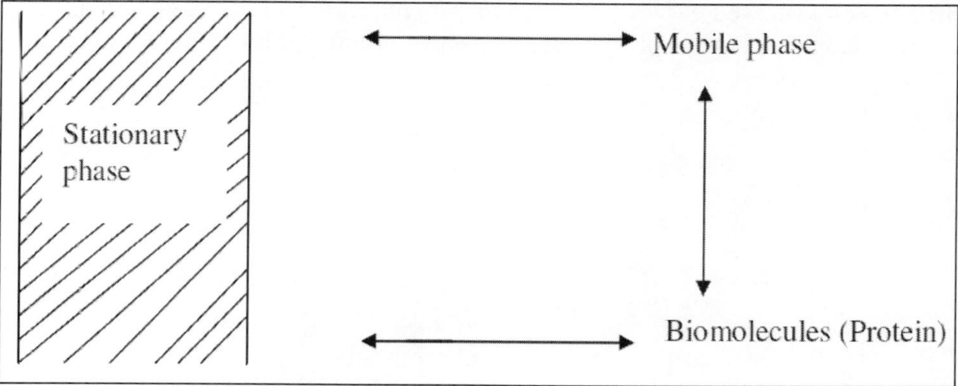

The **Partition** or **Distribution coefficient** (K_d) is the basis of chromatography

$$K_d = \frac{\text{Concentration in phase (A)}}{\text{Concentration in phase (B)}}$$

Where two A and B are two immiscible phases

K_d describes the way in which a compound distributes itself between two immiscible phases.

Method of Chromatography

Chromatography separation may be achieved by two basic techniques:

1. Column chromatography
2. Thin-layer or planar (paper) chromatography

Column Chromatography	*Thin-layer or Planar Chromatography*
Stationary phase Consists of a packed suitable matrix into a glass or metal column	**Stationary phase** Consists of a suitable matrix coated thinly onto a glass, plastic or metal foil plate
Mobile phase Any suitable solvent depending on the nature of product which is passed through the stationary phase either by gravity feed or by use of pressure	**Mobile phase** Mobile phase passes through the stationary phase through capillary action

Gel Filtration Chromatography or Molecular Exclusion (Permeation) Chromatography

This is based on separation of molecules on the basis of their shape and size. Molecules are passed down a column containing swollen particles of a gel. Small molecules get entrapped inside the gel whereas larger molecules are excluded from the cross-linked network. This technique requires a single mobile phase and isocratic elution. Ultraviolet adsorption spectrophotometer is needed for detection.

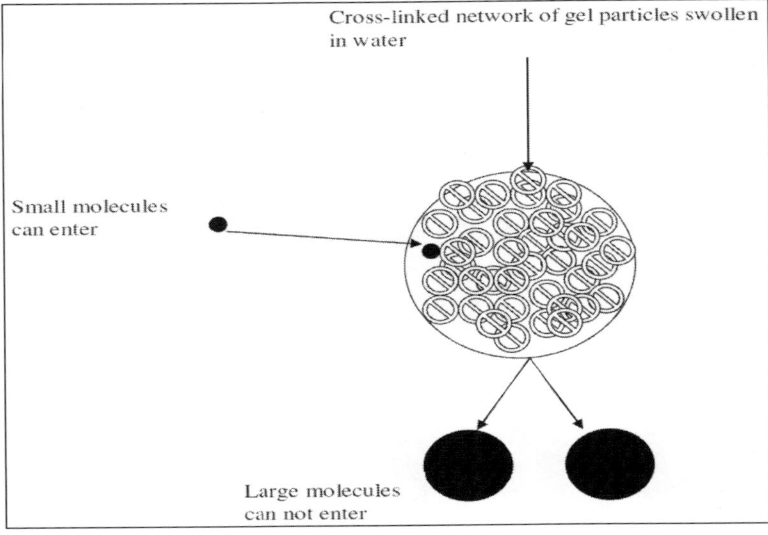

Column of sponge-like gel beads with pores works as a molecular sieve for separating the molecules on the basis of their size. Large molecules, which can enter the pores, will come out first with the mobile liquid. Smaller molecules enter the pores of gel beads and then pass through the column at a slower rate, hence appearing last in the effluent.

$$V_T = V_i + V_o + V_g$$

where,

V_T = Total volume of a column of gel

V_i and V_o = Volume of water inside and outside the gel particle, respectively

V_g = Volume of gel matrix

V_i can be calculated from a knowledge of the dry weight of the gel (a) and water regain (W_r)

$$V_i = a\,W_r$$

V_o is also known void volume

Void volume, is the volume of liquid required to elute compounds that are completely excluded from the gel grains.

V_e = the volume required to elute that compound from the column.

$$V_e = V_o + K_d\,V_i$$

K_d = distribution coefficient.

$$K_d = \frac{V_e - V_o}{V_i} = \frac{V_e - V_o}{a\,W r}$$

If,

K_d = 0, then $V_e = V_o$ then molecule is completely excluded from the gel.

K_d = 1, then $V_e = V_o + V_i$ then molecule is completely accessibility to the gel.

K_d > 1, then the adsorption of the compounds on the gel has occurred.

K_d values vary between 0 to 1.

Gel filtration chromatography can also be used to estimate the molecular mass of a protein. There is a linear relationship between the relative elution volume of a protein (V_e/V_0 where V_e is the elution volume of a given protein and V_0 is the void volume of the column that is the volume of the solvent space surrounding the beads) and logarithm of its molecular mass. Thus a 'standard' curve of V_e/V_0 against the log of molecular mass can be estimated using protein of known mass.

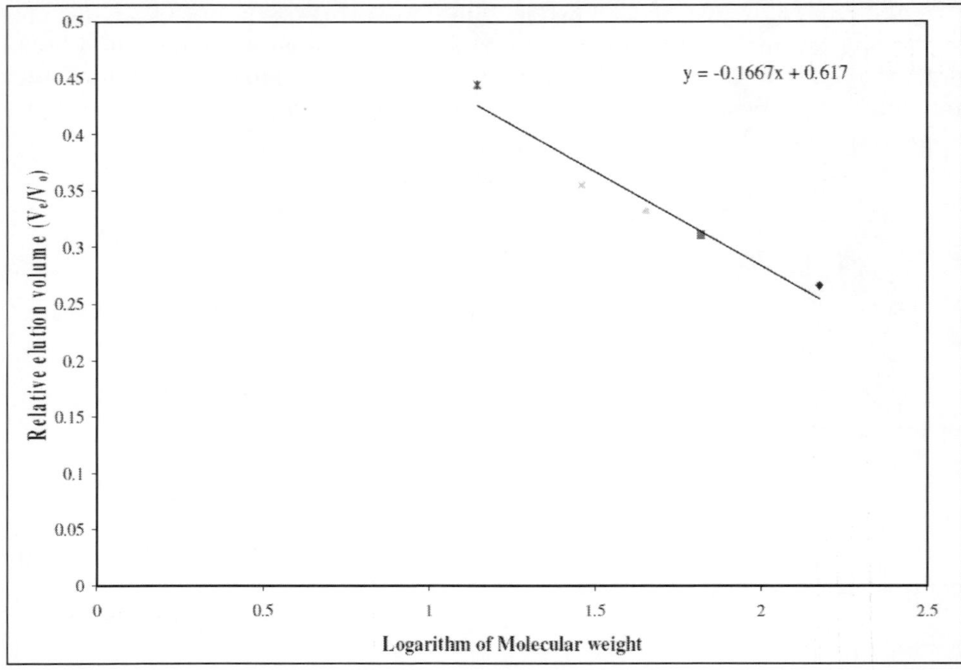

Some Gel Commonly Used for Exclusion Chromatography

Polymer	*Trade Name*
Dextran	SephadexSephacryl
Agarose	SepharoseBio-gel

Ion-exchange Chromatography

The basic principle of Ion exchange chromatography is separation of molecules depending on their overall charge. These can be of two types:

1. Cation exchangers (negatively charged groups): If a protein contains positive charge then columns containing negatively charged groups such as carboxymethyl (CM) or CM-Sephadex are used and this is termed as cation exchange chromatography.
2. Anion exchangers (positively charged groups): If a protein is negatively charged then columns containing positively charged groups like diethylaminoethyl (DEAE) are used and this is termed as anion exchange chromatography.

Affinity Chromatography

It is based on the interaction of protein with an immobilized ligand and is widely used for the purification of proteins from a complex mixture. The ligand can be any substrate analogue, specific antibody or inhibitor. This ligand is, first of all, attached to an inert matrix followed by addition of protein mixture. The target compound will bind to the ligand and all other proteins will pass through the column. Finally, the bound protein is detached from the ligand by changing the solvent conditions.

Separation and purification of biological molecule, on the basis highly specific interaction between pairs of biological materials is affinity chromatography.

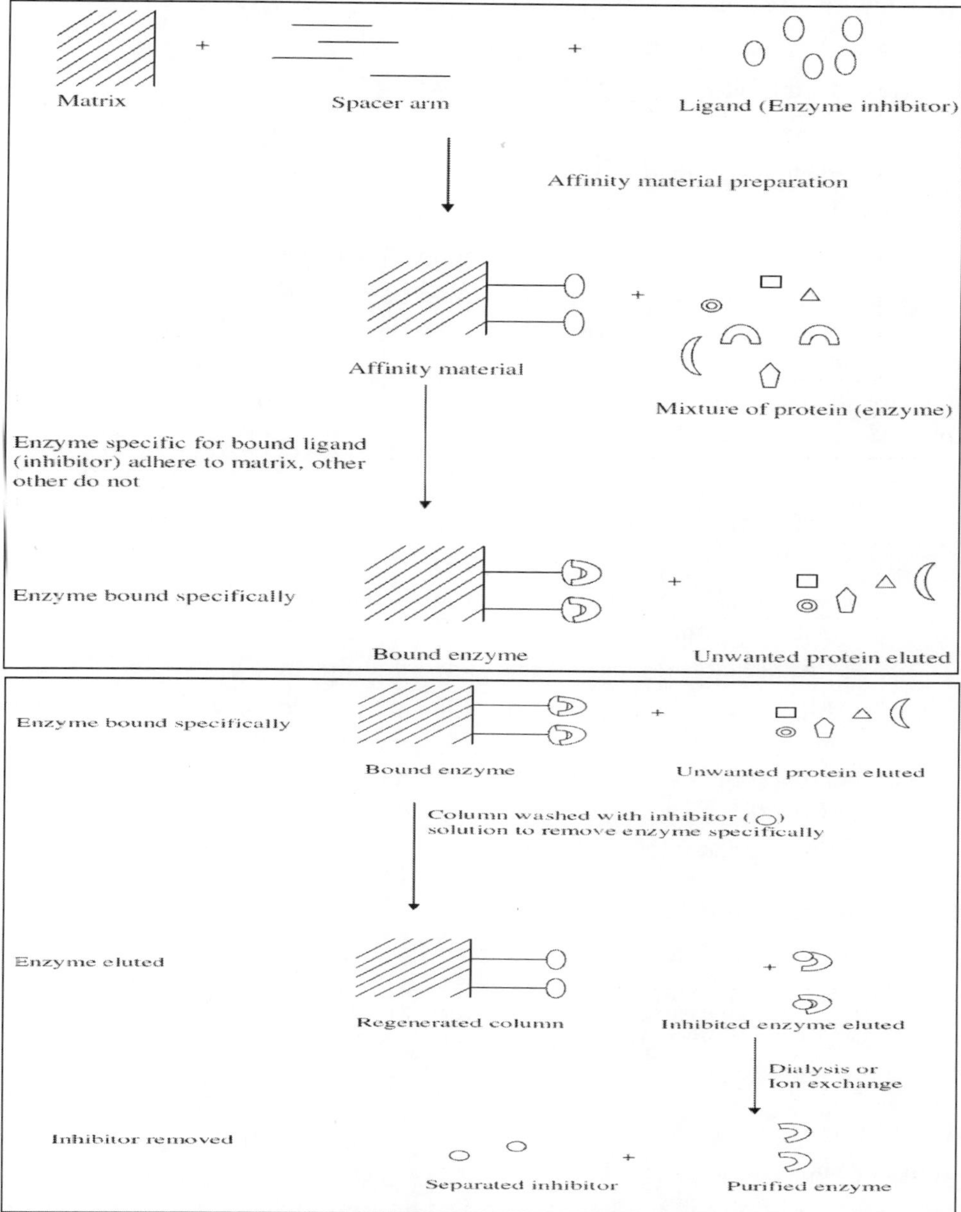

This technique exploits the unique and specific interaction that exists between biological molecules.

Enzyme – substrate (Molecule to be purified - ligand)

Molecule to be purified = Enzyme

Ligand = substrate

Enzyme – inhibitor

Molecule to be purified = Enzyme

Ligand = inhibitor

Antigen – antibody

Molecule to be purified = Antigen

Ligand = antibody

Ligand = Binding substance, which is immobilized to insoluble support (**matrix**)

Spacer arm = always inserted between matrix and ligand. But it should neither be too long (to avoid undesirable non specific adsorption) nor too short (to avoid steric hinderance)

Ligand and matrix are either attached by physical adsorption or attached by chemical bond.

Matrix

The ideal matrix for affinity chromatography must posses the following properties:

1. Contain suitable and sufficient group to which the ligand may be may be covalently coupled.
2. Must be stable under the condition of the attachment with the ligand.
3. Must be stable during binding of the macromolecule and its subsequent elution.
4. Interact only weakly with other macromolecules to minimize non-specific adsorption.
5. Exhibit good flow properties.

Commonly used Matrix

1. Cross-linked dextran (Sephacryl S)
2. Agarose (Sepharose, Bio-Gel A)
3. Polyacrylamide gel (Bio-Gel P)
4. Cellulose
5. Silica

Spacer Arm

Spacer arm possess a second functional group to which the ligand may be attached conventional organosynthetic procedures, which frequently involve the use of succinic anhydride and a water-soluble craboliimide.

Commonly Used Spacer Arm

1. 1,6 diamino hexane
2. 6-aminohexanoic acid

Ligand

Commonly used ligand in affinity chromatography

Ligand	*Affinity*
Avidin	Biotin-containing enzyme
Calmodulin	Calmodulin – binding protein
Proteins A and G	Immunoglobulins
Lysine	r RNA
5′AMP	NAD^+ dependent dehydrogenase
2′5′ADP	$NADP^+$ dependent dehydrogenase

4.5 Dialysis

It is a membrane separation operation used for the removal of low –molecular weight solutes such as organic acid and inorganic ions from a solution. Protein can be separated effectively from small molecules by this technique using cellophane (cellulose acetate, a semi permeable membrane). This membrane is selectively permeable to molecules up to approximately 10kDa whereas larger molecules are retained inside the dialysis bag.

4.6 Electrodialysis

It is also a membrane separation method where application of a direct electric current helps in separating the charged molecules from a solution. The membranes contain ion-exchange groups and have a fixed electrical charge. This method is very effective in the concentration of electrolytes and proteins.

Positively charged membranes (anion membranes; contain positively charged quaternary ammonium group-N_3R^+, chemically bound to the phenyl groups in the polystyrene) allow the passage of anions and repel cations; negatively charged membranes (cation membranes; contain negatively charged group, chemically bound to the phenyl groups in the polystyrene) allow the passage of cations and repel anions.

4.7 Microfiltration and Ultrafiltration

Microfiltration is a filtration process which removes contaminants from a fluid (liquid and gas) by passage through a micro porous membrane. A typical microfiltration membrane pore size range is 0.1 to 10 micrometres (μm). It uses low pressure (10-100 psig) process for separating larger size solutes from aqueous solutions by means of a semi-permeable membrane. Microfiltration is used for fermentation broth clarification and biomass clarification and recovery.

Ultrafiltration is a variety of membrane filtration in which hydrostatic pressure forces a liquid against a semipermeable membrane. In ultrafiltration, solution moves by pressure gradient. Suspended solids and solutes of high molecular weight are retained, while water and low molecular weight solutes pass through the membrane. This separation process is used in industry and research for purifying and concentrating macromolecular (10^3 - 10^6 Da) solutions, especially protein solutions. Ultrafiltration is also referred to as convection, is fluid flow through the membrane, forced by a difference in pressure on the two sides of the dialyzer (pressure gradient).

4.8 Electrophoresis

It is a technique used to purify proteins of different size and charge depending on their movement under the influence of an electric field.

Electrostatic force on charged particle = $q\,E$

Where, q is the charge on the particle; E is the intensity of electric field.

Drag force on the particle = $6\,\pi\,r\,\eta\,v$

Where, r is the radius of particle; η is the viscosity of the fluid; v is terminal velocity of the particle.

$$q\,E = 6\,\pi\,r\,\eta\,v$$

$$v = \frac{q\,E}{6\,\pi\,r\,\eta}$$

SDS PAGE

This is also known as denaturing gel electrophoresis. In SDS-PAGE, the proteins are denatured hence the separation is only dependent on their mass. The protein mixture is first treated with a reducing agent such as 2-mercaptoethanol or dithiothreitol to break all disulphide bonds. The commonly used denaturant used is strong anionic detergent SDS which gives the denatured proteins a large net negative charge that is proportional to its mass. The SDS/protein mixture is then applied to sample wells in the top of a polyacrylamide gel.

Native PAGE

This technique helps in purifying protein in native condition *i.e.* protein is not denatured. The basic different from SDS PAGE is that in this case SDS is not used.

Isoelectric Focusing

Isoelectric focusing electrophoretically separates proteins on the basis of their relative content of positively and negatively charged groups. When a protein is its pI, net charge is zero and hence it will not move in an electric field. In isoelectric focusing, polyacrylamide gel is used which has large pores and contains a mixture of polyampholyte (small multi-charged polymers that have many pI values). If an electric field is applied to the gel, the polyampholytes migrate and produced pH gradient. To separate proteins by isoelectric focusing, they are electrophoresed through such gel. Each protein will migrate through the gel until it reaches a position at which pH is equal to its pI.

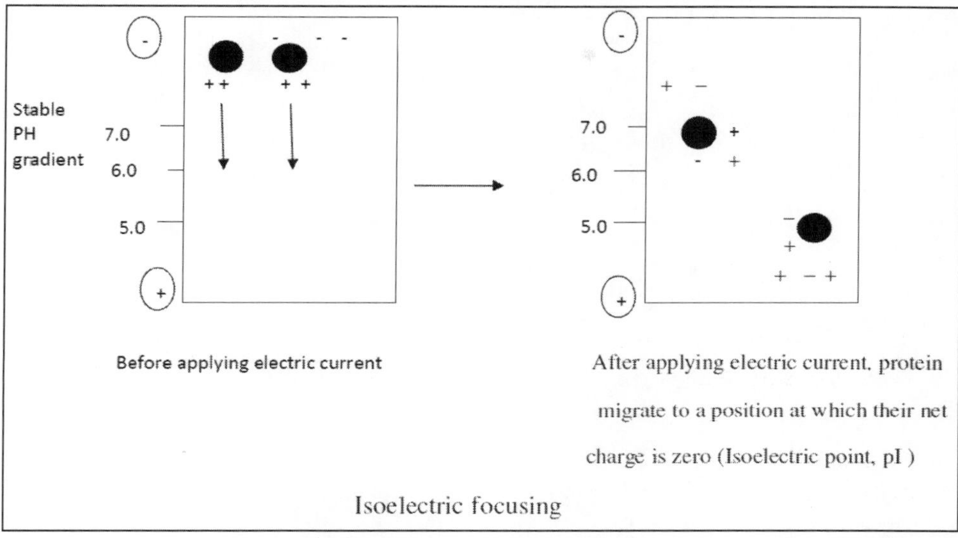

Isoelectric focusing

Two Dimensional Gel Electrophoresis

Isoelectric focusing can be combined with SDS-PAGE to obtain very high resolution separations in a procedure known as two dimensional gel electrophoresis. The protein sample is first subjected to isoelectric focusing in a narrow strip of gel containing polyampholytes. This gel strip is then placed on top of an SDS polyacrylamide gel and electrophoresed to produce two-dimensional pattern of spots in which the proteins have been separated in the horizontal direction on the basis of their pI, and in the vertical direction on the basis of their mass. The overall result is that proteins are separated both on the basis of their size and charge.

4.9 Reverse Osmosis

Osmosis is the movement of water molecules through a selectively-permeable membrane down a water potential gradient. More specifically, it is the movement of water across a selectively permeable membrane from an area of high water potential (low solute concentration) to an area of low water potential (high solute concentration).

The osmotic pressure is defined to be the pressure required to maintain an equilibrium, with no net movement of solvent. Osmotic pressure is a colligative property, meaning that the osmotic pressure depends on the molar concentration of the solute but not on its identity. The osmotic pressure (π) can be expressed as

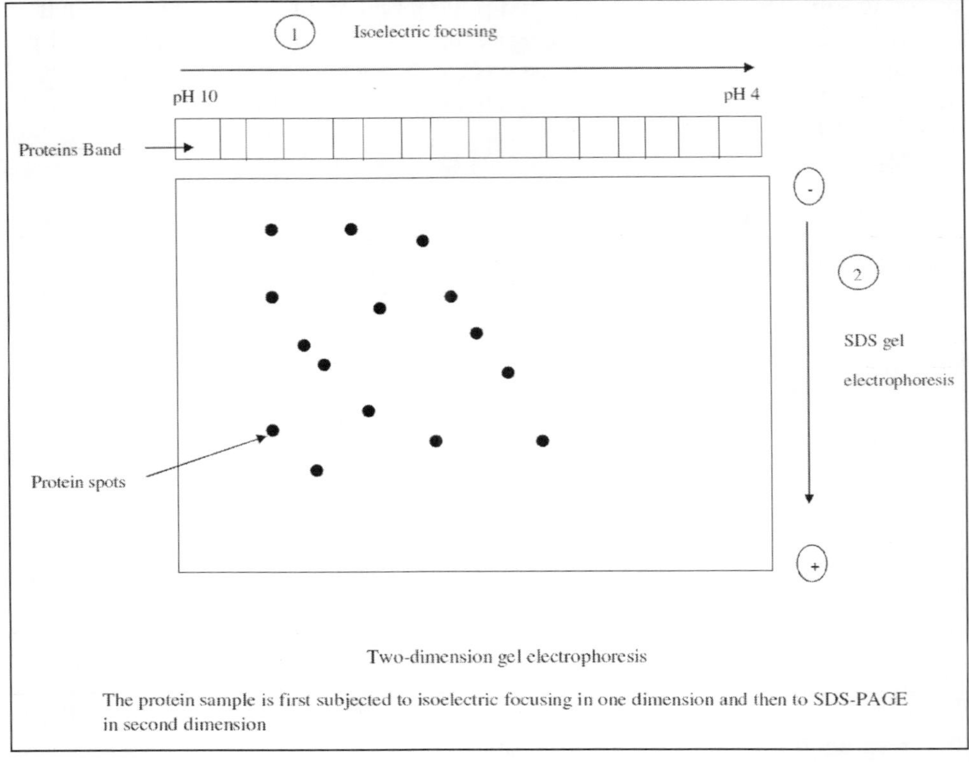

Two-dimension gel electrophoresis

The protein sample is first subjected to isoelectric focusing in one dimension and then to SDS-PAGE in second dimension

$$PV = n R T$$

$$P = \frac{n}{V} RT$$

$$\pi = CRT$$

Reverse osmosis is a separation process that uses pressure to force a solvent through a semipermeable membrane that retains the solute on one side and allows the pure solvent to pass to the other side. In reverse osmosis, a pressure is applied onto a solvent from a region of high solute concentration through a semipermeable membrane to a region of low solute concentration by applying a pressure in excess of the osmotic pressure.

The semi-permeable membrane used in reverse osmosis contains tiny pores through which water can flow. The small pores of this membrane are restrictive to such organic compounds as salt and other natural minerals, which generally have a larger molecular composition than water. These pores are also restrictive to bacteria and disease-causing pathogens.

5 Final Steps for Purification

The final steps in fermentation product purification are crystallization and drying.

5.1 Crystallization

It is usually the last step in producing highly purified products. It is carried out at low temperatures, which minimize thermal degradation of heat-sensitive materials. High-purify crystals are recovered by using batch Nutsche-type filter or centrifugal filter. The following equation is used for the filtration of crystal slurries; assuming the crystals are non compressible and the resistance of the filter medium is negligible.

$$\frac{dV}{dt} = K\frac{A\,\Delta P}{\Delta X}$$

where, V is liquid volume; K is the transfer coefficient; A is surface are; ΔP is pressure drop; ΔX is the thickness of crystal layer. Substituting W α V, where W is the solid concentration in the cake

$$\frac{dW}{dt} = K\frac{A\,\Delta P}{\Delta X}$$

Integration of above equation

$$t = K\frac{W^2}{\Delta P\,A^2}$$

5.2 Drying

The removal of solvent from purified wet product (crystal or dissolved solute) is usually achieved by drying. Before selecting drying conditions, due consideration should be given to the heat sensitivity and physical properties of the product. Most of the biological products are temperature sensitive, hence, gentle drying methods should be used. The major types of driers used for drying fermentation product are the following;

1. A vacuum-tray drier.
2. Freeze drying (lyophilization)
3. Rotary drum driers
4. Spray driers
5. Pneumatic conveyor driers

REFERENCES

1. Comprehensive Biotechnology, Moo-Young, Alan T. Bullm Howard Dalton, Panima Publication.
2. Bioseparations: Downstream Processing for Biotechnology, P.A. Belter *et al.*, John Wiley and Sons Inc.
3. Downstream Processing, J.P. Hamel, J.B. Hunter and S.K. Sikdar, American Chemical Society
4. Principles of Fermentation Technology by P.F. Stanbury, A. Whitaker, and S.J. Hall, Aditya Books (P) LTD.

5. Freitag R, Horváth C. Chromatography in the downstream processing of biotechnological products. Adv Biochem Eng Biotechnol. 1996;53: 17-59.

6. Biochemical Engineering and Biotechnology By Ghasem Najafpour.

7. Practical Biochemistry, Principles and Techniques, Keith Wilson and John Walker.

Chapter 17

Nanobiotechnology

*Akanksha Sharma[1], Sanchi Gupta[1] and Deepak Kumar[2]**

[1]Department of Botany, Central University of Jammu, Rahya-Suchani (Bagla), Jammu and Kashmir – 181 143, India

[2]Department of Botany, Institute of Science, Banaras Hindu University, Varanasi – 221 005, Uttar Pradesh, India

**e-mail: deepakkumar@bhu.ac.in*

ABSTRACT

Nanobiotechnology is an emerging field of nanotechnology. It is a multi-stratal way of amalgamating nanotechnology and biotechnology. This technique is based on the use of various nanoparticles as its structural and functional units. Various studies have been conducted on the size, chemical and physical properties of these nanoparticles. The synthesis of nanoparticles with diverse chemical composition, sizes, shape, structure and properties is being extensively studied. The unequalled size (about 1-100 nm) and properties of nanoparticles make them exceptionally potential in various fields of research and industrial sectors. Now a days, nanoparticles are widely explored for their commercial uses in various fields like medical, surface science, textile, molecular biology, semiconductor physics etc. This chapter gives a detailed description about the various types, properties and characteristics of nanoparticles. Apart from the traditional chemical and physical methods of nanoparticle synthesis, the modern-day eco-friendly approaches for the green synthesis of nanoparticles have also been elucidated. The diverse applications of nanoparticles are also enumerated in detail.

Keywords: *Bottom-up approach, Green synthesis, Nanobiotechnology, Metallic nanoparticles, Nanoparticles, Top-down approach, SEM, TEM, UV-vis spectroscopy.*

1. Introduction

"There's Plenty of Room at the Bottom:" the highly acclaimed and prophetic lecture delivered by **Nobel Laureate Richard P. Feynman (American physicist)** in the year 1959 at Caltech is extensively considered to be the genesis for the concept of 'Nanotechnology'. In his lecture, Feynman discussed about manipulating atoms to solve many fundamental problems of biology and in his own eccentric manner emphasized that, "We need to make the microscope 100 times more powerful so as to just look at the thing!". But even for a visionary like Feynman, it would be hard to believe that biological systems especially plants would be central to the synthesis of nanoparticles which are in many ways the protagonist in green nanotechnology.

Etymologically the word "Nano" comes from **nanos**, which in Greek means **dwarf**. According to the International System of Units *i.e.*, SI, one nanometer equals to one billionth of a meter or 0.000 000 001 m. Nano (symbolic "n") is a unit prefix denoting 10^{-9} meter. **Figure 17.1** highlights the three different forms of matter on the basis of size. The term 'Nanotechnology' and 'Nanoscience' pertains to the study and application of matter at nanoscale. The expected size of nanoparticles is estimated between **1 and 100 nanometers**. As earlier stated, Feynman is credited with introducing the broad conjectures of the world at atomic level but it was **Norio Taniguchi** belonging to the Tokyo Science University who for the first time used the term 'Nanotechnology' in his paper titled "On the basic concept of Nano-Technology," in 1974. Therefore, nanotechnology is defined as the ability to quantify, influence and synthesize things on an atomic or molecular scale.

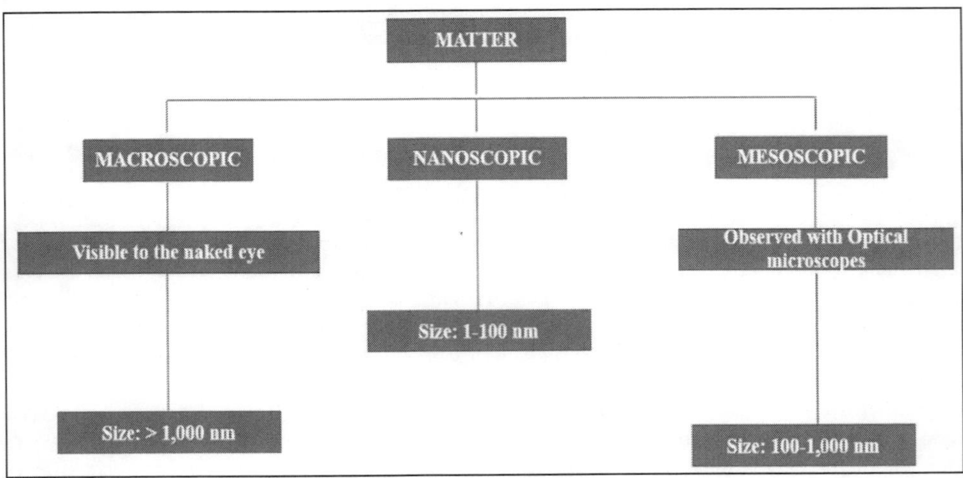

Figure 17.1: Size Differentiation of different Forms of Matter.

The terms 'nanoscience' and 'nanotechnology' as mentioned earlier, may not have the clearest of separation due to their various overlapping domains, resulting in some ambiguity. The major difference lies in the fact that nanotechnology implicitly involves the actual application whereas nanoscience mainly deals with the understanding of laws and observable phenomenon as supported by the Royal Society and Royal Academy of Engineering (2004) which have defined nanoscience as: "The study of phenomenon and manipulation of materials at atomic, molecular and macromolecular scales, where properties differ significantly from those at the larger scale" and nanotechnology as: "The design, characterization, synthesis and application of structures, devices and systems by controlling shape and size at nanometer scale". Since these nanoparticles have large surface area to volume ratio along with unique optical, electrical, thermal physical and chemical properties, they find a variety of applications in the areas of medicine, chemistry, energy, agriculture, information, communication, mechanics, heavy industry, optics, biotechnology, electronics, microbiology, consumer goods and environmental remediation. Nanobiotechnology is the science of producing and constructing devices. Now-a-days, maximum attention is being given to the synthesis of NPs with different chemical compositions, sizes and morphologies, and controlled disparities. In fact, biology or to be more precise molecular biology and biochemistry are associated with nanoscience, as many of the cellular structures like DNA, RNA and other sub-cellular organelles are of nanoscale, viruses too fall in this category.

2. Characteristics of Nanoparticles

The general characteristics of nanoparticles (NPs) include:

1. High surface area to volume ratio, when the particles get reduced, their surface to volume ratio increases dramatically, from that of bulk material. As the reactions take place on the surface of the particles, it thus, creates a large area as compared to that of bulk material with the same volume. It is very interesting to note that when a particle becomes nanosized, its chemical and physical properties are very much different from its macro counterparts. For example, gold as a noble metal is inert in its macroscale, whereas the same become extremely reactive and can be used as catalyst while being nanosized. This has important application for the design of catalytic agents. Another property of the materials that gets changed when converted to nanoscale is the melting point, for example melting point of gold is 1064°C, whereas a 1nm size particle would become liquid at room temperature. This observed trend in melting point is due to the size of the nanoparticles.
2. Nanoparticles exhibit Surface Plasmon Resonance (SPR) and Surface-Enhanced Raman Spectroscopy (SERS). Plasmon represents the collective oscillations of the free charges in a metal, when an external electric field in the form of light source is applied. Owing to the fact that electrons are electrically charged particles, which upon vibration can give rise to electric field. When the electric field is applied externally, it resonates. Also, the electric field from the vibrations of the free electrons resonate. This collective phenomenon results in Surface Plasmon Resonance (SPR) that occurs prominently on the surface of the metal.
3. Nanoparticles are bounded by an interfacial layer which may consist of organic and inorganic molecules, ions *etc.* Organic molecules that coat these inorganic nanoparticles are known as stabilizers, surface ligands, capping or passivating agents. This interfacial layer fundamentally affects the different nanoparticle properties.

A nanoparticle can be of various sizes. Nanodots for example, have zero dimension with fixed length, breadth and height at a single point. While, nano dots possess only one parameter and are one dimensional, graphene possesses both length and breadth and is two dimensional while carbon nanotubes are three dimensional as they have all the parameters such as length, breadth and height.

3. Classification of Nanoparticles

The nanoparticles can be generally classified into organic, inorganic and carbon based.

3.1 Organic Nanoparticles

These types of nanoparticles are biodegradable and non-toxic. These are commonly known as polymers. Particles like micelles and liposomes have a hollow core, therefore are called as nano capsules. These nano-capsules are thermal sensitive and can be sensitive to electromagnetic radiation as well. Nano-capsules being efficient and able to be injected easily in distinct parts of the body form an exemplary drug delivery system. This system is also known as targeted drug delivery. They have an extensive importance in the biomedical field. Examples include: Dendrimers, micelles, liposomes and ferritin *etc.*

3.2 Inorganic Nanoparticles

Inorganic nanoparticles constitute metal and metal oxide-based nanoparticles. They are further classified as:

Metal Based

These nanoparticles are synthesized from metals by destructive or constructive methods. It has been found that all the metals can be used to synthesize nanoparticles. Some of the examples of widely used metals for the synthesis of nanoparticles are gold (Au), aluminium (Al), copper (Cu), cadmium (Cd), cobalt (Co), iron (Fe), silver (Ag), lead (Pb) and zinc (Zn). Metal based nanoparticles possess various different properties like sizes as low as 10 to 100 nm, surface characteristics like high surface area to volume ratio, pore size, surface charge and surface charge density, crystalline and amorphous structures, shapes like spherical and cylindrical and color reactivity and sensitivity to environmental factors such as air, moisture, heat and sunlight.

Metal Oxides Based

The properties of corresponding metal associated counterparts can be altered using metal-oxide based nanoparticles. These are more commonly synthesized now-a-days, primarily because of their increased reactivity and efficiency. For example, in aerobic conditions, iron nanoparticles instantly oxidize and convert into Fe_2O_3 at room temperature. These oxidized nanoparticles have increased reactivity as compared to iron nanoparticles. The commonly synthesized nanoparticles are Cerium oxide (CeO_2), Aluminium oxide (Al_2O_3), Titanium oxide (TiO_2), Iron oxide (Fe_2O_3), Silicon dioxide (SiO_2), Magnetite (Fe_3O_4), and Zinc oxide (ZnO). Metal oxide-based NPs possess exceptional properties in contrast to their metal counterparts.

3.3 Carbon Based Nanoparticles

Nanoparticles synthesized completely from carbon are known as carbon-based nanoparticles. These are further classified into graphene, fullerenes, carbon nano tubes (CNT), carbon nanofibers, carbon black and sometimes activated carbon in nano size.

Graphene

It is a carbon allotrope with thickness of approximately 1 nm. The carbon atoms are arranged in a 2-D planar orientation resembling a hexagonal honeycomb structure.

Fullerenes

Fullerene (C_{60}) is another allotrope of carbon composed of carbon atoms bound together by double and single bond in sp2 hybridization. It exists in the forms of fully or partially enclosed spherical structure. The dimensions of the diameter range from 8.2 nm and 4-36 nm for single and multiple layered fullerenes respectively. Approximately it consists of around 28- 1500 carbon atoms.

Carbon Nano Tubes (CNT)

Carbon Nano Tubes (CNT) are woven into hollow cylinders forming nanotubes ranging from diameters around 0.7 nm to 100 nm for single and multiple layered CNT respectively. It structurally resembles the graphene nano foil, also having alike honeycomb structure of carbon atoms. Its length ranges can be as less as a few micrometers and may even maximally range up to several millimeters. The termini may be hollow or enclosed partially by a fullerene molecule.

Carbon Nanofiber

Carbon nanofibers are synthesized from graphene nano foils but unlike CNT they are woven into a cup or cone shaped structure instead of the traditional cylindrical tubes.

Carbon Black

It is a carbon based spherical amorphous substance with diameters ranging from 20-70 nm. It is often clumped together and forms agglomerates up to 500 nm in size because of the high interaction among the particles.

4. Properties of Nanoparticles

Nanoparticles can be of various different shape, size and structure. Their shape can range from tubular, spherical, spiral, cylindrical, conical, flat, hollow core, *etc.* to irregular. Their size can range from 1 nm to 100 nm. They may have smooth or uneven surface. The amorphous or crystalline nanoparticle may be single or multiple crystal solids which may either be free or clumped together. Mainly, zinc, alginate, titanium, gold, copper, silver and magnesium *etc.* are involved in nanoparticle synthesis.

Physical properties of nanoparticles include their light penetration, reflection abilities and optical properties such as the absorption and reflection properties, color of the NP and UV absorption when NPs are adsorbed on a surface or in the solution form. Mechanical properties such as tensile strengths, elasticity, flexibility and ductility also considerably determine their role and applications. Other nanoparticle properties like suspension, hydrophilicity, hydrophobicity, settling characteristics and diffusion play a crucial role in our day-to-day life. Nanoparticles have found their way in present thermal and electrical devices because of their electrical and magnetic properties like semi conductivity, conductivity and resistivity.

Besides physical properties, chemical properties also play an important role in deciding the role of nanoparticles in various industries. These chemical properties include stability and sensitivity of nanoparticles to heat, moisture, light and atmosphere along with their interactions with the target. Environmental and biomedical industries utilize the disinfective, antifungal, antibacterial, and toxicity-based properties of NPs. Anti-corrosive, flammability characteristics, oxidation, corrosive, reduction properties of the NPs also affect their individual roles.

5. Synthesis of Nanoparticles

Currently, nanoparticles are synthesized using two main approaches, called the **Bottom-up** and **Top-down approaches.** The top-down approach revolves around the principle of size reduction. Here, bulk material is converted into nanoparticles by mechanical and lithographic means such grinding. On the contrary, bottom-up approach, is mainly concerned with aggregation and assembly of smaller subunits to form a bigger structure *i.e.*, NPs are "grown" from smaller molecules called as reaction precursors via., chemical or biological synthesis. **Figure 17.2** portrays various NP synthesis methods for the bottom up and top-down approaches. Simpler structures such as atoms and molecules coalesce to form nanoparticles viz-a-viz the bottom-up approach. In contrast, nanoparticle synthesis via top-down technique relies on the principle of size reduction for NPs synthesis. In this technique, various chemical and physical methods are used to synthesize nanoparticles from an appropriate starting material.

Conventional physical and chemical NP synthesis techniques such as pyrolysis and attrition have many limitations like low synthesis rate, large energy requirement, high cost of manufacturing and defective surface formation. Chemical methods for NPs synthesis such as sol gel technique and chemical reduction employ the use of harmful substances such as sodium borohydride and hydrazine hydrate. Additionally, these precursor compounds release toxic by-products causing hazardous and undesirable effects on animals and plants along with the ecosystem. Different chemical and physical methods for the synthesis of nanoparticles are enlisted in **Figure 17.3.**

The bottom-up method for NPs synthesis is mainly preferred over the top-down method as it allows us to alter the shape, size and structure of the nanoparticles synthesized by varying the reaction conditions such as pH and temperature along with the concentration of precursor molecules. Therefore, both biological and chemical nanoparticles synthesis mechanisms rely on the bottom–up approach.

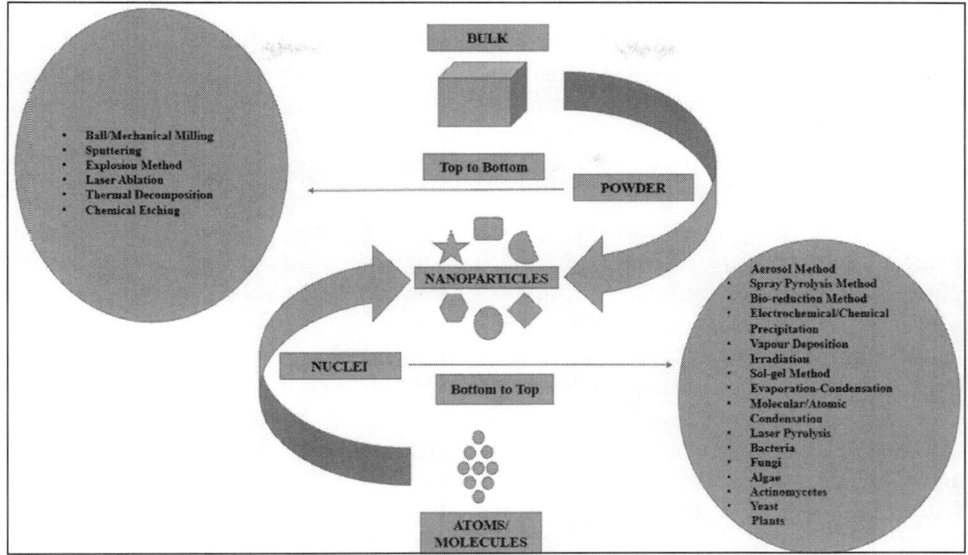

Figure 17.2: Various Top-down and Bottom-up Approaches for Nanoparticle Synthesis.

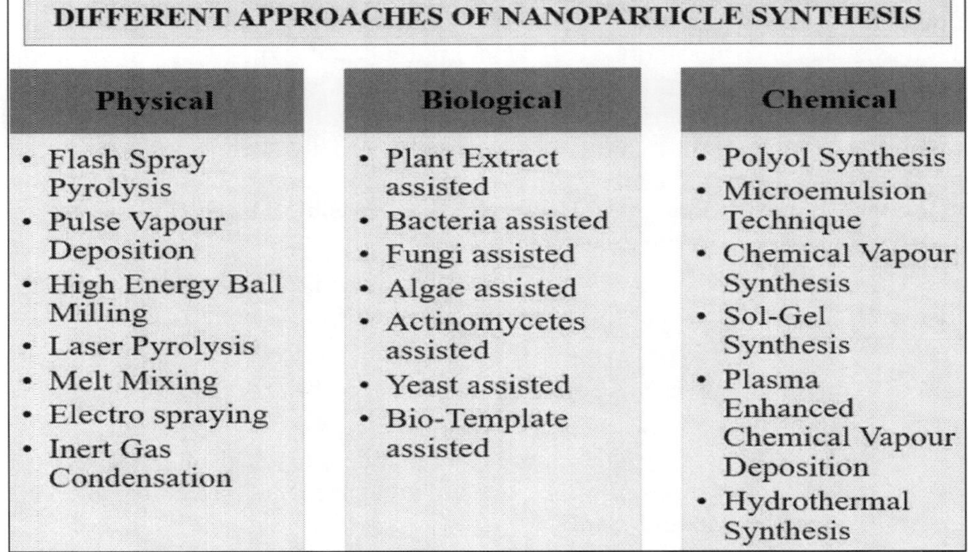

Figure 17.3: Different Chemical and Physical Methods for the Synthesis of Nanoparticles.

Since, the mechanical processes involved in top-down approaches may affect the outer surface of NPs, these approaches are not widely used in NP synthesis. This is because damaged surface reduces the efficiency of NPs, owing to the fact that properties of NPs mainly depend on their surface chemistry.

Chemical and physical approaches of NP synthesis require use of harmful chemicals which may additionally lead to non-eco-friendly byproducts. Thus, alternative method like green synthesis of NPs is being utilized today. Various plant parts especially leaves are now a days used for cost effective metal NP synthesis. This process is based on the principle of bio- reduction of metal ions.

5.1 Biological Synthesis of NPs

Over the past years, various biological units including: bacteria, algae, diatoms, yeast, plants, fungi and even human cells have exhibited the conversion of inorganic metal NPs to metal ones. This transformation takes place with the help of the reducing abilities of the metabolites and proteins already existing in these entities. Microorganisms being environmentally safe, fuel efficient and least toxic with least energy consumption are proven to be a feasible means for the physiochemical synthesis of NPs. In previous years, extensive studies have been carried out for the synthesis of metal NPs via. various microorganisms like fungi, bacteria like actinomycetes and yeasts using various intracellular as well as intracellular pathway. Current studies have revealed the use of bacteria like *Weissella oryzae, Pseudomonas deceptionensis* and *Bacillus methylotrophicus* for the synthesis of gold and silver NPs. In addition to using bacteria, myco-synthesis is an unequivocal method for the reliable as well as simple synthesis of NPs with the help of fungi. Most fungi (*Trichderma viride, Aspergillus niger, Fusarium solani, Aspergillus oryzae etc.*) comprising of various significant metabolites having immense potential for bioaccumulation as well as unexacting downstream processing are convenient for systematic and cost-effective synthesis of NP. Furthermore, yeast, actinomycetes and virus-mediated synthesis of stable and well functionalized nanoparticles is also possible. Additionally, the inexpensive cultivation, less time-consuming synthesis time, safety and the capability to enhance the quantity of synthesis eventually make plants an alluring method for the synthesis of NPs. However, environmental sustainability, economic viability and social adaptability along with the accessible parochial resources are an important aspect for the green synthesis of NPs.

The methods for biological synthesis of NPs are considered far more beneficial than the traditional chemical and physical methods. These benefits of the biological synthesis of NPs over the traditional ones are discussed below:

1. Environment- friendly and tidy method since the use of harmful chemicals is eluded.
2. Cost effective since the presence of mobile biological constituents does not requires the need of capping and reducing agents. These enzymes are competent enough to do so.
3. Small NPs can be constructed despite the synthesis is at large scale.
4. Power efficient since external experimental factors such as high pressure and high energy are futile.

5.1.1 Nanoparticle Synthesis by Bacteria

Bacteria are extensively used now-a-days for the biological synthesis of nanoparticles. *Bacillus* species has been employed to synthesize Ag nanoparticles extracellularly, with dimensions ranging from 10-20 nm. *Pseudomonas stutzeri* AG259 exhibits accumulation of silver nanoparticles in its periplasmic space. It is isolated from silver mines. Synthesis of AgNPs using *Shewanella oneidensis,* a metal reducing bacterium has been studied in detail. When the bacteria were cultured in silver nitrate solution, small and nearly monodispersed Ag-NPs were formed. The silver nanoparticles exhibited characteristics like hydrophobicity and stability along with an increased surface area. The synthesis of stable, monodispersed Au NPs using a novel strain of *Marinobacter Pelagius* and Ti NPs using strains of the bacterium *Lactobacillus* has also been reported.

5.1.2 Nanoparticle Synthesis by Fungi

Many studies on fungal species such as *Aspergillus oryzae*, *Aspergillus niger* and *Fusarium solani* have proclaimed to synthesize silver nanocrystals. For extracellular synthesis of NPs, the use of *Pleurotus sajor* caju has also been described. *Trichoderma viride* can be used to synthesize spherical nanoparticles while stable Ag hydrosols can be synthesized using *Fusarium oxysporum*. The efficiency of *Phoma glomerata* over *P. aeruginosa*, *E. coli* and *S. aureus* has been studied extensively. Also, some studies have been conducted to use the same for the synthesis of silver NPs. The genus *Penicillium* is considered as the most competent fungus as far as silver nanoparticle synthesis is concerned.

The synthesis of nanoparticles by fungi can be intracellular or extracellular depending on the position of the nanoparticles synthesized. This is further explained in detail below:

- ☆ **Intracellular synthesis of nanoparticles by fungi:** Here, ions are transported inside the cells of the microbe eventually resulting in the formation of the NPs using the enzyme present. The size of NPs formed intracellularly is quite reduced than those formed extracellularly. The size range varies according to the entities nucleating internally in the cell.
- ☆ **Extracellular synthesis of nanoparticles by fungi:** As extracellular synthesis lacks any unnecessary redundant cellular constituent; it is used widely when compared to the intracellular synthesis of NPs. Mostly, fungi are engaged in the synthesis of NPs via extracellular pathways due to their major secretory constituents ie. The enzymes. These components play a major role in the capping and reduction of NPs.

5.1.3 Nanoparticle Synthesis by Yeast

Koushik *et al.* (2003), reported a yeast strain MKY3 (silver-tolerant) imbuing it aqueous silver nitrate. Under enforced environmental surroundings, the establishment of 2-5 nm Ag NPs was detected. Synthesis of cadmium NPs using *Candida glabrata* and *Schizosaccharomyces pombe* have also been proclaimed. The use of an extremophilic strain of yeast, extracted from acid mine damage for the synthesis of Ag and Au NPs has also been reported. Moreover, a pelagic yeast namely *Rhodosporidium diobovatum* is also exploited to synthesize stable lead sulfide NPs via intracellular pathways for synthesis of NPs.

5.1.4 Plant Mediated NPs Synthesis

Plants are the major photosynthetic organisms of Earth, trapping almost about 75 per cent of the Sun's solar energy and converting it into chemical energy in the form of simple sugars such as glucose and other carbohydrates. Being the primary producers on this planet, plants have a high rate of biomass synthesis. Thus, plants and plant products are more sustainable and scalable for synthesis of nanoparticles over other biological systems like fungi, bacteria and algae which require expensive laboratory conditions for their growth, decreasing their feasibility for large scale nanoparticle synthesis. Also, plants are considered a better alternative for the synthesis of NPs. Green synthesis is preferred over chemical and physical approaches of NPs synthesis because it does not use toxic chemicals and makes use of the already existing capping agents produced naturally by plants. Metallic NPs synthesis using plant extracts is a single step technique. On the contrary, the capacity of microorganisms to synthesize nanoparticles may be lost because of random mutations over the course of time.

Plants and plant products are being used in various medicinal practices and allied fields. Additionally, many of these natural products directly act as potent drugs. Various secondary metabolites, enzymes, proteins, amino acids, vitamins, polysaccharides and organic acids are responsible for nanoparticle synthesis. These compounds are environmentally benign, yet complex. This leads to the greener approach of nanoparticle synthesis, which is comparatively a newer field of nanotechnology. **Figure 17.4** shows the various plant parts used for nanoparticle synthesis.

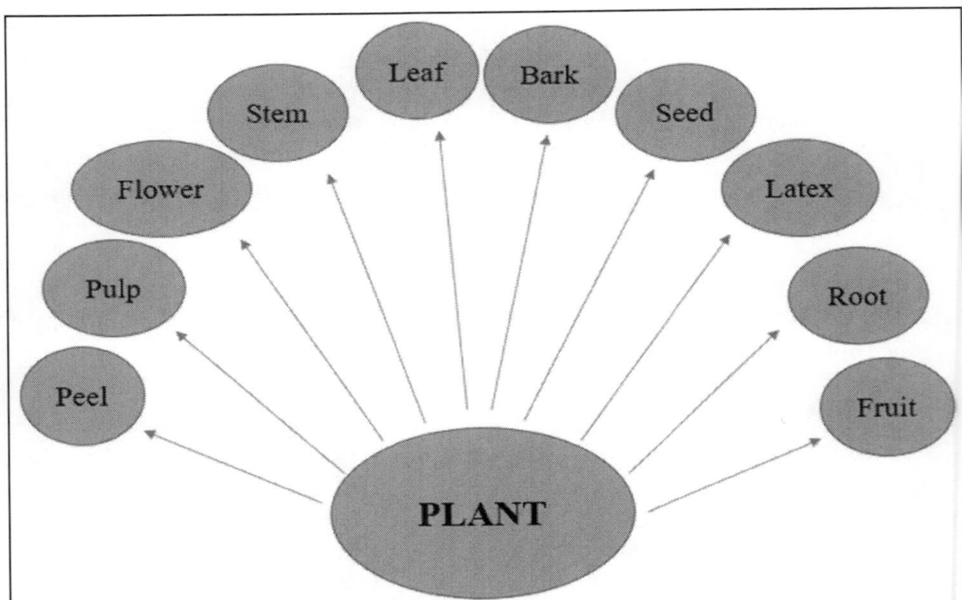

Figure 17.4: Plant Parts Used for Nanoparticle Synthesis.

Many plant species are reported to be used conveniently for the systematic as well as swift synthesis of Ag NPs via extracellular methods. Leaf extracts of *Azadirachta indica* Juss., *Aloe vera* (L.) Burm., *Cymbopogon flexuous* (Nees ex Steud) Watson., *Tamarindus indica* (L.), *Hibiscus rosa sinenesis* (L.), *Chenopodium album* (L.), *Cinnamomum camphora* (L.) Presl., fruit extracts of *Embelica officinalis* (L.), apiine extracted from *Lawsonia inermis* (L.), have been shown to synthesize silver (Ag) nanoparticles. **Table 17.1** lists few of the plants that are reported to be involved in nanoparticle synthesis. *Geranium* extract, *Azadirachta* indica leaf extract, sundried *Cinnamomum camphora*, and *Aloe vera* plant extracts have been exploited extensively for the synthesis of silver and gold NPs. *Plumeria rubra* plant latex, *Murraya koenigii* leaf extract and *Szyygium aromaticum* bud extract have also been used for the NP

Table 17.1: List of Plants Reported for Nanoparticle Synthesis

Plant Name	*Plant Part Used*	*Type of Nanoparticle Synthesized*	*Size (nm)*	*Shape*
Acalypha indica	Leaf	Ag	20-30	Spherical
Allium cepa	Bulb	Ag	-	-
Aloe vera	Leaf	Ag/Au	15	Spherical
Areca catechu	Nut	Ag	18.2-24.3	Spherical
Azadirachta indica	Leaf	Ag/Au	30	Spherical
Azadirachta indica	Leaves	Zn	-	-
Camellia sinensis	Leaf	Ag/NiO	30-40	Spherical
Carica papaya	Peel	Ag	10-30	Spherical
Citrullus colosynthis	Roots, Fruits and leaves	Ag	-	Spherical
Cycas sp.	Leaves	Ag	2-6	Spherical
Desmodium trifolium	Leaf	Ag	5-20	Spherical
Dryopteris crassirhizoma	Rhizome	Ag	5–60	Spherical
Emblica officinalis	Leaves	Ag	40	Spherical
Emblica officinalis	Fruits	Au	-	Spherical
Euphorbia prostrate	Leaves	Ag	52	Spherical, rod
Grewia flaviscens	Leaves	Ag	50-70	Spherical
Hibiscus rosa-sinensis	Petals	Ag	~ 18.79	Spherical
Jatropha curcas	Seed	Ag	-	Spherical
Jatropha gossypifolia	Stem	Ag	-	Spherical
Mangifera indica	Leaves	Ag,Au	20	Spherical
Ocimum sanctum	Leaf	Ag/Au	4-30	Spherical, hexagonal, triangular
Oryza sativa	Husk	Ag	-	Spherical
Pelargonium graveolens	Leaf	Ag/Au	16-40	Decahedral, isohedral, crystalline

Plant Name	Plant Part Used	Type of Nanoparticle Synthesized	Size (nm)	Shape
Pinus resinosa	Bark	Pd	16-20	-
Piper beetle	Leaves	Ag	3-37	Spherical
Prunus serotina	Fruit	Ag	20-80	Spherical
Rhazya stricta	Root	Ag	20	Spherical
Salmalia malabarica	Gum	Ag	7 ± 2	Spherical
Syzigium cumini	Seed	Ag	93	Spherical
Terminalia arjuna	Leaves	Ag	-	-

synthesis. The presence of intrinsic reducing agents like eugenol and carbazoles in the extract simulatenously is held responsible for this synthesis. In another study, AgNPs were synthesized using *Syzygium cumini* seeds extract as reducing agent. An average size of approximately 93 nm is observed for the resulting NPs synthesized. Anti-oxidant properties of the green synthesized NPs were found to be greater than that of seed extract of *S.cumini*. the leaf extracts of *Mirabilis jalapa* have also been exploited for the synthesis of gold NPs. Recently, the seed extract of *Pongamia pinnata* has been used for the green synthesis of silver nanoparticles. Spherical silver NPs were synthesized using leaf extract of *Aloe vera* and *Azadirachta indica* with an average size of 15nm and 30 nm respectively. Synthesis of Ag-NPs is not only restricted to leaf extract but other plant parts are also equally potent. Root extract of *Rhazya stricta* were used for the synthesis of AgNPs which were monodispersed and showed antibacterial properties. Addition of xylitol further enhanced the rate of reaction mainly due to the capping properties exhibited by it. Changes in pH plays a very important role in controlling and regulating the size and shape of the nanoparticle synthesized. The shape and size of nanoparticles synthesized using plants can be controlled and modulated by changing the pH. Members of the Lamiaceae family such as *Vitex negundo, Plectranthus amboinicus* and *Anisochilus carnosus* showed the formation of NPs with different shapes and sizes such as hexagonal, quasi-spherical, spherical and rod-shaped with agglomerates. It was hence, concluded that the size of the nanoparticle synthesized decreases when the concentration of the plant extract is increased simultaneously.

5.1.4.1 Mechanism of Plant Mediated Synthesis

Though various plants are exploited for the green synthesis approach, the exact procedure of nanoparticle synthesis via plant extracts is still a matter of debate in the scientific community. Despite the uncertainty surrounding the mechanism, there seems to be a common consensus that secondary metabolites and other molecules found in plant extracts plays an important role in reducing the metal salts.

Pelargonium graveolens leaf extract when manifested to silver nitrate solution showed that the size of NPs formed via extracellular synthesis varies from 16 nm to 40 nm. It was assumed that the Ag NPs were formed as a result of the presence of protein, terpenoids and other bio-organic compounds present in the leaf extract.

These components are believed to be involved in the capping and bio-reduction of NPs formed. To further elucidate the role of these secondary metabolites, when silver nitrate solution was made to react with *Desmodium trifolium* extract, silver nanoparticles were synthesized at room temperature. The study concluded that the synthesis of H^+ ions together with NAD during glycolysis eventually leads to the development of silver nanoparticles. Synthesis of Ag-NPs form *Cycas* leaf extract indicated the role of various phytochemicals like glutathione's, polyphenols, ascorbates and metallothionein's in the formation of Ag-NPs. Among them glutathione have a crucial role in plants during metal stress whereas metallothionein have the ability to bind to heavy metals via the thiol group present in their cystine residues.

It is well noted that flavonoids play a vital role in the synthesis of metallic nanoparticles. Flavonoids are known to chelate and reduce metal ions. This tautomeric conversion of flavonoids from enol to keto form liberates reactive hydrogen species which further behaves as a reducing agent for NP synthesis. Carbonyl group of flavonoids also influences metal NP synthesis because carbonyl group can chelate metal ions at three positions involving carbonyl and hydroxyl groups. These groups are known to reduce a number of metal ions including Fe^{3+}, Al^{3+} and Cu^{2+}. It is also known that terpenoids come into play during the reduction of metal salts. Terpenoids having alcohols, ketones, amines, carboxylic acids and aldehydes as their functional groups were found to play a vital role in stabilizing these newly formed metal NPs. Saponins are triterpenes known for their soap like properties whereas sterols constitute another class of triterpenes and are important constituents of cell membrane. Both these terpenoids are known to stabilize nanoparticles due to their hydrophobic interaction with the biomolecules present on the surface of metallic NPs. Interestingly, the amino acid tryptophan has strong reductive abilities for the synthesis of Au^+ NPs among other amino acids. As per reports, the reducing behavior of the metal ions is conferred with the polyol constituents present in the plant extracts. Also, the heterocyclic components which are water soluble help in stabilizing the NPs synthesized.

Since, leaf is the site of photosynthesis, the end product *i.e.*, is glucose is bound to be found in the leaves along with various other sugars. It is reported that sugars act as good reducing agents of metal salts reducing them to NPs. Glucose is a strong reducing agent. Monosaccharide may undergo tautomeric transformations from ketone to an aldehyde thus, acting as a strong anti-oxidants as seen in the case of fructose. The ability of disaccharides and polysaccharides to reduce metal salts depends mainly on the individual monosaccharide constituents, to form an open aliphatic chain and provide access to an aldehyde. Also, glycosides are sugar derivatives where the sugar moiety is bound to another functional group via. a glycosidic bond. Both sugars and glycosides play an important role in reducing metal salts primarily through their carbonyl group. The reduction takes place via. the tautomeric transformation of enol to keto forms in case of aldose sugars.

Though it has been proved that the already existing phyto-chemicals in the plant have appropriate redox properties which helps to systematically reduce these meta precursors and convert them into corresponding NPs but the exact mechanism of this conversion has not been explicated in much detail as of now. Tannins of alfalfa have been used to reduce metal salt as tannins related with alfalfa, resulted in the formation of radical tannins "R" which further with the help of pH reduced the metal ion. Similarly, the structure of the iron-polyphenol complex nanoparticles (Fe-P NPs), produced from the *Eucalyptus* leaves has also been studied. The polyphenols present in *Eucalyptus* extract are responsible for the reduction of Fe^{3+} to Fe^{2+}, thereby creating a reduction potential. Water soluble, polar heterocyclic components and the polyol compounds are respectively responsible for stabilizing and reducing the synthesized nanoparticles.

5.2 Nanoparticle Synthesis using Microbes Vs. Plants

Microbes take more time to reduce metal ions as compared to plants which can synthesize nanoparticles in less than a few minutes or several hours depending on the type of plant used and the phytochemical quantities used. The major limitation of microbe-mediated nanoparticle synthesis is the indispensable requirement of sterile conditions aided by expertise technicians, thereby, increasing the synthesis expenses. Moreover, easy accessibility of plants in nature, is another reason for them as a preferential bioresources than the microbes for the synthesis of nanoparticles.

6. Limitations of Green Synthesis

NPs synthesized via biological methods have higher chances of contamination by pathogenic bacteria throughout the purification process, rendering these NPs unfit for medical applications. Moreover, the toxic effects of metallic nanoparticles including the biogenic nanoparticles have also been reported. These include nephrotoxicity and neurotoxicity. These NPs bind to the free acetylcholine enzyme (AChE) and the enzyme-substrate (AChE-acetylcholine) complex. AgNPs synthesized using chemical or biological method sowed equal toxicity whether *in vivo* or *in vitro*.

7. Characterization of Nanoparticles

Nanoparticles are required to be characterized well after synthesis. There are a number of characterization techniques namely, UV-visible spectroscopy, X-ray diffraction, Electron Microscopy such Scanning electron microscopy (SEM), Transmission electron microscopy (TEM), Atomic force microscopy (AFM), Fourier transform infrared (FTIR) spectroscopy, and Zeta potential that are commonly used.

7.1 UV-visible Spectroscopy

Optical property is one of the important aspects for the characterization of NPs. UV-Vis spectroscopy analysis is a significant method to determine the synthesis of NPs in aqueous medium. On absorption of visible light, UV- visible absorption spectroscopy is referred to as **colorimetry**. Since, it is based on the principle of electron excitation from the molecular bonding to the molecular antibonding orbital, it is also known as **electronic spectroscopy**. A monochrome beam of light is made to pass initially via. a light absorbing liquid medium and then through a blank solution. The comparison of its percent transmittance (per cent T) in both the cases forms the basis of adsorption spectroscopy.

Given equation is used to calculate optical density or absorbance (A):

$$A = \log \frac{Io}{I}$$

where,

Io: Intensity of incident light

I: Intensity of transmitted light

Beer-Lambert's Law describes the relation between concentration (c) and absorbance (A) of the absorbing medium. According to this law, the amount of incident light adsorbed by all the solute molecules is fixed irrespective of their concentration in a non-absorbing medium. Beer-Lambert's Law can be given as:

$$A = xcl$$

where,

x: The molar extinction co-efficient.

l: Length of solution the light passes through (cm)

Using UV-Vis absorption spectroscopy, the optical properties of any liquid medium can be easily determined. A light beam is passed across the sample solution followed by measurement of the absorbed light. Subsequently using the obtained absorbance value, concentration of the solution using Beer-Lambert Law can be determined. In a UV-Vis scan, absorbance can be calculated at every wavelength ranging from 200 to 1100 nm. The optical measurement of UV visible spectrophotometer has different absorbance peak for different solutions.

7.2 Scanning Electron Microscopy (SEM)

Scanning Electron Microscopy (SEM) mainly allows us to study the external features of the synthesized particle along with size and shape. SEM gives a very high resolution of the surface morphology. The principle of SEM is same as that of an optical microscope, except that it quantifies the scattered electrons from the sample in place of photons. Velocity of electrons can be increased by the application of an electric field thereby, reducing their wavelength than any one of the photons. Relying on this principle, SEM can magnify images up to 200 times greater than the simple optical microscope which offers a resolution of 250 nm and more owing to the diffraction hinderances. Unlike optical microscope which uses visible light for magnification, SEM uses a beam of electrons to resolve the sample. Since, the wavelength of an electron beam is much smaller than that of visible light, diffraction hinderances in case of SEM are reduced to a great extent thereby, offering finer resolution. Primary electron sources in SEM are the field and thermionic electron emissions. Initially, the electron beam is initiated, focused and subsequently allowed to traverse across the sample in a raster fashion. This electron beam is then made to traverse across different electromagnetic lenses to obtain much finer resolution by demagnifying and focusing the beam. SEM chamber is a low vacuum chamber with length and pressure commonly reaching up to 1 m and 10^{-4} torr respectively. This helps to obtain an appropriate electron mean free path.

7.3 Transmission Electron Microscopy (TEM)

The Transmission Electron Microscopy (TEM) works on the principle similar to that of the light microscope. A beam of electrons is made to pass through the sample and the association between electrons and atoms are used to carry out various studies. Since the wavelength of electrons is lesser than that of light, the optimal resolution thus obtained is far better than light microscope. Hence, the images obtained from TEM divulge the minute details about the internal structures. There are three vital systems required for TEM:

1. An Electron Gun
2. The image-producing system
3. The image recording system

The electron gun produces a beam of electrons. The condenser present focuses this beam on the objects. Further, the image producing system, including the specimen stage, objective lens, projector lens and intermediate focus the passing electrons and result in the formation of a highly magnified image. The electronic image formed is further converted and processed with the help of an image recording system which consists of a fluorescent screen for viewing and a digital camera as well. Along with these, a vacuum system along with its gauges, valves and power supply is also required.

8. Applications of Nanoparticles in Nanobiotechnology

The use of nanoparticles has increased exponentially over the past decade. They are being widely used in pharmacology, electronics, sensors, optics and imaging. Nanoparticles are preferably being used as Drug Delivery System (DDS) over other conventional methods. **Figure 17.5** showcases the two different forms of nanoparticles used in drug delivery systems. Surface interaction with ligands along with fluorescent properties forms the pre-requisite for drug delivery.

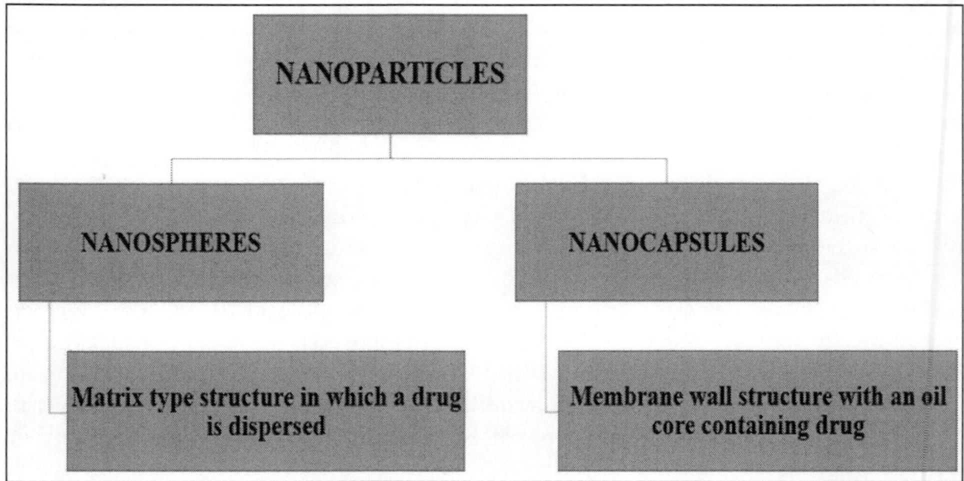

Figure 17.5: Different Forms of Nanoparticles Used in Drug Delivery Systems.

Moreover, they are ideal transporters for bio-molecules such as proteins, DNA or RNA. Nanoparticles not only protect these macromolecules from damage and deterioration but also aid in their transportation across the plasma membrane. Guarded transportation of these bio-molecules forms the basis for the use of nanoparticles in gene therapy and protein-based therapeutic treatment.

Recent advances in optics, chemical industries, optoelectronic devices, photo electrochemical applications and space industries have led to an increased dependence on nanoparticles. For example, the formation of nanometer sized geranium quantum dots can easily be regulated for the novel opto-electronic devices like light emitters and single electron transistors. Au NPs are being used for tumor deletion, drug delivery and genetic diagnosis. Iron oxide NPs are being used for magnetic responsive drug delivery, magnetic resonance imaging, cell labeling, tissue repair and immunoassays. Copper and palladium nanoparticles are being used in batteries, optical devices and formation of polymers. Zinc and titanium NPs are lately being used in skin industry due to their non-toxicity; they are used as UV blocking agents and for self-cleansing properties. **Table 17.2** enlists different nanoparticles used by industries in various consumer products.

Table 17.2: Use of different Nanoparticles in Various Sectors of ZIndustry

Sl.No.	*Industries*	*Nanoparticles Used*
1.	Medicine	Carbon, silver, gold, diamond, clay, hydroxyapatite, titanium dioxide, silicon dioxide, zirconium dioxide, aluminium oxide and ytterbium trifluoride
2.	Agriculture	Calcium, silver, iron, silicon dioxide, zinc potassium, boron, phosphorus, zinc oxide and molybdenum
3.	Construction	Clay, carbon, calcium hydroxide, titanium dioxide, silver, silicon dioxide, aluminium oxide, calcium carbonate calcium silicate hydrate and aluminium phosphate cerium(IV) oxide
4.	Food	Diamond, silver, silicon dioxide, zinc oxide and titanium dioxide
5.	Home appliance	Zinc, zinc oxide, platinum, gold, copper, manganese, calcium silver, clay, titanium dioxide, silicon dioxide, palladium and carbon
6.	environment	Gold, selenium, carbon, clay, silver, titanium dioxide, carbon and manganese oxide
7.	Automotive	Tungsten, calcium carbonate, zinc oxide, diamond, disulfide silicon dioxide, clay, titanium dioxide, calcium sulfonate, copper, cobalt oxide, boron, boron nitride, zirconium dioxide, tungsten, γ-aluminium oxide, Silver, palladium, carnauba, platinum, cerium(IV) oxide, aluminium oxide and silver
8.	Textile	Gold, silver, silicon dioxide, carbon, clay, titanium dioxide, gold, copper sulfide and polyethylene terephthalate
9.	Petroleum	Tungsten, diamond, disulfidezinc oxide, clay, silicon dioxide, boron, boron nitride, titanium dioxide, silver, tungsten, γ-aluminium oxide, molybdenum disulfide, carbon and γ-aluminium oxide
10.	Cosmetics	Silver, gold, titanium dioxide, zinc oxide, carbon, silicon dioxide, kojic acid, sodium silicate, clay and hydroxy acid
11.	Renewable Energies	Clay, titanium, graphite, palladium, zirconium(IV) oxide-yttria stabilized, tungsten disulfide, silicon dioxide, clay, carbon, gd-doped-cerium(IV) oxide, nickel(II) oxide, nickel cobalt oxide, rhodium, sm-doped-cerium(IV) oxide, silver and barium strontium titanate

Sl.No.	Industries	Nanoparticles Used
12.	Electronics	Silver, silicon dioxide, aluminum and palladium
13.	Printing	Toner
14.	Sports and fitness	Gold, silver, carbon, clay and titanium dioxide

Owing to the anti-bacterial properties of AgNPs, they are commonly used to disinfect water, home appliances and medical equipment. Silver NPs are not only effective against bacteria but also certain viruses and other eukaryotes. Interestingly, this property has significantly increased the use of AgNPs in various textile industries. Fibers are coated onto Ag NPs to prepare nanocomposite silver fibers. As such, cotton nanocomposite silver fibers showed strong anti-bacterial reaction particularly against *Escherichia coli.*

According to many recent studies, iron nanoparticles (NPs) can be a potential source for environmental remediation. Owing to the reactivity of nanoscale zero-valent iron (nZVI) having a greater surface area to volume ratio, the interest in employing it for environmental remediation is increasing.

Drawbacks of physical and chemical approaches of nanoparticle synthesis over the green synthesis method:

1. nZVIs formed using conventional methods show high reactivity and coalesce together to form agglomerates thereby, causing a reduction in their reactivity.
2. Unfit for use in medical appliances that use nonpolar organic solvents.
3. Iron oxide nanoparticles synthesized by conventional methods suffer a loss in their dispersal and magnetic properties on exposure to air.

8.1 Applications of Nanobiotechnology in Plant Sciences

Nanobiotechnology has recently become an emerging discipline in the field of plant sciences. Although the trends in the development of this field in plant sciences are not that pleasant but some measures are being taken to develop well organized systems to ameliorate germination of seed and its growth along with the plant's ability to hoist various biotic and abiotic stresses. Lately, the field has attained an burgeon curiosity to observe the use of nanomaterials as a channel of agrochemicals and various biomolecules thus resulting in the improved crop yield. Genetic engineering, biosensing and transportation of agrochemicals are some of the other latest approaches in the field of nanobiotechnology.

9. Summary and Conclusion

In the last few decades, the field of nanotechnology has been progressing rapidly, offering huge scope and prospect to overcome the restriction of several unresolved challenges. Expertise from diverse fields like material science, bioinformatics, biomedical, electronics and even computer science are incorporating their proficiency to understand the complex phenomenon involved in the synthesis especially through biological mediated processes. Development of the biologically important materials by systematic arrangement of the materials in nanoscale level is one of the emerging areas of research in this regard. This offers a viable option of establishing novel nanostructured products with enhanced properties owing to its high surface to volume ratio, suitable for drug delivery, bio-imaging and sensing. One of the main intentions of nanotechnology involves the development of new therapeutic substances suitable for pharmaceutical and biomedical purposes. Chemical and physical approaches adopted for the synthesis of metal NPs are common and old practices. But these methods are associated with high-cost chemicals that are toxic and hazardous to both human health and environment. Therefore, biological methods of NP synthesis were studied widely that are capable of replacing synthetic reducing and stabilizing agents. Biological methods of synthesis of NPs involve different micro and macroscopic organisms such as plants, algae, fungi and bacteria. It is reported that the speed of NP synthesis using plant systems is faster than in the micro-organisms and the NPs so formed are also comparatively more stable. Moreover, as the plants are existing abundantly over the earth, procurement of plant parts for the synthesis of NPs offer a great deal of scope in the wide-scale synthesis of NPs. Employment of plant extract has unfurled a new era in fast and harmless synthesis of metal NPs. Green chemistry synthesis methods or the biological methods for the synthesis of nanoparticles have many benefits over the other chemical and physical methods. They are safe, eco-friendly, cheap and do not use harmful compounds. Moreover, in green synthesis, the active biological components such as phytochemicals and enzymes work as capping and reducing, thereby, aiding their wide-scale synthesis. Though there are still some limitations in using plants as a source of NPs such as large polydispersity, poor stability *etc.* but the overall cost to benefit ratio is bound to supersede all such hurdles.

REFERENCES

1. Ahmad N, Sharma S, Singh VN, Shamsi SF, Fatma A and Mehta BR (2011) Biosynthesis of silver nanoparticles from *Desmodium trifolium*: A novel approach towards weed utilization. *Biotechnology Research International*, 1-8

2. Ahmed S and Ikram S (2015) Silver nanoparticles: One pot green synthesis using *Terminalia arjuna* extract for biological application. *Journal of Nanomedicine and Nanotechnology*, 6(4)

3. Awad MA, Mekhamer WK, Merghani NM, Hendi AA, Ortashi KMO, Al-Abbas F and Eisa NE (2015) Green synthesis, characterization and Antibacterial activity of silver/polystyrene nanocomposite. *Journal of Nanomaterials*, 943821: 1-6

4. Chandran SP, Chaudhary M, Pasricha R, Ahmad A and Sastry M (2006) Synthesis of Gold Nanotriangles and Silver Nanoparticles using *Aloe vera* plant extract. *Biotechnology Program*, 22: 577-583

5. Banerjee J and Narendhirakannan RT (2011) Biosynthesis of Silver Nanoparticles from *Syzygium cumini* L. seed extract and evaluation of their in vitro antioxidant activities. *Digest Journal of Nanoparticles and Biostructures*, 6(3): 961-968

6. Christy AJ and Umadevi M (2012) Synthesis and characterization of monodispersed silver nanoparticles. *Advances in Natural Sciences: Nanosciences and Nanotechnology*, 3(035013): 1-4

7. Dowling A, Clift R, Grobert N, Hutton D, Oliver R, O'neill O, *et al.* (2004) Nanoscience and nanotechnologies: opportunities and uncertainties. *A report by the Royal Society and the Royal Academy of Engineering, London*, 3-116

8. Ealias AM and Saravanakumar MP (2017) A review on the classification, characterization, synthesis of nanoparticles and their application. *IOP Conference Series: Materials Science and Engineering*, 263: 1-16

9. Feynman RP (1959) *There's Plenty of Room at the Bottom. Engineering and Science*, 23(5): 22-36

10. Hasan SA (2015) Review on Nanoparticles: Their Synthesis and Types. *Research Journal of Recent Sciences*, 4: 1-3

11. Gayathri S and Daniel RR (2012) A plant- mediated synthesis of Silver and Gold nanoparticles and their characterization using aqueous leaf extract of selected medicinal plants. *International Journal of Current Research*, 4(12): 509-514

12. Herlekar M, Barve S and Kumar R (2014) Plant-Mediated Green Synthesis of Iron Nanoparticles. *Journal of Nanoparticles*, 1-9

13. Ingale AG and Chaudhari AN (2013) Biogenic Synthesis of Nanoparticles and Potential Applications: An Eco- Friendly Approach. *Journal of Nanomedicine and Nanotechnology*, 4: 165

14. Iravni S (2011) Green synthesis of metal nanoparticles using plants. *Green Chemistry*, 13: 2638-2650

15. Iravani S, Korbekandi H, Mirmohammadi SV and Zolfaghari B (2014) Synthesis of silver nanoparticles: chemical, physical and biological methods. *Research in Pharmaceutical Sciences*, 9(6): 385–406

16. Jha AK and Prasad K (2010) Green synthesis of silver nanoparticles using *Cycas* leaf. *International Journal of Green Nanotechnology: Physics and Chemistry*, 1(2): 110-117

17. Katas H, Moden NZ, Lim CS, Celesistinus T, Chan JY, Ganasan P and Abdalla SI (2018) Biosynthesis and Potential Applications of Silver and Gold Nanoparticles and Their Chitosan-Based Nanocomposites in Nanomedicine. *Journal of Nanotechnology*, 1-13

18. Khandel P, Yadav RK, Soni DK, Kanwar L and Shahi SK (2018) Biogenesis of metal nanoparticles and their pharmacological applications: present status and application prospects. *Journal of Nanostructure in Chemistry*, 8: 217-254

19. Kokila T, Ramesh PS and Geetha D (2016) Biosynthesis of AgNPs using *Carica Papaya* peel extract and evaluation of its antioxidant and antimicrobial activities. *Ecotoxicology and Environmental Safety*, 134: 467-473

20. Krishna IM, Reddy GB, Veerabhadram G and Madhusudhan A (2016) Eco-friendly green synthesis of silver nanoparticles using *Salmalia malabarica*:

synthesis, characterization, antimicrobial, and catalytic activity studies. *Applied Nonoscience*, 8(1-2): 173-186

21. Lee JH, Lim JM, Velmurugan P, Park YJ, Park YJ, Bang KS and Oh BT (2016) Photobiologic-mediated fabrication of silver nanoparticles with antibacterial activity. *Journal of Photochemistry and Photobiology*, 162: 93-99
22. Makarov VV, Love AJ, Sinitsyna OV, Makarova SS, Yaminsky, Taliansky ME and Kalinina ON (2013) "Green" Nanotechnologies: Synthesis of Metal Nanoparticles Using Plants. *Acta Naturae*, 6(20): 35-44
23. Nayak D, Ashe S, Rauta PR and Nayak B (2015) Biosynthesis, characterization and antimicrobial activity of silver nanoparticles using *Hibiscus rosa-sinensis* petals extracts, *IET Nanobiotechnology*, 9: 288-293
24. Palanisamy K, Kalaiselvi PA, Gabriel M, Thangavel J and Sundaram L (2014) *Emblica officinalis* leaf extract mediated green synthesis of silver nanoparticles against human pathogens. *World Journal of Pharmacy and Pharmaceutical Science*, 3(3): 2019-2032
25. Pattanayak M and Nayak PL (2013) Ecofriendly synthesis of iron nanoparticles from various plants and spices extract. *International Journal of Plant, Animal and Environment Sciences*, 3(1): 68-78
26. Prasad K, Jha AK and Kulkarni AR (2007) Lactobacillus assisted synthesis of titanium nanoparticles. *Nanoscale Research Letter*, 2: 248-250
27. Rajan A, Vilas V and Philip D (2015) Catalytic and antioxidant properties of biogenic silver nanoparticles synthesized using *Areca catechu* nut. *Journal of Molecular Liquids*, 207: 231-236
28. Sadia Saif, Arifa Tahir and Yongsheng Chen (2016) Green Synthesis of Iron Nanoparticles and Their Environmental Applications and Implications. *Nanomaterials (Basel)*, 6(11): 1-26
29. Shankar SS, Ahmad A and Sastry M (2003) Geranium leaf assisted biosynthesis of silver nanoparticles. *Biotechnology Program*, 19(6): 1627-1931
30. Sharma M, Singh A and Ankit (2014) Biological Synthesis of Nanoparticles Using Bacteria and Their Applications. *American journal of pharmatech research*, 4: 38-61
31. Shenton W, Douglas T, Young M, Stubbs G and Mann S (1999) Inorganic organic nanotube composites from template mineralization of tobacco mosaic virus. *Advanced Materials* 11(3); 253-256
32. Singh P, Kim YJ, Zhang D and Yang DC (2016) Biological synthesis of nanoparticles from plants and microorganisms. *Trends in Biotechnology*, 34(7): 588-599
33. Subedi SK (2014) An introduction to nanotechnology and its implications. *The Himalayan Physics*, 5(5): 78-81
34. Toumey C (2009) Plenty of room, plenty of history. *Nature Nanotechnology*, 4: 783–784

35. Tran QH, Nguyen VQ and Le AT (2018) Silver Nanoparticles: synthesis, properties, toxicology, applications and perspectives. *Advances in natural science: Nanoscience. Nanotechnology*, 4: 1-20

36. Yeh YC, Creran B and Rotello VM (2012) Gold Nanoparticles: Preparation, properties and applications in nanobiotechnology. *Nanoscale*, 4(6): 1871-1880

Chapter 18

Pharmaceutical Biotechnology and Drug Design

Ritu Pasrija

Department of Biochemistry, Maharshi Dayanand University, Rohtak, Haryana, India
e-mail: ritupasrija@yahoo.com

ABSTRACT

Pharmaceutical Biotechnology is the discipline that encompasses all proficiencies required for conducting research in inventing, developing and registering of biological drugs. Pharma firms apply bioengineering procedures in finding lead compounds and formulating drugs, including- recombinant technology, gene therapy, pharmacogenomics and genetic analysis. Along with that, drug designing is severely dependent on handling and altering organisms, generally at molecular level. All these procedures provide initial inputs in formulating drugs, studying the best administration routes, possible side-effects, release and metabolism of new remedial drugs, mediators for medicinal investigations and in gene therapy for rectifying the signs of heritable disorders.

Besides drug development, the pharmaceutical companies also need to deal with many ethical issues in healthcare practices, following strict standards and procedures in conducting laboratory experiments, as well as clinical trial on patients and launching of drugs. This chapter is an attempt to provide initial clarity about various procedures required for introducing new products in the market.

Keywords: *Pharmaceutical biotechnology, Drug designing, Recombinant technology, Gene therapy, Computer aides drug design (CADD), Toxicology, Pharmacokinetics and pharmacodynamics (PK-PD), Novel therapies, Chemoinformatics.*

Pharmaceutical Sciences

It is an interdisciplinary study, involving- design, pathway, delivery, and disposal of drugs. This branch is further divided into four main subdivisions:

1. **Pharmacology:** this branch deals with composition of drugs, their uses, affected biochemical pathways and physiological consequences on living creatures.
2. **Pharmaceutical chemistry:** involves designing of new drugs, so as to optimize their pharmacokinetics and pharmacodynamics. This branch is also known as Medicinal Chemistry.
3. **Pharmaceutics:** the branch which entails with devising the formulation for best delivery and stability of drug, its pharmacokinetics and acceptance inside the patient's body.
4. **Pharmacognosy:** the study of drugs derived from natural resources like plants and their various parts.

Sources of Drugs

Various drugs can be derived from either nature (natural source), synthetic or semi-synthetic in origin. The various possible sources are:

1. **Plants Origin:** Since ancient time, humans depend on medicinal qualities of the plants. One such example is turmeric, used for application on wounds for its anti-bacterial and anti-fungal properties *etc.* Different parts of plants including- leaves, fruits, barks, roots, seeds, stem, wood, bulb, blossoms *etc.* are utilized for their medicinal properties.
2. **Animal Origin:** Medicines are obtained from animals as well, either derived from their bodily discharges, liquid or glands. These include- heparin, insulin, cod liver oil, thyroxin, adrenaline, beeswax, musk, enzymes, antitoxins and sera are acquired from them.
3. **Microbes:** Some life-saving drugs, including the antibiotics are microbial in origin. *e.g.*, penicillin is acquired from *Penicillium chrysogenum*, amphotericin B from *Streptomyces nodosus*, streptomycin from *Streptomyces griseus etc.*
4. **Marine Origin:** Fishes and marine microorganisms, including- corals and sponges, yield many biologically compounds with exhilarating anti-viral, anti-inflammatory and antitumor properties. A fungus *Leptosphaeria oraemaris* (Pleosporaceae) is useful for obtaining leptosphaerin and has anti-cancer activity.
5. **Minerals:** It is well known that human body needs many trace elements to sustain homeostasis in organs and are prescribed specific mineral-based drugs. Like iron deficiency results in anemia and ferrous sulfate can compensate the reduced levels *etc.*
6. **Synthetic derivative:** At times, a man-made drug is manufactured from biochemical production to form a new compound. Bulk of drugs are synthesized through this method only. The drugs include- acetylsalicylic acid (aspirin or ASA) and paracetamol *etc.* This method offers the advantage of higher yields with good purity.

7. **Semi-synthetic Sources:** These drugs are neither absolutely natural nor solely man-made, but rather are created by chemically amending ingredients of natural origin. This modification increases its effectiveness, with minimizing the negatives, like ampicillin is obtained by modifying penicillin structure *etc.*
8. **Recombinant Drugs:** These drugs are developed by advent in molecular biology and recombinant DNA technology. Examples- Hepatitis B vaccine and insulin *etc.*

The drugs obtained from various sources need to be optimized for their effectiveness, which is controlled by compounds size and fluidity, which ensure persistent drug delivery. This gives rise to the field of micromeritics and rheology.

Micromeritics

It is the discipline and expertise of small particles. The information, manipulation of the dimension and choice of particle size are of substantial significance because these are associated to the physical and biological properties as a drug. It is well known that as the particle size decreases, the surface area increase and expressed in μm (micrometer) or micron (μ), which is equivalent to 10^{-6} m. The particle size alters the drug release from various dosage forms, administered from different routes. In pill and capsule production, effective particle size is critical in attaining the mandatory flow. Thus, magnitude range is much needed during tablet synthesis. The graph between the number/weight of particles, against the size range is called frequency distribution curve and come under micromeritics, which has following applications:

1. **Release and dissolution-** Element dimension and expanse regulate the drug discharge. A greater surface area ensures better interaction of the drug with the bodily fluids and improves drug dissolution.
2. **Absorption and drug action-** It is easily understandable that rapid dissolution would result in superior drug performance.
3. **Physical firmness -** The particle size influences suspensions formation, as a smaller particle size provide better physical stability.
4. **Good flow properties**: Good flow properties of dissolved particles are crucial factors in tablets and capsules manufacturing.

Particle sizes are estimated by techniques like- **(1)** Sedimentation (range: 0.08-300 μm); **(2)** Optical microscopy (0.2-100 μm); **(3)** Particle volume measurement (range: 0.5-300 μm); and **(4)** Sieving (40-9500 μm).

Viscosity and Rheology: Viscosity of a liquid dictates its fluidity. "Heavy" or "thick" liquid like oils have high viscosity and water has very low viscosity. The fluid viscosity isn't permanent and vary, like temperature changes alters the fluidity. This branch of science where materials behavior and flow are studied, comes under rheology. Its measurement is done with rheometers. Water, honey, oil and toothpaste also have their own rheological properties. Many liquids contain a combination of dispersed phase and distributed particles, like milk contain oil dispersed in liquid.

Here liquid is the dispersion medium and dispersed material varies in sizes, which can be used to categorize dispersed system, as shown below.

Table 18.1: Particle Size Used for Categorization of Dispersed Systems

Category	*Size-Range*	*Properties*	*Features*	*Examples*
Molecular dispersions	Smaller than 1 nm	The solutes are homogeneously distributed in dispersion medium or solvent	Invisible under electron microscope; undergo rapid diffusion	A molecular mixture of gases, electrolytes
Colloidal dispersion	1 nm - 0.5 µm	Solute particles are small to be separated under gravity or centrifugal forces	Visible in electron microscope, Diffuse very slowly	Milk is an emulsion of fat and some other substances in water
Coarse dispersion	Bigger than 0.5 µm	These are dissimilar dispersed systems in which particles sediment fast under gravity, filtration or other forces	Observable underneath microscope, Don't diffuse	Particles of sand, generally pharmaceutical emulsions and suspensions, red blood cells

Both particle size and flow affect the drug delivery system, which deals with the rate at which drug is released in body over a specified period of time. Well-ordered discharge maintains persistent drug levels in the target sites of body. There are different forms of drug discharge systems.

1. Dissolution Controlled Systems

The drug is released slowly from a gradually softening matrix or by covering with slowly suspending substances. It can be done through, either- (a) encapsulation dissolution, where drug molecules are either compressed in a gradually softening substances like cellulose, waxes, polyethylene glycols (PEG) *etc.* The thickness of the outer coat and its solubility mediate regulated flow; or (b) Matrix systems, in which drug is spread in a rate controlling medium, such as hydrogenated castor oil, beeswax *etc.* Here, the medicine dissolution is regulated by fluid penetration into the matrix or by adjusting the porosity.

2. Diffusion Controlled Systems

These are dependent on discharge rate of drug, which is dependent on dispersal through inert water unsolvable membrane barricade. There are mainly two forms of diffusion devices. (a) Reservoir diffusion system and (b) Matrix diffusion system, and are shown in Figure 18.1.

3. Dissolution and Diffusion-Organized Release Systems

The drug core is bounded by a slightly solvable case. Openings produced due to dissolution, allow entrance of aqueous medium into the inside, ending in drug suspension. Mixture of ethyl cellulose with methyl cellulose is used to make such a system. Beside them, the chemical kinetics also influence reaction rate.

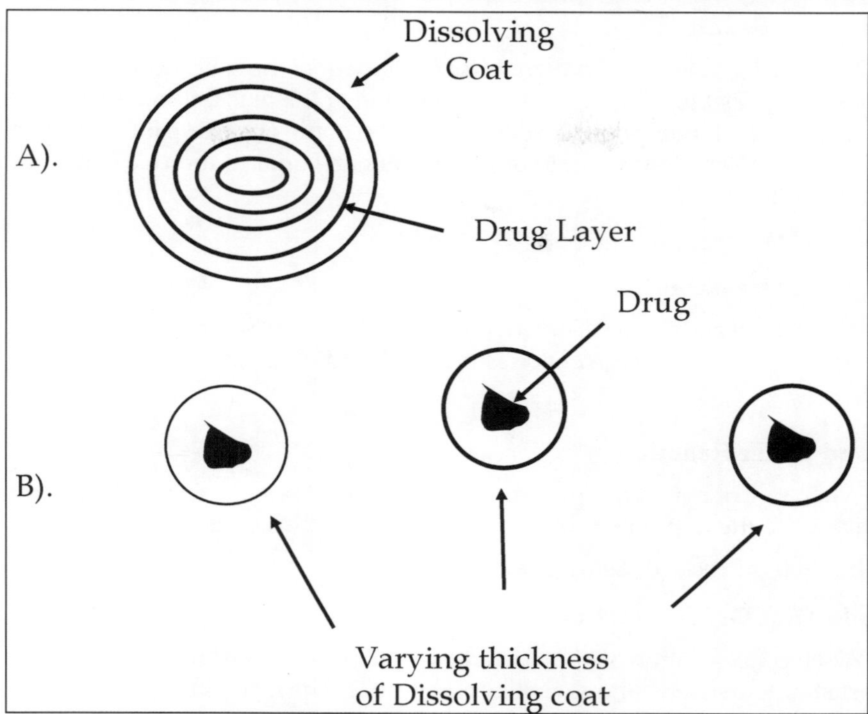

Figure 18.1: Types of Diffusion-Coordinated Systems: (A) Reservoir Diffusion System and (B) Matrix Diffusion System.

Chemical Kinetics is an analysis of factors which influence the rate of these chemical reactions. The chemical reaction rate refers to the velocity with which reactants undergo chemical change. It can be done either by following the reactant (utilization) or product (accumulation) concentration, over a particular period of time, as shown in Figure 18.2. Depending upon the factors affecting the reaction rate, the reaction can be either-

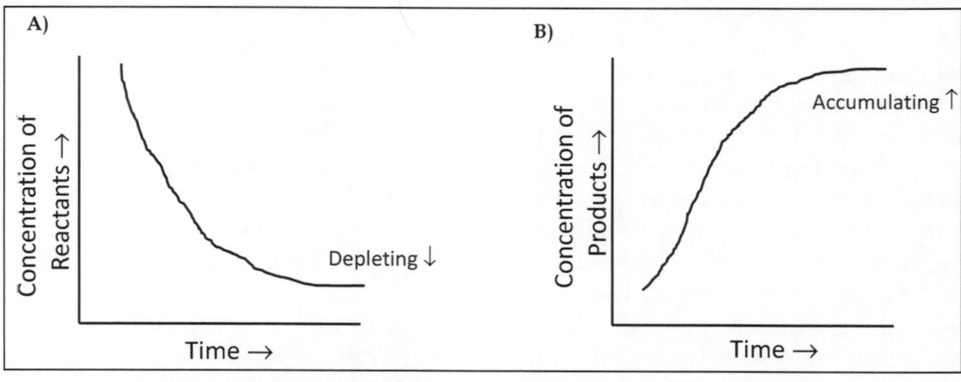

Figure 18.2: (A) Reactant's Utilization Plotted against Time, and (B) Products Accumulation Plotted against Time.

Zero Order Reaction

The reaction rate is zero, when it is independent of the concentration of reacting species. It is possible, when only a small portion of the reactant molecules are able to react from the larger pool, like decomposition of nitrous oxide into nitrogen and oxygen This means that the rate of the reaction is equal to the rate constant, and given by following equation:

$$-da/dt = k$$

First Order Reaction

When the reaction rate is positively regulated by the first power of the dilution of a single reactant, the conversion is first and written as:

$$-dc/dt = kc$$

Second Order Reaction

When rate of reaction is proportionate to second power of the dilution of a one reactant or to the first power of the intensity of two reactants.

If A + B = Produce then, $dx/dt = (a - x)(b - x)$

Pseudo First Order Reaction

When concentration of one reactant is in surplus, then its concentration change almost stays persistent, and rate obeys first order. The factors that affect the rate of reaction are- solvent, temperature, ionic strength, light, *etc.* The hydrolysis reactions (acid or base catalyzed) are common examples of pseudo first order reactions.

Drugs and Pharmaceutical Science

Drugs are envisioned for use in the identification, therapy, alleviation, treatment, or avoidance of diseases. There are many factors which affect the drug activity and studied in **biopharmaceutics**, which is the analysis of the physical and chemical properties of a drug, and its dosage structure, duration of drug action, including co-constituents and mode of manufacture. Drugs are taken in a variety of forms such as solids (capsules, tablets), fluids, (suspensions, emulsions) or semi-solids (balms, ointments) *etc.* The functioning of drug is supported by discharge of the active pharmaceutical ingredient (API) from the medicine. The drug can be taken through various route of administration like intravenous, oral, subcutaneous or transdermal, *etc.* In this process, some part of the medicine is soaked at place of entry and some portion spread into the frame. After this only, drug reaches at the intended location in body. Thus, it is crucial to evaluate the drug quantity available in the body (*in-vivo*) after administering the drug product, which might vary with different routes of administration. Like, same quantity of intravenous injected isoproterenol increases the heart rate but orally route fails to do so. In the body, drug is metabolized which mediate its disposal. So, duration for which drug is available in the body, it should be able to perform its function. It is recorded that various physicochemical properties of drug substances affect its effectiveness, including- drug solubility and dissolution speed, stability, surface area, particle size, salt formula of the drug, pKa of the drug, lipophilicity, and gastrointestinal pH, *etc.*

Thus, to maintain the effective concentration of drug, the dosage form characteristics becomes crucial, like- disintegration, dissolution and dissolution time (tablets/ capsules), excipients, type of dosage form, product age and storage conditions *etc.* Besides them, the Patient-Related Factors, including- their age, gastric emptying time and pH, intestinal transit time and enzymes, blood flow and presence of other Foods and Fluids affect drug action. All these variables require extensive in-vitro testing and gave way to develop particulate technology.

Particulate Technology

It is related with particle size, dosage forms, compaction and powder flow *etc.*

Particle Size

It is understood that physicochemical (particle size and shape) and biopharmaceutical properties of drug constituents and dosage shapes are subjective to the particle size. Particle size affects the:

a) Degree of suspension and bioavailability of API.
b) Medicine discharge is persistent or regulated.
c) The distribution, deposition, assimilation rate and clearance time.
d) Flow and compaction
e) Grittiness of solid elements in edible tablets *etc.*

Compaction

In spite of varied routes of administration, oral, is still the most popular route, due to simplicity of administration, production, accurate dosing and patient compliance. For tablets manufacture, compaction is an indispensable manufacturing stage, mainly includes solidity (*i.e.,* decline of powder quantity under consideration and particle reorganization), and depends on the physical-technical properties of drugs.

Powder Flow

Tablets are manufactured by filling the tablet cast with powders and thus flow of powder decides weight, hardness, and content uniformity of tablets. Thus, an understanding of powder flow is crucial during mixing, packaging, and transportation. Several methods are exercised to measure the powder flow including- measuring texture, angle of repose, Carr's compressibility index, Hausner ratio, avalanching determination, bulk density, caking strength and dielectric imaging *etc.*

Dosage Forms

Drugs/medicines are given in the form of either simple solutions or complex formulations with appropriate additives/excipients. The excipients help in various ways in solubilization, suspension, thickening, preservation, emulsification, control dissolution, enhance the compaction and flavoring drug materials to form numerous medicines or dose forms. Solutions act faster than suspensions, which operate quicker than capsules and tablets. Variations in dosage forms alter the bioavailability features and therapeutic performance. Some considerations, like- ensuring that the drug constituent must be in liquid form before it can be taken up via gastrointestinal (GI) tract and into body fluids, increase their absorption.

Dosage Form Designs

Drug manufacturing involves considering multiple factors and studies under dosage form design, discussed below:

1. **Particle size and surface area:** Size distribution and particle size reduction increase the specific surface, dissolution and absorption degree, dosage form content, consistency, and steadiness. The fine material, in micrometer or sub-micrometer (nanometer) structure, dissolves at faster rates resulting in improved drug absorption by passive diffusion.
2. **Solubility:** Relatively insoluble compounds exhibit erratic absorption. Sometimes, drugs previously in solution/liquid dosage forms undergoes precipitation in the GI region, and amending bioavailability.
3. **Dissolution:** During dissolution, the dose in the surface layer dissolves, heading to forming the diffusion zone, followed by passing of drug through the dissolving fluid and getting absorbed.
4. **Partition coefficient, pKa:** A molecule partition coefficient between an oil and a water phase (log P) provides a degree of the lipophilicity of a molecule, which predicts drug's ability to cross biological membrane.
5. **Crystal properties and polymorphism:** Most drug substances occur in more than single form, which display separate molecular packaging preparations in the crystal lattice, called polymorphism. Diverse polymorphs can be formulated by maneuvering of settings of crystallization such as temperature solvent, speed of cooling *etc.*
6. **Stability:** The drug's stability and compatibility with the other ingredients is well considered during packaging. Chemical changes involving additives should be vigilantly supervised to enhance stability of formulation.
7. **Organoleptic properties:** Many drug substances are unpalatable in their natural state and may involve the addition of appropriate flavors or/and colors. It improves color or complement a flavor.
8. **Other drug properties:** Ensuring chemical and physical stability of dosage forms is crucial. Hygroscopic drugs command little moisture production conditions and need to evade water during formulation. Weakly flowing formulations may compel the addition of flow agents (*e.g.*, fumed silica).
9. **Compactability of drug substances** inspect the tableting potential of the material during compaction and may necessitate modification to the formulation or processing settings.
10. **Therapeutic considerations in Design:** Need for systemic/or oral therapy, and whether the medication will be consumed in crisis situations, requires consideration. Patients expecting earnest respite from angina pectoris, position pills of nitroglycerin sublingually for quick drug assimilation into the blood.

Development of Drug Delivery System in Biopharmaceuticals

Biopharmaceuticals are manufactured by biotechnology methods. They have biological origin involving live organisms or their components, like- protein, nucleic acid (generally used for in-vivo diagnostic purpose). Biotechnology made large-scale production of existing substances possible, for example, insulin in the field of diabetes treatment, Interferon b (relapsing MS) Interferon g (granulomatous), TPA (heart attack). Currently, almost 77 FDA approved protein drugs are available in the market. Out of these, almost 66 are recombinant proteins. Due to their proteinaceous nature, these proteins are not easy to deliver via the oral route and generally injected using IV route, so novel drug delivery methods are developed and discussed below:

a) **Polymeric release:** It reduces regularity of doses; drug is stable inside polymer. Choice of polymers depends on its bio-degradability, bio-stability, non-toxicity and release. Polyphosphoesters, polyanhydrides, and polylactides fit in to these criteria, as they are degraded by hydrolysis and enzymes.

b) **Microsphere encapsulation:** involves encapsulating protein in small porous particles for sustained release.

c) **Polymer Scaffolds:** Integrate drug into matrix polymer and protects the drug from proteolytic enzymatic degradation and release (diffusion) occurs over prolonged duration through polymer.

d) **Magnetic Targeted Carriers (MTCs):** Microparticles of iron and activated carbon are used as carriers, to adsorb the drug into these MTCs and transported. They serve as delivery vehicles for site-specific targeting. FeRX Incorporation (San Diego) is the leader in the development in this innovative technology and latest drug trials show the drug remains for 28-days at the targeted site.

e) **Liposomes:** Spherical vesicles with a phospholipid bilayer. Bleomycin captured in temperature sensitive liposomes results in heightened antineoplastic action and lessened side-effects.

f) **Hydrogel's Based Drug Delivery:** Hydrogels are 3-D systems of hydrophilic polymers that are insoluble. These expand due to changes in pH, temperature, solvent composition, ionic strength, pressure, application of electric fields *etc.*

g) **Oral Protein Delivery:** Buccal aerosol delivery system is formulated with selection of stabilizers and additives to avert denaturation and stabilize aerosols.

h) **Patch Delivery:** Patches could be muco-adhesive or transdermal in nature. The Ethyl cellulose layer shields medicines from proteolytic mortification.

i) **Oral Delivery by Microsphere** for nasal release of proteins

Biosimilar

The biosimilar medication is alike biological drug, previously approved. The active component of a biosimilar is comparable to the single biological recommended medicines. Thus, both are similar but not identical. Biosimilars are not generics. They are also called as Second entry biologicals, Biogenerics, Subsequent Entry Biologicals, Off-patent biotech products or follow-up biologics.

Genomics and Proteomics in Drug Discovery

Drug Discovery is a long and costly procedure. It takes almost 15 years and US$500 million, for any pharmaceutical company to develop a drug from its discovery to marketplace. During this process, almost 40 per cent compounds don't even reach market launch due to either poor pharmacokinetics or preclinical toxicity. Drug development involves variety of studies in different fields, including genomics and proteomics. These methods aid in detecting novel genes and proteins, as well as calculating their expression or allocating functions. A comparison of gene and protein expression between diseased and normal cells (control) or cells treated with drugs suggest the effectiveness and harmfulness of compounds under study. Thus, these branches are helpful in identifying new drugs and their effects, which would-be crucial in optimizing the selection of lead compound for forecasting their success or closure.

Genomics

Deals with analysis of genes and their purpose. It involves recognising the genome structure and mapping of genes by sequencing the DNA and comparing human and other genomes to find possible new drug targets. Genome is relatively static, while **Proteomics** encompasses protein analysis involving bioinformatics tools to comprehend structure and posttranslational modifications of the protein under study. It is not-static like genomics and keep on changing with environmental variations inside/outside the cell.

Role in Drug Discovery and Development

Drug discovery starts with target identification and validation, which involves structural analysis of potential ligand binding sites and subsequent docking (landing) of small potential drug molecules on them. Further confirmation requires extensive biochemical assays and lead optimization to correct any probable cytotoxicity. Its role can be estimated from the fact that nucleic acid sequences comparison with Basic Local Alignment Search Tools (BLAST) of tumour necrosis factor (TNF)-induced cell death-inducing ligand was exposed by examining homologs of the TNF family proteins in the database. Similarly, genome of pathogenic organisms reveals the information about species specific genes, virulence and toxins genes and common genes.

In a likewise manner, comparison of fluorescent labelled protein levels in normal and diseased tissue (comparative proteomics) is possible. The proteomic changes in a disease can be identified with techniques like 2-dimensional (2D)-gel electrophoresis and Mass spectrometry (MS) *etc.* Together, both disciplines contribute in our perception of cell functioning and drug discovery.

Biopolymers in Pharmaceutical Industry and Packaging

Polymers are long chain molecules connecting many smaller molecules called monomers. Polymers are used extensively in our daily life, including pharmaceutical industry, where they are used for manufacturing of bottles, syringes, vials and also in drug formulations. Three primary mechanism for drug release, namely: diffusion, degradation, water penetration (swelling). Any of these mechanisms can occur in a given release system. Several criteria are used for their classification-

1. Classification, Based on the Source

a) **Natural:** These exist in nature as such and also called as biopolymers, like- rubber, silk and cellulose *etc.*

b) **Semi-Synthetic:** are obtained after modification of natural polymers by chemical treatment, like cellulose nitrate, methyl cellulose *etc.*

c) **Synthetic**: are manmade and synthesized in the laboratory, like polyethylene and polyvinyl alcohol.

2. Based on the Type of Polymerization

a) **Addition Polymer:** When linear monomer is added one after another. *e.g.* Polystyrene polyethylene, and polypropylene.

b) **Condensation Polymers**: They are formed after intermolecular reactions between bifunctional or polyfunctional monomer molecule having sensitive functional groups, such as -COOH, –OH, -NH_2. *e.g.*- polyesters.

3. Based on the Degradability

a) **Biodegradable:** They degrade naturally in the body. *e.g.*- polylactic acid (PLA), PGA, polycaprolactone (PCL).

b) **Nonbiodegradable:** They are not degraded naturally in the body. *e.g.*- polyethylene vinyl acetate (PVA), cellulose acetate (CA).

Packaging is a technique that facilitates shuttling of a drugs and devices from its manufacture to consumer. It protects the drugs from external factors which can affect the period of maintaining shelf life of the product and minimizing environment impact. Packaging industry continuously undergoes designing advanced materials with minimal possible ecological impacts. Packaging might involve either natural substances like polysaccharides, but cyclic olefin copolymer (COC) is most frequently tamper-resistant packaging material and is a remarkable alternative to a damped polyvinyl chloride (PVC).

Good Lab Practices (GLP)

GLP is a superiority management structure for research laboratories and establishments for certifying quality, consistency, trustworthiness, reproducibility and reliability of commodities under improvement for human or animal consumption and environment safety. It is done through non-clinical safety tests, including toxicity tests and ensures correct planning, execution, reporting and archival of data. Its inclusion is spread to drugs manufacturing, medical devices, food additives, color or animal food additives, food packaging, other non-pharmaceutical products or ingredients, biological products. These practices were initially launched in 1972 in New Zealand and Denmark. United States adopted them in 1978 after some false reporting of data scandal. In 1992, OECD (Organization for Economic Co-operation and Development), an intergovernmental organization, having representatives form 29 countries, along with European Union (EU) devised the principles of GLPs. WHO (World Health Organization) has a booklet in place for suitable GLP's as well.

GLP ethics include:

1. **Organization and Personnel management** accounts for almost 15 per cent of regulations. Management responsibilities include adoption of good science practices like designing of experiments, experimentation, use of controls and proper documentation of results and variables. Thus, organization need to supply adequate space, facilities and resources, their maintenance along with proper training to the staff for experimentation, their documentation and disposal. GLPs also recommend appointing a Study Director for preparation of protocol (Standard Operating protocol or SOP), planning and implementation of the same.
2. **Quality assurance** is required for integrity of the studies. It is done by witnessing and review the entire process and thus ensuring implementation of the compliance system. Quality Assurance Personnel is appointed for this role, as well as for audits and inspections. All these data are used for making audit reports.
3. **Facilities** should be of suitable size and rooms; its building and position must meet the requirements of the study. It is done to diminish interruption that would obstruct the study, safeguarding archives and proper disposal. Facilities for Test and Reference Items should be in place too.
4. **Equipment, reagents and materials:** All the Apparatus, including computerized systems for the production, storing and recovery of data should be suitably located. Apparatus should be clean and calibrated as per SOP's. Chemicals and Reagents should be properly labelled and stored.
5. **Test systems:** Apparatus used for Physical/Chemical data generation must be positioned appropriately, after proper designing and location setup. Similarly, storing and usage of biological test systems should be done to ensure guarantee quality of data. Cleaning, sanitation and free of contamination should be ensured as well.
6. **Test and reference items:** refer to records of receipt, handling, storage and expiry date maintenance. Storage containers should be labeled with adequate information. Stability and storage of test and references should be safeguarded.
7. **Standard operating procedures:** All test facilities should have written SOP's, edited and approved to ensure quality and integrity of data

generated. SOPs should be there for test and reference items, apparatus maintenance, cleaning and calibration, record keeping, reagents preparation, storage and retrieval and QC.

8. Enactment of study involves Study Design and Conduct of work.
9. Reporting of results.
10. Archival – refers to Storage of documentations and Reports.

Pharmacodynamics (PD)

It involves the relationship between dose and drug effect. The molecular interactions of drugs with their receptors, control the consequences of drugs on the human body. The degree of firmness binding between two is expressed in terms of affinity or dissociation constant (Kd), which is the drug dilution at which at least 50 per cent of receptors are engaged with drug. Numerous receptors occupied with drug drives the cumulative effect of receptor occupancy. Two important parameters of drug effect are- efficacy and potency. Potency (EC_{50}) of a drug is expressed as the concentration at which the drug provokes 50 per cent of its maximal response. Efficacy (E_{max}) is the highest outcome of a drug when all accessible rectors are occupied.

Besides this, the effect of drug or its side effects is also dependent on dosing regimen. Thus, clinical pharmacology tries to exemplify the extent of drug effects from a specified quantity, time taken for desired outcome, as well as duration of these outcomes. At one point of time, drug quantity can be assessed but before and after the sampling time also drug gets continuously metabolized and requires complex models for time effect on doses. These studies are covered under Clinical Pharmacology and precisely deals with pharmacokinetics or PK (the time track of drug dilution in the biological fluids) and pharmacodynamics or PD.

Pharmacodynamic Models and Biomarkers

Pharmacodynamic (PD) models and biomarkers are molecular pointers of drug's outcome on the intention site of the person. It is used to assess the relationship between drug routine, focused outcome and reaction, and thus is critical in deciding the fate of lead compounds, drug combinations and regimes to be followed. These studies are done in PK/PD models, which considers- (1) the route of drug administration, absorption, metabolism, and elimination; (2) the anticipated outcome of drug. It relies on ordinary differential calculations, which define the adjustment in drug levels as it journeys across the body after administration. Different routes of administration (oral, intravenous, subcutaneous, *etc.*), the drug affect the absorption, distribution, metabolism and effect/elimination (ADME). These are also known as principles of drug distribution and effectiveness studies. Along this journey, body struggles to remove the drug from system, and thus requires multiple doses. The equations for calculation are:

dD/dt = administration – absorption - elimination

dD/dt = absorption – binding to the target + release from target – elimination

The equation requires values, which is calculated my measuring the drug concentrations at multiple time intervals. To exclude the variations, it is done on small set of patients. Here, a PD model defines the connection among drug concentration and outcome, independent of time. Thus, pharmacokinetics models explains the association between quantity and concentration, portrayed as the concentration vs. time profile for each dosage. The effectiveness of a drug decides its dosing regimen and the time course of drug concentration in the body is the study of PK. When both PK and PD are combined, it becomes a PKPD model. This acknowledges the drug influence to be linked straight to the time after a given dosage. As routes affect the PK/PD values, thus they need to be studies in detail.

Routes of Administration

Drugs introduced via intramuscular, respiratory, subcutaneous routes, passes directly into the blood-stream from absorbing tissues. Intravenous route is the truly direct among all, whereas in the oral route, drug action includes the transit time in the GI tract, followed by absorption. The different administration routes affect absorption of drugs.

a) **Oral route:** It is the easiest, most accessible, preferred and harmless means of drug administration. It involves drug assimilation through the epithelial tissue and mucosa sheath of the GI tract. A few drugs, soften in the mouth for speedy absorption or for local impact due to poor absorption by this route.

b) **Rectal route:** Drugs are generally directed for neighboring rather than systemic effects. Drugs are solid forms intended for introduction into body cavities (usually rectal but also vaginal and urethral), where they soften, discharging the drug. This route is also specified for drugs deactivated by the GI fluids when given orally or when the oral route is excluded, for instance when a patient is unconscious or vomiting.

c) **Parenteral route:** A drug inserted via a syringe into the body at different sites and is parenteral. The three main parenteral routes are intramuscular (i.m), subcutaneous (s.c.) and intravenous (i.v). It is preferred for rapid absorption and in emergency situations like unconsciousness, incapable to undertake oral medication, or when drugs are subdued, disabled or inadequately orally absorbed.

d) **Topical route:** Drugs are smeared to the skin, for local action. This route is also exploited for transdermal patches supplying drug for systemic distribution (*e.g.*, glyceryl trinitrate patches for the prophylaxis and management of angina). Drugs smeared to the skin for local effect include antifungals, antiseptics, anti-inflammatory agents, as well as skin ointments for protective effects. *e.g.*, creams and pastes.

e) **Respiratory route:** The lungs is an outstanding site, when the drug is dispensed in gaseous, aerosol mist form. Drug particles delivered through this route have 0.5-1μm diameter.

Dosage Forms for Various Routes

The preferred form of dosage for various routes are tabulated below.

Table 18.2: Various Routes of Administration and Dosage Forms

Administration Route	*Dosage Forms*
Oral	Solutions, syrups, suspensions, emulsions, gel, powders, granules, capsules, tablets
Parenteral	Injections (Solutions, suspensions, emulsion forms), implants, irrigation and dialysis solutions.
Rectal	Suppositories, ointments, creams, powders, solutions.
Topical	Ointments, creams, pastes, lotions, gels, solutions, topical aerosols, transdermal patches
Nasal	Nasal Aerosols (Solutions), inhalations
Eye	Solutions, ointments, solutions
Ear	Solutions, suspensions, ointments, creams.
Respiratory/Lungs	Aerosols (Solutions, suspension, powder form), inhalations, sprays and gases.
Nasal	Nasal Aerosols (Solutions), inhalations

Plasma Concentration of Drug

Effectiveness of a drug product changes with the drug concentration at the directed body site after administration. If with quantity of drug, we additionally contemplate the capacity of the compartment, it gives the theory of drug concentration. It is defined as the amount of drug in plasma (if the concentrations in all tissues are the same as the plasma concentration), and expressed as mg/L. If we uninterruptedly measure the concentration of a drug in the plasma after an intravenous dose and then plot these plasma drug concentrations against the times they are obtained, the curve shown in Figure 18.3. It should be understood that retrieving targeted tissues or fluids to measure drug levels is not feasible, so, plasma is collected, with the anticipation that it correlates with concentration at the targeted sites. The degree and amount to which a drug is accessible to mediate its function, like binding to a receptor or take part in a biochemical reaction at target tissue, refers to its bioavailability. Bioavailability is ascertained by associating plasma readings of a drug with path of administration. The graph between plasma concentrations of the drug versus time, gives the value of area under the curve (AUC), which reflets the bioavailability for absorption. In case of two drugs, if they show similar bioavailability and analogous period to achieve peak blood concentrations, they are said to be bioequivalent.

However, it is seen that variances in concentration due to diffusion of structurally dissimilar drugs at different sites is feasible, along with local metabolism and efflux. To avoid this, innovative methods have been established to calculate drug quantities at the target site. On example to measure drug in the cerebrospinal fluid (CSF) involves lumbar puncture. Other options include micro dialysis (for following blood–brain barrier), invasive bronchiolar lavage, radiology and urine analysis.

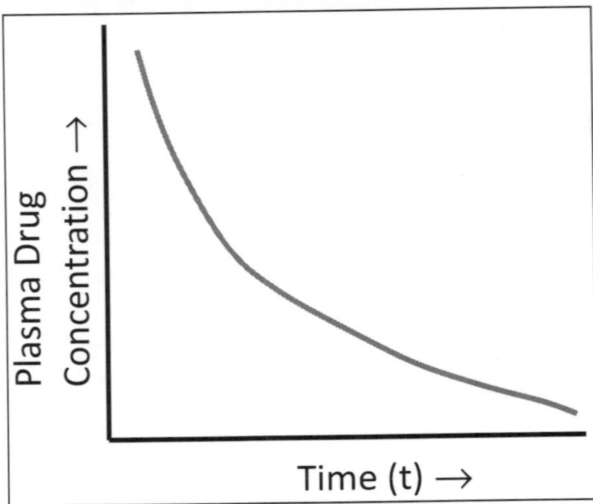

Figure 18.3: The Curve Showing Drug Metabolism and Excretion with Time, Leading to Reduced Plasma Concentration.

Even after all these studies, sometimes patients develop **adverse drug reactions (ADR)**, which is the harmful and unintended drug response and occurs at doses generally used for healing, identification, or treatment. Although ADR's can be predictable (generally mild, like diarrhea, nausea, dizziness) at times but sometimes, serious adverse reactions can even result in seizures, hospitalization, disability or death of patients. These could be either due to faulty drug regimens, allergy, overdose, combining alcohol and drug intake, intolerance or taking reacting medicines. Still, genetic factors (idiosyncrasy), age, underline diseases, lifestyles could be other possible reasons for ADR related complications. Some drug can cause birth defects, so USA FDA recommend grading risk and doing extensive drug testing before launch. These testing is done on animals for any possible toxicology or genotoxicology. They come under Toxicology Studies, which is the science to investigate potential harmful effects of chemicals/drugs. In these studies, animals have been used since historical times. Like early Greek scientists- Aristotle (384 – 322 BC) and Erasistratus (304 – 258 BC), conducted trials on live animals, which again gained popularity in 20th century after Sulfanilamide drug intake related multiple deaths (USA in 1937), where poisonous diethylene glycol (DEG) was used as a solvent. This drug launch didn't have any animal testing and public outcry made FDA to include safety testing of drugs on animals, beforehand their marketing and launch. Many other incidences are documented in history, which underlines the need for such testing.

Introduction to Preclinical Drug Developments

The drug development progression is classically divided into three main phases: discovery, preclinical development, and clinical trial. Once a compound with therapeutic index is shortlisted, it has to undergo pre-clinical testing. Preclinical progress incorporates the actions that connects drug discovery in the research labs to commencement of human clinical trials. It narrows down focus from several hits to the identification a lead candidate. The studies on model organisms like rodent, or nonrodent mammalian models are also included at this level to understand the pharmacokinetic (PK) profile, drug safety, and recognize any possible toxicity patterns. Animal studies help in calculating the drug's average dwelling duration in the body, which actually is a measure of absorption, distribution, metabolism, and excretion properties (ADME). For specialized treatment like neurological system-based medication designing, compound has to pass through the blood-brain barrier (BBB) *e.g.*, Alzheimer's disease. Besides that, toxicology studies rule out any possible adverse effects, deadliness, and thus define the therapeutic index, which is crucial in clinical studies. These pre-clinical studies require approval from regulatory authorities and are done under their supervision, by following rigid guidelines and GLP.

Drug Testing in Animals

Many pharma companies across the globe investigate the safety, effectiveness and any possible toxicity of their drugs on animals, like- rats, mice, rabbits, monkeys, guinea pig and dogs *etc.*, before future human use. In numerous studies, it was seen that pharmacological effects are same in humans, as in animals, Investigators exercise animal testing to acquire signs about how the ailment regresses in the body, after treatment. Also, various variables like genetics, diet and environment can affect the therapy and is also possible in animal testing. Over the years, it has facilitated the progress of many life-saving therapies for both humans and animals. It is unavoidable as there is no substitute mode for examining a whole living organism. Different model organisms have been developed for disease research including-digestive, neurological, infectious, genetic, connective tissue, and chronic diseases *etc.* Besides this, the toxicity of drugs is tested to assess the benefit vs. risk ratio of drugs and consumer care products. Toxic effect in other species help in predicting unpleasant effects in man. Thus, risk estimation is done by evaluation of toxic doses in model organism, with predicted curative dosage in man and is expressed in terms of therapeutic index.

Therapeutic Index = Maximum tolerated dose/Minimum curative dose

Certain toxicity tests such as mutagenicity, teratogenicity, carcinogenicity, reproductive toxicity, neurotoxicity immunotoxicity, *etc.* evaluate different type of toxicity. Toxicity tests needs to be executed in various laboratories and the similar outcomes must be obtained. It is done at pre-clinical testing level. Sometimes, alternative test methods (non-animal systems) are used that reduce, refine and replace animal use (3Rs). There are several diverse types of toxicity tests: acute toxicity tests, sub chronic (Repeated-Dose Toxicity Testing) and chronic toxicity (carcinogenicity). Acute toxicity is expressed in terms of LD_{50} or lethal dose 50, introduced by Trevan (1927), for insulin testing. It is the quantity of the drug that kills 50 per cent of the test animals. However, it was modified in 2002 to a fixed dose procedure, to reduce the number of animals involved. Sometimes, the toxicity can also damage the genetic information within a cell causing mutations, and is called genotoxicology. The DNA mutilation can be in the form of breaks in DNA (single strand or double strand, Ds breaks), failure of excision repair, point mutations, and chromosomal anomalies *etc.* The Ames Test (Bacterial Reverse Mutation Assay), Comet Assay and in-vitro or in-vivo tests are done to examine the lead compounds capacity to cause DNA damage.

Recent advance in pharmacology has led to the concept of **pharmacogenetics,** which implies to the variability in response to drug therapies in people. It is a fast-growing area in clinical medicine and voice about the genetic and non-genetic factors that affect our response to treatments. This study gained momentum and suggested personalized medicine, especially after complete sequencing and annotation of Human Genome Project (HGP) in 2003. It is proved that personalized medicine improves both diagnosis and treatment. Pharmacogenomics emphasizes on identifying patients, who would be responsive/non-responsive to treatment, develop interactions, generate side- effects, by examining the genetic predisposition and single nucleotide polymorphism (SNP) mapping in DNA. Like Tamoxifen, (commercially sold as Nolvadex) is an estrogen receptor modulator and used in breast cancer treatment, only if person is positive for estrogen receptor (ER +ve). Similarly, polymorphisms in genes of human leukocyte antigen (HLA) system, on chromosome 6, alters the immune response and metabolism of drugs. Many other drugs effectiveness have been found related to the genotype and often studied under genome-wide association studies (GWAS).

This preclinical phase ends with report submission to regulatory authority and after scrutinizing the results, phase I clinical trials permission can be given to the drug developing companies/organizations.

Biological and Novel Therapies

Many therapies under development for safe and efficacious novel formulations of biologics, vaccines and cancer therapy therapies are either genuinely novel and have never been earlier used in treatment.

Biological or biologic therapy is a healing method designed to re-establish the capacity of the body's guard system to combat infection and ailment. It often implicates the use of substances called biological response modifiers (BRMs), produced by either microbes, animals or humans, in small quantities (*e.g.*, antibody, interferon, interleukins, hormones, growth factors *etc.*) to retort sickness. Using various laboratory techniques, it is possible to synthesize these BRMs in greater quantities for treatment of diseases, including cancer, rheumatoid arthritis and Crohn's disease. Depending on the agent, biological therapies can be given various routes like- oral, intravenously *etc.*

Types of Biological Drugs, Depending on their Mechanism

1. **Biologic with enzymatic or regulatory activity:** include insulin, interferons, interleukins, streptokinase, *etc.*
2. **Biologic with special targeting activity:** Tumor Necrosis Factor (TNF) antagonists, which specifically block this proinflammatory cytokine in Crohn's Disease; monoclonal antibodies-based therapy *etc.*

3. **Vaccines:** They are used for either protecting against a foreign agent (Human Papilloma virus, HPV); treating against an autoimmune disease (anti Rh IgG) or treating cancer (Non-Hodgkin's Lymphoma) *etc.*
4. **Diagnostic Biologics:** Imaging agents labelled anti-Prostate serum antigens; antibodies against HIV (ELISA) *etc.*

Interferons (IFN)

Enhance the immune system activity against cancer cells. It also acts straight on cancer cells to slow their growth. They are naturally occurring proteins that were originally known for their capacity to impart resistance in cells against viral entry. Later, other roles were identified as well. The different IFN are put in separate categories:

1. Interferon alfa (IFN-α),
2. Interferon beta (IFN-β)
3. Interferon gamma (IFN-γ)

The functions attributed to interferons include- antiviral, anti-proliferative, controller of differentiation, inhibitor of angiogenesis, modulator of lipid metabolism, antitumoral, and immune-regulator *etc.* For activities, IFNs need to bind to their cognate cell receptors (paracrine), which are of two separate sets: type I and type II. IFN-alfa and beta binds to type I receptors, while IFN-gamma binds to type II receptors. Neutralizing antibodies bind to IFN molecules and results in loss of IFN-related side effects.

Interleukins (IL)

The interleukins are a type of polypeptides, originally entitled on their ability to umpire interactions between leukocytes. The interface between IL and effector cells is mediated by binding to cell-surface receptors. *e.g.* IL-2 activates T-cells proliferation, improves the performance of other immunocompetent cell, such as NK cells and B-cells. However, interleukins are immune molecules that can be used to treat particular diseases and cancers. *e.g.*, IL-2 promotes the development and action of specific immune cells that distinguish and terminate cancer cells.

Growth Factors

Growth factor are a group of structurally and evolutionarily related proteins that stimulate the cell growth. They act as signaling molecules between cells. They include: cytokines and hormones, which binds on exclusive target cells receptors. *e.g.*, GM-CSF (Granulocyte macrophage colony-stimulating factor) is a cytokine that works as a white blood cell growth factor, which promotes stem cells to produce monocytes and granulocytes.

Gene Therapy and Immunotherapy

Gene therapy and immunotherapy are both types of treatment for cancer and other diseases. Few rare inherited diseases are caused by a single mutant gene and gene therapy replace faulty genes in the body that are responsible for the disorder.

The examples include Sickle Cell anemia, Hemophilia, Cystic fibrosis *etc.* Today, most gene therapy is performed in clinical trials, but approved for few disorders.

Immunotherapy, on the hand, is a strategy aimed at improving the ability of the body's immune system to identify and attack cancer cells. Scientists have initial idea that specialized cell, like T lymphocytes can fight cancer cells successfully, but more often fails to recognize tumor cells or fight them effectively. So, if drugs can incite the immune response to recognize cancer cells and remove them, is a new idea and called immunotherapy. One form of immunotherapy makes use of genetically modified T cells. CAR-T cell therapy uses a patient's own T-lymphocytes, which are genetically altered in a lab to synthesize a protein called a chimeric antigen receptor (CAR). When these personalized T cells are returned to the patient, the CAR enables the T cells to seek out and destroy the cancer cells wherever they are found in the body. The first CAR T-cell treatment, called tisagenlecleucel or Kymriah, was approved in August 2017 to treat a form of leukemia, the FDA called it the "first gene therapy" in the United States.

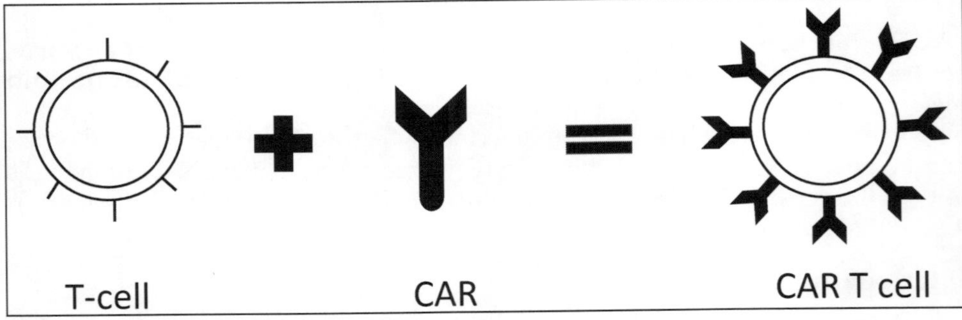

Figure 18.4: Chimeric Antigen Receptor (CAR) T-cell Therapy. T cells are collected from the patient's blood and are genetically engineered in the laboratory so that they recognize the cancer cells as targets.

Novel Targets for Anti-cancer Drugs

Generally, the anticancer agents target, one of these pathways:

1. Tyrosine protein kinase inhibitors
2. **EGF receptor inhibitor:** Geftinib Inhibits EGFR tyrosine kinase activity by blocking the ATP binding site
3. Angiogenesis inhibitors
4. Proteasome inhibitor
5. **Monoclonal antibody:** Rituximab is a chimeric monoclonal antibody against, which is primarily surface the immune system B cells. Cancer cells express a variety of antigens, which are targeted by monoclonal antibodies, and has gained popularity. Thus, needs to be discussed in detail.

Actually, in early 1970s, Kohler and Milstein developed Hybridoma technology, which led to the concept of monoclonal antibody. Merging of B-lymphocytes from an injected mouse with murine cancer cell lines, lead to hybrids. EGFR (Epidermal growth factor) is commonly expressed by colorectal cancer cells. Cetuximab, a chimeric monoclonal antibody precisely blocking epidermal growth factor receptor. **Monoclonal antibodies** are employed as vehicles to supply radiation or cancer drugs to cancerous cells as part of a biological therapy regimen. This contrasts with conventional non-biologic pharmaceutical drugs, which are manufactured in a laboratory via chemical processes, without using parts of living beings. Biologic therapies are often taken together with older non-biologic therapies. For example, somebody with rheumatoid arthritis might still continue taking methotrexate, while adding an additional biologic treatment.

Bio Reductive Drugs

Bio reductive drugs are dormant prodrugs that undergo metabolic reduction into potent functional cytotoxins under special conditions, including low oxygen tension (hypoxia) or presence of elevated reductases in certain tumors. *e.g.*, Mitomycin C is such a bio reductive drug. This could be the reason behind their specificity and limited toxicity. The other cytotoxic compounds (like radiation) show better activity with bio reductive drugs. Tirapazamine (TPZ) is a bio reductive drug that exhibits greatly enhanced cytotoxicity in hypoxic tumor cells, which are frequently radiation-resistant Four groups of compounds exist in this concept of drugs: quinones, nitroaromatics, aliphatic and heteroaromatic N-oxides.

Cancer Vaccines

There are therapeutic vaccines that can prevent healthy people from getting certain cancers caused by viruses. Like chicken pox vaccine, viral vaccines also only work if a person gets the vaccine before they are infected with the virus. Thus, they are included in immunotherapy. Right now, two types of vaccines are approved by the U.S. Food and Drug Administration (FDA) for cancer prevention, including human papillomavirus (HPV) which causes cervical, vaginal and anal cancers; and Hepatitis B virus which results in Liver cancer.

Drug Development in the Past Decade

In earlier days, drug discovery was done through random inspection of higher plants for therapeutic properties, like opium, reserpine, senna, belladonna, ephedrine, *etc.*, However, the Penicillin discovery and later its modifications resulted in better derivatives (Penicillin G, Penicillin V, Methicillin, Carbenicillin, Oxacillin, Amoxicillin *etc.*). This led to opening an era of synthesis of compounds with remedial potential, which gave some good lead compounds and later its optimization resulted in good candidates for scale-up. The Sulfanilamide development shares a similar story like many others such drugs. Later, the approach was more rational and considered the organic structure and related potency in consideration. NMR and X-ray crystallography enabled the study of structures of ligands and targets. The penultimate in the list are genetic engineering and recombinant DNA technologies, which led to discovery of insulin as well. However, most recent are computer aided discovery and discussed next.

Computational Drug Discovery

It is actually Computer-Aided Drug Designing (CADD), which uses computational methods to determine, improve and evaluate the compounds as potential drugs. These approaches are based on structure-activity relationships (SAR) and ligands binding approximation is done on target sites (enzymes, receptors, ion channels and transporters). The reference compounds 2D and 3D structures can aid in estimation of pharmacophores (important groups involved in binding) and quality and intensity of its interactions. These are officially called as 'docking' and followed by energy minimization tools. Various such software's are FLIPDock, AutoDock 4 and Vina, SwissDock, UCSF DOCK, SWISS MODEL, EADock, LOMETS, HADDOCK 2.2, FIND SITE, PatchDock and ClusPro *etc.* These are high throughput methods to screen a library of structures for ant potential desired activity. The energy minimization is also done through computer servers like, YASARA, KoBaMIN and 3-D REFINE. Many of these are freely available and easy to download. The lead optimization includes ascertaining quantitative structure-activity relationships (SAR). The CYP inhibition and metabolism studies gives initial idea about their safety and efficacy and is done by software like Gastroplus, Swiss ADME *etc.* All these in-silico work constructs the road for lab work, including *in-vitro*, followed by *in-vivo* work.

CADD (Computer-Aided Drug Designing)

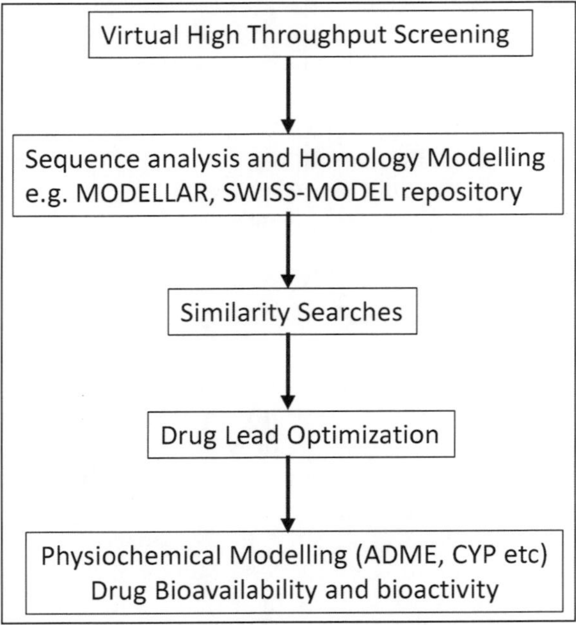

Figure 18.5: The Flow Chart, Showing Step-wise Development in CADD.

Thus, it can be summarized that calculating the relationship between SAR is supportive in drug discovery, generate large amounts of data. Interpolation, if done carefully can generate novel analogues. However, it should be kept in mind that incorrect associations may develop sometimes. Additionally, data generated don't assist in designing of experiments and their feasibility. Therefore, QSAR may not always choose the best compounds, and chances of errors exist. The different physicochemical parameters/settings of experiments are dynamic, with separate variables and cross-correlated at times, which may not be efficiently tapped by computers and software. Conclusively, it is accepted that drug designing is a complex, multi-disciplinary and intellectually intensive process.

Web Based Cheminformatics System for Drug Discovery

Cheminformatics deals with computational analysis for analysing and managing the data concerning chemical and molecular structures of potential compounds, to be developed as future drugs. In other words, it is an *in-silico* technique or scientific study, performed virtually on computers *via* various software and simulations. The processing of the useful information and statistics, allows the creation of relationship curve between chemical structure, properties, and subsequent molecular action. It is opposite of normal course of drug discovery, that involves choosing an ailment, followed by probing for potential compounds/molecules for therapeutic intervention and generally involves different stages of investigation, to ascertain effectiveness without any toxicity. On the other hand, cheminformatics radically speedup the discovery process, in which use of software's to estimate and envisage structures is fundamental. The advantage of latter lies in the fact that results are accurate, reduce both time, as well as cost and virtual-screening can separate out certain compounds during initial trials only, which otherwise aren't compatible and thus avoid the hassle of their physical examination. The compounds are classified and categorised on their solubility, cross-reactivity and possible toxicity. In this strategy, High throughput screening (HTS) is a classic technique to examine a large quantity of diverse molecules in an automated screening process, for either stimulatory or inhibitory effects. It is automated, efficient and uses advanced robotics for precise screening, like ligand-receptor interactions. The online databases of compounds, and software can compute chemical relations which are compared to other online libraries to improve screening in the future.

Hit-to-Lead Optimization

Hit-to-Lead optimization explores the chemistry and biology of hits to focus efforts on the most promising starting points so that development time and costs are saved. As discussed, high-throughput screening (HTS) identifies lead compounds, but it is seen that mere screening is not enough and more work is required to convert hits into lead compounds, otherwise most lead compounds are likely to fail in subsequent preclinical and clinical testing. It should be understood that the physical and chemical properties of a drug need to be fully realised to work out the mechanism of drug molecule absorption, distribution metabolism, excreted and toxicity (called *in-silico* ADMET). Hit to lead (H2L) implicates integrating medicinal chemistry and ADME/Tox studies, generating focused collections nearby encouraging hits and using for generation of structure activity relationship (SAR). Thus, integration of chemistry, biology, and computational studies can maximize the synergy of their efforts and help in developing new drugs.

Polypharmacological Approach in Drug Discovery

Polypharmacology is based on the concept of 'one-drug/agent, multiple-targets' (or SMAT) hypothesis in drug discovery. These are multi-targeting drugs (MTDs), which have ability to display an adequate extent of specificity towards multiple targets. Even drug combinatorial therapy also comes under the same umbrella. However, utmost care should be taken as drug molecules might interact with multiple unintended targets and might lead to adverse reactions. This strategy has potential in treating bacterial infections, epilepsy, cancer and psychiatric disorders. One such multi-target drug is aspirin, which is mostly suggested to relieve pain or control fever, but also has anti- inflammation and anti-clotting activity. Like that, sildenafil initially developed for hypertension and heart disease prevention but also has secondary property in treating erectile dysfunction.

REFERENCES

1. Buda V, Baul B, Andor M, *et al.*, Solid-State Stability and Kinetics of Degradation for Candesartan–Pure Compound and Pharmaceutical Formulation. Pharmaceutics 2020; 12: 86.
2. Bullock TNJ. Fundamentals of Cancer Immunology and Their Application to Cancer Vaccines. Clinical and Translational Science 2021; 14: 120–31.
3. Kelly C, Mir F. Economics of biological therapies. British Medical Journal 2009; 339: b3276.
4. Krishna EH, Gupta VRM, Krishna M, Jyothi S, Dasari R. Preparation and evaluation of sodium CMC zaltoprofen spherical agglomerates for direct compression. Journal of Pharmacy Research 2013; 6: 61–7.
5. Lyu J, Wang S, Balius TE, *et al.*, Ultra-large library docking for discovering new chemotypes. Nature 2019; 566: 224–9.
6. Mahato R. I., Narang. Ajit S. In Pharmaceutical Dosage Forms and Drug Delivery, 3rd edition: CRC Press.; 2018
7. Maheshwari R, Todke P, Kuche K, Raval N, Tekade RK. Chapter 17 Micromeritics in Pharmaceutical Product Development. In: Tekade RK, ed. Dosage Form Design Considerations. Advances in Pharmaceutical Product Development and Research. Academic Press, 2018; 599–635.
8. Melief CJM, Hall T van, Arens R, Ossendorp F, Burg SH van der. Therapeutic cancer vaccines. Journal Clinical Investigation 2015; 125: 3401–12.
9. Oliver K., Heribert W. In Pharmaceutical Biotechnology: Drug Discovery and Clinical Applications, 2nd Edition. Wiley-Blackwell; 2012.
10. Palucka K, Ueno H, Banchereau J. Recent Developments in Cancer Vaccines. The Journal of Immunology 2011; 186: 1325–31.

11. Price G, Patel DA. Drug Bioavailability. In: StatPearls [Internet]. Treasure Island (FL): StatPearls Publishing; 2021.

12. Soleimani B, Murray K, Hunt D. Established and Emerging Immunological Complications of Biological Therapeutics in Multiple Sclerosis. Drug Safety 2019; 42: 941–56.

13. Umashankar, V. and Gurunathan, S. Chemoinformatics and its Applications. In General, Applied and Systems Toxicology (eds B. Ballantyne, T.C. Marrs, T. Syversen, D.A. Casciano and S.C. Sahu). Wiley Online Library; 2011

14. Xu J, Hagler A. Chemoinformatics and Drug Discovery. Molecules 2002; 7: 566–600.

15. Yadlapalli JSK, Albayati ZAF, Breen PJ, Dobretsov M, Penthala NR, Hendrickson HP, Crooks PA. A pharmacokinetic study of morphine-6-O-sulfate in rat plasma and brain. Drug Development research. 2021 Jan 11. doi: 10.1002/ddr.21785.

Chapter 19

Stem Cells and Gene Therapy

Suvarna Chatterjee[1,2], Rizwanul Haque[2] and Syed Shadab Raza*[1,3]

[1]Laboratory for Stem Cell and Restorative Neurology, Department of Biotechnology, Era's Lucknow Medical College Hospital, Era University, Sarfarazganj, Lucknow – 226003, Uttar Pradesh, India
[2]Department of Biotechnology, Central University of South Bihar, Gaya – 824 236, Bihar, India
[3]Department of Stem Cell Biology and Regenerative Medicine, Era University, Sarfarazganj, Lucknow – 226003, Uttar Pradesh, India
**e-mail: drshadab@erauniversity.in*

ABSTRACT

For patients with a range of disorders, stem cell and gene therapy are the most cutting-edge treatments currently available. Fresh hope for repairing and replacing damaged cells and tissues was born with discovering stem cells capable of multiplying indefinitely in culture and differentiating into many other cell types under unfavorable conditions. The characteristics of stem cells that provide treatment for some incurable diseases, and some therapies, especially those derived from adult stem cells, are already in clinics. On the other hand, gene therapy can be described as a collection of strategies for treating disease by altering gene expression or correcting mutant/defective genes by administering DNA or RNA to cells. Gene therapy is currently only available as part of a clinical trial. Basic stem cell biology, gene therapy, and their applications in different diseases are covered in this chapter. To brief, it includes topics on embryonic, adult, and induced pluripotent stem cells, stem cell therapy for various disorders, gene therapy, methods of gene delivery, vehicles employed in gene delivery, and the use of gene delivery in human diseases.

Keywords: *Stem cells, Gene therapy, Regenerative medicine, Adult stem cells, Embryonic stem cells, Induced pluripotent stem cells, Viral transfer.*

Introduction

At the onset of a trailblazing technological revolution, the scientific and the medical community have reached novel solutions to various acute and chronic diseases that are much more effective and less hazardous than ever before. And one such solution is the practice of Regenerative medicine. Regenerative medicine takes a new approach to treat disease by replacing, engineering, or renewing cells, tissues or organs to restore normal function. Interestingly, as regenerative medicine focuses on the replacement and regeneration of tissues or organs, the premise is to mitigate the symptoms of the conditions so that the body can heal itself in due course, leading to a substantial increase in the quality of life of patients. The biomedical approaches within regenerative medicine incorporate gene therapy, stem cell transplantation, and tissue engineering.This chapter will emphasize the use of stem cells and gene therapy technologies as new tools under the domain of regenerative medicine. Stem cell and gene therapy are novel therapeutic branches of modern medicine. In stem cell therapy, whole cells are infused or transplanted, while, in gene therapy, either a specific gene or gene material is delivered.To elaborate, given their unique regenerative abilities, stem cells can repair, restore or recreate functional tissues through various mechanisms: bystander effect, reducing apoptosis and inflammation, modulating the immune system, and integrating into the tissues. These properties make stem cells a viable treatment option for a variety of medical conditions. Likewise, as the name signifies, gene therapies are a technique that modifies a person's genes to treat or cure disease. If a defective gene causes a required protein to be faulty or absent, gene therapy may restore the protein's function by introducing a normal copy of the gene.

Stem Cell Definition

Stem cells are the undifferentiated cell of a multicellular organism. They can give rise to more cells of the same type from which certain other kinds of cells arise by differentiation.

Stem Cells Properties

1. Stem cells are undifferentiated cells found in our bodies that can replicate indefinitely and differentiate into cells with unique functions.
2. Stem cells provide a constant supply of new cells that make up an organism's various tissues and organs.
3. Stem cells can give rise to cells of mesoderm, ectoderm, and endoderm.
4. They are the first cell lineage cells in all tissues found in both embryonic and adult organisms.
5. Stem cells are classified as embryonic and adult stem cells, depending on their origin (Table 19.1).
6. Induced pluripotent stem cells (iPSCs) are a new type of stem cells obtained by reprogramming animal and differentiated human cells.
7. Depending on their role, stem cells may be totipotent, multipotent, or pluripotent (Table 19.2).

Table 19.1: Stem Cell Types Based on Origin

Embryonic Stem Cells	*Adult Stem Cells*	*Induced Pluripotent Stem Cells*
Origin	**Origin**	**Origin**
Inner cell mass of the blastocyst of embryo	Adult tissues, such as Bone Marrow, Adipose tissue, Brain, Kidney etc.	Reprogramming of somatic cells (with c-Myc, Klf-4, Oct-3/4 and Sox-3)
Strength	**Strength**	**Strength**
☆ Pluripotent (3 germ layer) in nature ☆ Ability to Self-renewal ☆ Can give rise to whole embry	☆ Multipotent cells ☆ Ability to Self-renew ☆ Typical lineage committed cells	☆ Totipotent (3 germ layer and trophoblast) ☆ Self-renewal ☆ Cells unique to patients

Table 19.2: Stem Cell Types Based on Function

Cell Type	*Function*	*Examples*
Totipotent	Ability to differentiate into all cell types and functional organism	Cells from early(1-3) days embryo
Pluripotent	Ability to differentiate into all cell types but cannot form a functional organism	Embryonic stem cells
Multipotent	Ability to differentiate into closely related family of cells	Hematopoietic stem cell, Mesenchymal stem cells, Dental pulp stem cell, fetal tissue *etc.*
Oligopotent	Ability to differentiate into few cell types	Lymphoid or myeloid stem cell
Unipotent	Ability to only produce cells of their own type, though having property to self-renew.	Muscle stem cells

Stem Cell Types

Embryonic Stem Cells

Embryonic stem cells are pluripotent cells originating from the inner cell mass of an early-stage pre-implantation embryo (Figure 18.1A). This stage reaches at 4-5 days after fertilization, and at this stage, the embryo is known as a blastocyst, which comprises 50–150 cells. Pluripotency, or the capacity to give rise to cell types consisting of all embryo and adult tissues when differentiated, and immortality, or unlimited proliferation, are characteristics of embryonic stem cells.

Adult Stem Cells

Adult stem cells are undifferentiated cells found in fully developed specific tissues and can only produce a limited number of cell types (Figure 18.1B). They play a vital role in tissue repair and regeneration. Adult stem cells' primary function is to keep tissues in a state of homeostasis. Adult stem cells are usually kept in a dormant state, but when cells are lost, or tissue is injured, they can be stimulated to proliferate and differentiate into the desired cell form.

A

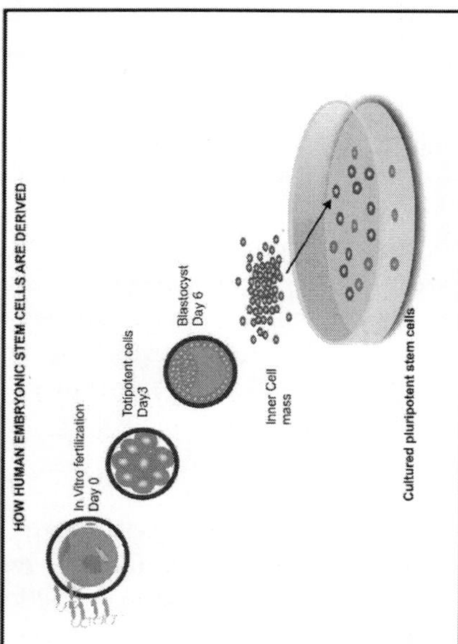

B

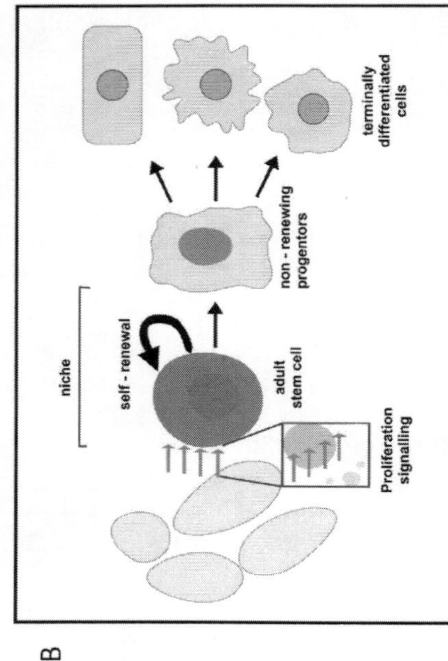

C

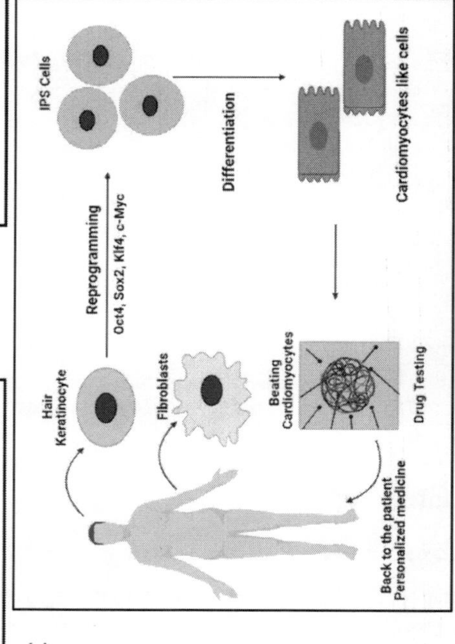

Figure 19.1: Represents the Technique to Generate Embryonic Stem Cells in Laboratory Condition (A). Fig B represents Adult stem cells, undifferentiated cells found throughout the body that multiplies by cell division to replenish dying cells and regenerate damaged tissue. Fig C represents the Pluripotent stem cells toolbox for Heart disease modeling. Image creation: BioRender.com

Induced Pluripotent Stem Cells

Induced Pluripotent Stem Cells (iPSCs) (Figure 18.1C) are a type of pluripotent stem cell that can be generated directly from adult cells. Induced pluripotent cells were first described in 2006 by Japanese physician and researcher Shinya Yamanaka and colleagues. Since its discovery, the iPSCs have been used to treat certain diseases, such as heart diseases, inborn metabolic diseases, Autism Spectrum Disorders, and Glioma.

Types of Adult Stem Cells Based on Origin and their Uses

Mesenchymal Stem Cells

Mesenchymal stem cells (MSCs) are a non-hematopoietic cell population characterized as fibroblast-like adherent cells. MSCs have immunomodulatory properties as well as trophic activity. They have long and thin bodies and very prominent nuclei and can be differentiated into neuronal cells, adipocytes, osteocytes, chondrocytes, and myocytes, *etc*. They can be isolated from the adipose tissues, bone marrow, umbilical cord, molar cells, *etc*. MSCs have been used to treat various disorders, including cardiovascular diseases, cerebrovascular disorders, bone and cartilage repair, and autoimmune diseases, to name a few.

Hematopoietic Stem Cells

Hematopoietic stem cells are immature cells that can develop into all types of blood cells, including white blood cells, red blood cells, and platelets. These cells are found in the peripheral blood and the bone marrow. They are often used after high-dose chemotherapy to improve hematologic conditions and cure malignant diseases.

Neural Stem Cells

Neural stem cells (NSCs) are undifferentiated cells originating in the central nervous system. NSCs can give rise to offspring cells that grow and differentiate into neurons and glial cells. These stem cells are found in two brain zones, namely, the dentate gyrus (part of the hippocampus) and the sub ventricular zone (SVZ). These cells are widely employed in brain cellular therapy after an injury or disease.

Dental Pulp Stem Cells

They are a diverse group of cells isolated from the permanent third molar pulp of humans. These are multipotent cells that can differentiate into odontoblasts, neural cells, adipocytes, and other cell types, depending on microenvironmental factors. These stem cells are similar to MSCs, except that DPSCs can transform into dentin-forming odontoblast-like cells. They proliferate quickly into dental pulp tissue and pulp complex, hence treating infected or damaged pulp tissues. Due to ease of isolation, they have become a cell of choice to treat various diseases.

Epidermal Stem Cells

Epidermal stem cells are responsible for the everyday regeneration of the different layers of the epidermis. These stem cells are found in the basal layer of the epidermis. These rejuvenating cells can self-renew indefinitely. These cells can be used in cellular regeneration, wound healing, and dermal neoplasm formation in addition to natural skin homeostasis.

Pancreatic Stem Cells

The pancreatic stem cells are multipotent stem cells originating from the developing fore-gut endoderm. They can differentiate into lineage-specific progenitors that are responsible for the development of the pancreas. They give rise to both the exocrine and endocrine cells. Exocrine cells constitute the acinar cells and the ductal cells which produce digestive enzymes. The endocrine cells form the alpha cells that secrete glucagon, beta cells that make insulin, and delta cells that secrete somatostatin.

Applications of Stem Cells at Clinics

Stem cell therapies are no longer considered science fiction now. Since the first bone marrow transplantation in 1957, stem cell transplantation has been around for more than 60 years. In *vitro* non-expanded and expanded stem cells, adult stem cells, and induced pluripotent stem cells (iPSCs) are currently used in clinical trials. With the first use of iPSCs in treating ophthalmological infections by Japanese research, the patient-specific stem cells are available for various diseases. Though, except for hematopoietic stem/progenitor cells for hematological applications, the current clinical results with stem cells are somewhat disappointing. Summarized are a few stem cell applications:

Stem Cell Therapy for Heart Repair

The heart muscle is nourished and kept pumping by a constant supply of oxygen-rich blood. A blockage in an artery interrupts blood flow during a heart attack. In this case, stem cells with the ability to differentiate into a range of heart cell types may be able to restore and regenerate damaged heart tissue. Cardiac progenitor cells and bone marrow mononuclear cells have been used in clinical trials of the damaged heart. Acute myocardial infarction, advanced coronary artery disease, and chronic heart failure patients will benefit from stem cell therapy to improve myocardial perfusion and contractile efficiency.

Stem Cell Therapy for Neurological Disorders

Neurological disorders encompass various diseases affecting the central and peripheral nervous systems, which are the leading cause of disease burden globally. Cells from infants, adults, aborted fetuses, embryos, umbilical cord, menstrual blood, amniotic fluid, and placenta have all shown promising therapeutic results in pre-clinical settings of neurological diseases or injuries. Stem cell therapy is widely practiced in non-clinical settings for Parkinson's disease, Alzheimer's disease, spinal cord injury, stroke, *etc.*

Stem Cell Therapy for Diabetes Mellitus

Replacement of usable insulin-producing pancreatic cells with pancreas or islet-cell transplants is the mainstay of diabetes mellitus treatment. Researchers are looking into ways to generate cells, such as islet expansion, encapsulated islet xenografts, human islet cell lines, and the use of stem cells.The ability to generate beta cells from embryonic stem cells, adult stem cells, and the induced pluripotent stem cells has recently made considerable progress in this area. A good example of adult stem cells converting into pancreatic cells is MSCs, after infusion, producing exocrine and endocrine-functioning pancreatic cells.

Stem Cell Therapy for Autoimmune Diseases

An autoimmune disease is a disorder in which your immune system mistakenly attacks your own body. In Autoimmune disorders, anti-inflammatory, immunosuppressive, and immunomodulating medicines are often prescribed. Nonetheless, some patients develop resistance to standard treatment. In such cases, the use of large doses of drugs necessitates bone marrow reconstitution. This has sparked interest in the use of hematopoietic stem cells in the treatment of autoimmune diseases.Adult stem cells, such as MSCs, have been used extensively in the treatment of autoimmune disorders in addition to hematopoietic stem cells in recent years.

Identification of Stem Cells

Due to their extraordinary complexities, precision, validity, and lack of specific molecular markers, our understanding of stem cell recognition in the therapeutic application is minimal. Despite our lack of understanding of marker functions, their distinct expression patterns and timing provide us with a valuable method for identifying and isolating stem cells. Stem cells are widely identified through various markers: genes and their protein products. Functional assays, which are considered the gold standard for identifying and treating stem cells, may also be used to identify them. While functional assays are the best way to identify stem cells, molecular markers provide a systematic way to identify a stable and robust stem cell population.

Here, we have summarized a couple of markers used in identifying and isolating embryonic and adult stem cells.

Embryonic Stem Cells: Klf4, c-Myc, Oct4, Sox2, and Nanog, Sall4, Dax1, Essrb, Tbx3, Tcl1, Rif1, Nac1, and Zfp281, NANO, TRA-1-60, and SSEA4 *etc.*

Adult Stem Cells

Neural Stem Cells: CD133, CD15, GCTM-2, PSA-NCAM, CD24, ABCG2, FGF R4, Musashi-1 (Msi1) and Nestin *etc.*

Mesenchymal Stem Cells: CD10, CD13, CD73, CD105, and CD271, CD140b, HER-2/erbB2 (CD340), and frizzled-9 (CD349).

Bone Marrow Mesenchymal Stem Cells: STRO-1, CD29, CD73, CD90, CD105, CD146, Oct4, and SSEA4, it is noteworthy that BMMSC do not express CD14 and CD34.

Dental Pulp Stem Cells: CD44, CD73, CD90, and CD105 *etc.*

Potential Benefits of Stem Cell Therapy

Stem cell therapy uses stem cells to solve the issues happening in the human body caused due to cell malfunction or degeneration. A few of the benefits are enlisted below:

1. Advances in this area have paved the way for developing other cell-based therapies for diseases that are resistant to traditional treatments.
2. Since stem cells originate in one's own body, there is no risk of catching any disease from stem cell therapy.
3. Stem cell treatment can speed up recuperation times for patients with severe wounds or those recuperating from surgical procedures.
4. Stem cell therapy is non-invasive and can be delivered with the help of ultrasound or fluoroscopy devices.
5. Stem cell therapy is much less stressful to patients and comes with far fewer risks of complications.
6. In most cases, only biological materials derived from the patient's body are used in stem cell treatments. When opposed to other forms of therapies, this decreases the chance of body rejection.

Disadvantages of Using Stem Cell Therapy

- Immune suppression may be needed for stem cell treatments because the patient's immune system may attack the stem cells.
- Pluripotency in specific stem cells could complicate obtaining a particular cell type because not all cells in a population divide equally. Undifferentiated cells can, as a result, produce undesirable tissues.
- Pluripotency, especially in embryonic stem cells, foetal stem cells, and induced pluripotent stem cells, is linked to tumour development after transplantation in specific stem cells.
- Ethical concerns surround the use of embryonic stem cells or induced pluripotent stem cells.
- Stem cell therapy is expensive, and not everybody who needs it can afford it.

Ethics in Stem Cell Transplantation

The ethical concerns about stem cells have primarily cantered on their source. Human embryonic stem cell therapy holds great promise for curing incurable diseases such as spinal cord injury, ALS, Alzheimer's, Parkinson's, and other neurological disorders. Medical procedures that kill human embryos when stem cells are destroyed are morally unacceptable. Similarly, Stem Cells isolated from the foetal tissue require ethical permission. As isolating stem cells from the foetus, the foetus has to be killed, which has a right to exist as a human being.

Following transplantation, specific stem cells form tumours. Teratoma is cancerous tumours with a benign appearance. ESCs and iPSCs have shown a high rate of teratoma formation, though the rate of teratoma formation in human iPSCs is reported higher than ESCs.

Gene Therapy

Gene therapy involves the transfer of genetic material into the appropriate cells. It primarily involves genetic manipulations in animals or humans, like in the case of mutated genes. It is a method for treating, curing, or preventing disease by altering gene expression patterns. It is mainly experimental, and it may affect somatic or germ cells.To summarize, gene therapies can operate in a variety of ways:

- Introducing a new or updated gene into the body to better cure a disease
- Replacing a disease-causing gene with a safe copy of the gene
- Inactivating a disease-causing gene that is not working properly

Gene Therapy at Clinics

Human gene therapy seeks to modify or manipulate a gene's expression or alter the biological properties of living cells for therapeutic use. The idea is to modify the genetic information of the patient's cell that is responsible for a disease and then return that cell to normal conditions. Both inherited genetic diseases and acquired disorders can be treated with gene therapy. Examples of these disorders are primary immune deficiencies, where gene therapy has been able to fully correct the presentation of patients and cancer, where the gene therapy is still at the experimental stage.

Gene Therapy Process

One of the most critical obstacles in the process is releasing the gene into the cell. Thus, a molecular carrier known as a "vector" is used to release the gene, which must be very precise, efficient in releasing one or more genes of the sizes required for clinical applications. Should be able to get purified in large amounts and high concentrations to be manufactured and made available on a large scale.Once injected into the patient, the vector should not cause allergic reactions or inflammation; instead, it should improve normal functions, correct deficits, or prevent harmful activities. Also, it should be safe not only for the patient but also for the community and the professionals who work with it. Finally, the vector should express the gene for the duration of the patient's life.

Gene Therapy Approaches

Gene therapy treatment is broadly divided into Somatic and germline cell gene therapy. Somatic cell gene therapy involves obtaining non-reproductive cells from a person with a genetic disease and then introducing a normal gene into the defective cell. Germline therapy takes place in the reproductive cells. It entails the genetic alteration of germ cells, which will be passed on to future generations. A comparative analysis is provided in Table 19.3.

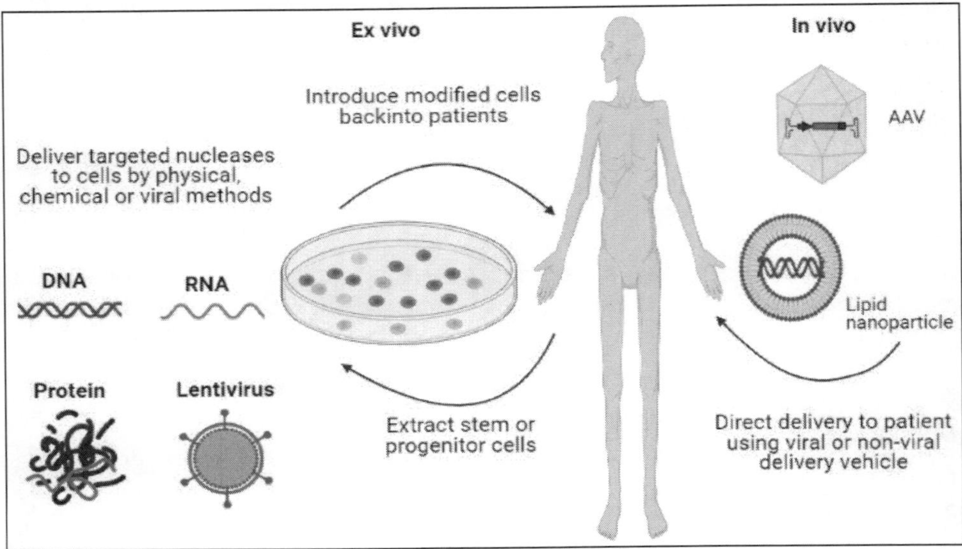

Figure 19.2: Diagram Depicts the Mode of Therapeutic Gene-Editing Strategies and Gene Delivery, including Viral Vectors, such as Lentivirus, AAV, and Non-viral Vectors, such as Liposomes, into the Human.Viral or non-viral vectors containing nucleases are directly injected into the body for *in vivo* gene editing. For *ex vivo* gene editing, the target cells are isolated and gene-edited through viral or non-viral vectors containing nucleases, following the gene-edited cells are expanded and re-injected into the body. Image created by: BioRender.com

Gene Delivery Methods

To introduce the gene of interest into the desired cell, a variety of gene therapy products are available, such as:

- **Plasmid DNA:** Genetically modified therapeutic genes can be delivered to human cells using Plasmid DNA.
- **Viral vectors:** Since viruses have the inherent ability to deliver genetic material into cells, viruses may be used as vectors (vehicles) to transport therapeutic genes into human cells after being modified to suppress their ability to cause infectious disease.
- **Bacterial vectors:**Bacteria may be engineered to avoid infection and then used as vectors (vehicles) to deliver therapeutic genes into human tissues.
- **Human gene-editing technology:** Gene editing aims to either disrupt dangerous genes or restore mutated genes.
- **Cellular gene therapy products obtained from patients:** Cells are taken from the patient, genetically modified (often with the aid of a viral vector), and then returned to the patients.

Table 19.3

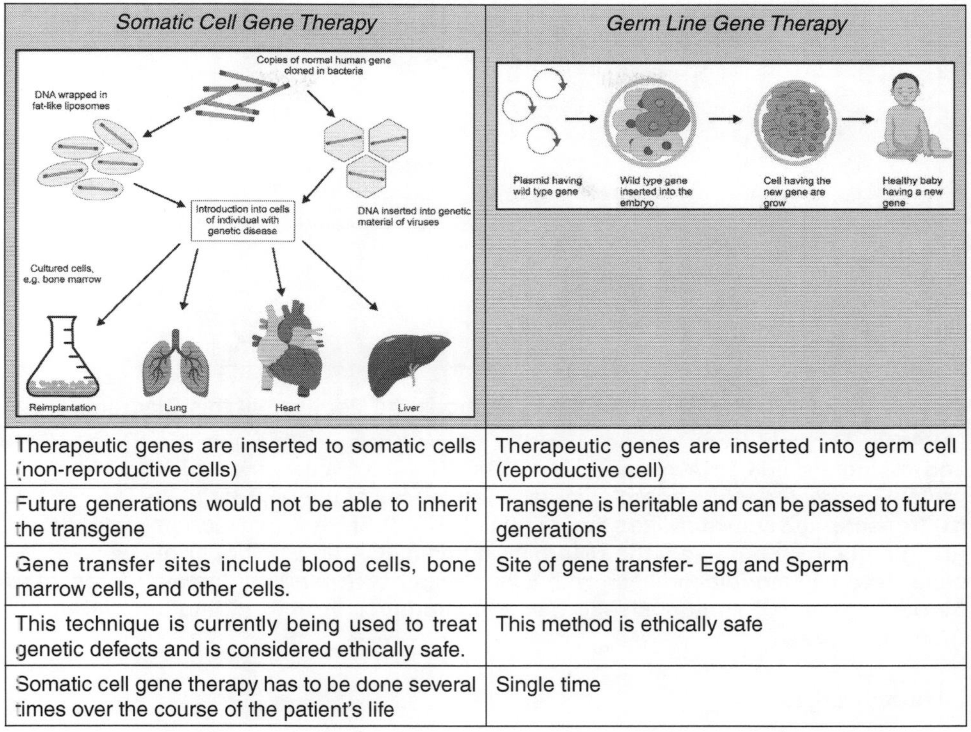

Somatic Cell Gene Therapy	*Germ Line Gene Therapy*
Therapeutic genes are inserted to somatic cells (non-reproductive cells)	Therapeutic genes are inserted into germ cell (reproductive cell)
Future generations would not be able to inherit the transgene	Transgene is heritable and can be passed to future generations
Gene transfer sites include blood cells, bone marrow cells, and other cells.	Site of gene transfer- Egg and Sperm
This technique is currently being used to treat genetic defects and is considered ethically safe.	This method is ethically safe
Somatic cell gene therapy has to be done several times over the course of the patient's life	Single time

*Image created by: BioRender.com

Gene Editing Technology for Gene Therapy

Gene editing technologies allow genetic material to be added, removed or altered at particular locations in the genome. In gene editing, a mutant gene is edited, deleted, or substituted at the genome level. There have been several approaches to genome editing. A few of them are discussed below (Figure 19.3):

CRISPR-Cas9 Technology

CRISPR-Cas9 is a novel technology that allows scientists to modify parts of the genome by deleting, adding, or changing DNA sequences. Cas9 enzymes, together with CRISPR sequences, form the basis of technology. CRISPR (clustered regularly interspaced short palindromic repeats) is a family of DNA sequences found in prokaryotic organisms, including bacteria and archaea. Cas9 (CRISPR-associated 9) is an enzyme that uses CRISPR sequences as a guide to recognize and cleave specific strands of DNA that are complementary to the CRISPR sequence.

Advantages

- ✰ Relative simplicity and versatility
- ✰ Highest efficiency

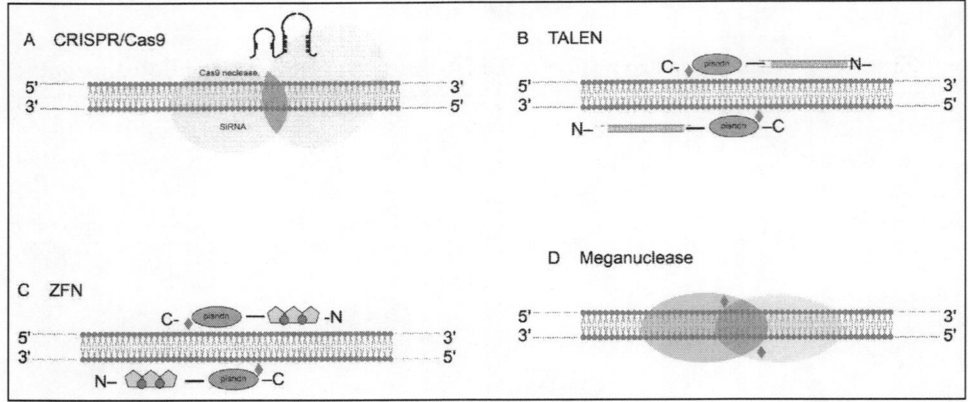

Figure 19.3: The Genome Editing Methods are Depicted in this Diagram.

(A) A Cas9 protein (shown in light gold) with two nuclease domains (HuvC and HNH) and a single guide RNA make up the CRISPR/Cas9 framework (sgRNA). The Cas9 protein is directed to the complementary sequences of the DNA target by the sgRNA. (B) Transcription activator-like effector nuclease (TALEN) has two monomers, and light green rectangles represent the DNA bind domain. (C) The zinc finger nuclease (ZFN) comprises two monomers, each with a zinc finger DNA-binding domain represented by pentagons. (D) Meganuclease has a homodimer structure. Image created by: BioRender.com

Disadvantages

- ✰ Off-target effects
- ✰ It may result in genomic instability
- ✰ Target selection limited by requirement for PAM sequence

Transcription Activator-like Effector Nucleases (TALENs)

Restriction enzymes called transcription activator-like effector nucleases (TALENs) are designed to cut unique DNA sequences. A DNA-recognition transcription activator-like effector (TALE) and a DNA nuclease domain make up TALENs. They function by identifying a particular sequence to edit genes.

Advantages

- ✰ TALENs have the potential to target any part of the genome
- ✰ TALENs have less off-target consequences, meaning they are less likely to cause mutations elsewhere in the genome

Disadvantages

- ✰ TALENs is more costly than CRISPR-Cas9 technology
- ✰ Sensitive to off-target methylation
- ✰ Relatively low efficiency
- ✰ This method necessitates considerably more effort than those dedicated to sequence design and cloning

Zinc-Finger Nucleases

Zinc finger nucleases are a type of DNA-binding protein that allows targeted genome editing by causing double-strand breaks in DNA at user-specified locations. Double-strand breaks are required for site-specific mutagenesis because they activate the cell's natural DNA-repair mechanisms, such as homologous recombination and non-homologous end-joining (NHEJ). These processes are harnessed by using well-established, field-proven methods to produce precisely tailored genomic edits, resulting in cell lines with targeted gene deletions, integrations, or modifications.

Advantages

- ☆ Rapid disruption of, or integration into, any genomic loci
- ☆ Irreversible and heritable mutations
- ☆ Works in a wide range of mammalian somatic cell types
- ☆ Screening does not necessitate antibiotic selection

Disadvantages

- ☆ Expensive, laborious and time consuming in making constructs
- ☆ Target only one site each time
- ☆ Low efficiency

Meganucleases

Meganucleases, also known as homing endonucleases, have a large recognition site (double-stranded DNA sequences of 12 to 40 base pairs). They are "molecular DNA scissors" that can efficiently induce homologous recombination, produce mutations, and change reading frames by replacing, eliminating, or modifying sequences in a highly targeted manner.

Advantages

- ☆ Less toxic than Zinc finger nucleases because their DNA sequence identification is rigorous
- ☆ Very precise in nature

Disadvantage

- ☆ It is expensive and time-consuming to create sequence-specific enzymes for all possible sequences

Now the below sections will deal with a few viral and non–viral gene delivery vectors:

Viral Vectors

Adeno-associated Virus (AAV)

- ☆ Small, single-stranded DNA
- ☆ Belong to parvovirus family

Advantages

- Constitutive in nature that is protein is expressed all the time, even when not required
- Very prolonged-expression
- Infect both dividing and non-dividing cell

Disadvantages

- Insert size is limited to 4.5kb
- Low information capacity

Example: Haemophilia treatment

Retrovirus Vector

- Single-stranded RNA animal viruses
- Belong to Retroviridae
- Insert capacity for transgene < 7-8kb

Advantages

- Low immunogenicity
- Broad cell tropism of infectivity
- Prolonged expression

Disadvantages

- Transfect only proliferating cells
- Difficult targeting of viral infection

Example: Rous sarcoma virus

Lentiviral Vector

- They are the type of retrovirus
- Linear single-strand RNA
- Insert size capacity, upto 10kb

Advantages

- Infect both proliferating and non-proliferating cells
- Stable gene expression

Disadvantages

- Not safe enough for gene therapy

Example: Human Immunodeficiency Virus

Herpes Virus Vector

- It belongs to the Herpesviridae family

- ☆ Double-stranded DNA virus
- ☆ They have a large insert size capacity, *i.e.*, >20kb

Advantages

- ☆ Generation of high viral titers.

Disadvantages

- ☆ They are non-integrating; so long term expression of transferred genes is not possible
- ☆ Possibility of toxicity

Example: Herpes Simplex Virus vector type.

Non-viral Gene Transfer

Injection of naked DNA

Advantages

- ☆ The simplest method of gene transfer
- ☆ Easy to produce as no special skill is needed

Disadvantages

- ☆ Cellular uptake of naked DNA is relatively inefficient
- ☆ Requires a large amount of DNA
- ☆ Inefficient delivery and the resulting transient transgene expression

Physical Method

Gene Gun

In this process a particles of gold or tungsten are coated with DNA and then shot through inert gas into young cells or embryos.

Advantages

- ☆ Does not use toxic chemicals
- ☆ Higher expression rate

Disadvantage

- ☆ Gene expression is for short-term and also low
- ☆ Reproducibility problems
- ☆ May cause cell damage

Electroporation

A brief electric field (of 10-20 kV/cm) is applied to cells in this technique, resulting in pores in the cell membrane through which plasmid DNA is transferred. After the electric shock, the cell membrane repair mechanisms rapidly close the gaps in the membrane.

Advantages

- ☆ Very efficient and works across a broad range of cell types
- ☆ Promotes competence
- ☆ Simple and safe method

Disadvantages

- ☆ High voltage can inflict permanent tissue damage due to its high temperature
- ☆ Difficulty to access with electrodes at treatment sites

Sonoporation

- ☆ Sonoporation, or ultrasound-mediated gene delivery, is a minimally invasive, non-viral, and clinically translatable form of gene therapy.This method is less invasive than other physical gene delivery methods and has a better safety profile than viral vectors.

Advantages

- ☆ A simple and reliable method
- ☆ High expression

Disadvantages

- ☆ Expensive instrument and the problem of availability

Hydrodynamic

- ☆ Here high-pressure DNA solution is pumped into the veins or through the catheter. A hydrodynamic capillary effect is employed to manipulate cell permeability.

Advantages

- ☆ Simple and safe method
- ☆ Efficient transfection

Disadvantages

- ☆ Volumes too large, so difficult to use in humans at present
- ☆ Surgical procedure may be required for localized gene delivery

Sonication

- ☆ A sound wave creates pores in a cell membrane which allows the entry of genetic material.

Advantages

- ☆ Allows uptake of large molecules such as DNA into the cell
- ☆ Suitable for the introduction of foreign genes in mammalian cells

Disadvantages

- ☆ Involvement of expensive instrument

Chemical Method

Liposomes Mediated Transfer

Colloidal drug delivery mechanisms are known as liposomes. Liposomes can be categorized into three categories as per their charges- cationic, anionic, or neutral. Cationic lipids (liposomes) have a positive charge interacting with the negatively charged cell membrane, resulting in the delivery of the DNA directly into the target site.

Advantages

- ☆ Nucleic acid preservation
- ☆ Efficacy at low concentrations
- ☆ Optimal transport for active compounds with a short half-life

Disadvantages

- ☆ Short gene expression time and low transgene expression level
- ☆ Difficult to transfect the targeted gene (selected cells)

Calcium-Phosphate Transfer

The formation of a calcium phosphate-DNA precipitate is used to introduce DNA into mammalian cells. Calcium phosphate aids the binding of DNA to the cell surface. DNA can enter the cell via endocytosis. This method is widely used to generate stable transformants by transfecting a variety of cell types.

Advantages

- ☆ Simple
- ☆ Low cost
- ☆ Stable and long-lasting expression

Disadvantages

- ☆ The frequency is limited
- ☆ Low transfection rate

DAE-Dextran Mediated DNA Transfer

Diethylaminoethyl (DEAE)-dextran is a polycationic derivative of the carbohydrate polymer dextran. It was the very first chemical vector used for DNA delivery.

Advantages

- ☆ Simplicity
- ☆ Reproducibility
- ☆ Low cost

Disadvantages

- ✰ Cytotoxicity
- ✰ Poor transfection performance
- ✰ Limitation to transient transfections

Gene Therapy for Heart disease

In heart disease, gene therapy can place a normal copy of the gene into the human cell with the end goal of correcting the disease. Researchers have the resources to target particular genes and pathways that play a role in cardiovascular diseases thanks to sequencing the human genome and the advancement of gene transfer vectors and delivery systems. Early clinical trials have shown promising efficacy in several attempts, with few side effects in all of them. Preclinical studies suggest that myocardial gene transfer can improve angiogenesis with VEGF or FGF, increase myocardial contractility.

Gene Therapy for Diabetes Mellitus

Diabetes mellitus is a medical disorder that results in high blood glucose levels due to insulin deficiency or resistance. Type 1 and type 2 diabetes are the two most common types of diabetes.A cell deficiency causes type 1 diabetes. Insulin resistance is a hallmark of type 2 diabetes and is often accompanied by a secretory defect in insulin-producing cells. As both type 1 and type 2 diabetes are linked to a loss of cell mass, gene therapy aimed at the cell and insulin replacement may be used to treat both types of diabetes. It is suggested that using a suitable promoter and insulin gene construct, non-insulin-producing cells could be converted to insulin-producing cells. In both type 1 and type 2 diabetes, these replacement cells may restore insulin production. Though noteworthy, promoter constructs that respond to glucose are the only way to regulate insulin gene transcription.

Gene Therapy for Neurological Disorders

Targeted gene therapy has advanced to the point that it can now be used to treat various neurological conditions using multiple modalities ranging from exogenous gene expression to endogenous gene suppression. Highly specific viral vector designs, plasmid transfection, nanoparticles, polymer-mediated gene delivery, engineered microRNA, and in vivo clustered regulatory interspaced short palindromic repeats (CRISPR)-based therapeutics have been the subject of recent technical advances for improved gene sequence delivery to the central nervous system. Recent clinical studies have demonstrated encouraging safety and efficacy in diseases like Parkinson's disease, Alzheimer's disease, spinal muscular atrophy, autism spectrum disorder, and amyotrophic lateral sclerosis.

Gene Therapy for Cancer

New genes can be introduced into a cancerous cell or surrounding tissue through gene transfer to cause cell death or slow cancer development. This treatment method is very adaptable, and clinical trials have used a wide variety of genes and vectors with positive results. These therapies can be used alone or in conjunction with current treatments to help make cancer a more manageable disease as they develop. Suicide gene therapy, oncolytic viral therapies, anti-angiogenesis, and gene therapy vaccines are just a few of the gene therapy techniques that have been developed. Combining gene therapy with traditional treatments like chemotherapy, radiotherapy, and immunotherapy has increased clinical effectiveness. Altogether preclinical and experimental trials have yielded very positive results.

Gene Therapy for Autoimmune Disorders

Advances in our understanding of autoimmune diseases' immunological and molecular basis have made gene therapy a viable treatment option for those suffering from these diseases. Gene therapy's ultimate goal is to improve patient outcomes by restoring and preserving immune tolerance to specific autoantigens. Via effective delivery and expression of therapeutic genes inappropriate cells, gene therapy for autoimmune disorders aims to control the levels of pro-inflammatory cytokines or molecules and lymphocyte penetration to the affected sites. Several gene therapy-mediated clinical trials for Multiple Sclerosis, Rheumatoid Arthritis, Arthritis, and other disorders have been initiated, with more in the works.

Advantages and Disadvantages of Gene Therapy

Gene therapy can prevent diseases from being passed down across generations. A disease can be prevented, and the quality of life improved by using gene therapy. In cases where there is no cure, gene therapy has the potential to save many lives. The best part of it is that it can be done outside of the body. It may be beneficial in treating a wide range of diseases, including Leber congenital amaurosis, a rare type of blindness, CNS disease. It can also be efficiently used in cancer treatment. Further, it may be used in conjunction with cell therapy. Since it can produce lifelong effects, this procedure is usually long-lasting.

Gene therapy can cause adverse immune system reactions. There is a chance that gene therapy approaches could target the wrong cells, resulting in new diseases. Gene therapies can induce tumours. The gene therapy treatment is fraught with incompatibility problems. Since the effects of gene therapy may be transient, humans may develop resistance to it. Gene therapy raises several legal concerns. It is a costly treatment that not everyone can afford.

Ethical Considerations of Gene Therapy

Gene therapy is the deliberate alteration of genetic material in a patient's cells to achieve a therapeutic result. While gene therapy is still in its early stages as a clinically viable therapeutic modality, a review of the ethical issues is beneficial in many ways because it includes ethical concepts applicable across the board in clinical medicine. Ethics in gene therapy involves examining moral conflicts, codes, and other patterns of received morality.

Future Perspectives of Stem Cell and Gene Therapy

Stem cells have given us a lot of hope and sparked a lot of excitement because they can massively expand the number and types of patients that may benefit from transplants and provide cell replacement therapy for chronic diseases. The advancements made in this area have laid the groundwork for curing diseases that have been resistant to traditional treatment. To determine the most successful stem cell source and protocol for intervention to redress pathologies we still don't fully understand, a balanced approach in the basic and preclinical sciences is needed. It is important to recognize that the only way to know if a stem cell selection and delivery procedure is successful is to perform a clinical trial. If investment grows over the next decade, we can see translation happen far faster and more generally.Over the next ten years, scientific due diligence will be needed to increase the effectiveness of stem cell therapy and the number of patients who benefit. With epigenetic or patient-specific pluripotent cell lines developed through standardized production, new methods of diagnosis and high-throughput therapeutic screening will emerge. This will make a basic understanding of growth, physiology, and pathology, and pharmacologic screening of stem cells much more straightforward.

In terms of the future of gene therapy, advances in gene transfer efficiency into target cells and the conservation of expression from the appropriate transferred gene must occur before gene therapy can become the strategy of choice in a wide range of clinical settings. New gene therapy applications will be the subject of efforts, in addition to advances in delivery and expression technologies. These include, but not limited to:

1. The identification and use of new resistance genes that can effectively protect the organ of interest from hazardous agents.
2. Intracellular immunization with therapeutic genes for use in adoptive immunotherapies against various life-threatening infectious diseases (*e.g.*, cytomegalovirus).
3. The use of homologous recombination to fix or substitute faulty genes, enabling the treatment of dominantly inherited diseases.

REFERENCES

1. Quesenberry PJ, Stein GS, Forget BG, Weissman SM. Stem Cell Biology and Gene Therapy. ISBN: 9780471223955.
2. Clevio N, Liliana M, CarlosM. A Handbook of Gene and Cell Therapy. ISBN: 978-3-030-41333-0
3. Mohamed AR, Mariam N. Stem Cells and Cell Therapy. ISBN 978-94-007-7196-3
4. Abdelalim EM. Recent Advances in Stem Cells: From Basic Research to Clinical Applications. ISBN: 9783319332680
5. Nobrega C, Mendonca L, Matos CA. A Handbook of Gene and Cell Therapy. ISBN: 9783030413323

Chapter 20

Intellectual Property Rights (IPR), Biosafety and Bioethics

Machiavelli Singh[1]* *and Babita Khosla*[2]

[1]*Amity Institute of Biotechnology, Amity University Haryana, Gurugram (Manesar) – 122 413, Haryana, India*

[2]*Department of Environmental Sciences, Maharshi Dayanand University, Rohtak – 124 001 , Haryana, India*

**e-mail: msingh2@ggn.amity.edu*

ABSTRACT

Ethical questions and Intelligence quotient have surrounded the development of biotechnology right from the start. On the national and international level, bioethical committees have been set up to clarify the boundaries of what is acceptable in biotechnology development and application. The care with which bioethics are addressed is likely to have an influence on the marketability of products derived from biotechnology, since it will finally be the consumers who decide the prospects of the biotechnology markets. To assess, evaluate, prove, validate, and authenticate one must keep biosafety measures in terms of check to ensure the safety on exploitation of biological system or processes towards the service of mankind including individuals, community, and environment. Keeping in view to protect the rights of innovators and creators towards lifelong incentives to gain along with freedom to operate via global outreach in service of mankind is a much challenging and strategic task for humanity. In the present chapter, developments of the intellectual property system in India, evaluation of an Intellectual Property Regime, new dimensions and introduction to bioethics and the importance of biosafety management with key to the conscious responsible operation of biotechnology is discussed.

Keywords: *IPR, Patent, Copyright, Trademark, Geographical indication, TRIPS, WIPO, Bioethics, Biosafety, Containment, Cartagena protocol.*

Intellectual Property Rights (IPR)

In 21st century the intellectual property system has become a tool for harnessing the power of knowledge and creations of mind for development in the artistic, scientific and technological fields worldwide. The dynamics of economic, social, cultural and political factors in a democratic dialogue shape the evolution of intellectual property system. The vitality of accumulated knowledge through creative ideas and its innovative interpretation leads to recognition of intellectual property (IP) as an important asset. Intellectual primarily focuses on intelligence as either a professional or an individual capacity, genius that lies in the personality. As a substantive or adjective, it refers to the work product of such persons or to an aspect of something where learning, erudition, informed and critical thinking is the focus. The property is something that can be owned, possessed, and expressed with legal belongingness with evidence either in tangible or intangible form. It's the transformation of artistic, literary and scientific creations into a tangible asset which is known as intellectual property. The rights which provide the protections to these are intellectual property rights (WIPO, 2004). Intellectual property rights are the basic rights given to the respective person over the creations of their minds, thoughts and idea transformed into a tangible representative form. These give the creator an exclusive right over the use of his/her creation for the certain period (WIPO, 2004).

Intellectual Property (IP)

Intellectual property, very broadly, means the legal rights which result from intellectual activity in the industrial, scientific, literary, and artistic fields. Countries have laws to protect intellectual property for two main reasons. One is to give statutory expression to the moral and economic rights of creators in their creations and the rights of the public in access to those creations. The second is to promote, as a deliberate act of Government policy, creativity and the dissemination and application of its results and to encourage fair trading which would contribute to economic and social development (WIPO, 2003).

Intellectual Property is defined in an all-pervasive sense in Article 2 (viii) of the Convention Establishing the World Intellectual Property Organization (WIPO) signed at Stockholm on July 14, 1967, to include the rights relating to literary, artistic and scientific works; performances of performing artists. Intellectual property rights as a collective term includes the following independent IP rights which can be collectively used for protecting different aspects of an inventive work for multiple protection: -Scientific discoveries, the remaining area mentioned in the WIPO Convention, are not the same as inventions. The Geneva Treaty on the International Recording of Scientific Discoveries (1978) defines a scientific discovery as "the recognition of phenomena, properties or laws of the material universe not hitherto recognized and capable of verification" (Article 1(1) (i)). Inventions are new solutions to specific technical problems. Such solutions must, naturally, rely on the properties or laws of the material universe (otherwise they could not be materially or "technically" applied), but those properties or laws need not be properties or laws "not hitherto recognized." An invention puts to new use, to new technical use, the said properties, or laws, whether they are recognized ("discovered") simultaneously with the making of the invention or whether they were already recognized ("discovered") before, and independently of, the invention (WIPO, 2004)

History and Development of Intellectual Property Law and Recognition in India

Intellectual Property Right in India was adopted from the west. The Indian Trade and Merchandise Marks Act 1884 was the first Indian Law regarding IPR. The first Indian Patent Law was enacted in 1858 followed by series of Acts being passed. They are Indian Patents and Design Act in 1911 and Indian Copyright Act in 1914, Indian Trade and merchandise Marks Act and Indian Copyright Act have been replaced by Trademarks Act 1958 and Copyright Act 1957 respectively (Ganguli, 2003). After Independence in 1948, the Indian Government appointed the first committee to review the prevailing Patents and Designs legislation. In 1957, Government appointed Justice Rajgobala Ayyangar Committee (RAC) to revise the Patent Law Rajagobala Ayyangar Committee submitted its report on 1959, the report tried to balance the constitutional guarantee of economic and social justice enshrined in the preamble of the constitution. This report outlined the policy behind the Indian Patent System (Prabhu *et al.*, 2012).

The conceptualization of the patent system was based on medium providing an opportunity of acquiring exclusive rights in an invention, stimulates technical process by encouraging research and innovation, inducing an inventor to disclose discoveries, reward for developing inventions and facilitate to invest capital in new lines of production which motivate the research and development culture.

1. Patent

A patent is an exclusive right granted by a country to the owner of an invention to make, use, manufacture, and market the invention, provided the invention satisfies certain conditions stipulated in the law. Exclusive right implies that no one else can make, use, manufacture, or market the invention without the consent of the patent holder. This right is available for a limited period. Despite the ownership of the rights, the use or exploitation of the rights by the owner of the patent may not be possible due to other laws of the country which has awarded the patent. These laws may relate to health, safety, food, security *etc.* Further, existing patents in similar area may also come in the way. A patent in the law is property right and hence, can be gifted, inherited, assigned, sold or licensed. As the right is conferred by the State, it can be revoked by the State under very special circumstances even if the patent has been sold or licensed or manufactured or marketed in the meantime. The patent right is territorial in nature and inventors/their assignees will have to file separate patent applications in countries of interest, along with necessary fees, for obtaining patents in those countries (WIPO, 2004). A new chemical process or a drug molecule or an electronic circuit or a new surgical instrument or a vaccine is a patentable subject matter provided all the stipulations of the law are satisfied.

The Indian Patent Act

The first Indian patent laws were first promulgated in 1856. These were modified from time to time. New patent laws were made after the independence in the form of the **Indian Patent Act 1970**. The Act has now been radically amended to become fully compliant with the provisions of TRIPS. The most recent amendment was made in 2005 which were preceded by the amendments in 2000 and 2003. While the process of bringing out amendments was going on, India became a member of the Paris Convention, Patent Cooperation Treaty and Budapest Treaty. The salient and important features of the present **The Patent (Amendment) Act 2005 and Rules 2006** in force are described in the patentability subject matter section 5.2 below (The Patent Act, 2005).

Patentability Subject Matter

A clear definition has now been provided for an invention, which makes it at par with definitions followed by most countries. Invention means a new product or process involving an inventive step and capable of industrial application. New invention means any invention or technology which has not been anticipated by publication in any document or used in the country or elsewhere in the world before the date of filing of patent application with complete specification *i.e.*, the subject matter has not fallen in public domain or it does not form part of the state of the art. Inventive step means a feature of an invention that involves technical advance as compared to existing knowledge or having economic significance or both and that makes the invention not obvious to a person skilled in the art "capable of industrial application means that the invention is capable of being made or used in an industry"

Novelty

An invention will be considered novel if it does not form a part of the global state of the art. Information appearing in magazines, technical journals, books, newspapers *etc.* constitutes the state of the art. Oral description of the invention in a seminar/conference can also spoil novelty. Novelty is assessed in a global context. An invention will cease to be novel if it has been disclosed in the public through any type of publications anywhere in the world before filing a patent application in respect of the invention. Therefore, it is advisable to file a patent application before publishing a paper if there is a slight chance that the invention may be patentable. Prior use of the invention in the country of interest before the filing date can also destroy the novelty. Novelty is determined through extensive literature and patent searches. It should be realized that patent search is essential and critical for ascertaining novelty as most of the information reported in patent documents does not get published anywhere else. For an invention to be novel, it need not be a breakthrough. No invention is small or big. Modifications to the existing state of the art, process, or product or both, can also be candidates for patents provided these were not earlier known. In a chemical process, for example, use of new reactants, use of a catalyst, new process conditions can lead to a patentable invention. Any innovation proved physically is considered for be new patent registration provisionally.

Inventiveness (Non-obviousness)

A patent application involves an inventive step if the proposed invention is not obvious to a person skilled in the art *i.e.*, skilled in the subject matter of the patent application. The prior art should not point towards the invention implying that the practitioner of the subject matter could not have thought about the invention prior to filing of the patent application. Inventiveness cannot be decided on the material contained in unpublished patents. The complexity or the simplicity of an inventive step does not have any bearing on the grant of a patent. In other words, a very simple invention can qualify for a patent. If there is an inventive step between the proposed patent and the prior art at that point of time, then an invention has taken place. A mere 'scintilla' of invention is sufficient to find a valid patent. It may be often difficult to establish the inventiveness, especially in upcoming knowledge areas. The reason is that it would depend a great deal on the interpretative skills of the inventor and these skills will really be a function of knowledge in the subject area.

Industrial Applicability

An invention must possess utility for the grant of patent. No valid patent can be granted for an invention devoid of utility. The patent specification should spell out various uses and manner of practicing them, even if considered obvious. If you are claiming a process, you need not describe the use of the compound produced thereby. Nevertheless, it would be safer to do so. But if you claim a compound without spelling out its utility, you may be denied a patent.

Non Patentable Inventions

An invention may satisfy the conditions of novelty, inventiveness, and usefulness but it may not qualify for a patent under the following situations:

(i) An invention which is frivolous, or which claims anything obviously contrary to well established natural laws *e.g.*, different types of perpetual motion machines.

(ii) An invention whose intended use or exploitation would be contrary to public order or morality or which causes serious prejudice to human, animal or plant life or health or to the environment *e.g.*, a process for making brown sugar will not be patented.

(iii) The mere discovery of a scientific principal or formulation of an abstract theory *e.g.*, Raman effect and Theory of Relativity cannot be patented.

(iv) The mere discovery of a new form of a known substance which does not result in enhancement of the known efficacy of that substance or the mere discovery of any new property or new use of a known substance or the mere use of a known process, machine or apparatus unless such a known process results in a new product or employs at least one new reactant. For the purposes of this clause, salts, esters, polymorphs, metabolites, pure form, particle size, isomers, mixtures of isomers, complexes, combinations and other derivatives of known substance shall be considered to be the same substance unless they differ significantly in properties with regard to efficacy.

(v) A substance obtained by a mere admixture resulting only aggregation of the properties of the components thereof or a process for producing such' substance.

(vi) The mere arrangement or rearrangement or duplication of features of known devices each functioning independently of one another in a known way. If you put torch bulbs around an umbrella and operate them by a battery so that people could see you walking in rain when it is dark, then this arrangement is patentable as bulbs and the umbrella perform their functions independently.

(vii) A method of agriculture or horticulture. For example, the method of terrace farming cannot be patented.

(viii) Any process for medical, surgical, curative, prophylactic, diagnostic, therapeutic or other treatment of human beings, or any process for a similar treatment of animals to render them free of disease or to increase economic value or that of their products. For example, a new surgical technique for hand surgery for removing contractions is not patentable.

(viii) Inventions relating to atomic energy;

(ix) Discovery of any living thing or non-living substance occurring in nature;

(x) Mathematical or business methods or a computer program per se or algorithms;

(xi) Plants and animals in whole or any part thereof other than microorganisms but including seeds, varieties and species and essentially biological processes for production and propagation of plants and animals;

(xii) A presentation of information;

(xiii) Topography of integrate circuits;

(xiv) A mere scheme or rule or method of performing mental act or method of playing games;

(xv) An invention which, in effect, is traditional knowledge or which is aggregation or duplication of known component or components.

Computer program per se as such has not been defined in the Act but would generally tend to mean that a computer program without any utility would not be patentable. Protection of seeds and new plant varieties is covered under the Protection of Plant Varieties and Farmers Act of India 2001 (PPVFR Act of India, 2001), which is discussed under section 12 of the chapter. Similarly, topography of integrated circuits (*e.g.*, mother boards of electronic and digital gadgets) as well as protection of undisclosed information can be protected by the means of trade secrets and non-disclosure agreements.

Term of the Patent

Term of the patent will be 20 years from the date of filing for all types of inventions.

Provisional Specification

A provisional specification is usually filed to establish priority of the invention in case the disclosed invention is only at a conceptual stage and a delay is expected in submitting full and specific description of the invention. Although, a patent application accompanied with provisional specification does not confer any legal patent rights to the applicants, it is, however, a very important document to establish the earliest ownership of an invention. The provisional specification is a permanent and independent scientific cum legal document and no amendment is allowed in this. No patent is granted based on a provisional specification.

Complete Specification

It may be noted that a patent document is a techno-legal document and it has to be finalized in consultation with an attorney. Submission of complete specification is necessary to obtain a patent. Complete specification must be submitted within 12 months of filing the provisional specification. This period can be extended by 3 months. It is not necessary to file an application with provisional specification before the complete specification. An application with complete specification can be filed right at the first instance.

Examination, Grant and Working of Patent

Compulsory License

Any time after three years from date of sealing of a patent, application for compulsory license can be made provided following conditions

1. Reasonable requirements of public have not been met
2. Patented invention is not available to public at a reasonably affordable price
3. Patented invention is not worked in India

Application outside India; and (b) either no direction has been given under the secrecy clause of the Act or all such directions have been revoked. among other things, reasonable requirements of public are not satisfied if working of patented invention in India on a commercial scale ***is being prevented or hindered by importation*** of patented invention.

Applicant's capability including risk taking, ability of the applicant to work the invention in public interest, nature of invention, time elapsed since sealing, measures taken by patentee to work the patent in India will be considered. In case of national emergency or other circumstances of extreme urgency or public noncommercial use or an establishment of a ground of anti-competitive practices adopted by the patentee, the above conditions will not apply. A patentee must disclose the invention in a patent document for anyone to practice it after the expiry of the patent or practice it with the consent of the patent holder during the life of the patent.

Timeline for Filing a Patent Application

Filing of an application for a patent should be completed at the earliest possible date and should not be delayed. An application filed with provisional specification, disclosing the essence of the nature of the invention helps to register the priority by the applicant.

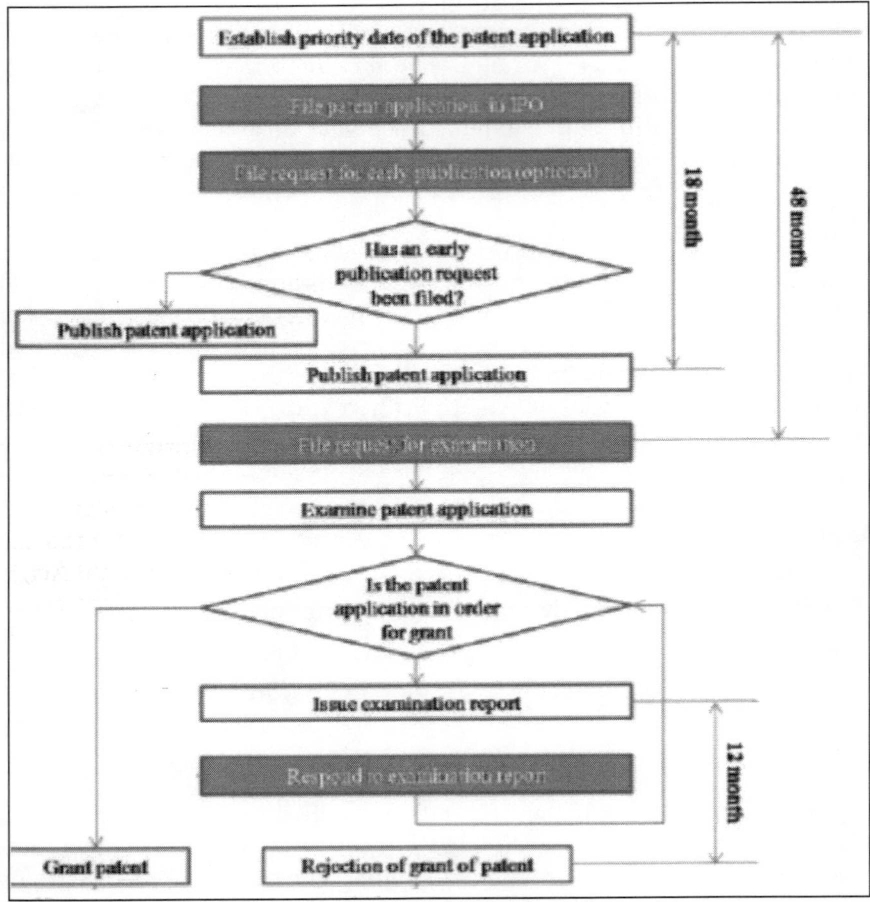

Figure 20.1: The Patent Filing Process and Timeline in India (Puttaiah, 2014).

Patenting of Microbiological Inventions

The Indian Patent Act has now a specific provision regarding patenting of microorganisms and microbiological processes. It is now possible to get a patent for a microbiological process and products emanating from such processes.

As it is difficult to describe a microorganism on paper, a system of depositing strain of microorganisms in some recognized depositories was evolved way back in 1949 in USA. An international treaty called "Budapest Treaty" was signed in Budapest in 1973 and later on amended in 1980. India became a member of this Treaty, with effect from December 17, 2001. This is an international convention governing the recognition of deposits in officially approved culture collections for the purpose of patent applications in any country that is a party to this treaty. Because of the difficulties and virtual impossibility of reproducing a microorganism from a description of it in a patent specification, it is essential to deposit a strain in a culture collection centre for testing and examination by others.

An inventor is required to deposit the strain of a microorganism in a recognized depository, which assigns a registration number to the deposited microorganism. This registration number needs to be quoted in the patent application dealing with the microorganism. Obviously a strain of microorganism is required to be deposited before filing a patent application. It may be observed that this mechanism obviates the need of describing a microorganism in the patent application. Further, samples of strains can be obtained from the depository for further working on the patent. There are many international depositories in different countries such as ATCC, DSM *etc.* which are recognized under the Budapest Treaty. The Microbial Type Culture Collection (MTCC) at Institute of Microbial Technology (IMTEC), Chandigarh is the first Indian depository set up under the Budapest Treaty.

2. Copyright

Copyright is a right, which is available for creating an original literary or dramatic or musical or artistic work. Cinematographic films including soundtrack and video films and recordings on discs, tapes, perforated roll or other devices are covered by copyrights. Computer programs and software are covered under literary works and are protected in India under copyrights. The Copyright Act, 1957 as amended in 1983, 1984, 1992, 1994 and 1999 governs the copyright protection in India. The total term of protection for literary work is the author's life plus sixty years. For cinematographic films, records, photographs, posthumous publications, anonymous publication, works of government and international agencies the term is 60 years from the beginning of the calendar year following the year in which the work was published. For broadcasting, the term is 25 years from the beginning of the calendar year following the year in which the broadcast was made (The Copyright Act, 2005). Copyright gives protection for the expression of an idea and not for the idea itself. For example, many authors write textbooks on physics covering various aspects like mechanics, heat, optics *etc.* Even though these topics are covered in several books by different authors, each author will have a copyright on the book written by him/her, provided the book is not a copy of some other book published earlier. India is a member of the Berne Convention, an international treaty on copyright. Under this Convention, registration of copyright is not an essential requirement for protecting the right. It would, therefore, mean that the copyright on a work created in India would be automatically and simultaneously protected through copyright in all the member countries of the Berne Convention. The moment an original work is created, the creator starts enjoying the copyright. However, an undisputable record of the date on which a work was created must be kept. When a work is published with the authority of the copyright owner, a notice of copyright may be placed on publicly distributed copies. The use of copyright notice is optional for the protection of literary and artistic works. It is, however, a good idea to incorporate a copyright notice. As violation of copyright is a cognizable offence, the matter can be reported to a police station. It is advised that registration of copyright in India would help in establishing the ownership of the work. The registration can be done at the office of the Registrar of Copyrights in New Delhi. It is also to be noted that the work is open for public inspection once the copyright is registered (The Copyright Act, 2005). Computer program in the Copyright Act has been defined as a set of instructions expressed in words, codes, schemes or any other form, including a machine-readable medium, capable of causing a computer to perform a particular task or achieve a particular result. It is obvious that algorithms, source codes and object codes are covered in this definition. It is advisable to file a small extract of the computer program at the time of registration rather than the full program. It is important to know that the part of the program that is not being filed, would remain a trade secret of the owner but would have to be kept well-guarded by the owner. It may be noted that computer programs will become important in the area of medicines when one talks about codification of DNA and gene sequencing. Generally, all copyrightable expressions embodied in a computer program, including screen displays, are protectable. However, unlike a computer program, which is a literary work, screen display is considered an artistic work and therefore cannot be registered through the same application as that covering the computer program. A separate application giving graphical representation of all copyrightable elements of the screen display is essential. In the digital era, copyright is assuming a new importance as many works transacted through networks such as databases, multimedia work, music, information *etc.* are presently the subject matter of copyright (WIPO, 2004).

Coverage Provided by Copyright

(i) Literary, dramatic and musical work. Computer programs/software are covered within the definition of literary work.

(ii) Artistic work

(iii) Cinematographic films, which include soundtrack and video films.

(iv) Recording on any disc, tape, perforated roll or other device.

Infringement of Copyright

Copyright gives the creator of the work the right to reproduce the work, make copies, translate, adapt, sell or give on hire and communicate the work to public. Any of these activities done without the consent of the author or his assignee is considered infringement of the copyright. There is a provision of 'fair use' in the law, which allows copyrighted work to be used for teaching and research and development. In other words making one photocopy of a book for teaching students may not be considered an infringement, but making many photocopies for commercial purposes would be considered an infringement. There is one associated right with copyright, which is known as the 'moral right', which cannot be transferred and is not limited by the term. This right is enjoyed by the creator for avoiding obscene representation of his/her works.

Computer Program

A Computer includes any electronic or similar device having information processing capabilities. Computer program means a set of instructions expressed in words, codes, schemes or any other form, including a machine-readable medium, capable of causing a computer to perform a particular task or achieve a particular result. It is now possible to have copyrights both on object code and source code. Generally, all copyrightable expressions embodied in a computer program, including screen displays, are protectable. However, unlike a computer program, which is a literary work, screen displays are artistic work and cannot therefore be registered in the same application as that covering the computer program. A separate application giving graphic representation of all copyrightable elements of the screen display is necessary.

In the case of a program made in the course of author's employment under a contract of service or apprenticeship, the employer shall, in the absence of any agreement to the contrary, be the first owner of the copyright. However, works created by third parties on commission do not automatically vest the copyright in the commissioning party. If the third party is an independent contractor, it is essential for the commissioning party to obtain the copyright through a written deed of assignment. It is a common misconception that the copyright automatically belongs to the commissioning party. Thus, it is only where the developer is an employee creating the work under a contract of service that the rights belong to the employer.

Transfer of Copyright

The owner of the copyright in an existing work or prospective owner of the copyright in a future work may assign to any person the copyright, either wholly or partially in the following manner.

i. For the entire world or for a specific country or territory; or
ii. For the full term of copyright or part thereof; or
iii. Relating to all the rights comprising the copyright or only part of such rights.

3. Trademarks

A trademark is a distinctive sign, which identifies certain goods or services as those produced or provided by a specific person or enterprise. Trademarks may be one or combination of words, letters, and numerals. They may also consist of drawings, symbols, three dimensional signs such as shape and packaging of goods, or colours used as distinguishing feature. Collective marks are owned by an association whose members use them to identify themselves with a level of quality. Certification marks are given for compliance with defined standards. (Example ISO 9000.). A trademark provides to the owner of the mark by ensuring the exclusive right to use it to identify goods or services, or to authorize others to use it in return for some consideration (payment).

Well-known trademark in relation to any goods or services, means a mark which has become so to the substantial segment of the public which uses such goods or receives such services that the use of such mark in relation to other goods or services would be likely to be taken as indicating a connection in the course of trade or rendering of services between those goods or services and a person using the mark in relation to the first-mentioned goods or services (The Trademark Act, 2004).

Service Marks

The Indian Act of 1958 did not have any reference to service marks. Service means service of any description that is made available to potential users and includes the provision of services in connection with the business of industrial or commercial matters such as banking, communication, education, financing, insurance, chit funds, real estate, transport, storage, material treatment, processing, supply of electrical or other energy, boarding, lodging, entertainment, amusement, construction, repair, conveying of news or information and advertising. Marks used to represent such services are known as service marks.

Certification Trademarks and Collective Marks

A certification trademark means a guarantee mark which indicates that the goods to which it is applied are of a certain quality or are manufactured in a particular way or come from a certain region or use some specific material or maintain a certain level of accuracy. The goods must originate from a certain region rather from a particular trader. Certification marks are also applicable to services and the same parameters will have to be satisfied. Further these marks are registerable just like any other trademark. AGMARK used in India for various food items is a kind of certification mark although it is not registered as a certification mark; the concept of certification mark was not in vogue at the time of introduction of AGMARK (Prabhu, 2012).

A collective mark means a trademark distinguishing from those of others, the goods or services of members of an association of persons (not being a partnership within the meaning of the Indian Partnership Act, 1932), which is the proprietor of the mark.

Term of a Registered Trademark

The initial registration of a trademark shall be for a period of ten years but may be renewed from time to time for an unlimited period by payment of the renewal fees.

4. Protection of Geographical Indications

Indications which identify a good as originating in the territory of a member or a region or a locality in that territory, where a given quality reputation or other characteristics of the good is attributable to its geographical origin. The concept of identifying GI and protecting them is a new concept in India, perhaps in most developing countries, and has come to knowledge in these countries after they signed the TRIPS Agreement. It may be noted that properly protected GI will give protection in domestic and international market. Stipulations of TRIPS would be applicable to all the member countries. According to TRIPS, GI which is not or cease to be protected in its country of origin or which has fallen into disuse in that country cannot be protected. Homonymous GI for wines will get independent protection. Each state shall determine conditions under which homonymous indications will be differentiated from each other. Principles of national treatment and fair competition are applicable. TRIPS provide for seizure of goods bearing false indications of GI. TRIPS provide for refusal or invalidation of registration of a trademark containing a GI with respect to goods not originating in the territory indicated. The Geographical Indications of Goods (Registration and Protection) Act, 1999 along with Geographical Indications of Goods (Registration and Protection) Rules 2002 are in force.

The term GI has been defined as "Geographical Indications", in relation to goods, means an indication which identifies such goods as agricultural goods, natural goods or manufactured goods as originating, or manufactured in the territory of a country, or a region or locality in that territory, where a given quality, reputation or other characteristics of such goods is essentially attributable to its geographical origin and in case where such goods are manufactured goods one of the activities of either the production or of processing or preparation of the goods concerned takes place in such territory, region or locality, as the case may be (The GI Act, 2004).

Applicants for GI's Registration

Any association of persons or producers or any organization or authority established by or under any law for the time being in force representing the interest of the producers of the concerned goods, who are desirous of registering geographical indication in relation to such goods shall apply in writing to the Registrar in such' form and in such manner and accompanied by such fees as may be prescribed for the registration of the geographical indication. It should be significantly distinguishable from known designs or combination of known designs. It should not comprise or contain scandalous or obscene matter.

Punishment for Falsifying GI

A sentence of imprisonment for a term between six months to three years and a fine between fifty thousand rupees and two lakh rupees is provided in the Act. The court may reduce the punishment under special circumstances.

Term of GI protection

The registration of a GI shall be for a period of ten years but may be renewed from time to time for an unlimited period by payment of the renewal fees.

5. Industrial Design

We see so many varieties and brands of the same product (*e.g.* car, television, personal computer, a piece of furniture *etc.*) in the market, which look quite different from each other. If the products have similar functional features or have comparable price tags, the eye appeal or visual design of a product determines the choice. Even if the similarities are not close, a person may decide to go for a more expensive item because that item has a better look or color scheme.

What is being said is that the external design or color scheme or ornamentation of a product plays a key role in determining the market acceptability of the product over other similar products. If you have a good design that gives you an advantage, then you must have a system to protect its features otherwise there would be wide scale imitation (WIPO, 2004). Design as per the Indian Act means the features of shape, configuration, pattern, ornament or composition of lines or colors applied to any article - whether in two dimensional or three dimensional or in both forms - by any industrial process or means, whether manual, mechanical or chemical, separate or combined, which in the finished article appeal to and are judged solely by the eye; but it does not include any mode or principle of construction or anything which is in substance a mere mechanical device. In this context an article means any article of manufacture and any substance, artificial, or partly artificial and partly natural; and includes any part of an article capable of being made and sold separately. Stamps, labels, tokens, cards, *etc.* cannot be considered an article for the purpose of registration of design because once the alleged design *i.e.*, ornamentation is removed only a piece of paper, metal or like material remains and the article referred to ceases to exist. An article must have its existence independent of the designs applied to it. So, the design as applied to an article should be integral with the article itself. In India the registration is covered under The Design Act 2000 along with Design Rules 2001 (The Design Act, 2004).

The Essential Requirements for the Registration of Design

1. The design should be new or original, not previously published or used in any country before the date of application for registration. The novelty may reside in the application of a known shape or pattern to a new subject matter. However, if the design for which the application is made does not involve any real mental activity for conception, then registration may not be considered.
2. The design should relate to features of shape, configuration, pattern or ornamentation applied or applicable to an article. Thus, designs of industrial plans, layouts and installations are not registrable under the Act.
3. The design should be applied or applicable to any article by any industrial process.

   Normally, designs of artistic nature such as painting, sculptures and the like which are not produced in bulk by any industrial process are excluded from registration under the Act.
4. The features of the designs in the finished article should appeal to and are judged solely by the eye. This implies that the design must appear and should be visible on the finished article, for which it is meant. Thus, any design in the inside arrangement of a box, money purse or almirah may not be considered for showing such articles in the open state, as those articles are generally put in the market in the closed state.
5. Any mode or principle of construction or operation or anything, which is in substance a mere mechanical device, would not be a registrable design. For instance, a key having its novelty only in the shape of its corrugation or bend at the portion intended to engage with levers inside the lock it is

associated with, cannot be registered as a design under the Act. However, when any design suggests any mode or principle of construction or mechanical or other action of a mechanism, a suitable disclaimer in respect thereof is required to be inserted on its representation, provided there are other registrable features in the design.

6. The design should not include any trademark or property mark or artistic works. trademarks under this Act.

Duration of the Tegistration of a Design

The total term of a registered design is 15 years. Initially the right is granted for a period of 10 years, which can be extended, by another 5 years by making an application and by paying a fee of Rs. 2000/- to the Controller before the expiry of initial 10 years period. The proprietor of design may make the application for such extension even as soon as the design is registered.

6. The Protection of Plant Varieties and Farmer's Right (PPV and FR) Act of India

Plant genetic resources (PGRs) are the foundation for the development of a food and nutritionally secure society. In addition, plants have many uses, including feed, fibre, medicine and industrial applications. PGRs were treated as the 'heritage of mankind' and were shared freely among nations, till the concerns for conservation of biological diversity were raised by the Convention on Biological Diversity (CBD), which came into force in 1993. The conservation and sustainable utilization and access to biological diversity were considered as national sovereignty by CBD. Consequently, many issues regarding the rights of the conservers, users, breeders, farmers and intellectual property have emerged (Brahmi *et al.*, 2004).

In order to provide for the establishment of an effective system for the protection of plant varieties, the rights of farmers and plant breeders and to encourage the development of new varieties of plants it has been considered necessary to recognize and to protect the rights of the farmers in respect of their contributions made at any time in conserving, improving and making available plant genetic resources for the development of new plant varieties. The Govt. of India enacted "The Protection of Plant Varieties and Farmers' Rights (PPV and FR) Act, 2001 and Rules 2003" adopting sui generis system. Indian legislation is not only in conformity with International Union for the Protection of New Varieties of Plants (UPOV), 1978, but also have sufficient provisions to protect the interests of public/private sector breeding institutions and the farmers. The legislation recognizes the contributions of both commercial plant breeders and farmers in plant breeding activity and also provides to implement TRIPS in a way that supports the specific socio-economic interests of all the stakeholders including private, public sectors and research institutions, as well as resource-constrained farmers.

To implement the provisions of the Act the Department of Agriculture and Cooperation, Ministry of Agriculture established the Protection of Plant Varieties and Farmers' Rights Authority on 11th November, 2005.

The main objectives of the PPV and FR Act, 2001 framed are as under:

1. To establish an effective system for the protection of plant varieties, the rights of farmers and plant breeders and to encourage the development of new varieties of plants.
2. To recognize and protect the rights of farmers in respect of their contributions made at any time in conserving, improving and making available plant genetic resources for the development of new plant varieties.
3. To accelerate agricultural development in the country, protect plant breeders' rights; stimulate investment for research and development both in public and private sector for the development of new plant varieties.
4. Facilitate the growth of seed industry in the country which will ensure the availability of high quality seeds and planting material to the farmers.

The breeder shall be required to deposit the seed or propagating material including parental line seeds of registered variety to the Authority. An applicant has to submit a fixed amount of seed sample (breeder seed) with prescribed germination percentage, physical purity and phyto-sanitary standards. The applicant shall also submit along with the seed/propagating material and the seed quality test report. The seed samples received by the Authority will be properly tested for its purity and germination. A part of the seed sample sent to the test centre for conduct of distinct, uniform and stability (DUS) tests and a part of is kept by the Authority in the National Gene Bank to maintain the seed samples of the registered varieties for their entire period of protection.

The duration of protection of registered varieties is different for different type of crops which are as below:

1. Trees and vines - 18 years.
2. For other crops - 15 years.
3. For extant varieties (means a variety available in India) notified - 15 years from the date of notification under section 5 of the Seeds under section 5 of the Seeds Act, 1966 Act, 1966.

Management of IPR in Publicly Funded Institutions in India

The aims of publicly funded institutions such as universities, colleges, autonomous bodies and public sector undertakings are multifaceted and are not purely driven by economic considerations but they are primarily driven by considerations of social obligations and political objectives and will of a nation. India has stuck to these aims since the independence. On one hand the above approach has helped us in creating a pool of highly educated population and also building an inherent strength in research and development and core competency in basic industries like steel, power, fertilizers *etc.* However on the other hand, an insulated system breeds complacency, which blunts the spirit of innovation and fire for being ahead of others. Globalization has taught us many new lessons by opening our eyes to the existing and forthcoming ground realities, which cannot be shunned away just because we do not happen to like them.

In order to maintain a continuous stream of new ideas and experimentation, public private partnership in R and D would need to be nurtured to arrive at a win-win situation. Therefore all publicly funded institutions and agencies will have to come to terms with the new ground realities and take positive steps to direct research suitably to generate more intellectual property rights, protect and manage them efficiently in respect of such institutions, especially related to their management and funding sources. It has been observed that educational and R and D institutions are being asked to generate their own funds and depend less and less on block grants by central or state governments. In respect of public sector undertaking (PSU) the message has been to generate more and more revenue from the available resources. The Central Government was quick to understand the importance of innovations and new ideas for adjusting to new streams of paradigm shifts. The Government also realized that the journey is not going to be smooth, easy or straight forward in the absence of indigenous knowledge about new paradigms among scientists, technologists and policy makers.

B. Bioethics and Biosafety

Bioethics is the study of moral choices arising from human involvement with life which may include an assessment of benefits and risks related to human interventions, especially with new technologies, and looks at balancing pursuit of individual autonomy with the duties of justice. Bioethics demands that technology assessment be thorough, and include assessment of the impact upon societies and individuals (Macer, 1997)

Biosafety in a broader term is used in reference to policy frameworks and actions for assessment and management of the safe application of modern biotechnology, frequently referred to as genetic engineering. Concepts of safety are applied with respect to hazards that modern biotechnology may pose to human and animal health as well as to the environment. The risks include related non-technology concerns of a social, ethical or political nature (Persley and Doyle, 1999). In this context therefore, biosafety is a concept that is being applied to regulate situations in which products of biotechnology are introduced into the environment directly as genetically modified crops, animals and microbes or through derived products such as food, cosmetics, drugs and other biologicals.

Bioethics is basically documented as our concern and values that we realise while directly or indirectly connecting with the biological system, what we perceive from our experience and thought is that there are at least three ways to express bioethics (Macer, 1998):

1. **Descriptive bioethics** is the way people view life, their moral interactions and responsibilities with living organisms in their life. Everyone already has their own bioethics, and this evolves through our life and experience.
2. **Prescriptive bioethics** is to tell others what is ethically good or bad, or what principles are most important in making such decisions. It may also

be to say something or someone has rights, and others have duties to them. We may re-examine our own bioethics and change, and also offer advice to our society on how to change.

3. **Interactive bioethics** is discussion and debate between people, groups within society, and communities about descriptive and prescriptive bioethics. In a global society the richness of interactive bioethics should improve, but it can only do so if we are tolerant of others.

There are a set of principles or ideals which people use as a common ground for bioethics. They include the autonomy of individuals to make choices, while respecting the choices of others, justice. In all things we do, the ideal is to avoiding doing harm, and trying to do good.

1. Biosafety Guidelines

The World Health Organization (WHO) has long recognized that safety and, in particular, biological safety are important international issues. WHO issued the the Laboratory biosafety guidelines in form of manual in 1983, 1993 and safety information 1997 and followed by last updated 2004. The manual encouraged countries to accept and implement basic concepts in biological safety and to develop national codes of practice for the safe handling of pathogenic microorganisms in laboratories within their geographical borders. Since then, many countries have used the expert guidance provided in the manual to develop such codes of practice. WHO continues to provide international leadership in biosafety by addressing biological safety and security issues facing us in the current millennium. The clear instructions on risk assessment, safe use of recombinant DNA technology and transport of infectious materials. Recent world events COVID-19 pandemic has revealed new threats to public health through deliberate misuse and release of microbiological agents. The protection of microbiological assets from theft, loss or diversion, which could lead to the inappropriate use of these agents to cause public health harm lead to the introduction of the biosecurity concept. WHO Laboratory biosafety practices are helpful to nations that accept the challenge to develop and establish national codes of practice for securing microbiological assets, yet ensuring their availability for clinical, research and epidemiological purposes (WHO, 2004).

2. Risk Groups

The World Health Organization have internationally classified and made to the relative hazards of infective microorganisms by risk group (WHO Risk Groups 1, 2, 3 and 4). This risk group classification is to be used for laboratory work only. The factors used to determine which risk group an organism falls into is based upon the characteristics of the organism, such as below:

- Pathogenicity
- Infectious dose
- Mode of transmission
- Host range

- ☆ Availability of effective preventive measures
- ☆ Availability of effective treatment.

These classifications presume ordinary circumstances in the research laboratory or growth in small volumes for diagnostic and experimental purposes. The four levels of risk have been defined as follows:

Risk Group 1 (no or very low individual and community risk)

A microorganism that is unlikely to cause human or animal disease.

Risk Group 2 (moderate individual risk, low community risk)

A pathogen that can cause human or animal disease but is unlikely to be a serious hazard to laboratory workers, the community, livestock or the environment. Laboratory exposures may cause serious infection, but effective treatment and preventive measures are available and the risk of spread of infection is limited.

Risk Group 3 (high individual risk, low community risk)

A pathogen that usually causes serious human or animal disease but does not ordinarily spread from one infected individual to another. Effective treatment and preventive measures are available.

Risk Group 4 (high individual and community risk)

A pathogen that usually causes serious human or animal disease and that can be readily transmitted from one individual to another, directly or indirectly. Effective treatment and preventive measures are not usually available.

3. Containment

Containment facilities for different Risk Groups as per the recommendations of World Health

Organization (DBT, 1990). The term "Containment" is used in describing the safe methods for managing infectious agents in the laboratory environment where they are being handled or maintained.

Purpose of containment: To reduce exposure of laboratory workers, other persons, and outside environment to potentially hazardous agents.

Types of Containment

Biological Containment (BC)

In consideration of biological containment, the vector (plasmid, organelle, or virus) for the recombinant DNA and the host (bacterial, plant, or animal cell) in which the vector is propagated in the laboratory will be considered together. Any combination of vector and host which is to provide biological containment must be chosen or constructed to limit the infectivity of vector to specific hosts and control the host-vector survival in the environment. These have been categorized into two levels; one permitting standard biological containment and the other even higher that relates to normal and disabled host-vector systems respectively.

Physical Containment (PC)

The objective of physical containment is to confine recombinant organisms thereby preventing the exposure of the researcher and the environment to the harmful agents. Physical containment is achieved using i) Laboratory Practice, ii) Containment Equipment, and iii) Special Laboratory Design. The protection of personnel and the immediate laboratory environment from exposure to infectious agents, is provided by good microbiological techniques and the use of appropriate safety equipment, (Primary Containment).

The protection of the environment external to the laboratory from exposure to infectious materials, is provided by a combination of facility design and operational practices, (Secondary Containment).

Elements of Containment

The three elements of containment include laboratory practice and technique, safety equipment and facility design.

i) Laboratory Practice and Technique

- Strict adherence to standard microbiological practices and techniques
- Awareness of potential hazards
- Providing/arranging for appropriate training of personnel
- Selection of safety practices in addition to standard laboratory practices if required
- Developing of adopting a biosafety or operations manual which identifies the hazards

ii) Safety Equipment (Primary barriers)

Safety equipment includes biological safety cabinets and a variety of enclosed containers (*e.g.*, safety centrifuge cup). The biological safety cabinet (BSC) is the principal device used to provide containment of infectious aerosols generated by many microbiological procedures. Three types of BSCs (Class I, II, III) are used in microbiological laboratories. Safety equipment also includes items for personal protection such as gloves, coats, gowns, shoe covers, boots, respirators, face shields and safety glasses, *etc.*

iii) Facility Design (Secondary barriers)

The design of the facility is important in providing a barrier to protect persons working in the facility but outside of the laboratory and those in the community from infectious agents which may be accidentally released from the laboratory. There are three types of facility designs: viz, the Basic Laboratory (for Risk Group I and II), the Containment Laboratory (for Risk Group III) and the Maximum Containment Laboratory (for Risk Group IV).

4. Biosafety Levels

It consists of a combination of laboratory practices and techniques, safety equipment and laboratory facilities appropriate for the operations performed and the hazard posed by the infectious agents. The guidelines for Microbiological and Biomedical Laboratories suggest four Biosafety levels in incremental order depending on the nature of work. Additional flexibility in containment levels can be obtained by combination of the physical with the biological barriers. The proposed safety levels for work with recombinant DNA technique take into consideration the source of the donor DNA and its disease-producing potential. These four levels correspond to (BSL1<BSL2<BSL3<BSL4) facilities approximate to 4 risk groups assigned for etiologic agents.

These levels and the appropriate conditions are enumerated as follows: The classification of organisms according to risk group is not meant to establish the actual handling of biological hazards in the laboratory setting. For example, the risk group system does not consider the procedures that are to be employed during the manipulation of a particular organism. Containment levels are selected to provide the end-user with a description of the minimum containment required for handling the organism safely in a laboratory setting. In addition to the inherent characteristics of each organism as described under different section, the containment system includes the engineering, operational, technical and physical requirements for manipulating a particular pathogen. These containment levels are applicable to facilities such as diagnostic, research, clinical, teaching and production facilities that are working at a laboratory scale. There are four (4) biosafety or containment levels are described as follows (DBT, 1990).

1. **Biosafety Level 1** is suitable for work involving well-characterized agents not known to cause disease in healthy adult humans, and of minimal potential hazard to laboratory personnel and the environment.
2. **Biosafety Level 2** is like Level 1 and is suitable for work involving agents of moderate potential hazard to personnel and the environment.
3. **Biosafety Level 3** is applicable to clinical, diagnostic, teaching, research, or production facilities in which work is done with indigenous or exotic agents which may cause serious or potentially lethal disease because of exposure by the inhalation route.
4. **Biosafety Level 4** is required for work with dangerous and exotic agents which pose a high individual risk of aerosol-transmitted laboratory infections and life-threatening disease.

The relation of risk groups to different biosafety levels, type of work, practices and equipment required are described in the matrix form in Table 20.1.

5. Biological Safety Cabinets (BSC)

Laboratory techniques may produce aerosols, which can contain hazardous research materials, such as infectious agents that laboratory workers could inhale. Biological safety cabinets (BSC) are one type of primary barrier to contain potentially infectious research materials to prevent exposure of laboratory personnel and contamination of the general environment.

Table 20.1: Relation of Risk Groups to Biosafety Levels, Practices and Equipment's

Risk Group (RG)	*Biosafety Level (BSL)*	*Laboratory type*	*Laboratory Practices*	*Safety Equipment*
1	Basic – Biosafety Level 1	Basic teaching, research	Good Microbiological Techniques (GMT)	None; open benchWork
2	Basic – Biosafety Level 2	Primary health services. diagnostic, research	GMT plus protective clothing, biohazard sign	Open bench plus BSC for potential Aerosols
3	Containment – Biosafety Level 3	Special diagnostic, research	As Level 2 plus special clothing, controlled access, directional airflow	BSC and/or other primary devices for all activities
4	Maximum Containment – Biosafety Level 4	Dangerous pathogen units	As Level 3 plus airlock entry, shower exit, special waste disposals	Class III BSC, or positive pressures uits in conjunction with Class II BSCs, double-ended autoclave (through the wall), filtered air

Containment of hazardous aerosols in biological safety cabinets occurs by air barriers, physical barriers, and high-efficiency particulate air (HEPA) filtration. Air barriers provide containment by providing directional airflow from the laboratory, past the researcher, and into the cabinet via the work opening. Hazardous aerosols generated during experimental procedures inside the cabinet become captured and carried by the flow of air, and trap within HEPA filters. Some BSCs provide protection for experimental procedures by providing uniform, unidirectional HEPA filtered air, referred to as laminar airflow, continuously flowing over the work area. Laminar airflow minimizes turbulence inside the cabinet, allowing for immediate removal of contaminants generated by the procedures.

Classification of Biological Safety Cabinets

There are three classes of biological safety cabinets, designated as Class I, Class II, and Class III. Class I and II cabinets have a protective air barrier across the work opening that separates the laboratory researcher from the work area. Class II cabinets also provide a HEPA-filtered, clean work area to protect the experiment from room contamination. Class III cabinets have a physical barrier between the operator and the work area. Arm length rubber gloves sealed to glove ports on the cabinet provide the operator with access to the work area.

6. Implementation of Biosafety Guidlines

For implementation of the guidelines it is necessary to have an institutional mechanism to ensure the compliance of requisite safeguards at various levels. The guidelines prescribe specific actions that include establishing safety procedures for rDNA research, production and release to the environment and setting up containment conditions for certain experiments (DBT, 2017). The guidelines suggest compliance of the safeguards through voluntary as well as regulatory approach. In this connection, it is proposed to have a mechanism of advisory and regulatory bodies to deal with the specific and discretionary actions on the following:

a. Self-regulation and control in the form of guidelines on recombinant research activities; and
b. Regulation of large-scale use of engineered organisms in production activity and release of organisms in environmental applications under statutory provisions.

The institutional mechanism as proposed for implementation of guidelines and they are mainly consists of the following:

i. Recombinant DNA Advisory Committee (RDAC)
ii. Review Committee on Genetic Manipulation (RCGM)
iii. Genetic Engineering Approval Committee (GEAC)
iv. Institutional Biosafety Committee (IBSC)
v. Monitoring cum Evaluation Committee (MEC)
vi. State Biotechnology Coordination Committee (SBCC)
vii. District Level Committee (DLC)

Under Biosafety Research programme main emphasis is given to facilitate the implementation of biosafety procedures, rules and guidelines under Environment (Protection) Act 1986 and Rules 1989 to ensure safety from the use of Genetically Modified Organisms (GMOs) and products thereof in research and application to the users as well as to the environment. A three tier mechanism comprising Institutional Biosafety Committees (IBSC) at the Institute/company; the Review Committee on Genetic Manipulation (RCGM) in the Department of Biotechnology; and the Genetic Engineering Approval Committee (GEAC) in the Ministry of Environment and Forests (MoE and F) for granting approval for research and development activities on recombinant DNA products, environmental release of genetically engineered (GE) crops and monitoring and evaluation of research activities involving recombinant DNA technology has been established. Applications in pharma/agriculture sectors for import/export/transfer/exchange of GE materials including GE seeds, conduct of pre-clinical toxicity studies, evaluation of pre-clinical study reports and recommendations to DCGI for appropriate phase of clinical trials of new drug(s) or similar biologics, confined field trials on GE crops etc., were examined by the RCGM and appropriate decisions were taken. RCGM has taken several policy decisions on biosafety research on agricultural/bio-pharmaceuticals/industrial products (DBT, 2017).

7. The Cartagena Protocol on Biosafety

The Cartagena Protocol on Biosafety (hereafter referred to as 'the Protocol'), is an international agreement that was adopted on 29 January 2000 as a supplementary agreement to the Convention on Biological Diversity (CBD). It addresses the potential adverse effects on biodiversity, taking also into account risks to human health, of living modified organisms (LMOs), which are defined in the Protocol as any living organism that possesses a novel combination of genetic material obtained using modern biotechnology (CBD Secretariat, 2000). The term LMO is usually considered to be synonymous with GMO (genetically modified organism) or other similar terms, although precise definitions may vary. The Protocol focuses on trans-boundary movements and is therefore relevant to international trade in LMOs. While the Protocol deals exclusively with LMOs, its remit overlaps with that of other international bodies and agreements that deal to some extent with transgenic organisms. The relevant bodies and agreements to international trade are World Organization for Animal Health (OIE), the International Plant Protection Convention (IPPC), Organization for Economic Cooperation and Development (OECD) and the Codex Alimentarius Commission (Codex). It will be important for all countries that have ratified (hereafter referred to as 'the Parties') to consider the work done by these organizations on the particular issues for which they have specific responsibility.

The origin of the Cartagena Protocol dates to the 1992 United Nations Conference on Environment and Development, held in Rio de Janeiro. At that meeting, more than 178 governments adopted Agenda 21, which was a comprehensive action plan for dealing with ways in which human activities affect the environment; it included a chapter on 'environmentally sound management of biotechnology'. At the same meeting, the CBD was opened for signing.

The three principal objectives of this Convention are as follows:

- ☆ The conservation of biodiversity
- ☆ The sustainable use of its components
- ☆ The fair and equitable sharing of the benefits arising out of the utilization of genetic resources.

The one of the key issues addressed by the CBD is biosafety, i.e., the need to protect human health and the environment from the potential adverse effects of the products of modern biotechnology. At the same time, biotechnology is recognized as having great potential for the promotion of human well-being and for the sound management of the environment (CBD Secretariat, 2000). The CBD clearly recognizes these twin aspects of biotechnology and includes provisions for both the promotion of biotechnology and the development of procedures to ensure its safety, the objective of this Protocol is to contribute to ensuring an adequate level of protection in the field of the safe transfer, handling and use of living modified organisms resulting from modern biotechnology that may have adverse effects on the conservation and sustainable use of biological diversity, taking also into account risks to human health, and specifically focusing on transboundary movements. The scope of the Protocol is described in Article 4, and highlights this focus on transboundary movements: This Protocol shall apply to the transboundary movement, transit, handling and use of all living modified organisms that may have adverse effects on the conservation and sustainable use of biological diversity, taking also into account risks to human health.' The Protocol came into force in September 2003.

8. Good Laboratory Practice (GLP)

It refers to a system of management controls for laboratories and research organizations to ensure the consistency and reliability of results as outlined in the Organization for Economic Cooperation and Development (OECD) Principles of GLP and national regulations. GLP applies to non-clinical studies conducted for the assessment of the safety of chemicals to man, animals and the environment (WHO, 2009). The internationally accepted definition is as follows:

Good Laboratory Practice (GLP) embodies a set of principles that provides a framework within which laboratory studies are planned, performed, monitored, recorded, reported and archived. These studies are undertaken to generate data by which the hazards and risks to users, consumers and third parties, including the environment, can be assessed for pharmaceuticals, agrochemicals, cosmetics, food and feed additives and contaminants, novel foods and biocides. GLP helps assure regulatory authorities that the data submitted are a true reflection of the results obtained during the study and can therefore be relied upon when making risk/safety assessments.

Good Clinical Practice (GCP) is an international ethical and scientific quality standard for designing, conducting, recording and reporting trials that involve the participation of human subjects. Compliance with this standard provides public assurance that the rights, safety and well-being of trial subjects are protected, consistent with the principles that have their origin in the Declaration of Helsinki (ICH GCP Guideline).

Good Clinical Laboratory Practice (GCLP) applies those principles established under GLP for data generation used in regulatory submissions relevant to the analysis of samples from a clinical laboratory practice as defined in this document are complied with in their facility.

Biosafety Management

Although the responsibility for the safety of staff lies with the supervisors and directors of the microbiology laboratory, it can be advantageous to identify an individual(s) to specifically manage biological safety issues. In many laboratories, this role is either informally assigned to a qualified individual who performs these duties on a part-time basis (*e.g.*, senior microbiologist) or the role is shared by several individuals. This role can also be formally assigned to a dedicated Biological Safety Officer who has a working knowledge of the laboratory practices and procedures within the facility. The formation of an Institutional Biosafety Committee to oversee the facility's biological safety program can also be incorporated into the structure for the management of biological safety issues (in some institutions and universities, the requirement for an Institutional Biosafety Committee is mandatory). The Biological Safety Officer (or individual assigned to manage biological safety issues) should liaise with the Committee through regularly scheduled meetings and can present specific safety problems, concerns or policy/protocol improvements to be considered and addressed. The Committee is also available to the Biological Safety Officer for risk assessments, disputes about biological safety matters or other matters that may be of a biological safety nature. Careful consideration is to be given to the composition of the Institutional Biosafety Committee, which, when possible, should include several individuals with varying expertise, the Biological Safety Officer, at least one member of each of the research staff (researcher) and technical staff (technician), and a representative from management. Consideration should also be given to representation by a medical advisor. The structure for the management of biological safety issues within each facility should be determined locally and will vary according to the level of coordination and the associated resources necessary for implementation.

The determining factors include the size of the facility (staff and square footage), concentration of multiple laboratories in the facility, containment levels within the facility (level 2 laboratory, multiple level 3 laboratories), complexity of the processes (routine diagnostics, research, large scale, recombinant work), existence of shared laboratory space within the facility (multiple investigators, various organizations) and experimental or diagnostic animal activities within the facility.

Biological safety issues to be managed may include the following:

- ✰ Identifying training needs and assisting with the development and delivery of biosafety training programs, such as general biosafety, BSC use, animal biosafety, staff orientation and containment suite training.
- ✰ Performing risk assessments when required and developing recommendations for procedural or physical laboratory modifications.
- ✰ Auditing the effectiveness of the biosafety program and its associated management system on a regular basis.
- ✰ Participating in accident investigations and promoting the reporting of incidents within the facility or laboratory.
- ✰ Distributing new and relevant biosafety information to laboratory staff and maintaining liaison with support staff, housekeeping staff and contractors on matters related to facility biosafety.
- ✰ Coordinating and monitoring the decontamination, disinfection and disposal procedures for infectious materials in the facility or laboratory and coordinating emergency response activities.
- ✰ Coordinating the receipt, shipment and transport within the facility of infectious material according to the Workplace Hazardous Materials Information System (WHMIS) and Transportation of Dangerous Goods (TDG) regulations.
- ✰ Establishing a record keeping and secure storage system for all infectious material entering the facility.

Containment Level 3/4 laboratories may have the additional biosafety activities:

- ✰ Certification and recertification of the laboratory.
- ✰ Investigation and remediation of containment suite physical or operational failures.
- ✰ Access control to the containment suites.
- ✰ Liaison with applicable regulatory bodies, such as DBT, GEAC, RDAC.

REFERENCES

1. Brahmi P, Saxena S, Dhillon BS. The Protection of Plant Varieties and Farmers Rights Act of India. Current Science, 2004: 86(3): 392-398.
2. CBD Secretariat. Cartagena Protocol in biosafety to the Convention on Biological Diversity: text and annexes. 2000: Montreal www.biodiv.org/doc/legal/cartagena-protocol-en.pdf.
3. DBT. Recombinant DNA Safety Guidelines, Department of Biotechnology, Ministry of Science and Technology, Government of India. 1990
4. DBT. Regulations and Guidelines on Biosafety of Recombinant, DNA Research and Biocontainment, Department of Biotechnology, Ministry of Science and Technology, Government of India. 2017
5. Macer D. Bioethics is Love of Life, Christchurch N.Z.: Eubios Ethics Institute. 1998
6. Persley Gabrielle J, Doyle JJ. Biotechnology for Developing Country Agriculture: Problems and Opportunities Overview, Focus 2. Brief 1 of 10. IFPRI. Washington, DC USA. 1999
7. Prabhu LS, Suriyaprakash TNK, Kumar DK. Intellectual property rights and its development in India. Pharma Times 2012: 44(7): 19-22.
8. Puttaiah K. Indian patenting process timeline. 2014 (www.invntree.com)
9. The Copyright Act 1957 as amended up to 1999 along with Copyright Rules 1958 and International Copyright Order 1999: 2005
10. The Design Act 2000 along with Design Rules 2001; Universal Law Publishing Co. Ltd., New Delhi: 2004
11. The Geographical Indications of Goods (Registration and Protection) Act, 1999 along with Geographical Indications of Goods (Registration and Protection) Rules 2002; Universal Law Publishing Co. Ltd., New Delhi: 2004
12. The Patents Act, 1970 as amended by Patents (Amendment) Act 2005, Commercial Law Publisher (India) Private Ltd. 2005
13. The Protection of Plant Varieties and Farmers' Rights Act, 2001 along with Protection of Plant Varieties and Farmers' Rights Rules 2003; Akalank Publications, New Delhi. 2008
14. The Trademarks Act 1999 along with Trademarks Rules 2002; Commercial Law Publisher (India) Private Ltd. 2004
15. WHO. Handbook: Good Laboratory Practice (GLP): quality practices for regulated non-clinical research and development. 2009: 2
16. WHO. Laboratory Biosafety Manual. Geneva: World Health Organization 2004: 3: 5-105
17. WIPO. WIPO Intellectual Property Handbook, WIPO Pub. No. 2004: 489 (E)

Index